Fundamentals of Operative Dentistry
Second Edition

Fundamentals of
Operative Dentistry

A Contemporary Approach

Second Edition

Edited by

James B. Summitt, DDS, MS
Professor and Head
Division of Operative Dentistry
Department of Restorative Dentistry
University of Texas Health Science Center at San Antonio
San Antonio, Texas

J. William Robbins, DDS, MA
Clinical Professor
Department of General Dentistry
University of Texas Health Science Center at San Antonio
San Antonio, Texas

Richard S. Schwartz, DDS
Private Practice, Endodontics
San Antonio, Texas

Illustrations by

Jose dos Santos, Jr, DDS, PhD
Professor
Division of Occlusion
Department of Restorative Dentistry
University of Texas Health Science Center at San Antonio
San Antonio, Texas

Quintessence Publishing Co, Inc
Chicago, Berlin, London, Tokyo, Paris, São Paulo, Barcelona, Moscow, Prague, and Warsaw

Library of Congress Cataloging-in-Publication Data

Summitt, James B.
    Fundamentals of operative dentistry : a contemporary approach / James B. Summitt, J.
William Robbins, Richard S. Schwartz ; illustrations by Jose dos Santos, Jr.
    p. cm.
    On previous ed. the author Schwartz name appeared first.
    Includes bibliographical references and index.
    ISBN 0-86715-382-2
    1. Dentistry, Operative. I. Robbins, J. William. II. Schwartz, Richard S. III. Title.

RK501 .S436 2000
617.6'05--dc21   00-055278

© 2001 Quintessence Publishing Co, Inc

Quintessence Publishing Co, Inc
551 Kimberly Drive
Carol Stream, Illinois 60188
www.quintpub.com

Editor: Arinne Dickson
Production: Sue Robinson
Cover Design: Michael Shanahan

Printed in Singapore

Dedication

In the preface to the first edition of this textbook, special acknowledgment was given to Dr Miles R. Markley as one of dentistry's great leaders. On January 31, 2000, Dr Markley died at age 96. It is with great appreciation and admiration that we dedicate this edition to Dr Markley, in gratitude for his special gifts in analytical thinking and teaching and for his ability to motivate others to study and think scientifically and rationally. He had a tremendous professional and personal influence on the editors of this book and on countless others in our profession.

Regarded as the father of conservative dentistry, his philosophy dates from the early years of his practice in Denver, Colorado. In the early 1930s, he noted that some of his earlier restorations had unexpectedly failed after only a few years of service. He redesigned the cavity preparations he had learned in school to provide preparations that preserved sound tooth structure and tooth strength. He also incorporated philosophies of prevention and conservative nonsurgical treatment of dental caries.

In 1992, two of the contributors to this book (Drs Summitt and Osborne) were able to examine 20 of Dr Markley's patients who had been under his care since the 1930s and 1940s. Among that group of patients, only one tooth had been lost. All the patients credited Dr Markley with maintaining their healthy dentitions.

Miles Markley's innovations and philosophies have influenced every restorative dentist who is in practice today. He practiced for 52 years and continued his great interest and support of dentistry until his death. We should all follow Dr Markley's example of commitment, concern, and scientific basis in our practices.

To my wife and one love, Joanne, my terrific kids, Carrie and
J.B. (and his wife Minna), and three very important teachers,
Drs David Bales, Robert Cowan, and Aaron Wilson
JBS

To my favorite kids, Alyssa, Sarah, and Andrew,
and my wife and best friend, Brenda
JWR

To my wife, Jeannette, who has been my friend, advisor,
barber, mother of my child, and love of my life
for more than 25 years
RSS

Table of Contents

Preface   ix
Contributors   xi

1 Biologic Considerations   1
Jerry W. Nicholson

2 Patient Evaluation and Problem-Oriented Treatment Planning   26
Richard D. Davis

3 Esthetic Considerations in Diagnosis and Treatment Planning   56
J. William Robbins

4 Caries Management: Diagnosis and Treatment Strategies   70
J. Peter van Amerongen/Cor van Loveren/Edwina A. M. Kidd

5 Pulpal Considerations   91
Thomas J. Hilton/James B. Summitt

6 Nomenclature and Instrumentation   113
James B. Summitt

7 Field Isolation   149
James B. Summitt

8 Enamel and Dentin Adhesion   178
Bart Van Meerbeek/Satoshi Inoue/Jorge Perdigão/Paul Lambrechts/Guido Vanherle

9 Direct Anterior Restorations   236
David F. Murchison/Daniel C. N. Chan/Robert L. Cooley

10 Direct Posterior Esthetic Restorations 260
Thomas J. Hilton

11 Amalgam Restorations 306
James B. Summitt/John W. Osborne

12 Diagnosis and Treatment of Root Caries 365
Michael A. Cochran/Bruce A. Matis

13 Fluoride-Releasing Materials 377
John O. Burgess

14 Class 5 Restorations 386
Clifford B. Starr

15 Natural Tooth Bleaching 401
Van B. Haywood/Thomas G. Berry

16 Porcelain Veneers 427
J. William Robbins

17 Anterior Ceramic Crowns 451
Jeffrey S. Rouse

18 Esthetic Inlays and Onlays 476
J. William Robbins/Dennis J. Fasbinder

19 Cast-Gold Restorations 500
Thomas G. Berry/David A. Kaiser/Richard S. Schwartz

20 Conservative Cast-Gold Restorations: The Tucker Technique 526
Richard V. Tucker/Dennis M. Miya

21 Restoration of Endodontically Treated Teeth 546
J. William Robbins

Index 567

Preface

Dental educators and practicing dentists have, at times, been slow to respond to advances in dental materials and techniques. Operative dentistry, in particular, has often been influenced more by history and tradition than by science. Until recently, many restorative procedures taught in dental schools and practiced by dentists were based primarily on Dr G. V. Black's classic textbook, *A Work on Operative Dentistry,* published in 1908. The many advances in materials and instrumentation, linked with the development of reliable dental adhesives, have allowed us to modify many of Black's original concepts to more conservative, tooth-preserving procedures and to offer a much wider range of restorative options. Black was, indeed, one of dentistry's greatest innovators and original thinkers. Were he alive today, he would be leading the advance of new technology and innovation. We best honor his memory not by clinging to concepts of the past but rather by looking to recent scientific innovations and incorporating them into our practices and dental school curricula.

This textbook is about contemporary operative dentistry. It is a blend of traditional, time-proven methods and recent scientific developments. Whereas preparations for cast-gold restorations have changed relatively little over the years, preparations for amalgam and resin composite restorations are smaller and require removal of less sound tooth structure because of the development of adhesive technologies. While we still use many luting agents in the traditional manner, adhesive cements provide greater retention for cast restorations and allow expanded use of ceramic and resin composite materials. Many concepts of caries management and pulpal protec-tion have changed drastically as well. It is our hope that this textbook, which represents an ardent effort to present current concepts and the latest scientific evidence in restorative and preventive dentistry, will be helpful to students, educators, and practicing dentists during this time of rapidly developing technologies.

Several themes echo throughout this textbook. The first is the attempt to provide a scientific basis for the concepts described. The authors are clinically active, and many are engaged in clinical and laboratory research in the areas of cariology, restorative dentistry, and/or dental materials. Whenever possible, the diagnosis and treatment options described are based on current research findings. When conclusive evidence is not available, we have attempted to present a consensus founded on a significant depth of experience and informed thought.

A second theme reflected in the book is our commitment to conservative dentistry. The treatment modalities described involve the preservation of as much sound tooth structure as possible within the framework of the existing destruction and the patient's expectations for esthetic results. When disease necessitates a restoration, it should be kept as small as possible. When an extensive amount of tooth structure has been destroyed and remaining cusps are significantly weakened, occlusal coverage with a restoration may be the most conservative treatment. When portions of axial tooth surfaces are healthy, their preservation is desirable. In the conservative philosophy on which this book is based, a complete-coverage restoration (complete crown) is generally considered the least desirable treatment alternative.

The book describes techniques for the restoration of health, function, and esthetics of individual teeth and the dentition as a whole. Included are descriptions of direct conservative restorations fabricated from dental amalgam, resin composite, and resin-ionomer materials. Also detailed are techniques for partial- or complete-coverage indirect restorations of gold alloy, porcelain, metal-ceramic, and resin composite.

The second edition is broader and more in-depth than the first. Many existing chapters have been updated and expanded, and five new chapters have been added. A new chapter on esthetic considerations identifies the various components of esthetic diagnosis and provides a logical approach to treatment planning. Acknowledging the routine use of tooth bleaching in practices today, a detailed chapter on this treatment option was added, as were chapters on the diagnosis and treatment of root caries and on fluoride-releasing materials. A second chapter on cast-gold restorations presents the various preparation techniques as developed by Richard Tucker, the primary mentor of the famed Tucker Study Clubs. Finally, in light of recent research findings and an aging population exhibiting minimal tooth loss, the chapter on caries management was rewritten to reflect the changing strategies in this area. More color illustrations have been included to enhance the presentation of the clinical concepts of several key chapters.

The second edition has also undergone a change in editorship. Since publication of the first edition, Rick Schwartz has left the University of Texas faculty to practice endodontics full time. Because of this change in specialty, Jim Summitt and Bill Robbins together took on the major share of revising this textbook.

The primary objective in producing this book is to provide students and practitioners with current and practical concepts of preventive and restorative dentistry that will allow them to serve their patients well. It is our hope that the changes made in this edition will make the book more thorough and of greater benefit to those who use it.

Contributors

Thomas G. Berry, DDS, MA
Professor and Chairman
Department of Restorative Dentistry
University of Texas Health Science Center
   at San Antonio
San Antonio, Texas

John O. Burgess, DDS, MS
Professor and Chairman
Department of Operative Dentistry and Biomaterials
Louisiana State University Health Sciences Center
School of Dentistry
New Orleans, Louisiana

Daniel C. N. Chan, DDS, MS
Associate Professor and Head
Division of Operative Dentistry
Department of Oral Rehabilitation
Medical College of Georgia
School of Dentistry
Augusta, Georgia

Michael A. Cochran, DDS, MSD
Professor and Director
Graduate Operative Dentistry Program
Indiana University
School of Dentistry
Indianapolis, Indiana

Robert L. Cooley, DMD, MS
Associate Professor
Department of General Dentistry
University of Texas Health Science Center
   at San Antonio
San Antonio, Texas

Richard D. Davis, DDS
Department of Endodontology
Oregon Health Sciences University
School of Dentistry
Portland, Oregon

Dennis J. Fasbinder, DDS
Clinical Associate Professor
Director, AEGD
Department of Cariology, Restorative Sciences,
   and Endodontics
University of Michigan
School of Dentistry
Ann Arbor, Michigan

Van B. Haywood, DMD
Professor
Department of Oral Rehabilitation
Medical College of Georgia
School of Dentistry
Augusta, Georgia

Thomas J. Hilton, DMD
Associate Professor
Departments of Operative Dentistry and
   Biomaterials/Biomechanics
Oregon Health Sciences University
School of Dentistry
Portland, Oregon

Satoshi Inoue, DDS, PhD
Assistant Professor
Department of Operative Dentistry
Hokkaido University
School of Dentistry
Sapporo, Japan

David A. Kaiser, DDS, MSD
Professor
Department of Prosthodontics
University of Texas Health Science Center
  at San Antonio
San Antonio, Texas

Edwina A. M. Kidd, BDS, FDSRCS, PhD
Professor of Cariology
Division of Conservative Dentistry
The Dental School of Guy's, King's, and St. Thomas'
  Hospital
London, England

Paul Lambrechts, DDS, PhD
Professor
Department of Operative Dentistry and Dental Materials
Catholic University of Leuven
School of Dentistry, Oral Pathology,
  and Maxillofacial Surgery
Leuven, Belgium

Bruce A. Matis, DDS, MSD
Associate Professor
Department of Restorative Dentistry
Indiana University
School of Dentistry
Indianapolis, Indiana

Dennis M. Miya, DDS
Private Practice
Seattle, Washington

David F. Murchison, DDS
Assistant Chairman
Department of General Dentistry
Wilford Hall USAF Medical Center
Lackland Air Force Base
San Antonio, Texas

Jerry W. Nicholson, DDS, MA
Assistant Professor
Department of Restorative Dentistry
University of Texas Health Science Center
  at San Antonio
San Antonio, Texas

John W. Osborne, DDS, MSD
Professor and Director of Clinical Research
Department of Restorative Dentistry
University of Colorado Health Science Center
Denver, Colorado

Jorge Perdigão, DDS, MS, PhD
Associate Professor and Head
Division of Operative Dentistry
University of Minnesota
School of Dentistry
Minneapolis, Minnesota

Jeffrey S. Rouse, DDS
Private Practice
San Antonio, Texas

Clifford B. Starr, DMD
Clinical Associate Professor
Director, GPR and AEGD Residencies
Department of Operative Dentistry
University of Florida
College of Dentistry
Jacksonville, Florida

Richard V. Tucker, DDS
Private Practice
Ferndale, Washington

J. Peter van Amerongen, DDS, PhD
Associate Professor of Conservative Dentistry
Department of Cariology, Endodontology,
  Pedodontology
Academic Center for Dentistry Amsterdam
Amsterdam, The Netherlands

Guido Vanherle, MD, DDS
Professor
Department of Operative Dentistry and Dental
  Materials
Catholic University of Leuven
School of Dentistry, Oral Pathology,
  and Maxillofacial Surgery
Leuven, Belgium

Cor van Loveren, DDS, PhD
Associate Professor of Preventive Dentistry
Department of Cariology, Endodontology,
  Pedodontology
Academic Center for Dentistry Amsterdam
Amsterdam, The Netherlands

Bart Van Meerbeek, DDS, PhD
Associate Professor
Department of Operative Dentistry and Dental
  Materials
Catholic University of Leuven
School of Dentistry, Oral Pathology,
  and Maxillofacial Surgery
Leuven, Belgium

Biologic Considerations

Jerry W. Nicholson

Success in clinical dentistry requires a thorough understanding of the anatomic and biologic nature of the tooth, with its components of enamel, dentin, pulp, and cementum, as well as the supporting tissues of bone and gingiva (Fig 1-1). Dentistry that violates the physical, chemical, and biologic parameters of tooth tissues can lead to premature restorative failure, compromised coronal integrity, recurrent caries, patient discomfort, or even pulpal necrosis. It is only within a biologic framework that the materials, principles, and techniques that constitute operative dentistry are validated. This chapter presents a morphologic and histologic review of tooth tissues with emphasis on their clinical significance for the practice of restorative dentistry.

Enamel

Enamel provides a hard, durable shape for the functions of teeth and a protective cap for the vital tissues of dentin and pulp. Both color and form contribute to the esthetic appearance of enamel. Much of the art of restorative dentistry comes from efforts to simulate the color, texture, translucency, and contours of enamel with synthetic dental materials such as resin composite or porcelain. Nevertheless, the lifelong preservation of the patient's own enamel is one of the defining goals of the dentist.[6] Although enamel is ca-

pable of lifelong service, its crystallized mineral makeup and rigidity, as well as stress from occlusion, make it vulnerable to acid demineralization (caries), attrition (wear), and fracture (Fig 1-2). Compared to other tissues, mature enamel is unique in that, except for alterations in the dynamics of mineralization, repair or replacement is only possible through dental therapy.

Permeability

At maturity, enamel is about 90% inorganic hydroxyapatite mineral by volume. Enamel also contains a small amount of organic matrix, and 4% to 12% water, which is contained in the intercrystalline spaces and in a network of micropores opening to the external surface.[61,98] The micropores form a dynamic connection between the oral cavity and the systemic, pulpal, and dentinal tubule fluids.[5,168] When teeth become dehydrated, as from nocturnal mouth breathing or rubber dam isolation for dental treatment, the empty micropores make the enamel appear chalky and lighter in color (Fig 1-3). The condition is reversible with return to the "wet" oral environment. Various fluids, ions, and low-molecular weight substances, whether deleterious, physiologic, or therapeutic, can diffuse through the semipermeable enamel. Therefore, the dynamics of acid demineralization,[79,153] caries,[134] reprecipitation or remineraliza-

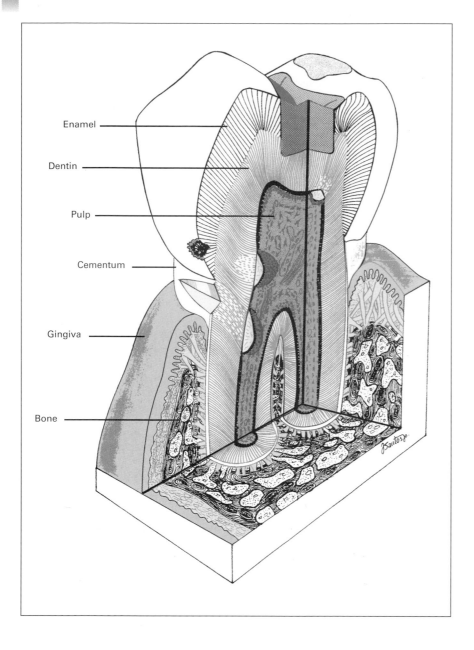

Fig 1-1 Component tissues and supporting structures of the tooth.

Enamel

Dentin

Pulp

Cementum

Gingiva

Bone

tion,[33,36,82] fluoride uptake,[41,102] and vital bleaching therapy[42] are not limited to the surface but are active in three dimensions.

Gradual coloration and improved caries resistance are two results of lifelong exposure of semipermeable enamel to the ingress of elements from the oral environment into the mineral structure of the tooth. The yellowing of older teeth may be attributed partly to accumulation of trace elements in the enamel structure[42] and perhaps to the sclerosis of mature dentin. Surface enamel benefits from incorporation of salivary or toothpaste fluoride to increase the ratio or conversion of hydroxyapatite to larger, more stable crystals of fluorohydroxyapatite or fluoroapatite.[41]

Therefore, with aging, color is intensified and acid solubility, pore volume, water content, and permeability of enamel are reduced.[38]

Clinical Appearance and Diagnosis

The dentist must pay close attention to the surface characteristics of enamel for evidence of pathologic or traumatic conditions. Key diagnostic signs include color changes associated with demineralization, cavitation, excessive wear, morphologic faults or fissures, and cracks (Fig 1-2).

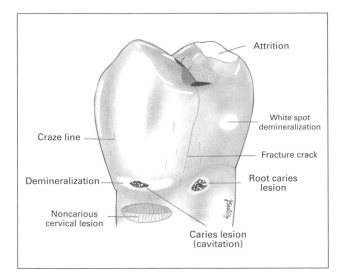

Fig 1-2 Observations of clinical importance on the tooth surface.

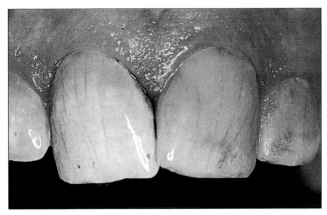

Fig 1-3 Color change resulting from dehydration. The right central incisor was isolated by rubber dam for approximately 5 minutes. Shade matching of restorative materials should be determined with full-spectrum lighting before isolation.

Color

Enamel is relatively translucent; its color is primarily a function of its thickness and the color of the underlying dentin. From approximately 2.5 mm at the cusp tips and 2.0 mm at the incisal edges, enamel thickness decreases significantly below deep occlusal fissures and tapers to a negligible thickness cervically at the junction with the cementum or dentin of the root. Therefore, the young anterior tooth has a translucent gray or slightly bluish enamel tint at the thick incisal edge. A more chromatic yellow-orange shade predominates cervically, where dentin shows through thinner enamel. Coincidentally, in about 10% of teeth, a gap between enamel and cementum at this juncture leaves vital, potentially sensitive dentin completely exposed.[100]

Anomalies of development and mineralization, extrinsic stains, antibiotic therapy, and excessive fluoride can alter the natural color of the teeth.[42] However, because caries is the primary disease threat to the dentition, color changes related to enamel demineralization and caries are critical diagnostic observations. The translucency of enamel is directly related to the degree of mineralization. Subsurface enamel porosity from carious demineralization is manifested clinically by a milky white opacity termed a *white spot lesion* when located on smooth surfaces (Figs 1-2, 1-4a, and 1-4b). In the later stages of caries, internal demineralization of enamel at the dentinoenamel junction (DEJ) imparts a whiteness or opacity seen through the more translucent overlying enamel. Subsurface cavitation imparts a blue or gray tint to the overlying enamel. With the advent of remineralization and sealant techniques, several authorities have suggested that invasive restorative procedures or replacement restorations should be initiated only if caries extension to dentin can be confirmed visually or radiographically.[21,39,108] Smooth surface enamel that is chalky white and roughened from prolonged contact with acidic plaque (Fig 1-4a) generally indicates that the patient has inadequate oral hygiene, has a cariogenic diet, and is at a higher risk for caries.

Cavitation

Unless prevention or remineralization can abort or reverse the carious demineralization, dentin is affected until the undermined enamel breaks away to create a "cavity"; a restoration must then be placed. Untreated, the cavitation expands to compromise the structural strength of the crown, and microorganisms infiltrate into deep dentin to jeopardize the vitality of the tooth. When the carious lesion extends gingival to the cementoenamel junction (CEJ), as in root caries (Fig 1-2), isolation, access, and gingival tissue response complicate the restorative procedure.

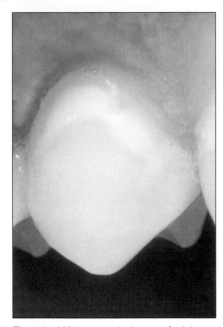

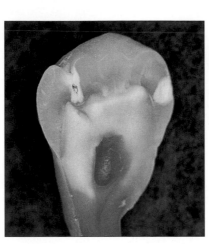

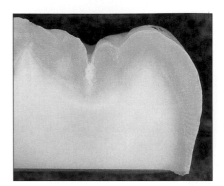

Fig 1-4a White spot lesion on facial surface of maxillary premolar.

Fig 1-4b Premolar with both an occlusal fissure caries lesion (Class 1), extending into the dentin, and a proximal smooth surface caries lesion (Class 2).

Fig 1-4c Sectioned molar with enamel caries lesion in deep occlusal fissure.

Wear

Enamel is as hard as steel,[30] with a Knoop Hardness Number of 343 (compared with a Knoop Hardness Number of 68 for dentin). However, enamel will wear because of attrition or frictional contact against opposing enamel or harder restorative materials, such as porcelain. Normal physiologic contact wear for enamel is as much as 29 µm per year.[83] Restorative materials that replace or function against enamel should have compatible wear, smoothness, and strength. Heavy occlusal wear is demonstrated when rounded cuspal contacts are ground to flat facets. Depending on factors such as bruxism, other parafunctional habits, malocclusion, age, and diet, cusps may be completely lost and enamel abraded away so that dentin is exposed and occlusal function compromised. However, the effects on vertical dimension from tooth wear may be offset by apical cementogenesis and tooth eruption. Cavity outline form should be designed so that the margins of restorative materials avoid critical, high-stress areas of occlusal contact.[22]

Faults and Fissures

Various defects of the enamel surface may contribute to the accumulation and retention of acidic plaque. Perikymata (parallel ridges formed by cyclic deposition of enamel) (Fig 1-5), pitting defects formed by termination of enamel rods, and other hypoplastic flaws are common, especially in the cervical area.[43] Limited linear defects or craze lines result from a combination of occlusal loading and age-related loss of resiliency but are not clinically significant. Organic films of surface pellicle and dendritic cuticles extending 1 to 3 µm into the enamel may play key roles in ion exchange[145] and in adhesion and colonization of bacterial plaque on the enamel surface.[63]

Of greater concern are the fissure systems on the occlusal surfaces, and often on other surfaces, of posterior teeth. A deep fissure is formed by incomplete fusion of lobes of cuspal enamel in the developing tooth.[130] The resulting narrow clefts provide a protected niche for acidogenic bacteria and the organic nutrients they require (Figs 1-4b, 1-4c, 1-6a, and 1-6b). Because of these fissure faults, 57.7% of total decayed, missing, and filled surfaces (DMFS) of schoolchildren in the United States occur on the occlusal surfaces; only 12.0% are found on the mesial and distal surfaces.[170] Altogether, pit and fissure defects are eight times more vulnerable to caries than are smooth surfaces.[63] Careful observation of enamel surrounding fissures for evidence of demineralization or cavitation is necessary to determine the need for restorative intervention.

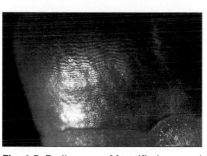

Fig 1-5 Perikymata. Magnified enamel surface morphology at cervical aspect of maxillary molar.

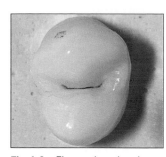

Fig 1-6a Fissured occlusal surface of maxillary premolar.

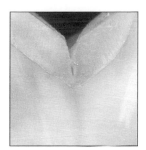

Fig 1-6b Cross section of fissure shown in Fig 1-6a.

Cracks

Although craze lines in the surface enamel are of little consequence, pronounced cracks that extend from developmental grooves across marginal ridges to axial surfaces, or from the margins of large restorations, may portend a coronal or cuspal fracture.[1] This defect is especially critical when the crack, viewed with cavity preparation, extends through dentin or when the patient has pain when chewing. A cracked tooth that is symptomatic or involves dentin requires a restoration that provides complete cuspal coverage.[155]

Crystal Structure

Enamel is a mineralized epidermal tissue. The organic matrix gel is first formed and then later partly digested by ameloblastic cells of the developing tooth organ. Calcium and phosphorus in the form of hydroxyapatite are seeded throughout the developing matrix and immediately begin to crystallize, enlarge, and supplant the organic matrix.

The majority of hydroxyapatite crystals, $Ca_{10}(PO_4)_6(OH)_2$, exist in an impure form in which ions or molecules are missing, or extrinsic substitutions occur to destabilize the crystal and make it more soluble. An important therapeutic exception is the incorporation of fluoride ion through systemic intake or topical application via remineralization dynamics.[102] In mature enamel, the closely packed, hexagonal crystals are 25 to 39 nm in thickness and 45 to 90 nm in width (Fig 1-7). Crystal length, whether columns of full enamel thickness or segmented units, is yet to be determined.[44] The matrix proteins, enamelins, and water of hydration form a shell, or envelope, around each crystal. Because the crystals are oriented perpendicular to the concave contours of the secreting ameloblastic cells, the crystal orientation gradually varies by as much as 70 degrees from the center of the cell (corresponding to the core center of the enamel rod) to the periphery[92] (Fig 1-8). The closely packed crystal deposition, repeated in a symmetric pattern, forms the basic structural units of enamel, the rods.

Enamel Rods

The enamel rods are described as keyhole- or mushroom-shaped, with a circular core, or head, 4 to 5 μm in diameter, in which the long axis of crystals runs approximately parallel to the rod. Cervically, the progressive disinclination of the crystals produced from the boundaries of adjacent ameloblasts forms a fan-shaped tail known as the interrod area (Fig 1-9). Except for a narrow, highly mineralized zone without rod structure both at the surface and at the DEJ, each rod runs the full thickness of the enamel. Because each row of rods is offset, the core of each rod is surrounded by the interrod substance of adjacent rods. As a result, the occlusal three-fourths of each core boundary is characterized by a junction of crystals meeting at acute angles. This interface, termed the *rod sheath*, is only increased intercrystalline space in which micropores and greater amounts of organic matrix are located.

The spacing and orientation of the crystals and amount of organic matrix make the enamel rod boundary and central core differentially soluble when exposed for a brief time to weak acids. Acid etchants remove about 10 μm of surface enamel and then preferentially dissolve either the rod core or periphery to form a three-dimensional, pitted surface with microporosities greater than 20 μm in depth[59,60,143] (Fig 1-10). The acid-treated enamel surface has a high surface energy, so that resin monomer flows into and intimately adheres to the etched depressions to poly-

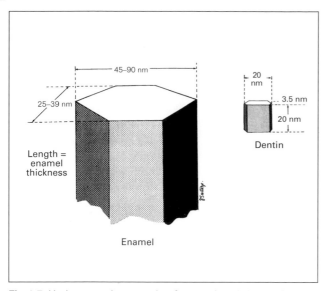

Fig 1-7 Hydroxyapatite crystals of enamel and dentin. Enamel crystal length may extend the full thickness of enamel. Dentin hydroxyapatite crystals are significantly smaller and thinner, and their surface-to-volume ratio (exposure) is greater.

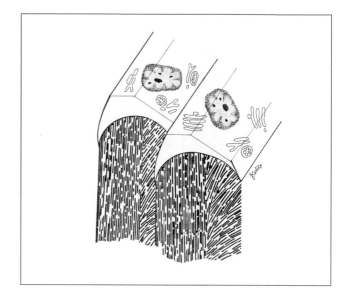

Fig 1-8 Ameloblastic formation of the enamel rod. Crystal orientation varies because crystals form perpendicular to the concave surface of the cell.

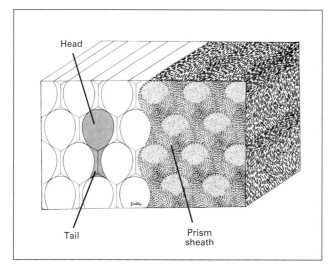

Fig 1-9 Enamel rods. Rod head (core) is formed from the center of a single ameloblast; its crystal direction is essentially parallel to the long axis. A combination of peripheries of several adjacent, hexagonal ameloblasts form the tail or interrod extension with divergent crystal orientation. A nearly perpendicular crystal interface around the rod head periphery results in greater intracrystalline space (formerly called the *prism sheath*).

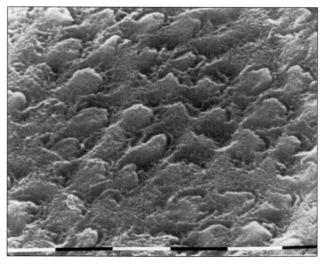

Fig 1-10 Scanning electron photomicrograph of an acid-etched enamel surface. Note the keyhole-shaped rods and uneven surface formed by the disparity in depth of rod heads and rod peripheries. (Bar = 10 μm.)

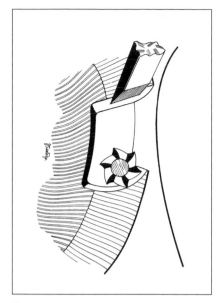

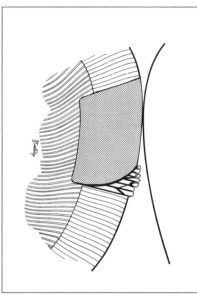

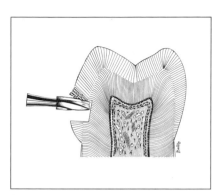

Fig 1-11a Coronal section through inter-proximal box cavity preparation. Use of a rotary bur, which may leave the proximal wall with an acute enamel angle and undermined enamel, requires careful planing.

Fig 1-11b Marginal defect, resulting from improper cavity wall preparation, leads to eventual loss of enamel at the restoration interface.

Fig 1-12 Buccal pit preparation of a molar that is cut perpendicular to the external facial, lingual, or approximal surface would not have occlusal walls oriented with the occlusal direction of the enamel rods.[41]

merize and form retentive resin tags.[58] Because there are 30,000 to 40,000 enamel rods/mm² and the etch penetration increases the bondable surface area 10- to 20-fold, micromechanical bonding of resin restorative materials to enamel is significant.[14,15] Transverse sections of enamel rods promote optimum tensile bond strengths to etched enamel of 19 to 20 MPa, compared to 11 MPa for longitudinal or parallel sections.[101] Acid-etch modification of enamel for restoration retention provides a conservative, reliable alternative to traditional surgical methods of tooth preparation and restoration.

The enamel rod boundaries form natural cleavage lines through which longitudinal fracture may occur. The fracture resistance between enamel rods is especially imperiled if the underlying dentinal support is pathologically destroyed or mechanically removed by a dental instrument (Figs 1-11a and 1-11b). Loss of enamel rods that form the cavity wall or cavomargin of a dental restoration creates a gap defect similar to an occlusal fissure. Leakage or ingress of bacteria and their products may lead to secondary caries.[74] Therefore, a basic tenet of cavity wall preparation is to bevel or parallel the direction of the enamel rods and to avoid undercutting them.[94]

However, a common precept, that cavity preparations should always be cut perpendicular to the external coronal surface, is not supported histologically. Each successive row of enamel rods runs a slightly different course in a wave pattern, both horizontally and vertically, through the inner half of the enamel thickness, and then continues in a relatively straight parallel course to the surface.[38] However, on axial surfaces and cuspal slopes, the path of each row terminates at an oblique angle to the surface rather than at a perpendicular tangent of 90 degrees (Fig 1-12). Starting at 1.0 mm from the CEJ, the rods on the vertical surfaces run occlusally or incisally at approximately a 60-degree inclination and progressively incline approaching the marginal ridges and cusp tips, where the rods are essentially parallel to the long axis of the crown. The rods beneath the occlusal fissures are also parallel to the long axis, but rods on each side of the fissure vary up to 20 degrees from the long axis.[46] Therefore, if cut perpendicular to the external surface, occlusal walls of preparations on axial surfaces might incorporate compromised enamel (Fig 1-12). An obtuse enamel-cavosurface angle would more closely parallel the rod direction and preserve the integrity of the enamel margin.

Considering the wide variation in direction of enamel rods and the structural damage caused by high-speed eccentric bur rotation, a finishing step of planing the cavosurface margin with hand or low-speed rotary instruments to remove any friable or fragile enamel structure is recommended.

Resilience

Although enamel is vulnerable and incapable of self-repair, its protective and functional adaptation is noteworthy. Carious demineralization, to the point of cavitation, generally takes 3 to 4 years.[126] Demineralization of enamel is impeded because the apatite crystals are 10 times larger than those in dentin[144] (see Fig 1-7). Enamel apatite crystals offer less surface-to-volume exposure and little space for acid penetration between the crystals. With preventive measures and exogenous or salivary renewal of calcium, phosphate, and especially fluoride, the dynamics of demineralization can be stopped or therapeutically reversed.

Enamel thickness and degree of mineralization are greatest at the occlusal and incisal surfaces where masticatory contact occurs.[28] If enamel were uniformly crystalline, it would shatter with occlusal function. A substructure, organized into discrete, parallel rods with a scalloped DEJ, minimizes the transfer of occlusal stress laterally and directs it anisotropically or unidirectionally to the resilient dentinal foundation.[147] The interwoven paths and interlocked keyhole morphology of the enamel rods help control lateral cleavage. As a functional adaptation to occlusal stress, the spiraling weave of rod direction is so pronounced at the cusp tips of posterior teeth that it is referred to as gnarled enamel. Finally, the further subdivision of enamel rods into distinct crystals separated by a thin organic matrix provides additional strain relief to help prevent fracture.[9]

Dentin

Function

The coronal (crown) dentin provides both color and an elastic foundation for enamel. Together with the radicular (root) dentin, which is covered with cementum, dentin forms the bulk of the tooth and a protective encasement for the pulp. As a vital tissue without vascular supply or innervation, it is nevertheless able to respond to thermal, chemical, or tactile external stimuli.

Support

Tooth strength and rigidity are provided by an intact dentinal substrate. Several investigators have reported that resistance to tooth fracture is significantly lower with increasing depth and/or width of cavity preparation.[8,99,165] A tooth with the deepest possible Class 1 amalgam preparation, that of an endodontic access preparation, retains only a third of the fracture resistance of an intact tooth.[132] To appreciate the magnitude of occlusal loading, mean maximum bite force of 738 N (166 lbs)[4,13] applied to an average contact area of 4 mm^2 distributed over 20 centric contacts[67] yields more than 26,744 psi. In vitro studies report that large mesio-occlusodistal preparations increase the strain or deflection of facial cusps by three times that of an intact tooth and decrease coronal stiffness by more than 60%.[91,133] Elastic deformation and excessive cuspal flexure are etiologic factors contributing to noncarious cervical lesions,[87] cervical debonding of restorations,[66] marginal breakdown,[127] fatigue failure, crack propagation, and fracture.[91] Removal and replacement of dental restorations over a patient's lifetime generally result in successively larger/deeper preparations. Therefore, to preserve coronal integrity, a conservative initial approach that combines localized removal of carious tooth structure, placement of a bonded restoration, and placement of sealant is recommended. If large preparations are required, the dentist should consider placement of an onlay or a crown.

Morphology

Dentin is composed of small apatite crystals embedded in a cross-linked organic matrix of collagen fibrils. The extended cytoplasmic processes of the formative cells, the odontoblasts, form channels or tubules traversing the full thickness of the tissue. Unlike enamel, which is acellular and predominantly mineralized, dentin is, by volume, 45% to 50% inorganic apatite crystals, about 30% organic matrix, and about 25% water. Dentin is pale yellow and slightly harder than bone. Two main types of dentin are present: (1) intertubular dentin, the primary structural component of the hydroxyapatite-embedded collagen

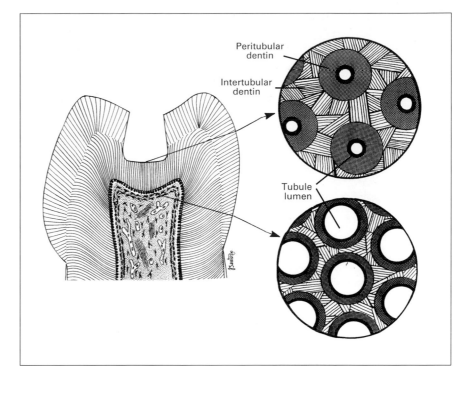

Fig 1-13 Dentin near the DEJ (outer) and near the pulp (inner) are compared to show relative differences in intertubular and peritubular dentin, and lumen spacing and volume.

Peritubular dentin

Intertubular dentin

Tubule lumen

matrix between tubules; and *(2)* peritubular dentin, the hypermineralized tubular wall.[161] The relative and changing proportions of mineralized crystals, organic collagen matrix, and cellular and fluid-filled tubular volume determine the clinical and biologic response of dentin. These component ratios vary according to depth of dentin, age, and traumatic history of the tooth.

Depth

Outer dentin (Figs 1-13 to 1-15). During formation of dentin, the odontoblastic cells converge from the dentinoenamel junction pulpally, creating a tapered channel surrounding their extended cytoplasmic processes. By secreting precursor collagen, these cells produce and nourish the developing dentinal matrix. In the first-formed dentin near the DEJ, the tubules of the outer dentin are relatively far apart and the intertubular dentin makes up 96% of the surface area.[119] Although the tubules are 0.8 μm in diameter and constitute about 4% of the surface area of outer dentin, there are as many as 20,000 tubules/mm².[53] In addition, there is extensive terminal branching of the tubules in the outer dentin along with regularly spaced connections, or canaliculi, between tubules, so that the cellular processes make up a highly interconnected system.[113] This interconnected structure may account for the paradox that superficial dentin, though furthest from the pulpal nerve receptors, is sensitive to a stimulus as localized as an explorer tip.

Inner dentin. The dentinal substrate near the pulp is quite different from that near the DEJ; these differences affect the permeability and bonding characteristics of the inner dentin. The formative odontoblast cells converge concentrically to terminate in a single, tightly packed layer at the wall of the pulp chamber. At the pulp-dentin interface, the number of odontoblasts (and therefore tubules) ranges up to 76,000/mm².[161] The tubule diameters are larger, 2.5 to 3.0 μm, and the distance between tubule centers within the inner dentin is half that of tubules at the DEJ. Thus, the intertubular matrix area is only 12% of the surface area, and the volume occupied by fluid-filled tubule lumens at the inner or predentin level is 22% of the surface, 20 times that at the DEJ.[48,53,98,123,161] Even though the tubule space is partially occluded by the cellular process, collagen, and mineral deposits, the dentin close to the pulp is still about eight times more permeable than the dentin near the DEJ.[31,116]

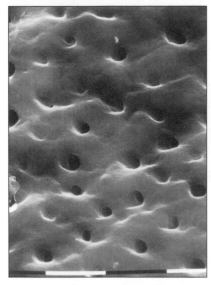

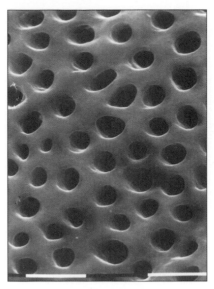

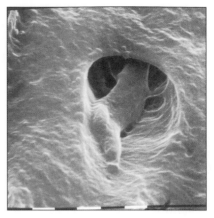

Fig 1-14a Scanning electron photomicrograph of tubules in outer dentin. All highly mineralized peritubular dentin has been removed in the specimen preparation. (Bar = 10 µm.)

Fig 1-14b Scanning electron photomicrograph of inner dentin. Compare to Fig 1-14a. All highly mineralized peritubular dentin has been removed in the specimen preparation. (Bar = 10 µm.)

Fig 1-14c Magnified tubule orifice with collagen matrix and odontoblastic process. (Bar = 1.0 µm.)

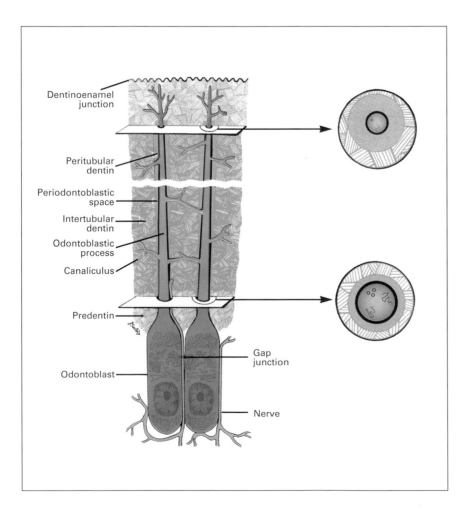

Fig 1-15 Odontoblastic cell, process, and tubule system through dentin. Continual deposition of peritubular dentin and minerals, accelerated by a chronic, noxious stimulus, gradually occludes the tubules peripherally. Note terminal branching and interconnections between odontoblastic cell processes and between cellular walls. Direct neural penetration of dentin is limited to less than 20% of the tubules, and then, rarely beyond the predentin.

Permeability

The permeability of dentin is directly related to its protective function (Fig 1-16). When the external "cap" of enamel or cementum is lost from the periphery of the dentinal tubules through caries, preparation with burs, or abrasion and erosion, the exposed tubules become conduits between the pulp and the external oral environment. Restored teeth are also at risk of toxic seepage through the phenomenon of microleakage between the restorative material and the cavity wall. No restorative material can provide a completely hermetic seal of the cavity wall.[7] Gaps of 10 μm or more may exist between newly placed amalgam and cavity walls,[19] and increased leakage at the cemental margins of resin-bonded restorations is commonly reported (Figs 1-17a and 1-17b).

Through capillary action, differential thermal expansion, and diffusion, fluids containing various acidic and bacterial products can penetrate the gap between tooth and restoration and initiate demineralization (secondary caries) of the internal cavity walls.[73,74] From this base, bacterial substances can continue by diffusion through permeable dentinal tubules to reach the pulp. Open tubule conduits to the external oral environment create a micropulpal exposure, putting the tooth at risk for pulpal inflammation and sensitivity.[11,25,120] The remaining dentinal thickness is the key determinant of the diffusion gradient.[116,120] Restorative techniques that incorporate varnishes, liners, or dentin bonding resin adhesives are effective to the extent that they provide reliably sealed margins and a sealed dentinal surface.

Sensitivity

Although sensitive to thermal, tactile, chemical, and osmotic stimuli across its 3.0- to 3.5-mm thickness, dentin is neither vascularized nor innervated, except for about 20% of tubules that have nerve fibers penetrating inner dentin by no more than a few microns. Therefore, attention has been focused on the odontoblast and its process as a possible stimulus receptor. This role is doubtful, however. Neither electron microscopy nor new research technologies have proven that the odontoblastic cellular process extends to the peripheral DEJ in mature dentin.[17,140,161] In addition, the cell membrane of odontoblasts is nonconductive, and there is no synaptic connection between the odontoblastic cell and the adjacent terminal branches of the pulpal nerve plexus. Finally, pain sensation re-

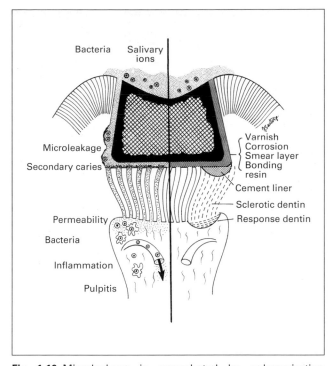

Fig 1-16 Microleakage is exacerbated by polymerization shrinkage, condensation gaps around the restorative material, and/or differences in thermal expansion. When microleakage is present, the tubule openings in dentin form a potential pathway between the oral environment and the pulp. Various restorative materials, together with the tooth's defenses of tubule sclerosis and reparative dentin, restrict the noxious infiltration.

mains even when the odontoblastic layer is disrupted.[162]

Brännström et al[10] proposed a theory based on the capillary flow dynamics of the fluid-filled dentinal tubules (Fig 1-18). Tubular fluid flow of 4 to 6 mm/s is produced by application of a stimulus, such as air evaporation, cold, or heat (ie, generated from a dental bur), or tactile pressure. The "current," or hydrostatic pressure, displaces the odontoblastic cell bodies and stretches the intertwined terminal branches of the nerve plexus to allow entry of sodium to initiate depolarization. Evidence supporting the hydrodynamic theory includes in vivo correlation of tubule patency with hypersensitive roots.[32] Also, Ahlquist et al[3] correlated intensity of pain with rapid hydrostatic pressure changes applied to the sealed, smear-free dentinal axial walls of cavity preparations. Therefore, the knowledge that permeable dentin is sensitive dentin may help the dentist avert postoperative discomfort associated with tooth restoration.[3]

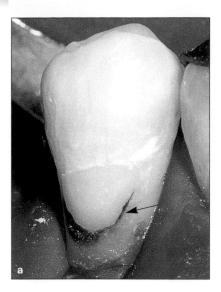

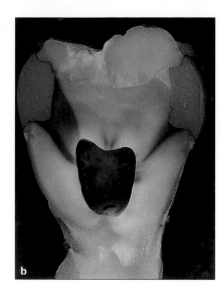

Fig 1-17a Failed resin composite restoration. Polymerization shrinkage and cervical debonding created a margin-wall gap defect, leading to microleakage and secondary caries. *(Arrow, cervical margin.)*

Fig 1-17b In vitro dye penetration reveals microleakage and diffusion through dentinal tubules.

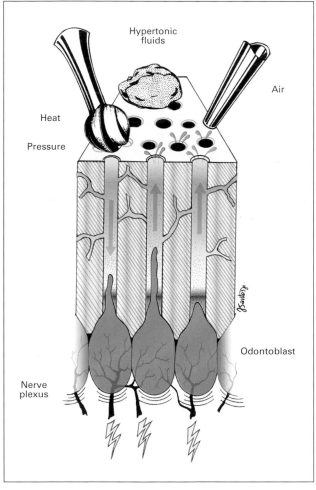

Fig 1-18 A hydrodynamic phenomenon explains the sensitivity of dentin, which is without significant innervation. Fluid dynamics of the tubules move the odontoblastic cell bodies and mechanically depolarize approximating nerve endings.

Substrate for Bonding

Early attempts to bond resins to etched dentin were relatively unsuccessful because of the variability of the dentinal substrate, the hydrolytic deterioration of the bonding agents, or interference by the smear layer, a tenacious, semipermeable film of organic and inorganic debris on the prepared dentinal surface. Many of the newer dentin bonding systems remove the smear layer, acid-etch the intertubular dentinal surface and peritubular walls to provide the porosity required for microretention, and penetrate and surround the exposed collagen fibrils. Hydrophilic bonding resin then forms a limited-depth interdiffusion or hybrid zone of resin and collagen/microetched dentin between the restorative resin composite and normal dentin.[104,105,166] Deeper levels of dentin offer an altogether different substrate for bonding that is wetter and less solid (see Figs 1-13 to 1-15). A positive pulpal pressure of 14 cm H_2O creates an outward flow of dentinal tubular fluid.[24] The odontoblastic process, mineral deposits, and intertubular collagen partially occlude the dentin tubule and provide some resistance to flow. When dentin is cut at deeper levels, flow is unimpeded, and the dentinal surface becomes wet, which can interfere with the adhesion of hydrophobic resin polymers. Not all bonding systems are equally effective in both deep and peripheral dentin.[40,125,128]

Another substrate variable that reduces bond strength is excessive sclerosis or hypermineralization of exposed root surface dentin characterized by a deeper yellow color and glossy surface. Aging and response to external stimuli are associated with tubule occlusion through continued mineralization.[96] These conditions are typical of long-standing root surface abrasion/erosion lesions.[35,167]

Physiologic and Tertiary Dentin

Primary dentin is formed relatively quickly until root formation is completed; the odontoblasts then become relatively quiescent. After this, the slowly formed dentin that continues to constrict the dimensions of the pulp chamber is termed *secondary dentin*. The morphology of the pulp chamber approximates the external tooth contours, but pronounced extensions, or pulp horns, into buccal cusps of premolars and mesiobuccal cusps of molars must be carefully avoided during cavity preparation in young teeth to prevent exposure. Perhaps in response to a mild occlusal stimulus, secondary dentin is preferentially deposited in the pulp horns and on the roof and floor of the pulp chamber so that, after many decades, the chamber becomes quite narrow occlusogingivally.[130] The dentist must allow for the size and location of the pulp chamber, for they may be deciding factors in the design of the preparation and placement of retentive features, such as pins.

Another physiologic or age-related process, perhaps mediated by the odontoblastic process, is the continual mineralization of tubule walls (see Fig 1 15). As a result, the peritubular dentinal wall progressively thickens and occludes the tubule lumen. Deposition of both peritubular and secondary dentin is considered physiologic, because reduction of the pulp chamber is found in unerupted teeth, and sclerosis is reported in radicular dentin in the premolars of 18 year olds.[157] However, with sufficient external stimulus or irritation, such as caries, attrition, or restorative procedures, the rate of dentin deposition can be accelerated. Unlike primary and secondary dentin, which are deposited uniformly, this added or tertiary dentin is localized to the affected area of the pulp-dentin complex. The tertiary dentin caused by an external stimulus that reactivates the dentinogenic activity of the pre-existing odontoblasts is termed *reactionary dentin*. If the odontoblasts are killed by a pernicious stimulus, the tertiary dentin generated by osteoblastlike replacement cells is termed *response dentin*.[161]

Sclerotic Dentin

With age, tubule lumens are gradually constricted by the continuing physiologic mineralization of the peritubular dentin. As with tertiary dentin, external stimuli can accelerate and augment the mineralization of the peritubular dentin or the tubular contents to make the dentin less permeable. Open tubules on exposed root surfaces predispose as many as one in seven adults to hypersensitivity.[56] Treatment modalities occlude the tubules, either by sealing the tubule orifice with bonded resin or by precipitating intratubular protein or crystals with application of fluoride or potassium nitrate compounds to the root surface.[52,136] When dentin is suddenly exposed by fracture or a lost restoration, plasma proteins are transported to the exposed tubules. Within 6 to 24 hours, a fibrinlike intratubular clot forms to constrain the hydrodynamic flow and diminish sensitivity.[118]

With initial enamel caries or microleakage, the outward flow of the dentinal fluid under positive pulpal pressure counteracts pulpal diffusion of endotoxins and acids.[122] As caries progresses, immunoglobulins are transported and concentrated in the tubular fluid and cellular processes within the dentin pulpal to the caries lesion.[2,115] Withdrawal, injury, or necrosis of the cytoplasmic contents leaves the tubule open to bacterial toxins and deeper invasion. However, calcium and phosphorus released by carious acid demineralization of the peripheral hydroxyapatite crystals reprecipitate deeper within the tubules, pulpal to the infected lesion. Platelike or rhomboid mineral crystals fill and barricade the open lumen[139] (Figs 1-19a and 1-19b). Also, accelerated mineralization, with constriction of the peritubular walls pulpal to the level of bacterial penetration, forms a protective confinement barrier, the sclerotic or translucent zone.[51,114,142]

With the protective response of stimulus-generated new or tertiary dentin, the in vitro permeability or hydraulic conductance of chronically carious dentin is reduced to only 7.6% of that recorded for normal dentin.[124] Thus, even a minimal width of remaining dentin below a deeply excavated carious lesion and restoration may transform into a protective impermeable barrier. One unfortunate consequence, however, is that sclerosed, insensitive dentin blocks painful warning symptoms that might alert the patient to the presence of caries.

Occasionally, with virulent bacteria and in young, permeable teeth, there is insufficient time for sclerosis. The tubules, empty and vulnerable, are described as

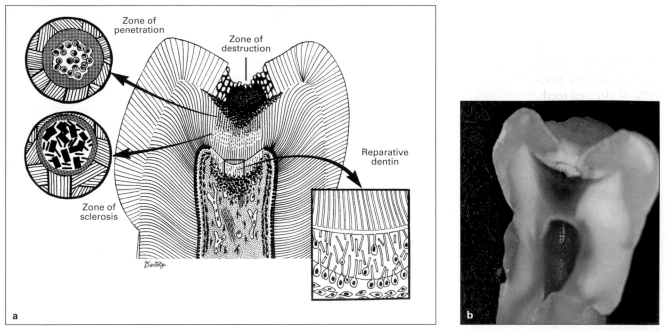

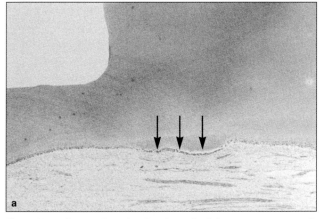

Figs 1-19a and 1-19b Carious response. Acid demineralization and enzymatic destruction of the collagen matrix lead to irreversible cavitation. (a) Bacteria fill and demineralize the lumens of the tubules peripherally, but dissolved minerals reprecipitate deeper to augment sclerosis and hypermineralization of subcarious dentin. Reparative dentin with irregular and noncontinuous tubules forms a final barricade against bacterial metabolites. (b) Note the lateral spread of the caries lesion at the DEJ and a hypermineralized sclerotic zone around the pulp.

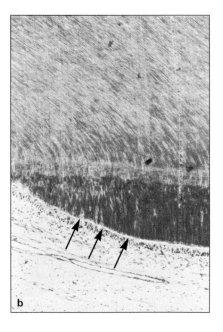

Fig 1-20a Reparative dentin deposited in response to microleakage and bacterial invasion under a dental restoration.

Fig 1-20b Reparative dentin deposited in response to infected primary and secondary dentin. (Courtesy of Dr Charles Cox, University of Alabama School of Dentistry.)

"dead tracts."[78] Fortunately, sclerosis is a predictable, protective dentinal response observed in more than 95% of carious teeth and often in conjunction with the production of tertiary or reparative dentin, another protective response that occurs in more than 63% of affected teeth.[151]

Reparative Dentin

Intense traumatic insult to the tooth, whether caused by bacterial penetration associated with caries, or heat and trauma from a dental bur, may be severe enough to destroy the supporting odontoblasts in the affected location (Figs 1-19a and 1-20). Within 3 weeks, fibroblasts or mesenchymal cells of the pulp are converted or differentiated to simulate the organization, matrix secretion, and mineralizing activities of the original odontoblasts. The matrix includes cellular and vascular components of the pulp and sparse, irregularly organized tubules. The rate of formation, the thickness, and the organization of the reparative dentin are commensurate with the intensity and duration of the stimulus.[161] Reparative dentin usually forms at a rate of about 1.5 µm/day, but the rate may be as high as 3.5 µm/day. At 50 days after trauma, a 70-µm thickness of reparative dentin has been reported.[149,150] The barrier protection of reparative dentin is superior because there is no continuity between the affected permeable tubules of the regular primary dentin and those within the reparative dentin. Nevertheless, some porosity defects have been reported in reparative dentin so that, with vital pulpal exposures, sterile technique and durable cavity liners/sealers are needed to preserve pulpal vitality.[27] But with reparative dentin, the tooth is able to compensate for the traumatic or carious loss of peripheral dentin with deposition of new dentin substrate and reduction of pulpal vulnerability from tubule permeability.

Unless the lesion is either arrested or removed and a restoration placed before it is about 0.5 mm from the pulp, the diffusion gradient of bacterial metabolites reaching the pulp can initiate a strong inflammatory response.[111] If the reparative dentin is breached to allow sufficient bacteria to overwhelm the vascular, inflammatory, and phagocytic defenses of the pulp, the result is pulpal necrosis.[78,134]

Pulp

The dental pulp, 75% water and 25% organic,[98] is a viscous connective tissue of collagen fibers and ground substance supporting the vital cellular, vascular, and nerve structures of the tooth. It is a unique connective tissue in that its vascularization is essentially channeled through one opening, the apical foramen at the root apex, and it is completely encased within relatively rigid dentinal walls. Therefore, it is without the advantage of an unlimited collateral blood supply or an expansion space for the swelling that accompanies the typical inflammatory response of tissue to injurious conditions. However, the protected and isolated position of the pulp belies the fact that it is a sensitive and resilient tissue with a great potential for healing.

The dental pulp fulfills several functions for the pulpodentin complex[129]: (1) formative, creating the primary and secondary dentin as well as the protective response of reactionary or reparative dentin; (2) nutritive, providing the vascular supply and ground substance transfer medium for metabolic functions and maintenance of cells and organic matrix; (3) sensory, transmitting afferent pain response (nociception) and proprioceptive response; and (4) protective, responding to inflammatory and antigenic stimuli and removing detrimental substances through its blood circulation and lymphatic systems.

Morphology

The pulpal tissue is traditionally described in histologically distinct, concentric zones: the innermost peripheral pulp core, the cell-rich zone, the cell-free zone, and the peripheral odontoblastic layer (Figs 1-21a to 1-21c).

The radicular and coronal pulp core is largely ground substance, an amorphous protein matrix gel surrounding cells, discrete collagen fibers, and the channels of vascular and sensory supply. The gel serves as a transfer medium, between widely spaced pulp cells and vasculature, for transport of nutrients and by-products. Terminal neural and vascular components, which divide and multiply extensively in the subodontoblastic zones, converge into larger vessels and trunks and together form a main trunk passing through the pulp core to or from the apical foramina. Both matrix and collagen components are formed and maintained by a dispersed network of interconnected fibroblastic cells.

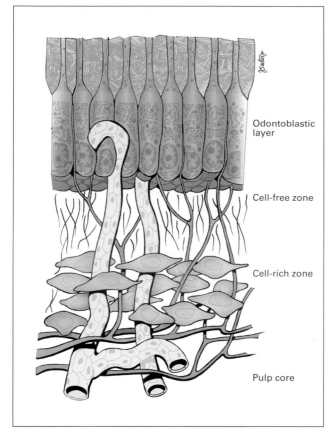

Fig 1-21a Pulpal histology. Odontoblastic layer, cell-free zone (filled with both nerve and vascular plexuses), cell-rich zone (fibroblasts), and pulp core.

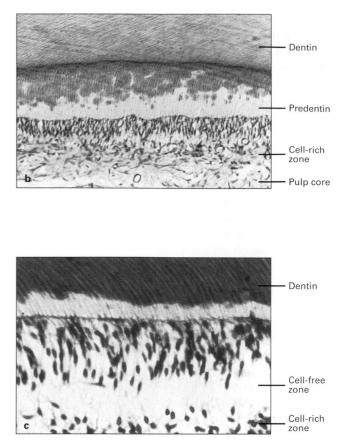

Figs 1-21b and 1-21c Photomicrographs of dentin and underlying pulpal tissues. (Courtesy of Dr Charles Cox, University of Alabama School of Dentistry.)

Fibrocytes and undifferentiated mesenchymal cells are particularly concentrated in the outer coronal pulp to form the cell-rich zone subjacent to the peripheral layer of odontoblastic cells. Functioning like troops in reserve, the mesenchymal cells and/or fibrocytes are capable of accelerated mitotic differentiation and collagen matrix production to serve as functional replacements for destroyed odontoblastic cells. They produce reparative dentin when bacteria or their by-products breach the permeable dentinal wall or a pulpal exposure occurs.[47,161,163] A dense and extensive capillary bed and nerve plexus form the cell-free zone, infiltrate the cell-rich zone, and separate it from the cellular bodies of the peripheral odontoblastic layer.

Vascular System

The circulatory system supplies the oxygen and nutrients that dissolve in and diffuse through the viscous ground substance to reach the cells. In turn, the circulation removes waste products, such as carbon dioxide, by-products of inflammation,[78] or diffusion products that may have permeated through the dentin before they accumulate to toxic levels[117] (see Fig 1-16). The equilibrium between diffusion and clearance may be threatened by use of long-acting anesthetics that contain vasoconstrictors such as epinephrine. An intraligamental injection of a canine tooth with 2% lidocaine with 1:100,000 epinephrine will cause pulpal blood flow to cease for 20 minutes or more.[77] Fortunately, the respiratory requirements of mature pulp cells are low so that no permanent cellular damage ensues.

Inflammation, the normal tissue response to injury and the first stage of repair, is somewhat modified by the unique location within the noncompliant walls of the pulp chamber. A stimulus producing cellular damage initiates neural and chemical reactions that increase capillary permeability so that proteins, plasma fluids, and leukocytes spill into the confined extracellular space, producing elevated tissue interstitial fluid pressure.[152] Theoretically, elevated extravascular tissue pressure could collapse the thin venule walls and start a destructive cycle of restricted circulation and expanding ischemia. However, the pulpal circulation is unique because it contains numerous arteriole "U-turns," or reverse flow loops, and arteriole-venule anastomoses, or shunts, to bypass the affected capillary bed.[158] Also, at the periphery of the affected area, where high tissue pressure is attenuated, capillary recapture and lymphatic adsorption of edematous fluids are expedited.[65] These processes confine the area of edema and elevated tissue pressure to the immediate inflamed area. Although tissue pressure at an area of pulpal inflammation is two to three times higher than normal, it quickly falls to nearly normal levels approximately 1.0 mm from the affected area.[159]

Another protective effect of elevated but localized pulpal tissue pressure is a vigorous outward flow of tubular fluid to counteract the pulpal diffusion of noxious solutes through permeable dentin.[55,95,122] However, an inflammatory condition and higher tissue pressure may also induce hyperalgesia, a lowered threshold of sensitivity of pulpal nerves. Thus, an afflicted tooth exposed to the added stress of cavity preparation and restoration may become symptomatic or hypersensitive to cold or other stimuli.[162]

Innervation

Dental nerves are either efferent autonomic C fibers to regulate blood flow or afferent sensory nerves derived from the second and third divisions of the fifth intracranial (trigeminal) nerve. Nerves are classified according to purpose, myelin sheathing, diameter, and conduction velocity. Although a few large and very high-conduction velocity A-ß (beta) nerves with a proprioceptive function have been identified, most sensory interdental nerves are either myelinated A-∂ (delta) nerves or smaller, unmyelinated C fibers.[162] The innervation of a premolar, for example, consists of about 500 individual A-∂ nerves that gradually lose their myelin coating and Schwann cell sheathing as they branch and form a sensory plexus of free nerve endings around and below the odontoblastic layer.[71] The A-∂ nerves have conduction velocities of 13.0 m/s and low sensitization thresholds to react to hydrodynamic pressure phenomena.[106,107] Activation of the A-∂ system results in a sharp, intense "jolt."

There are three to four times more of the smaller, unmyelinated C fibers, which are more uniformly distributed through the pulp. The conduction velocities of C fibers are slower, 0.5 to 1.0 m/s, and C fibers are only activated by a level of stimuli capable of creating tissue destruction, such as prolonged high temperatures or pulpitis. The C fibers are also resistant to tissue hypoxia and are not affected by reduction of blood flow or high tissue pressure. Therefore, pain may persist in anesthetized, infected, or even nonvital teeth.[37,160] The sensation resulting from activation of the C fibers is a diffuse burning or throbbing pain, and the patient may have difficulty locating the affected tooth.

The afferent transmission of painful sensations, commonly experienced although unreliable as a warning signal, may not be the primary protective function of pulpodentin innervation. Experimentally denervated teeth exposed to trauma suffer greater pulpal damage than innervated controls.[16] The initiation and coordination of the inflammatory cascade; the vascular, tissue, and tubular fluid dynamics; and the immunocompetent response are important protective functions of the neural components.[31,123,141]

Odontoblastic Layer

The peripheral cellular layer of the pulp, the odontoblasts, produce primary, secondary, and reactionary dentin. This layer may also regulate or influence tubular mineralization and sclerosis as a defense mechanism (see Fig 1-15).[73] Postmitotic and irreplaceable, the columnar cell bodies line the predentin wall of the pulp chamber in a single layer. From each cell, a single process extends into at least one third of the tubule and adjacent dental substrate that it formed. Each cell has an indefinite life span, but crowding from continued deposition of secondary dentin constricts the pulpal chamber to reduce the initial number of cells by half.[130] The odontoblastic cells are packed closely together, with both permanent and temporary junctions between the cellular membranes.[68,81,137] Just as the peripheral processes of the odontoblasts are physically interconnected, a third type of intercellular interface, a communicating junction, mediates transfer of chemical and electronic signals that permit coordinated response and reaction of the odontoblastic layer.[68,81,137] Thus, as an additional protective response, the integrity and spacing of the odontoblastic layer mediates the passage of tissue fluids and molecules between the pulp and the dentin. Routine operative procedures, such as cavity preparation and air drying of the cut dentinal surface, can temporarily disrupt the odontoblastic layer and may sometimes inflict permanent cellular damage.[12,164]

Restorative Dentistry and Pulpal Health

Surgical and restorative treatments generate considerable physical, chemical, and thermal irritation of the pulp. However, if the dentist uses an acceptable technique and achieves bacterial control, even a mechanical pulp exposure or use of acidic restorative materials poses few problems for pulpal health.[7,11,25,26,72,121,146] Although microleakage around restorations is ubiquitous, the fact that almost all pulps remain healthy is related to diminished virulence of the bacteria, relative impermeability of the dentin, and healing potential of the pulp.[78,103] But the capacity for pulpal healing is restricted by the effects of aging and by extensive and/or repeated restorative procedures. Two clinical reviews of patients who had received either a fixed prosthesis or single complete crowns reported that 6%[70] and 13%[45] of crowned teeth revealed some sign of pulpal necrosis requiring endodontic treatment.

Although pressure, desiccation, and surgical amputation of cellular processes accompany dental intervention, excessive heat generated by the friction of rotary instrumentation is considered the most damaging insult to the pulp. Heat may cause coagulation, extensive burn lesions, and temporary stasis of the pulpal circulation.[76,150] Studies of heat applied externally to enamel surfaces or cavity floors have produced equivocal results. Zach and Cohen[172] reported 15% irreversible pulpal necrosis after a 5.5°C increase of intrapulpal temperature and up to 60% necrosis after an 11°C rise. However, against prepared cavity walls of orthodontically condemned teeth with about 0.5 mm of remaining dentinal thickness, a 30-second heat application of 150°C (200°F) produced few symptoms, relatively minor pulpal changes, and no necrosis.[112] Interpretation of the studies indicates that the presence of a sufficient remaining dentinal thickness (0.5 mm or more) is a critical factor in limiting thermal conduction (providing insulation), just as it is in limiting dentinal permeability.[29,150]

Other in vitro studies have shown damaging temperature thresholds are possible if improper amalgam finishing and polishing techniques, such as continuous contact and excessive speed or pressure, are used.[57,64,154] Another study reported that 25 seconds of continuous contact of a rotating dental bur against a tooth without water coolant could produce a critical 6°C rise in intrapulpal temperature.[171] Therefore, an important safeguard to prevent the buildup of pulpal heat is use of a water coolant combined with intermittent instrument-tooth contact, especially during high-speed enamel or dentin reduction.[156] Another potential thermal threat to the pulp is from high-energy light-curing devices for polymerization of resin composites. These devices are capable of raising the pulpal chamber temperature as much as 8°C.[62] Other steps recommended to minimize pulpal damage associated with restorative procedures include the following[23]: use of sharp burs or single-use diamonds, use of concentrically rotating instruments, avoidance of overdrying and prolonged desiccation of cut dentin, and accurate fitting of provisional restorations.

Although the aged tooth is less permeable, some biologists suggest that it has less reparative potential. Age-related changes include reduced blood supply, a smaller pulp chamber, lower ratio of cells to collagen fiber, loss and degeneration of myelinated and unmyelinated nerves, loss of water from the ground substance, and increased intrapulpal mineralizations (denticles).[138,161] Restorative procedures easily tolerated in the younger patient may pose problems for the older patient. Nevertheless, the newer concepts of treatment, including preventive measures; improved restorative materials; reliable bonding and sealing of enamel fissures, margins, and dentinal tubules; and conservative tooth preparations should extend durability and biocompatibility of dental services.

Gingiva

The gingiva is that part of the oral mucosa that covers the alveolar bone, defines the cervical contours of the clinical crown, and seals the tooth root and periodontal structures from the external environment. A normal, healthy gingiva presents a scalloped marginal outline, firm texture, coral pink or normally pigmented coloration, and, in about 40% of the population, a stippled surface. A healthy, stable gingiva without hyperplastic, swollen, bleeding, or receding tissue is essential to both esthetic and restorative success.

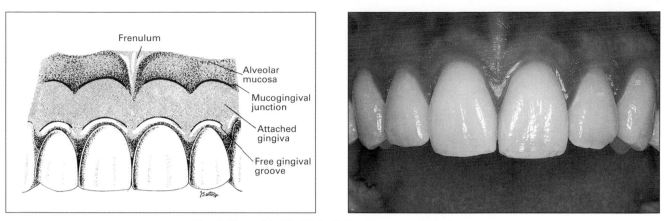

Figs 1-22a and 1-22b Clinically healthy, normal gingiva.

Gingivitis, an inflammatory soft tissue response to bacterial plaque, affects up to 44% of the adult population in the United States.[170] Gingival bacteria, associated with poor oral hygiene or defective restorations, can cause periodontal disease. Because periodontitis is a major cause of adult tooth loss, the status of the alveolar bone and soft tissues of the periodontium must be evaluated along with that of the teeth.

External Appearance

The two primary components of the gingival tissues are keratinized gingiva and alveolar mucosa (Figs 1-22a and 1-22b).[83,88] The keratinized gingiva includes both the attached gingiva and the marginal gingiva. Attached gingiva is firmly affixed to the periosteum of the alveolar bone and hard palate and to the supraalveolar cementum of the root. It extends coronally around the teeth to form the free gingiva, a scalloped, unattached cuff that also fills the gingival embrasure between adjacent teeth with a facial and lingual papilla. Attached and marginal gingiva are separated by an external free gingival groove in about 30% to 40% of the healthy adult population. The vertical width (height) of the keratinized gingiva (attached and marginal gingiva) is clearly measured from the mucogingival junction separating it from the alveolar mucosa, which is mobile, darker red, and nonkeratinized. The usual width of keratinized gingiva varies by location, from less than 2.0 mm on the lingual aspect of the mandibular incisors to 9.0 mm on the lingual aspect of mandibular molars.[84]

Histologically, the keratinized gingiva is composed of an underlying connective tissue, the lamina propria with an irregular boundary of projecting ridges supporting the oral epithelium. With attached gingiva, these layers are affixed directly to the periosteum. Oral epithelium in flexible areas, such as the cheek, overlays a vascular submucosal layer (Figs 1-23a and 1-23b). The epithelial layer is characterized by progressive strata in which the active mitotic cells of the basement membrane completely differentiate into scales of synthesized keratin protein as they migrate to the surface for desquamation.[148]

The significance of keratinized tissue in restorative dentistry is somewhat controversial. Lang and Löe[84] concluded that a minimum width of 2.0 mm of keratinized gingiva is required to prevent chronic gingival inflammation. However, several laboratory and clinical studies report that, with good oral hygiene, a healthy and stable gingival margin is possible even when the attached gingiva is minimal, missing, or remodeled.[34,97,157,169]

Dentogingival Junction

The complex of epithelial cell types and connective tissue forming the gingival attachment to the tooth and alveolar bone is called the *dentogingival junction* (Figs 1-23a to 1-23c).[18,49,90] Coronally, the keratinized marginal gingiva invaginates against the cervical enamel to form a partial or nonkeratinized epithelium–lined gingival sulcus with an average depth of 1.0 to 2.0 mm. A depth of more than 3.0 mm is generally considered pathologic and termed a *periodontal pocket*.[130]

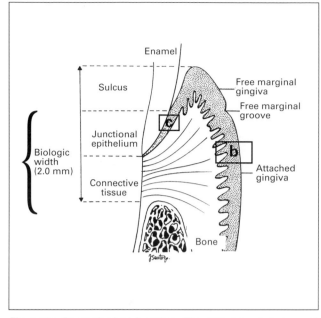

Fig 1-23a Dentogingival junction. The attachment tissues of the gingiva to the tooth and periosteum consist of superficial and deep connective tissues (see Fig 1-24) and three types of epithelium: masticatory keratinized epithelium (inset b, see Fig 1-23b), a nonkeratinized inner sulcus lining epithelium, and a junctional epithelium specialized for attachment to the tooth surface (inset c, see Fig 1-23c).

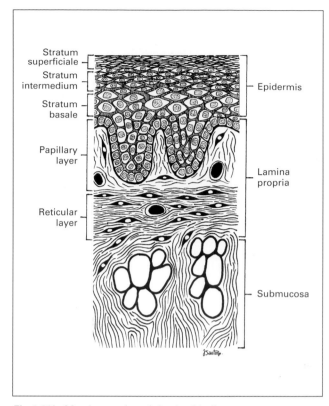

Fig 1-23b Masticatory keratinized epithelium.

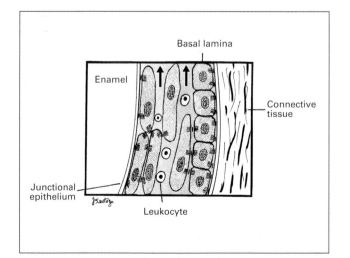

Fig 1-23c Maturing junctional epithelial cells and inflammatory cells from the connective tissue move coronally (arrows) to reach the base of the gingival sulcus and the gingival fluid.

From the base of the sulcus, which corresponds to the level of the CEJ in the young adult tooth, a layer of junctional epithelial cells forms an adhesive basement membrane seal against the cementum of the root. The thickness of the junctional epithelium narrows from 15 to 30 cells at the base of the sulcus to one to three cells apically. Over time, cumulative bacterial and mechanical irritation often result in a lower gingival level (longer clinical crown) and a corresponding increase in the width of the junctional epithelium.[54] Like other oral epithelial cells, the junctional epithelial cells exhibit high mitotic activity, and the cells migrate coronally to the base of the sulcus to be desquamated. An extensive vascular plexus underlies the junctional epithelial cells, which are widely spaced to facilitate the passage of vascular and inflammatory cells into the gingival fluid of the sulcus. Bacterial colonization within the sulcus is discouraged by the combination of a rapidly disrupted cellular base and the lavage and antibacterial action of the vascular transudate of gingival fluid.[75,86]

The supra-alveolar connective tissue and lamina propria of the gingiva are made up of dense interlaced bundles of collagen fibers supporting the gingiva and affixing it to the periosteum and cementum of the hard tissues (Fig 1-24). The fibers are classified by attachment and function into the following groups: *(1)* dentogingival, attaching the gingiva to the cementum; *(2)* alveologingival, affixing gingiva to alveolar bone; *(3)* transseptal, connecting interproximal cemental surfaces; *(4)* dentoperiosteal, from alveolar crest to cementum, an extension of the periodontal ligament; and *(5)* circular, around the tooth.[50]

Restorative Dentistry and Gingival Health

Although dental restorations with supragingival margins and physiologic contours would best sustain gingival health, apical extension of coronal caries lesions, root caries, tooth fracture, and esthetic considerations often dictate a subgingival placement of restorations. The relationship of plaque retention and local irritants to gingival inflammation is well documented.[18,89] Iatrogenic factors and restoration defects such as gingival overhangs, excessive axial contours, marginal defects, and surface roughness of the restorative materials may exacerbate or even cause localized gingival inflammation.[18] Elimination or control of restorative defects is essential. Nevertheless, a clinically acceptable periodontium is often maintained in the presence of less-than-perfect restorative dentistry, thereby implicating bacterial virulence and patient susceptibility as key etiologic cofactors.[80] Margins placed near the base of the sulcus are increasingly associated with problems of inflammation, bleeding, hyperplasia, gingival recession, and pathologic bacteria.[85,89,110] Assuming dental restorations and technique are of good quality, the most critical factors in preserving the health of the restorative-periodontal interface are the appropriate placement of the restorative margin, within the sulcus or supragingivally, and the preservation of the dentogingival junction, known clinically as the *biologic width*.[20,80,85,89,93,109,110,131,135]

Biologic Width

A histologic autopsy study of individuals of various ages and gingival levels revealed variations in depths of the sulcus and junctional epithelium, but the supra-alveolar connective tissue attachment consistently measured approximately 1.07 mm (see Fig 1-23a).[54] In health, the connective tissue and juntional epithelium occupy the space between the base of the sulcus

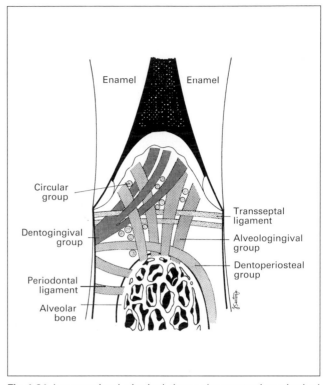

Fig 1-24 Interproximal gingival tissue demonstrating gingival collagen fiber groups: dentogingival, alveologingival, dentoperiosteal, circular (circumferential), and transseptal. (Modified from Ten Cate AR. Oral Histology, ed 4. St Louis: Mosby, 1994. Published with permission.)

and the alveolar crest and measure approximately 2.0 mm; this is termed the *biologic width*.[109] This dimension is assumed to be a physiologic minimum required to preserve the attachment and health of the supporting periodontium. Caries, tooth fracture, or operator error may create conditions in which the 2.0-mm biologic width is surgically traumatized or excised. Chronic and unsightly gingival inflammation and bone loss may occur as the body attempts to restore the biologic width to a more apical level.

In a review of clinical application,[80] Kois reported variability in the dentogingival complex and suggested that the location of the base of the sulcus is problematic because the junctional epithelium is readily penetrated with a probe. Therefore, under anesthesia, a periodontal probe should be used to measure, or "sound," the true dentogingival complex (biologic width + sulcus depth). The majority of midfacial depths from the free gingival margin to the alveolar bone level have a dimension of approximately 3.0 mm, but deviations are confirmed using a periodontal probe for sounding. With a 3.0-mm reading, predictable periodontal healing and health are assured, with the gingival margin of the restoration 0.5 to 1.0 mm apical to the free gingival margin. This preserves a 2.0- to 2.5-mm biologic width. If the biologic width cannot be maintained, prerestorative osseous surgery (crown lengthening) should be performed to reduce bone level and regain the 2.0 to 2.5 mm needed for the biologic width.[20,69,93]

References

1. Abou-Rass M. Crack lines: the precursor of tooth fractures—their diagnosis and treatment. Quintessence Int 1983;4:437–443.

2. Ackermans F, Klein JP, Frank RM. Ultrastructural localization of immunoglobulins in carious human dentine. Arch Oral Biol 1981;26:879–886.

3. Ahlquist M, Franzein O, Coffey J, Pashley D. Dental pain evoked by hydrostatic pressures applied to exposed dentin in man: a test of the hydrodynamic theory of dental sensitivity. J Endod 1994;20:130–137.

4. Anderson DJ. Measurement of stress in mastication. J Dent Res 1956;35:671–673.

5. Bartelstone HJ, Mandel ID, Oshry E, Seidlin SM. Use of radioactive iodine as a tracer in the study of the physiology of the teeth. Science 1947;106:132–133.

6. Bath-Balogh M, Fehrenback MJ. Illustrated Dental Embryology, Histology, and Anatomy. Philadelphia: WB Saunders, 1997:165.

7. Bergenholtz G, Cox CF, Loesche WJ, Syed SA. Bacterial leakage around dental restorations: its effect on the dental pulp. J Oral Pathol 1982;11:439–450.

8. Blaser PK, Lund MR, Cochran MA. Effects of designs of Class 2 preparations on resistance of teeth to fracture. Oper Dent 1983;8:6–10.

9. Boyde A. Enamel structure and cavity margins. Oper Dent 1976;1:13–28.

10. Brännström M, Johnson G, Linden LA. Fluid flow and pain response in the dentin produced by hydrostatic pressure. Odontol Rev 1969;20:15–16.

11. Brännström M, Vojinovic O, Nordenvall KJ. Bacteria and pulpal reactions under silicate cement restorations. J Prosthet Dent 1979;41:290–295.

12. Brännström M. Communication between the oral cavity and the dental pulp associated with restorative treatment. Oper Dent 1984;9:57–68.

13. Braun S, Bantleon HP, Hnat WP, et al. A study of bite force, part I: relationship to various physical characteristics. Angle Orthod 1995;65:367–372.

14. Buonocore MG. A simple method of increasing the adhesion of acrylic filling materials to enamel surfaces. J Dent Res 1955;34:849–853.

15. Buonocore MG. The Use of Adhesives in Dentistry. Springfield, IL: Thomas, 1975:75.

16. Byers MO, Taylor PE. Effect of sensory denervation on the response of rat molar pulp to exposure injury. J Dent Res 1993;72:613–618.

17. Byers MR, Sugaya A. Odontoblast processes in dentin revealed by fluorescent Di-I. J Histochem Cytochem 1995;43:159–168.

18. Carranza FA. Clinical Periodontology, ed 7. Philadelphia: WB Saunders, 1990:19–69.

19. Cassin AM, Pearson GJ, Picton DCA. Fissure sealants as a means of prolonging longevity of amalgam restorations. Clin Mater 1991;7:203–207.

20. Casullo DP. Periodontal considerations in restorative dentistry. In: Genco RJ, Goldman HM, Cohen DW (eds). Contemporary Periodontics, ed 7. St Louis: CV Mosby, 1990:629.

21. Chan DCN. Current methods and criteria for caries diagnosis in North America. J Educ Dent 1993;57:422–427.

22. Christensen GT. Alternatives for Class 2 restorations. Clin Res Assoc Newsletter 1994;18(5):1–3.

23. Christensen GT. Fixed prosthesis—avoiding pulp death. Clin Res Assoc Newsletter 1995;19(1):1.

24. Ciucchi B, Bouillaquet S, Holz J, Pashley D. Dentinal fluid dynamics in human teeth, in vivo. J Endod 1995;21:191–194.

25. Cox CF. Biocompatibility of dental materials in the absence of bacterial infection. Oper Dent 1987;12:146–152.

26. Cox CF, Keall CL, Keall HJ, Ostro E. Biocompatibility of surface-sealed dental materials against exposed pulps. J Prosthet Dent 1987;57:1–8.

27. Cox CF, Subay RK, Ostro E, et al. Tunnel defects in dentin bridges: their formation following direct pulp capping. Oper Dent 1996;21:4–11.

28. Crabb HS, Darling AI. The gradient of mineralization in developing enamel. Arch Oral Biol 1960;52:118–122.

29. Craig RG, Peyton FA (eds). Restorative Dental Materials, ed 5. St Louis: CV Mosby, 1975:47.

30. Craig RG. Restorative Dental Materials, ed 8. St Louis: CV Mosby, 1989:100.

31. Cuenin MF, Scheidt MJ, O'Neal RM, et al. An in vivo study of dentin sensitivity: the relation of dentin sensitivity and patency of dentin tubules. J Periodontol 1991;62:668–673.

32. Dai X-F, Ten Cate AR, Limeback H. The extent and distribution of intratubular collagen fibrils in human dentin. Arch Oral Biol 1991;36:775–778.

33. Dijkman A, Huizinga E, Ruben J, Arends J. Remineralization of human enamel in situ after three months: the effect of not brushing versus the effect of an F dentifrice and an F-free dentifrice. Caries Res 1990;24:263–266.

34. Dorfman HS, Kennedy JE. Gingival parameters associated with varying widths of attached gingiva [abstract 301]. J Dent Res 1981;60(special issue A):386.

35. Duke ES, Lindemuth J. Variability of clinical dentin substrates. Am J Dent 1991;4:241–246.

36. Edgar WM, Geddes DAM, Jenkins GN, et al. Effects of calcium gylcerophosphate and sodium fluoride on the induction in vivo of caries-like changes in human dental enamel. Arch Oral Biol 1978;66:1730–1734.

37. Edwall L, Scott D Jr. Influence of changes in microcirculation on the excitability of the sensory unit in the tooth of the cat. Acta Physiol Scand 1971;82:555.

38. Eisenmann DR. Enamel structure. In: Ten Cate AR (ed). Oral Histology—Development Structure and Function, ed 5. St Louis: CV Mosby, 1998:218–235.

39. Elderton RJ, Mjör IA. Changing scene in cariology and operative dentistry. Int Dent J 1992;42:165–169.

40. Elhabashy A, Swift EJ, Boyer DB, Denehy GE. Effects of dentin permeability and hydration on the bond strengths of dentin bonding systems. Am J Dent 1993;6:123–126.

41. Featherstone JDB, Ten Cate JM. Physicochemical aspects of fluoride enamel interactions. In: Ekstrand J, Fejerskov O, Silverstone LM (eds). Fluoride in Dentistry. Copenhagen: Munksgaard, 1988.

42. Feinman RA, Goldstein RE, Garber DA. Bleaching Teeth. Chicago: Quintessence, 1987.

43. Fejerskov O, Thylstrup A. Dental enamel. In: Mjör IA, Fejerskov O (eds). Human Oral Embryology and Histology. Copenhagen: Munksgaard, 1986:81–88.

44. Fejerskov O, Thylstrup A. Dental enamel. In: Mjör IA, Fejerskov O (eds). Human Oral Embryology and Histology. Copenhagen: Munksgaard, 1986:68–69.

45. Felton D. Long term effects of crown preparation on pulp vitality [abstract 1139]. J Dent Res 1989;69:1009.

46. Fernandes CP, Chevitarese O. The orientation and direction of rods in dental enamel. J Prosthet Dent 1991;65:793–800.

47. Fitzgerald M, Chiego DJ, Heys D. Autoradiographic analysis of odontoblast replacement following pulp exposure in primate teeth. Arch Oral Biol 1990;35:707.

48. Fosse G, Saele PK, Eide R. Numerical density and distributional pattern of dentin tubules. Acta Odontol Scand 1992;50:201–210.

49. Freeman E. Periodontium. In: Ten Cate AR (ed). Oral Histology—Development, Structure, and Function, ed 4. St Louis: CV Mosby, 1994:276–312.

50. Furseth R, Selvig KA, Mjör IA. The periodontium. In: Mjör IA, Fejerskov O (eds). Human Oral Embryology and Histology. Copenhagen: Munksgaard, 1986:136–137.

51. Fusayama T. Two layers of carious dentin; diagnosis and treatment. Oper Dent 1979;4:63–70.

52. Fusayama T. Etiology and treatment of sensitive teeth. Quintessence Int 1988;19:921–925.

53. Garberoglio R, Brännström M. Scanning electron microscopic investigation of human dentinal tubules. Arch Oral Biol 1976;21:355–362.

54. Gargiulo AW, Wentz FM, Orban B. Dimensions and relations of the dentogingival junction in humans. J Periodontol 1961;32:261–267.

55. Gerzina TMO, Hume WR. Effect of hydrostatic pressure on the diffusion of monomers through dentin in vitro. J Dent Res 1995;74:369–373.

56. Graf H, Galasse R. Morbidity, prevalence and intra-oral distribution of hypersensitive teeth [abstract 479]. J Dent Res 1977;56(special issue A):A162.

57. Grajower R, Kaufmann E, Rajstein J. Temperature in the pulp chamber during polishing of amalgam restorations. J Dent Res 1974;53:1189–1195.

58. Gwinnett AJ, Matsui A. A study of enamel adhesives. The physical relationship between enamel and adhesive. Arch Oral Biol 1967;12:1615–1620.

59. Gwinnett AJ. Morphology of the interface between adhesive resins and treated enamel surfaces as seen by scanning electron microscopy. Arch Oral Biol 1971;16:237–238.

60. Gwinnett AJ. Histologic changes in human enamel following treatment with acidic adhesive conditioning agents. Arch Oral Biol 1971;16:731–738.

61. Gwinnett AJ. Structure and composition of enamel. Oper Dent 1992;(suppl 5):10–17.

62. Hannig M, Bott B. In vitro pulp chamber temperature rise during composite resin polymerization with various light-curing devices. Dent Mater 1999;15:275–281.

63. Harris NO, Christen AG. Primary Preventive Dentistry, ed 3. Norwalk, CT: Appleton & Lange, 1991.

64. Hatton JG, Holtzmann DH, Ferrillo PJ, Steward GP. Effect of handpiece pressure and speed on intrapulpal temperature rise. Am J Dent 1994;7:108–110.

65. Heyeraas KJ. Interstitial fluid pressure and transmicrovascular fluid flow. In: Inoki R, Judo T, Olgart L (eds). Dynamic Aspects of Dental Pulp. London: Chapman and Hall, 1990.

66. Heymann HO, Sturdevant JR, Bayne SC, et al. Examining tooth flexure effects on cervical restorations: a two-year clinical study. J Am Dent Assoc 1991;122:41–47.

67. Hoffmann F, Eismann D. The total surface and number of occlusal contacts in static and dynamic occlusion. Bilt Udrux Ortodonata Jugosl 1991;24:71–78.

68. Holland GR. Membrane junctions on cat odontoblasts. Arch Oral Biol 1975;20:551.

69. Ingber JS, Rose LF, Coslet JG. The "biologic width"—a concept in periodontics and restorative dentistry. Alpha Omegan 1977;70(3):62–65.

70. Jackson CR, Skidmore AE, Rice RT. Pulpal evaluation of teeth restored with fixed prostheses. J Prosthet Dent 1992;67:323–325.

71. Johnsen DC, Harshabarger J, Rymer HD. Quantitative assessment of neural development in human premolars. Anat Rec 1983;205:431–439.

72. Kadehashi S, Stanley HR, Fitzgerald RJ. The effects of surgical exposures of pulps in germ-free and conventional rats. Oral Surg Oral Med Oral Pathol 1965;20:340–349.

73. Kidd EAM. Microleakage: a review. J Dent 1976;4:199–206.

74. Kidd EAM, Toffenetti F, Mjör IA. Secondary caries. Int Dent J 1992;42:127–138.

75. Kidera EJ, Mackenzie IC. Surface clearance of oral mucosa and skin [abstract 939]. J Dent Res 1981;60:544.

76. Kim S, Grayson A, Kim B, Schacter W. Effects of dental procedures on pulpal blood flow in dogs [abstract 268]. J Dent Res 1983;62:199.

77. Kim S. Ligamental injection: a physiological explanation of its efficacy. J Endod 1986;12(10):486–491.

78. Kim S, Trowbridge HO. Pulpal reaction to caries and dental procedures. In: Cohen S, Burns RC (eds). Pathways of the Pulp, ed 6. St Louis: CV Mosby, 1994.

79. Kirkham J, Robinson C, Strong M, Shore RC. Effects of frequency of acid exposure on demineralization/remineralization behavior of human enamel in vitro. Caries Res 1994;28:9–13.

80. Kois JC. The restorative-periodontal interface: biological parameters. Periodontol 2000 1996;11:29–38.

81. Koling A. Structural relationships in the human odontoblast layer, as demonstrated by freeze-fracture electron microscopy. J Endod 1988;14:239–246.

82. Lamb WJ, Corpron RE, More FG, et al. In situ remineralization of subsurface enamel lesion after the use of a fluoride chewing gum. Caries Res 1993;27:111–116.

83. Lambrechts P, Braem M, Vuylsteke-Wauters M, Vanherle G. Quantitative in vivo wear of human enamel. J Dent Res 1989;68:1752–1754.

84. Lang NP, Löe H. The relationship between the width of keratinized gingiva and gingival health. J Periodontol 1972;43:623–627.

85. Lang NP, Kiel RA, Anderhalden K. Clinical and microbiological effects of subgingival restorations with overhanging or clinically perfect margins. J Clin Periodontol 1983;10:563–578.

86. Lavelle CLB. Applied Oral Physiology, ed 2. London: Wright, 1988:86.

87. Lee WC, Eakle WS. Possible role of tensile stress in the etiology of cervical erosive lesions of teeth. J Prosthet Dent 1984;52:374–380.

88. Lindhe J, Karring T. The anatomy of the periodontium. In: Lindhe J (ed). Textbook of Clinical Periodontology, ed 2. Copenhagen: Munksgaard, 1989:19–69.

89. Löe H. Reactions of marginal periodontal tissues to restorative procedures. Int Dent J 1968;18:759–778.

90. Löe H, Listgarten M, Terranova V. Periodontal tissues in health. In: Genco R, Goldman H, Cohen D (eds). Contemporary Periodontics. St Louis: Mosby, 1990:3–55.

91. Lopes LM, Leitac JGM, Douglas WH. Effect of a new resin inlay/onlay system on cuspal reinforcement. Quintessence Int 1991;22:641–645.

92. Lyon DG, Darling AI. Orientation of the crystallites in the human dental enamel. Br Dent J 1957;102:438.

93. Malone WFP, Koth DL. Tylman's Theory and Practice of Fixed Prosthodontics, ed 8. St Louis: Ishiyaku EuroAmerica, 1989:10.

94. Marzouk MA, Simonton AL, Gross RD. Operative Dentistry—Modern Theory and Practice. St. Louis: Ishiyaku EuroAmerica, 1985:33–37.

95. Matthews B, Vongsavan N. Interactions between neural and hydrodynamic mechanisms in dentine and pulp. Arch Oral Biol 1994;39(suppl):87s–95s.

96. Mendis BRN, Darling AI. A scanning electron microscope and microradiography study of closure of human coronal dentinal tubules related to occlusal attrition and caries. Arch Oral Biol 1979;24:725–733.

97. Miyasato M, Crigger M, Egelberg J. Gingival condition in areas of minimal and appreciable width of keratinized gingiva. J Clin Periodontol 1977;4:200–209.

98. Mjör IA, Fejerskov O (eds). Human Oral Embryology and Histology. Copenhagen: Munksgaard, 1986.

99. Mondelli JH, Steagall L, Ishikiriama A, et al. Fracture strength of human teeth with cavity preparations. J Prosthet Dent 1980;43:419–422.

100. Muller CFJ, van Wyk CW. The amelo-cemental junction. J Dent Assoc South Afr 1984;39:799–803.

101. Munechika T, Suzuki K, Nishiyama M, et al. A comparison of the tensile bond strengths of composite resins to longitudinal and transverse sections of enamel prisms in human teeth. J Dent Res 1984;63:1079–1082.

102. Murray JJ, Rugg-Gunn AJ, Jenkins GN. Fluorides in Caries Prevention, ed 3. Boston: Wright, 1991.

103. Nagaoka S, Miyazaki Y, Liu HJ, et al. Bacterial invasion into dentinal tubules of human vital and nonvital teeth. J Endod 1995;21:70–73.

104. Nakabayashi N, Nakamura M, Uasuda M. Hybrid layer as a dentin-bonding mechanism. J Esthet Dent 1991;3:133–138.

105. Nakabayashi N, Pashley DH. Hybridization of Dental Hard Tissues. Chicago: Quintessence, 1998.

106. Narhi M, Hirvonen TK, Hakamura M. Responses of intradental nerve fibers to stimulation of dentin and pulp. Acta Physiol Scand 1982;115:173–178.

107. Narhi M, Virtanen A, Huopaniemi T, Hirvonen T. Conduction velocities of single pulp nerve fiber units in the cat. Acta Physiol Scand 1982;116:209–213.

108. National Institute of Dental Research. Oral Health of United States Children. Bethesda, MD: NIH, publication 89-2247, 1989.

109. Nevins M, Skurow HM. The intracrevicular restorative margin, the biologic width, and the maintenance of the gingival margin. Int J Periodont Restorative Dent 1984;4(3):30–39.

110. Newcomb GM. The relationship between the location of subgingival crown margins and gingival inflammation. J Periodontol 1974;45:151–154.

111. Nissan R, Segal H, Pashley D, Stevens R, Trowbridge H. Ability of bacterial endotoxin to diffuse through human dentin. J Endod 1995;21:62–64.

112. Nyborg H, Brännström M. Pulp reaction to heat. J Prosthet Dent 1968;19:605–612.

113. Nylen MU, Scott DB. An Electron Microscopic Study of the Early Stages of Dentinogenesis. Washington, DC: US Public Health Service, publication 613, 1958.

114. Ogawa K, Yamashita Y, Ichigo T, Fusayama T. The ultrastructure and hardness of the transparent layer of human carious dentin. J Dent Res 1983;62:7–10.

115. Okamura K, Maeda M, Nishikawa T, Tsutsui M. Dentinal response against carious invasion: localization of antibodies in odontoblastic body and process. J Dent Res 1980;59:1368–1373.

116. Outhwaite WC, Pashley DH. Effects of changes in surface area, thickness, temperature, and post-extraction time on human dentine permeability. Arch Oral Biol 1976;21:599–603.

117. Pashley DH. The influence of dentin permeability and pulpal blood flow on pulpal solute concentrations. J Endod 1979;5:355–361.

118. Pashley DH, Galloway SE, Stewart F. Effect of fibrinogen in vivo on dentin permeability in the dog. Arch Oral Biol 1984;29:725–728.

119. Pashley DH. Dentin: A dynamic substrate—a review. Scanning Microsc 1989;3:161–176.

120. Pashley DH, Pashley EL. Dentin permeability and restorative dentistry: a status report. Am J Dent 1991;4:5–9.

121. Pashley DH. The effects of acid etching on the pulpodental complex. Oper Dent 1992;17:229–242.

122. Pashley DH, Matthews WG. The effect of outward forced convective flow on inward diffusion in human dentine in vitro. Arch Oral Biol 1993;38:577–582.

123. Pashley DH. Dynamics of the pulpo-dentin complex. Crit Rev Oral Biol Med 1996;7:104–133.

124. Pashley EL, Talman R, Horner JA, Pashley DH. Permeability of normal verses carious dentin. Endod Dent Traumatol 1991;7:207–211.

125. Pashley EL, Tao L, Matthews HG, Pashley DH. Bond strengths to superficial, intermediate and deep dentin in vivo with four dentin bonding systems. Dent Mater 1993;9:19–22.

126. Pitts NG, Kidd EAM. Some of the factors to be considered in the prescription and timing of bitewing radiographs in the diagnosis and management of dental caries: contemporary recommendations. Br Dent J 1992;172:225–227.

127. Powell GL, Nicholls JI, Shurtz DE. Deformation of human teeth under the action of an amalgam matrix band. Oper Dent 1977;2:64–69.

128. Prati C, Pashley DH, Montanari G. Hydrostatic intrapulpal pressure and bond strength of bonding systems. Dent Mater 1991;7:54–58.

129. Provenza DV, Seibel W. Oral Histology—Inheritance and Development, ed 2. Philadelphia: Lea & Febiger, 1986:291–292.

130. Provenza DV. Fundamentals of Oral Histology and Embryology, ed 2. Philadelphia: Lea & Febiger, 1988.

131. Ramfjord SP. Periodontal considerations of operative dentistry. Oper Dent 1988;13:144–159.

132. Reeh ES, Douglas WH, Messer HH. Stiffness of endodontically-treated teeth related to restoration technique. J Dent Res 1989;68:1540–1544.

133. Reeh ES, Messer, HH, Douglas WH. Reduction in tooth stiffness as a result of endodontic and restorative procedures. J Endod 1989;15:512–516.

134. Reeves R, Stanley HR. The relationship of bacterial penetration and pulpal pathosis in carious teeth. Oral Surg Oral Med Oral Pathol 1966;22:59–65.

135. Richter WA, Ueno H. Relationship of crown margin placement to gingival inflammation. J Prosthet Dent 1973; 30:156–161.

136. Scherman A, Jacobsen PL. Managing dentin hypersensitivity: what treatment to recommend to patients. J Am Dent Assoc 1992;123:57–61.

137. Seltzer S, Bender IB. The Dental Pulp, ed 3. Philadelphia: Lippincott, 1984:86.

138. Seltzer S, Bender IB. The Dental Pulp, ed 3. Philadelphia: Lippincott; 1984:324–348.

139. Shimizu C, Yamashita Y, Ichigo T, Fusayama T. Carious change of dentin observed on longspan ultrathin sections. J Dent Res 1981;60:1826–1831.

140. Sigal MJ, Aubin HE, Ten Cate AR. An immuno cytochemical study of the human odontoblast process using antibodies against tubulin, actin, and vimentin. J Dent Res 1985; 64:1348–1355.

141. Silverman JI, Kruger L. An interpretation of dental innervation based on the pattern of calcitonin-gene-related peptide (CGRP) immunoreactive thin sensory axons. Somatosensory Res 1987;5:157–175.

142. Silverstone LM, Mjör IA. Dental caries. In: Hörsted-Bindslev P, Mjör IA (eds). Modern Concepts in Operative Dentistry. Copenhagen: Munksgaard, 1988:46–53.

143. Silverstone LM, Saxton CA, Dogon IL, Fejerskov O. Variation in pattern of acid etching of human dental enamel examined by scanning electron microscopy. Caries Res 1975; 9:373–383.

144. Simmelink JW. Histology of enamel. In: Avery JK (ed). Oral Development and Histology. Baltimore: Williams & Wilkins, 1987:143.

145. Slomiany BL, Murty VL, Zdebska E, et al. Tooth surface-pellicle lipids and their role in the protection of dental enamel against lactic-acid diffusion in man. Arch Oral Biol 1986;31:187–191.

146. Snuggs JM, Cox CF, Powell CS, White K. Pulpal healing and dentinal bridge formation in an acidic environment. Quintessence Int 1993;24:501–510.

147. Spears IR, van Noort R, Crompton RH, et al. The effects of enamel anisotrophy on the distribution of stress in a tooth. J Dent Res 1993;72:1526–1531.

148. Squier CA, Hill MW. Oral mucosa. In: Ten Cate AR (ed). Oral Histology—Development, Structure and Function, ed 4. St Louis: CV Mosby, 1994:389–431.

149. Stanley HR, White CL, McCray L. The rate of tertiary (reparative) dentin formation in the human tooth. Oral Surg Oral Med Oral Pathol 1966;21:180–189.

150. Stanley HR. Human Pulp Response to Restorative Dental Procedures. Gainesville, FL: Storter, 1981.

151. Stanley HR, Pereira JC, Spiegel E, et al. The detection and prevalence of reactive and physiologic sclerotic dentin, reparative dentin and dead tracts beneath various types of dental lesions according to tooth surface and age. J Oral Pathol 1983;12:257–289.

152. Stenvik A, Iverson J, Mjör IA. Tissue pressure and histology of normal and inflamed tooth pulps in Macaque monkeys. Arch Oral Biol 1972;17:1501–1511.

153. Stephan RM. Changes in hydrogen-ion concentration on tooth surfaces and in carious lesions. J Am Dent Assoc 1940;27:718–723.

154. Stewart GP, Bachman TA, Hatton JF. Temperature rise due to finishing of direct restorative materials. Am J Dent 1990;4:23–28.

155. Sugars DA, Sugars DC. Patient assessment, examination and diagnosis, and treatment planning. In: Sturdevant CM, Roberson TM, Heymann HO, Sturdevant JR (eds). The Art and Science of Operative Dentistry, ed 3. St Louis: CV Mosby, 1995:196–197.

156. Swerdlow H, Stanley HR. Reaction of human dental pulp to cavity preparation. J Prosthet Dent 1959;9:121–131.

157. Tai J, Soldinger M, Drelangel A, Pitaru S. Periodontal response to long-term abuse of the gingival attachment by supracrestal amalgam restorations. J Clin Periodontol 1989;16:654–659.

158. Takahashi K, Kishi Y, Kim S. A scanning electron microscope study of the blood vessels of dog pulp using corrosion resin casts. J Endod 1982;8:131–135.

159. Tonder KJ, Kvinnsland I. Micropuncture measurement of interstitial tissue pressure in normal and inflamed dental pulp in cats. J Endod 1983;9:105–109.

160. Torebjork HE, Hallin RG. Perceptual changes accompanying controlled preferential blocking of A and C fiber responses in intact human skin nerves. Exp Brain Res 1973;16:321–332.

161. Torneck CD. Dentin-pulp complex. In: Ten Cate AR (ed). Oral Histology—Development, Structure, and Function, ed 5. St Louis: Mosby, 1998:150–196.

162. Trowbridge HO. Intradental sensory units: physiological and clinical aspects. J Endod 1985;11:489–498.

163. Trowbridge HO, Kim S. Pulp development, structure, and function. In: Cohen S, Burns RC (eds). Pathways of the Pulp, ed 6. St Louis: CV Mosby, 1994:296–336.

164. Turner DF, Marfurt CF, Sattleberg C. Demonstration of physiological barrier between pulpal odontoblasts and its perturbation following routine restorative procedures: horseradish peroxidase tracing study in the rat. J Dent Res 1989; 68:1262–1268.

165. Vale WA. Cavity preparations. Ir Dent Rev 1956;2:33–41.

166. Van Meerbeek B, Dhem A, Goret-Nicaise M, et al. Comparative SEM and TEM examination of the ultrastructure of the resin-dentin interdiffusion zone. J Dent Res 1993;72: 495–501.

167. Van Meerbeek B, Braem M, Lambrechts P, Vanherle G. Morphological characterization of the interface between resin and sclerotic dentin. J Dent 1994;22:141–146.

168. Wainwright WW, Lemoine FA. Rapid diffuse penetration of intact enamel and dentin by carbon 14 labeled urea. J Am Dent Assoc 1950;41:135–145.

169. Wennström JL. Lack of association between width of attached gingiva and development of soft-tissue recession. A five-year longitudinal study. J Clin Periodontol 1987;14: 181–184.

170. White A, Caplan DJ, Weintraub JA. A quarter century of changes in oral health in the United States. J Educ Dent 1995;59:19–57.

171. Zach L, Cohen G. Thermogenesis in operative techniques. J Prosthet Dent 1962;12:977–984.

172. Zach L, Cohen G. Pulp response to externally applied heat. Oral Surg Oral Med Oral Pathol 1965;19:515–530.

2 Patient Evaluation and Problem-Oriented Treatment Planning

Richard D. Davis

Excellence in dental care is achieved through the dentist's ability to assess the patient, determine his or her needs, design an appropriate plan of treatment, and execute the plan with proficiency. Inadequately planned treatment, even when well-executed, will result in less-than-ideal care. The process of identifying problems and designing the treatment for those problems is the essence of treatment planning and the focus of this chapter.

As an integral part of comprehensive dental care, treatment planning for the restoration of individual teeth must be done in concert with the diagnosis of problems and treatment planning for the entire masticatory system. The objective of this chapter is to present a problem-oriented approach to treatment planning for restorative dentistry. This approach begins with a comprehensive patient evaluation and gradually narrows its focus to the restoration of individual teeth. Emphasis is placed on the decision-making processes involved in identifying problems related to restorative dentistry, assessing the demands of the oral environment, and selecting the materials and operative modalities best suited to the treatment of these problems.

The Problem-Oriented Treatment Planning Model

Treatment planning is generally accomplished with either a treatment-oriented model or a problem-oriented model. In the treatment-oriented model, the dentist examining the patient finds certain intraoral conditions and mentally equates those problems to the need for certain forms of treatment. The examination findings are summarized in the form of a list of needed treatments, which then becomes the treatment plan. The problem-oriented model requires that the examination lead to the formulation of a list of problems. Each problem on the list is then considered in terms of treatment options, each of which has different advantages and disadvantages. The optimal solution for each problem is then chosen, and after sequencing, this list of solutions becomes the treatment plan.

For patients with only a few, uncomplicated problems, the outcomes are similar, whether the treatment plan is problem based or treatment based. In more complex cases, problems are often interrelated, and the solution to one problem may affect the treatment needed to resolve other problems. In these instances, the process of identifying and listing the individual problems enables the dentist to think through each problem and consider the treatment options without getting lost in the magnitude of the overall task.

The problem-oriented approach is designed to direct the dentist's attention to a systematic evaluation of the patient, so that no problems are overlooked, either in diagnosis or in treatment planning. It prevents tunnel-vision syndrome, in which obvious pathoses are focused on at the expense of less obvious but equally important problems.

The treatment planning process includes the following steps: A thorough evaluation of the stomatognathic system is completed, problems requiring treatment are identified, and an integrated treatment plan is designed. Given all the problems, the clinician visualizes the state of the dentition after the anticipated removal of seriously compromised and nonrestorable teeth. Having pictured the remaining sound dentition, the dentist visualizes the optimal state to which the patient's dentition can be restored. The clinician then details the treatments needed to achieve this optimal result. The process of "planning in reverse," starting with the end result in mind, often enables the clinician to identify previously unforeseen problems and add them to the problem list. The orthograde plan (planning treatment based on existing problems) and the retrograde plan (planning in reverse, starting from the desired end result) are combined and then coordinated such that the treatment for each problem on the problem list is consistent with the desired optimal treatment goal. This list of treatment steps is then sequenced.

Problem List Formulation

The dentist initially evaluates the patient from a subjective standpoint, first ascertaining the chief complaint and the patient's goals of treatment. A medical history and a dental history are then elicited. The objective portion of the assessment consists of a categorical evaluation of the patient, beginning with vital signs and an extraoral head and neck examination and progressing through a thorough intraoral evaluation. The examination procedures are standardized and routinely completed in the same order and fashion to simplify the procedure and to ensure that crucial steps are not omitted. Related nonclinical portions of the evaluation include examinations of radiographs, diagnostic casts, and photographs.

The objectives of the examination are to distinguish normal from abnormal findings and to determine which of the abnormal findings constitute problems requiring treatment. From the findings of the initial examination, a problem list is established. If the problems are listed under categorical headings (eg,

periodontal problems, endodontic problems), the dentist is unlikely to omit problems. This list is dynamic and can be modified as new problems arise.

Problem-Oriented Planning

In the next phase of treatment planning, the dentist considers the various problems with which the patient presents and uses clinical judgment to estimate which teeth have a sufficiently favorable prognosis to retain and which teeth, if any, should be removed. Mental imaging is used to visualize the state of the dentition after the removal of nonsalvageable teeth. The dentist then formulates a mental image of the optimal condition to which the patient can be rehabilitated. This visualization requires that the dentist decide which teeth need to be replaced, as well as which form of prosthodontic replacement and restorative treatment is most appropriate. Once this optimal condition has been visualized, the dentist lists each procedure required to achieve the desired end result. A treatment solution is then proposed for each problem on the problem list, planning each individual solution to coincide with the final visualized optimal treatment objective.

If the treatment plan for any of the individual problems conflicts with the optimal treatment plan, either the treatment for the individual problem or the optimal treatment goal must be altered until they are coincident. When the clinician believes that, in consideration of all the problems and proposed treatments, the optimal treatment objective is feasible, this list of individual treatments becomes the unsequenced treatment plan.

Treatment Sequencing

The final step in treatment planning, sequencing the treatment, is completed by arranging the solutions to the various problems in a set order (see box).

Chief complaint
Medical/systemic care
Emergency care
Treatment plan presentation
Diagnostic procedures
Disease control
Reevaluation
Definitive care
Maintenance care

The proposed treatment sequencing follows the logic of the medical model, so disease is treated in the priority of importance to the patient's overall health. This method of sequencing ignores the common technique of treating by specialty, where, for example, all the periodontal care is provided, followed by the endodontic care, which is followed by the restorative care.

The patient's *chief complaint* should be addressed at the outset of treatment, even if only via discussion, and even if definitive treatment of this problem will be deferred.

The *medical/systemic care phase* includes aspects of treatment that affect the patient's systemic health. These take precedence over the treatment of dental problems and must be considered before dental problems are addressed. This most commonly includes medically related diagnostic tests and consultations. An example is the investigation of the status and control of a patient's hypertension or diabetes.

Problems addressed in the *emergency care phase* include those involving head and neck pain or infection. They are treated before routine dental problems but after acute problems involving the patient's systemic health. Clinical judgment is exercised to determine the relative importance of systemic problems and dental emergency problems. A review of this topic is found in the text by Little and Falace.[40]

The *treatment plan presentation* (and acceptance of the treatment plan) should precede all nonemergency dental care. Presentation and discussion of the proposed treatment are the basis of informed consent and must not be overlooked. In addition to the primary or optimal treatment plan, the dentist should be prepared to present alternative plans that may be indicated based on extenuating circumstances, such as patient finances or the therapeutic response of teeth crucial to the success of the plan.

Procedures needed to provide additional diagnostic information for treatment planning purposes are accomplished in the *diagnostic phase*. This includes treatment beyond the diagnostic procedures accomplished during the initial examination. It encompasses such items as the use of an occlusal appliance to assess comfort or discomfort in the masticatory apparatus or to determine needed changes in vertical dimension of occlusion; it may also include the use of an interim removable partial denture to evaluate modifications in esthetics. Diagnostic procedures may be used at various stages in treatment, whenever additional information is needed to determine which form of treatment is optimal.

The *disease control phase* consists of treatment designed to arrest active disease. Examples include endodontic treatment to control infection, periodontal treatment to control inflammation, and restorative care, linked with behavior modification, to control caries. Treatment in this phase is aimed at the control of active disease, so that the disease processes would not progress even if no treatment beyond disease control were provided.

The *reevaluation phase* consists of a formal reassessment, during which the dentist decides if all factors, including, for example, the patient's treatment goals, oral hygiene, and response to periodontal therapy warrant continuing with the original treatment plan. This is an important phase of treatment because it provides a predetermined point at which both patient and clinician may elect to alter or even discontinue treatment.

The *definitive care phase* is the final phase of treatment preceding maintenance. Many of the procedures accomplished within the disease-control phase, such as removal of carious tooth structure and placement of direct restorations, achieve both disease control and definitive restoration; however, a number of procedures that go beyond the treatment of active disease are possible. These include procedures designed to enhance function and esthetics, such as orthodontics, prosthodontics, and cosmetic restorative procedures. Treatment sequencing for most of these modalities is beyond the scope of this text. A detailed and comprehensive review of treatment sequencing is provided by Barsh.[5]

Maintenance care is an ongoing phase designed to maintain the results of the previous treatment and prevent recurrence of disease. The maintenance phase generally focuses on the maintenance of periodontal health; the prevention, detection, and treatment of caries; and the prevention of dental attrition.

Dental History and Chief Complaint

The key to successful treatment planning lies in identifying the problems present and formulating a plan that solves each problem, so that each phase of treatment is designed to lead to the final, optimal treatment goal. The dentist who follows this approach begins by listening carefully to the patient and asking relevant questions. A thorough dental history serves as a guide for the clinical examination.

The dental history is divided into three components: the chief complaint, dental treatment, and symptoms related to the stomatognathic system. The chief complaint is addressed first and is recorded in the dental record in the patient's own words. By discussing the patient's chief concern at the outset, the dentist accomplishes two important goals. First, the patient feels that his or her problems have been recognized and the doctor-patient relationship begins positively; second, by writing out the chief complaint, the dentist is assured that it will not be omitted from the problem list. It is not uncommon to encounter a patient who has a multitude of significant dental problems but only a minor chief complaint. If the dentist focuses too quickly on the other problems and omits a discussion of the chief complaint, the patient may question the dentist's ability and desire to resolve the patient's chief concern.

A brief history of past dental treatment can provide useful information. The number and frequency of past dental visits reflects the patient's dental awareness and the priority placed on oral health. The dentist should elicit information about the past treatment of specific problems, as well as the patient's tolerance for dental treatment. All of this information can be of use in fashioning the treatment plan.

Questions about previous episodes of fractured or lost restorations, trauma, infection, sensitivity, and pain can elicit information that will alert the dentist to possible problems and guide him or her in the clinical and radiographic examination. Patients may not volunteer this information; hence specific questions regarding thermal sensitivity, discomfort during chewing, gingival bleeding, and pain are warranted. When there is a history of symptoms indicative of pulpal damage or incomplete tooth fracture, specific diagnostic tests should be performed during the clinical examination.

Clinical Examination

For the purpose of restorative treatment planning, the intraoral assessment involves an examination of the periodontium, dentition, and occlusion. Specific diagnostic tests may be performed as indicated, and a radiographic examination is completed. Each portion of the evaluation should be completed before another aspect of the examination is begun. The findings from each area are placed under the appropriate heading in the problem list. Duplication is common, because

some problems are noted in the evaluation of more than one system. For example, gingival bleeding and periodontal inflammation resulting from a restoration's impingement on the periodontal attachment would be noted in both the periodontal examination and the evaluation of the existing restorations. At this stage, such duplication of effort is acceptable in the interest of completeness.

The following sections describe the intraoral examination used to establish the restorative dentistry problem list (see box).

Elements of the Clinical Examination

1. Evaluation of the dentition
   a. Assessment of caries risk and plaque
   b. Caries diagnosis
   c. Assessment of the pulp
   d. Evaluation of existing restorations
   e. Evaluation of the occlusion and occlusal contours
   f. Assessment of nonocclusal contours
   g. Assessment of tooth integrity and fractures
   h. Evaluation of esthetics
2. Evaluation of the periodontium
   a. Assessment of disease activity
   b. Evaluation of the structure and contour of bony support
   c. Mucogingival evaluation
3. Evaluation of radiographs
4. Evaluation of diagnostic casts

Evaluation of the Dentition

Plaque and Caries Risk

An assessment of caries risk (see Chapter 4) should be accomplished, and the presence of plaque should be documented with a standardized plaque index. The O'Leary index, for example, is a simple, effective measure of plaque accumulation.[49] The use of such an index permits an objective assessment of plaque accumulation. The determination of baseline caries risk and plaque levels at the time of initial examination provides a basis for communication with the patient and other dentists and permits assessments of changes over time. This is important information in establishing a prognosis for restorative care and provides criteria for deciding whether treatment should progress beyond the disease-control phase into the definitive rehabilitation stage.

The levels and location of plaque should be established at the outset of the examination. At the conclusion of the examination appointment, the patient can be given a toothbrush and floss and instructed to clean the teeth as well as possible. Reassessment immediately after the cleaning will establish the patient's hygiene ability and reveal the nature of hygiene instructions needed. A patient who sincerely tries to remove plaque but is unsuccessful in certain areas requires instruction in technique, whereas the patient who demonstrates effective hygiene while in the office but consistently presents with high plaque levels has a problem with motivation. This information is important in designing the treatment plan. A plan requiring a great deal of patient participation and compliance would not be appropriate for a patient with inadequate motivation. Alternatively, a motivated patient who is teachable may well be suited to such a plan.

One of the most reliable indicators of future caries activity is the presence of an existing or recently treated carious lesion.[18] Patients demonstrating active caries may be candidates for an evaluation that entails more than simply a determination of levels and location of plaque. Both a diet survey and a specific plaque assessment are useful in determining the patient's susceptibility to caries and the caries-related prognosis for restorative treatment.

Diet has been shown to be one of the most significant factors in caries risk. A review of more than 100 studies by van Palenstein Helderman et al[76] demonstrated that the frequency and duration of refined carbohydrate exposure is more predictive of caries occurrence than *Streptococcus mutans* counts. Using a diet survey, the patient itemizes *all* food and drink intake for a specified period (generally 1 week). From this diary, the dentist can identify the contribution of specific dietary habits to the patient's caries risk and can direct the patient's attention to these areas. The identification and management of episodic sugar and carbohydrate intake (snacking), as well as overall carbohydrate consumption, should be the focus of dietary intervention.[45]

Because the character of the microflora determines the cariogenicity of the plaque, for patients at high risk of developing caries, periodic assessment of the number of cariogenic bacteria present in the plaque can indicate alterations in the caries susceptibility of the patient.[75] Commercial systems designed to quantify salivary levels of *S mutans* are available. Although higher levels of *S mutans* are not consistently indicative of caries activity, a low level has proven to be an accurate indicator of low caries risk. By monitoring the levels at baseline and over time, the dentist can assess the effectiveness of caries management measures.

Once plaque assessments have been completed, an examination of other areas can be accomplished. The visual examination of the dentition should be conducted in a dry field, with adequate lighting, using a mirror and explorer. Ideally, the dentist will employ some form of magnification to aid in the examination. A number of products providing 2 to 4 times magnification are commercially available. Some magnifying lenses attach to eyeglasses and can be removed, while others are built directly into the lenses of specially constructed eyeglasses (see Chapter 6). The use of magnification, with adequate lighting, significantly enhances the ability of the clinician to detect subtle signs of disease. If the presence of plaque and calculus partially obscures the dentition, debridement must be completed to accomplish a thorough examination.

Detection of Caries Lesions

The terms *carious lesion* and *caries lesion* are both acceptable to describe the effect of the caries process on a tooth, and both terms will be used interchangeably throughout this textbook.

Caries lesions may be classified by location into two broad categories: smooth-surface and pit and fissure caries lesions. Smooth-surface lesions include proximal caries, root caries, and lesions on other smooth surfaces. Detection of caries lesions involves both clinical (visual and tactile) and radiographic examinations.

Pit and fissure caries lesions. Pit and fissure caries lesions are generally found in areas of incomplete enamel coalescence. These areas are most commonly found on the occlusal surfaces of posterior teeth, the lingual surfaces of maxillary anterior teeth, and the buccal pits of molar teeth. Because pit and fissure lesions may begin in small enamel defects that lie in close approximation to the dentinoenamel junction, they may be difficult to detect. Pit and fissure lesions must be extensive to be detected radiographically, generally appearing as a crescent-shaped radiolucency immediately subjacent to the enamel[79] (Figs 2-1a to 2-1c).

Tactile examination, with firm application of a sharp explorer into the fissure, has been the clinical technique most commonly used by dentists in the United States to locate pit and fissure lesions.[14] A sticky sensation felt on removal of the explorer has been the classic sign of pit and fissure caries. Clinical

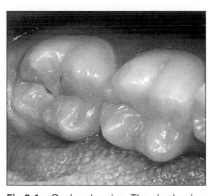

Fig 2-1a Occlusal caries. The shadowing around the stained pits in the second molar indicates the presence of carious dentin at the base of the fissure.

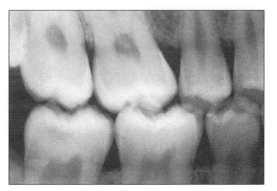

Fig 2-1b The caries lesion shown in Fig 2-1a extends well into dentin.

studies, however, have shown this method to be unreliable, producing many false-positive and false-negative diagnoses.[3] In addition, an explorer can cause cavitation in a demineralized pit or fissure, precluding the possibility of remineralization.[3,7,19,22]

Visual observation, with magnification, of a clean, dry tooth has been found to be a reliable, nondestructive method of detecting pit and fissure caries lesions.[3,19,22] Pit and fissure lesions appear as a gray or gray-yellow opaque area that shows through the enamel (Fig 2-1a). Fiberoptic transillumination may be helpful in visualizing pit and fissure and other types of caries lesions. A variety of new technologies are being evaluated for detection of caries lesions.

When the presence of pit and fissure lesions is uncertain and the patient will be available for recall evaluations, a sealant may be placed over the suspect area. Clinical investigation by Mertz-Fairhurst et al,[46] indicates that sealed caries lesions have little potential for progression. Placement of sealants in fissures over known carious dentin cannot be recommended at present, however. The risk of sealant loss in a patient known to have carious dentin makes this an injudicious practice. Mertz-Fairhurst et al[46] found the placement of a conservative amalgam or resin composite restoration, followed by placement of a resin fissure sealant over the margins of the restoration and remaining fissures, to be a predictable and relatively conservative treatment for such lesions.

Smooth-surface caries lesions. Of the three types of smooth-surface caries, proximal lesions are the most difficult to detect clinically. Generally inaccessible to both visual and tactile examination, proximal caries lesions in posterior teeth are usually detected radiographically. Proximal lesions in anterior teeth may be

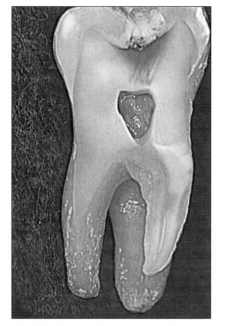

Fig 2-1c The typical pattern of an occlusal caries lesion in cross section.

diagnosed radiographically or with a visual examination using transillumination (Fig 2-2). Root caries lesions located on facial or lingual surfaces of the roots present few diagnostic problems. When root-surface lesions occur proximally, however, they are not readily visible on clinical examination and are generally detected through the radiographic examination (Fig 2-3). Smooth-surface caries lesions occurring on enamel in nonproximal areas are not difficult to detect clinically. Occurring on the facial and lingual enamel surfaces, they are most commonly found in patients with high levels of plaque and a cariogenic diet and are readily accessible to visual and tactile examination.

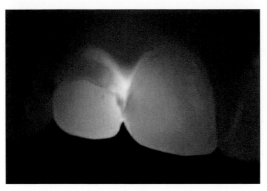

Fig 2-2 Proximal caries lesion is detected in an anterior tooth with the use of transillumination.

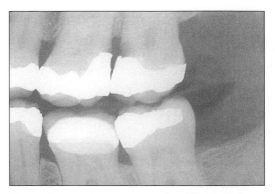

Fig 2-3 Root caries that would be difficult to detect in a routine clinical examination is revealed in a radiograph.

Dental Pulp

Evaluation of pulpal vitality in every tooth is not warranted; however, each tooth that will undergo extensive restoration, as well as all teeth that are critical to the plan of treatment and teeth with pulps of questionable vitality, should be tested.

The application of cold is a valuable method of vitality testing. A cotton pellet saturated with an aerosol refrigerant spray, such as tetrafluoroethane, is placed on the tooth to determine its vitality. A similar test can be performed by placing a "pencil of ice" (made by freezing water inside a sterilized anesthetic cartridge) against a tooth. Skin refrigerants present minimal risk to teeth and restorations; however, carbon dioxide snow and dry ice should be used with caution, because they are extremely cold (–78°C) and can damage enamel or ceramic restorations through thermal shock.[2]

An additional vitality test involves the use of an electric pulp tester. While it can provide information regarding pulp vitality, this test has limitations; it cannot be used in a wet field or on teeth with metallic proximal surface restorations unless measures are taken to insulate adjacent teeth. Furthermore, the numeric scale of the instrument does not reflect the health of the pulp or its prognosis. The electric pulp tester is merely a means of determining whether the tissue within the pulp senses electrical current. A high score may be due to the presence of a partially necrotic pulp or extensive reparative dentin, or it may be the result of poor contact between the tooth and the pulp tester.

When the results of pulp tests are not congruent with the clinical impression, additional tests are indicated. When neither thermal nor electric pulp tests

provide a clear picture of pulp vitality and a restoration is indicated, the preparation can be initiated without the use of anesthetic. This is termed a *test cavity*. If pain or sensitivity is elicited when dentin is cut with a bur, pulpal vitality is confirmed. The restoration may then be completed after administration of local anesthetic.

When a posterior tooth has received endodontic treatment, placement of a complete–cuspal-coverage restoration is generally indicated to prevent fracture.[61] When an anterior tooth has received endodontic treatment, the least invasive form of restoration that satisfies the esthetic and functional needs of the patient is indicated.[71] If sufficient enamel and dentin remain for support, a bonded restoration, such as a resin composite or a ceramic veneer, is the preferred choice. If there is insufficient support for such a restoration after removal of carious tooth structure or defective restorations or following endodontic access preparation, a ceramic or metal-ceramic crown is the restoration of choice. A post is indicated only when a crown is needed and there is insufficient tooth structure to provide support for the crown.[71] When a post is needed, preparation of a small post space preserves dentin and provides optimal fracture resistance for the tooth[69] (see Chapter 21).

Pulp vitality should be determined prior to restorative treatment. It is professionally embarrassing to discover that a recently restored tooth was nonvital prior to restoration and subsequently became symptomatic, requiring endodontic treatment and a replacement restoration.

It is advantageous to ascertain the pulpal prognosis of a tooth prior to restorative treatment. At times this may be difficult, however. When pulpal prognosis is uncertain or guarded, it is often best to perform endodontic therapy before extensive restorative treatment. If the endodontic treatment is completed before restorative care, the repair or replacement of a recently completed large restoration may be avoided.

Planning for endodontic treatment and presenting it as part of the original treatment plan is generally more acceptable to the patient than presenting this treatment option after treatment has begun. An added benefit is that the endodontic prognosis can be established before the dentist commits to restorative care.

When endodontic therapy is required, the feasibility of completing the endodontic procedures should be determined early in the course of treatment. The more critical the tooth is to the overall success of the treatment, the more important it becomes to complete the necessary endodontic treatment early in the treatment schedule. It is poor planning to rely on a tooth in the treatment plan when that tooth cannot be successfully treated with endodontics.

Endodontic diagnosis can be challenging. A thorough discussion of this subject can be found in the text by Cohen and Burns.[17]

Existing Restorations

In the course of the intraoral examination, existing restorations must be evaluated to determine their serviceability. The following general criteria are used to evaluate existing restorations: *(1)* structural integrity, *(2)* marginal opening, *(3)* anatomic form, *(4)* restoration-related periodontal health, *(5)* occlusal and interproximal contacts, *(6)* caries, and *(7)* esthetics.

Structural integrity. An evaluation of the structural integrity of a restoration involves determining whether it is intact or whether portions of the restoration are partially or completely fractured or missing. The presence of a fracture line dictates replacement of the restoration. If voids are present, the dentist must exercise clinical judgment in determining whether their size and location will weaken the restoration and predispose it to further deterioration or recurrent caries.

Marginal opening. Few restorations have perfect margins, and the point at which marginal opening dictates replacement of the restoration is difficult to determine. For amalgam restorations, it has been demonstrated that marginal ditching neither implies the presence nor necessarily portends the development of caries lesions.[33] Therefore, the existence of marginal ditching does not dictate the replacement of

amalgam restorations. Because the margins of amalgam restorations become relatively well sealed from the accumulation of corrosion products, a general guideline has been to continue to observe the restoration unless signs of recurrent caries are present. An accumulation of plaque in the marginal gap is also an indication for repair or replacement of an amalgam restoration. It has been suggested that noncarious marginal gaps in amalgam may be repaired with a resin sealant to enhance the longevity of the restoration.[66] The long-term clinical efficacy of this method has yet to be documented, but there is some recent in vitro evidence of its benefit.[58]

For restorations that do not seal by corrosion, a marginal gap into which the end of a sharp explorer may penetrate should be considered for repair, or the restoration should be replaced. This is especially true for resin composite restorations, because bacterial growth has been shown to progress more readily adjacent to resin composite than to amalgam or glass-ionomer materials.[67] An increased susceptibility to caries has been reported in resin composite restorations whose marginal gaps exceeded 100 to 150 μm (see Figs 2-6a and 2-6b).[50]

The presence of a marginal gap is less critical for restorations with anticariogenic properties (eg, glass-ionomer cement). Both in vitro[64] and in vivo[29,54,72] studies have shown that tooth structure adjacent to glass-ionomer restorations is less susceptible to caries than that adjacent to either resin composite or amalgam restorations. Consequently, restorations with anticariogenic properties should not generally be replaced because of marginal ditching, but rather when frank caries has occurred or when some other defect indicates the need for treatment. In anterior teeth, this is indicated when the tooth structure adjacent to the marginal gap becomes carious or by marginal staining that is esthetically unacceptable.

Anatomic form. Anatomic form refers to the degree to which the restoration duplicates the original contour of the intact tooth. Common problems include overcontouring, undercontouring, uneven marginal ridges, inadequate facial and lingual embrasures, and lack of occlusal or gingival embrasures. Many restorations exhibit one or more of these problems yet adequately serve the needs of the patient and do not require replacement. The critical factor in determining the need for replacement is not whether the contour is ideal but whether pathoses have resulted, or are likely to result, from the poor contour.

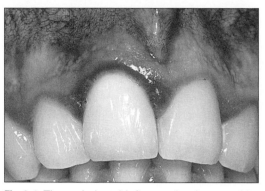

Fig 2-4 The periodontal inflammation is caused by the encroachment of the crown margins into the periodontal attachment area of the maxillary central incisors.

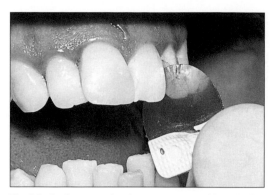

Fig 2-5 An interproximal contact–smoothing device is useful for removing irregularities that impede that passage of floss.

Restoration-related periodontal health. Examination of restorations must include an assessment of the effect that existing restorations have on the health of the adjacent periodontium. Problems commonly encountered in this area are *(1)* surface roughness of the restoration, *(2)* interproximal overhangs, and *(3)* impingement on the zone of attachment, called the biologic width (the area, approximately 2 mm in the apicocoronal dimension, occupied by the junctional epithelium and the connective tissue attachment) (see Fig 1-23a).

All three of these phenomena can cause inflammation within the periodontium.[44,68,77] If restorations extend vertically or horizontally beyond the cavosurface margin in the region of the periodontal attachment or impinge on the biologic width, the health of the periodontal tissue should be assessed (Fig 2-4). If other local etiologic factors have been removed, and periodontal inflammation persists in the presence of these conditions, treatment should be initiated. In the case of overhanging restorations, pathosis may be eliminated and the restoration may be made serviceable simply by removing the overhang. If the periodontal inflammation fails to resolve, the restoration should be replaced. In the case of biologic width impingement, space for a healthy periodontal attachment must be gained through surgical crown lengthening or a combination of orthodontic-forced eruption and surgical crown lengthening.

Inflammatory changes suggestive of biologic width violations are common on the facial aspects of anterior teeth that have been restored with crowns. On occasion, however, evaluation of the marginal areas reveals inflammation even when an adequate space

remains between the coronal margin and the periodontal attachment apparatus, leaving the clinician puzzled as to the cause of the problem. If periodontal inflammation persists in the apparent absence of local etiologic factors, including biologic width impingement, the dentist should evaluate the entire cervical circumference of the restoration. Inflammatory changes on the facial aspect of a restoration are sometimes a manifestation of interproximal inflammation. Further evaluation may reveal an interproximal violation of biologic width from which the inflammatory reaction has extended to the more visible facial area.

Even in the absence of impingement on biologic width, open or rough subgingival margins can harbor sufficient bacterial plaque to generate an inflammatory response. Gingival inflammation around a crown may also be due to an allergic reaction to a material in the crown. Nickel alloy in the casting often causes such reactions. During the assessment of existing restorations or the planning of future restorations, the location of margins is an important consideration. Supragingival margins result in significantly less gingival inflammation than do subgingival margins.[41] Supragingival margins should be the goal when overriding concerns (eg, esthetics or requirements for resistance and retention) do not contraindicate their use.

Occlusal and interproximal contacts. All interproximal contacts should be assessed with thin dental floss by the dentist. In addition, the patient should be queried regarding any problems encountered in the passing of floss through the contacts during home hygiene procedures. Contacts that do not allow the smooth passage of floss must be altered, or the restoration must

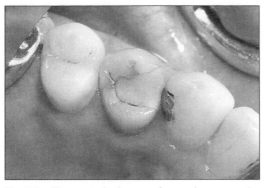

Fig 2-6a The marginal gap of a resin composite restoration is stained. Note the shadow indicating that caries has affected the dentin.

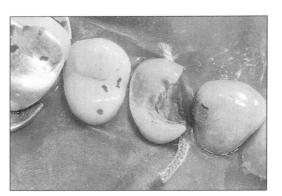

Fig 2-6b Removal of the restoration reveals that there is extensive carious dentin.

be replaced, to permit the use of floss. The use of an interproximal contact–smoothing device is often effective in eliminating roughness that impedes the passage of floss (Fig 2-5).

Contacts that are open or excessively light should be evaluated to determine whether pathosis, food impaction, or annoyance to the patient has resulted. When any of these problems is present, steps should be taken to alleviate them. Generally, the placement or replacement of a restoration is required to establish an adequate proximal contact.

When an open contact is found, an attempt should be made to determine its cause. If occlusal contacts have moved a tooth, and a restoration is to be placed to close the proximal contact, the occlusal contacts must be altered to prevent the open contact from recurring after the placement of the new restoration.

The occlusal contacts of all restorations should be evaluated to determine whether they are serving their masticatory function without creating a symptomatic or pathogenic occlusion. In the absence of periodontally pathogenic bacteria, traumatic occlusion has not been found to initiate loss of periodontal attachment.[78] In the presence of periodontal pathogens in a susceptible host, however, occlusal trauma has been found to accelerate the loss of attachment.[39] Existing restorations located in teeth exhibiting significant attachment deficits should be examined closely for the presence of hyperocclusion. Restorations whose occlusal contacts are creating primary occlusal trauma should be altered or replaced, as necessary, to resolve the problem. Restorations that are in significant infraocclusion may permit the supraeruption of teeth and should be considered for replacement.

Caries. The evaluation for carious tooth structure around existing restorations focuses on an examination of the margins. The dentist must use a combination of visual, tactile, and radiographic examinations to detect the presence of caries lesions. A radiolucent area surrounding a radiopaque restoration or the presence of soft tooth structure generally indicates a caries lesion and warrants either repair or replacement of the restoration.

Discoloration in the marginal areas is a sign that is more difficult to interpret. It often indicates leakage of some degree. In nonamalgam restorations without anticariogenic properties, discoloration that penetrates the margin often indicates the need for replacement of the restoration (Figs 2-6a and 2-6b). This is not a definite indication, however, and clinical judgment is required. In restorations with anticariogenic properties, leakage and stain may be observed with less concern for caries, leaving esthetics as the primary consideration. This is not to imply that restorative materials with caries-resistance properties are immune to caries. Caries lesions have been documented adjacent to glass-ionomer restorations.[47] If the tooth structure adjacent to the margin of a restoration appears to be carious (either with undermined enamel or frank cavitation), rather than simply discolored, the restoration should be replaced.

In the case of amalgam restorations, the decision to replace a restoration with discoloration in the adjacent tooth structure is less clear because corrosion products may discolor a tooth, even in the absence of caries, especially when little dentin is present. When there is no apparent communication between the cavosurface and the stained area and when the discol-

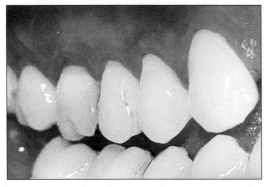

Fig 2-7 The shadow in the mesiofacial aspect of the maxillary first molar is caused by amalgam that shows through the translucent enamel. No caries is present.

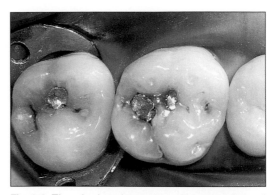

Fig 2-8 The shadow located on the mesiolingual cusp adjacent to the larger occlusal amalgam restoration on the maxillary right first molar indicates the presence of carious dentin.

oration is primarily gray, then metal "show through" is suspected and observation is warranted (Fig 2-7). When the discolored area appears yellow or brown and appears to communicate with the cavosurface, replacement of the restoration is indicated (Fig 2-8).

Esthetics. The esthetic evaluation of existing restorations is highly subjective. When the functional aspects of a restoration are adequate, it is often best to simply inquire whether the patient is satisfied with the esthetic appearance of the existing restorations. If the patient expresses dissatisfaction with the appearance of a restoration, the dentist must determine whether improvement is feasible. Care should be taken to ascertain the reason that the original restoration had less-than-optimal esthetics. An underlying problem may preclude improvement of the original esthetic problem, and an equally unsatisfactory result may occur in the replacement restoration.

When replacing a restoration for esthetic reasons only, the dentist must carefully explain the risks (eg, endodontic complications) incurred in replacement.

Some of the more common esthetic problems found in existing restorations are *(1)* display of metal, *(2)* discoloration or poor shade match in tooth-colored restorations, *(3)* poor contour in tooth-colored restorations, and *(4)* poor periodontal tissue response in anterior restorations. (See Chapter 3 for further discussion of esthetic problems.)

Occlusion and Occlusal Wear

The occlusion can have significant effects on the restorative treatment plan. The following factors should be evaluated in the course of the occlusal

examination: *(1)* occlusal interferences between the occlusion of centric relation (CR) and that of maximum intercuspation (MI); *(2)* the number and position of occlusal contacts, as well as the stress placed on the occlusal contacts in MI; *(3)* the amount and pattern of attrition of teeth and restorations resulting from occlusal function and parafunction; *(4)* the interarch space available for placement of needed restorations.

Occlusal interferences. Most people have some difference between the positions of centric relation and maximum intercuspation and have no consequent pathosis, indicating that the existence of a discrepancy between these positions is not, in itself, an indication for occlusal equilibration. Findings from the occlusal examination that should be recorded in the restorative dentistry problem list and do warrant treatment with occlusal equilibration are the following: *(1)* signs and symptoms of occlusal pathosis resulting from discrepancies between the occlusion of centric relation and maximum intercuspation (eg, mobility, excessive wear of teeth in the areas of interference between CR and MI, or periodontal ligament soreness) and *(2)* the need to restore the majority of the posterior occlusion.

This second factor does not imply the restoration of the majority of the posterior teeth but rather the restoration of the majority of the occlusal contacts. For example, insertion of a three-unit fixed partial denture in the mandibular right quadrant and several large restorations in the maxillary left quadrant results in the restoration of the majority of the occlusal contacts for the posterior teeth. There is no reason to fabricate the occlusion of the new restorations to duplicate the interferences that existed preoperatively. In such a case, occlusal equilibration should be completed prior to the restorative treatment. Through adjustment of only a very few occlusal contacts on teeth not involved in restorations and subsequent fabrication of the new restorations in centric relation, the occlusions of CR and MI become coincident.

Occlusal contacts. The number and position of occlusal contacts in the maximum intercuspation position, the force of the occlusal load, and the manner in which opposing teeth occlude in excursive function strongly influence the selection of restorative materials, as well as the design of the preparation and restoration. As the number of missing teeth increases, the proportion of the occlusal load borne by each tooth increases. As occlusal stress increases, the dentist is forced to select the strongest of the available restorative materials and to design restorations to provide the greatest strength in the areas of maximum stress. Likewise, the greater the potential for the patient to function on the restorations in lateral excursions, the greater is the need for strength in the restorative material and the greater is the imperative to select a material that will function without causing injury to the opposing dentition.

Wear. Out of concern for the opposing dentition, the clinician must consider the abrasive potential of the various restorative materials available. Clinical abrasivity is a function of a number of physical properties; no single variable is predictive of abrasivity.[51] Hardness is a useful indicator, but the best predictor of wear is the relative clinical performance of the various materials. In clinical determinations of wear behavior, the amalgam in an amalgam-enamel wear couple exhibits only slightly greater wear than does an enamel-enamel wear couple. The amalgam causes less wear to the opposing dentition than does enamel.[34] The wear rate of resin composite depends on the nature of the resin composite. Microfilled resins exhibit wear behavior similar to that of enamel, while hybrid resins exhibit more wear and generate more wear to opposing enamel than does either amalgam or enamel.[42] Polished cast gold is more wear resistant than enamel or amalgam and generates minimal wear of opposing tooth structure.

Ceramic restorations exhibit little wear themselves, but have demonstrated a consistent ability to severely abrade the enamel of the opposing dentition[48] (Fig 2-9).

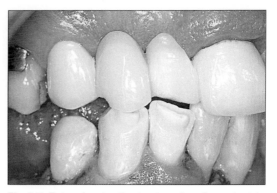

Fig 2-9 Extensive tooth structure has been lost in the mandibular teeth because of wear caused by the opposing porcelain fixed partial denture.

A newer generation of ceramic appears to have somewhat overcome this problem. In both in vitro and in vivo studies, Empress 2 (Ivoclar Williams) has been shown to cause virtually no wear of opposing enamel.[32,62,63]

Wear (attrition and abrasion) of the natural dentition is a normal clinical phenomenon. Only when wear becomes excessive is it deemed a problem. Wear may arise from a variety of causes. Excessive occlusal wear is caused primarily by occlusal parafunction. In these instances, facets on opposing teeth match well, indicating the predominant pattern of parafunctional activity. Because altering occlusal parafunctional habits is extremely difficult, prevention of excessive occlusal wear is accomplished with the use of an occlusal resin appliance (Figs 2-10a and 2-10b). The dentist should identify patients who demonstrate signs of excessive occlusal wear (especially those patients who exhibit these signs at an early age) and include occlusal appliance therapy in the treatment plan.

Occasionally, the presence of abrasive substances in the mouth is the cause of excessive occlusal wear. When the vocation or lifestyle of a patient frequently places him or her in contact with airborne abrasives, prevention of wear is difficult. Education of the patient and use of an occlusal resin appliance will decrease the occlusal abrasion; however, decreasing the patient's exposure to the causative agent is the only reliable means of eliminating the problem.

Another form of tooth loss that often mimics wear is caused by chemical erosion. Erosion can result from habits such as sucking lemons or from the introduction of gastric acid into the oral cavity, which can occur with repeated regurgitation. Gastro-esophogeal-

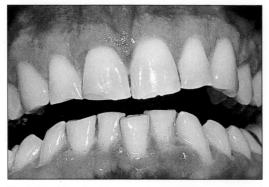

Fig 2-10a The significant occlusal attrition is caused by a habit of parafunctional grinding in a patient less than 30 years of age.

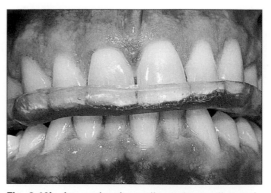

Fig 2-10b An occlusal acrylic resin appliance is used to minimize the abrasive trauma generated by the parafunctional grinding habit.

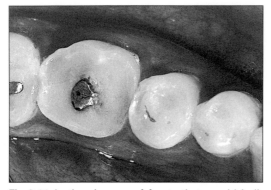

Fig 2-11 In the absence of facets that would indicate occlusal wear, significant loss of tooth structure is evidence of a chemical erosive process. Note both the amalgam restoration situated above the surrounding tooth structure and the smooth, glass-like character of the dentin.

reflux-disease, frequently referred to as GERD, occurs in the presence of an incompetent esophageal sphincter and is a common cause of acid-related erosion of the dentition. While the dentist may be the first to detect the signs of this condition, referral to a physician is in order to manage the disease.

Bulimia is another condition that may be first detected by the dentist. The frequent forced regurgitation associated with this disorder results in acidic dissolution of exposed tooth surfaces and can have devastating effects on the dentition.

Chemical erosion can be distinguished from mechanical wear by the location and character of the defects. Erosion lesions have a smooth, glassy appearance. When found on the occlusal surfaces of posterior teeth, these lesions are characterized by concave defects into which abrasive agents are unlikely to pene-

trate. Severely "cupped out" cusp tips and teeth that have restorations standing above the surrounding tooth structure are clinical findings commonly associated with chemical erosion (Fig 2-11).

Erosive lesions appearing primarily on the lingual surfaces of maxillary teeth and the occlusal surfaces of posterior teeth in both arches are characteristic of acid decalcification arising from gastric acid. Smooth lesions on the facial surfaces might be of chemical or mechanical origin. In instances of uncertainty, questions related to habits may elucidate the cause of mechanical abrasion, while a thorough history and medical evaluation may reveal the presence of acid-related erosion. When bulimia is the underlying problem, detection is often difficult. The dentist must be tactfully candid in discussing this possible etiology. Regardless of the cause of the loss of tooth structure, the primary cause should be determined and resolved before rehabilitative therapy is undertaken.

Interarch space. When the dentist determines that significant loss of occlusal tooth structure has occurred and pulpal sensitivity has arisen, or that teeth have been so weakened by abrasion or erosion as to be at risk for fracture, restorative treatment is indicated. The dentist must evaluate the occlusion at maximum intercuspation and determine whether sufficient space exists for the placement of the restoration. If inadequate space is available, the dentist must either gain space by surgical crown lengthening, shorten the opposing tooth, or select a different restorative option that requires less space. Recognition of the space inadequacy prior to tooth preparation is essential.

In those cases where generalized wear or erosion has taken place, resulting in the loss of an extensive amount of tooth structure, the dentist is faced with a significant restorative problem. In these instances, sufficient interarch space is often not available to restore the lost tooth structure without increasing the vertical dimension of occlusion. Increasing the vertical dimension of occlusion is a complex restorative process involving more than a consideration of the mechanics of individual tooth restoration. A description of treatment of this nature is beyond the scope of this text.

Nonocclusal Contours

Unlike changes in occlusal contours, the alteration of the axial contours of teeth is not due to tooth-to-tooth abrasion. Although it is generally due to erosion or toothbrush-related abrasion, occlusally generated stresses may contribute to this phenomenon in some instances. The term *abfraction* is applied to those noncarious lesions thought to have a combined cause of abrasion and occlusally induced tooth flexure.[30,37,80] Preventive treatment for cervical abrasion is directed at altering the habit causing the problem. Modification of toothbrushing habits and the use of minimally abrasive toothpastes with a neutral pH can reduce the rate of erosion and abrasion. If abfraction is suspected, treatment should include the nighttime wear of an occlusal resin appliance.

Noncarious cervical lesions should be included on the problem list to alert the patient to the problem and to ensure that the dentist addresses the cause and considers restorative treatment options. In the absence of symptoms, the extent of the lesion should be assessed, and restorative intervention should be a matter of clinical judgment. A prudent approach would be to restore the area when tooth loss has progressed to the point that the normal tooth contour could be replaced with restorative material without leaving the restorative material too thin to withstand functional and abrasive stresses.

Cracked-Tooth Syndrome

Cracked-tooth syndrome is a fairly common result of incomplete tooth fracture. Patients suffering cracked-tooth syndrome often experience cold sensitivity and sharp pains of short duration while chewing.[11,12,16,65]

Cracked-tooth syndrome may be found in restored or unrestored teeth.[31] In restored teeth, it is often associated with existing small to medium-sized restorations.[26,35] It has been reported to occur equally in both the maxillary and mandibular arches. In the maxillary arch, it has been reported to occur with similar frequencies in molars and premolars. In the mandibular arch, molars are the teeth most commonly found to be cracked.[13] Regardless of the location by arch, the cusps most commonly fractured are the nonfunctional cusps.[13] Often, patients with multiple cracked teeth have parafunctional habits or malocclusions that have contributed to the problem. Cracked-tooth syndrome is an age-related phenomenon; the greatest occurrence is found among patients between 33 and 50 years of age.[31]

Cracked-tooth syndrome is often difficult to diagnose. The patient is frequently unable to identify the offending tooth, and evaluation tools, such as radiographs, visual examination, percussion, and pulp tests, are typically nondiagnostic. The two most useful tests are transillumination and the "biting test."

Many teeth contain cracks and craze lines, most of which cause no symptoms; however, transillumination of a severely cracked tooth generally presents a distinctive appearance that permits the clinician to distinguish minor cracks from those deep enough to result in symptoms. When a tooth with a severe crack is transilluminated from either the facial or lingual direction, light transmission is interrupted at the point of the crack. This results in the portion of the tooth on the side away from the light appearing quite dark. The transition from bright illumination on one side of the tooth to darkness on the other is sudden rather than gradual, occurring abruptly at the point of the fracture.

The biting test is the most definitive means of localizing the crack responsible for the patient's pain. By having the patient bite a wooden stick, rubber wheel, or special device made for this test, the dentist is generally able to reproduce the patient's symptom and identify not only the fractured tooth but also the specific portion of the tooth that is cracked. Crunchy food, placed sequentially on suspect teeth, has also been suggested as a diagnostic aid.[1] Once the offending tooth has been identified, tooth preparation often allows visualization of the crack (Fig 2-12).

Where direct diagnostic methods prove unsuccessful, indirect methods may be used. An orthodontic band or sealant may be placed on suspected teeth to prevent separation of the crack during function. If the patient's symptoms subside, the diagnosis of cracked-tooth syndrome has been made.

In the treatment of incomplete tooth fracture, the tooth sections are splinted together with a cuspal coverage restoration.[26] This may include the use of an amalgam restoration, a crown, or an indirectly fabricated onlay of metal, ceramic, or resin composite. Because of their potential to lose bond integrity over time, bonded intracoronal restorations are presently not considered to be adequate for long-term resolution of the problem.[21,28]

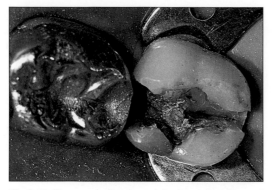

Fig 2-12 The mesiodistal crack in the pulpal floor of the mandibular right second molar caused sharp pain upon chewing. The tooth is to be restored with an onlay to splint the tooth together during function, to relieve the patient's symptoms, and to prevent propagation of the crack.

Esthetic Evaluation

In addition to an esthetic evaluation of existing restorations, an assessment of the esthetics of the entire dentition should be completed. Because dental esthetics is a subjective area, patients should be questioned about any dissatisfaction they may have regarding the esthetics of their dentition. In the absence of complaints by the patient, the impressions of the dentist regarding esthetic problems should be tactfully conveyed to determine whether the patient would like the esthetic problems addressed. The dentist who has studied dental esthetics is often better able than the patient to determine how cosmetic dental procedures might enhance the patient's appearance. If an agreement is reached between the patient and dentist as to the existence of specific esthetic problems, the problems should be included on the restorative dentistry problem list.

Commonly encountered esthetic problems that are related to or may be addressed by restorative dentistry include: (1) stained or discolored anterior teeth; (2) unesthetic contours in anterior teeth (eg, unesthetic length, width, incisal edge shape, or axial contours); (3) unesthetic position or spacing of anterior teeth; (4) carious lesions and unesthetic restorations; (5) excessive areas of dark space in the buccal corridors due to a constricted arch form; and (6) unesthetic color and/or contour of tissue adjacent to anterior restorations. This last problem includes excessive gingival display occasionally referred to as the "gummy smile." (See Chapter 3 for a thorough discussion of esthetic diagnosis.)

The restorative treatment of esthetic problems may range from conservative therapy, such as microabra-

sion or bleaching, to more invasive care, such as the placement of resin veneers, ceramic veneers, or complete-coverage crowns. Additionally, adjunctive periodontal, endodontic, or orthodontic procedures may be helpful, depending on the nature of the original problem. These procedures are discussed in subsequent chapters.

Evaluation of the Periodontium

From a restorative dentistry perspective, the periodontium must be evaluated primarily for two reasons: (1) to determine the effect that the periodontal health of the teeth will have on the restorative dentistry treatment plan and (2) to determine the effect that planned and existing restorations will have on the health of the periodontium.

Evaluation of the periodontium consists of a clinical assessment of attachment levels, bony topography, and tooth mobility; a qualitative assessment of tissue health; and a radiographic evaluation of the supporting bone. The assessment of attachment levels involves periodontal probing of the entire dentition with both a straight probe for determination of vertical probing depths and a curved probe to explore root concavities and furcation areas. Any bleeding induced by gentle probing should be noted. A variety of tests are available to aid in determining the presence and identity of periodontal pathogens; however, the most consistent clinical indicator of inflammation is bleeding on probing.[53] Bleeding on probing does not always indicate the presence of active periodontal disease, but active disease has been consistently found to be absent in the absence of bleeding on probing.[53]

The qualitative assessment of periodontal tissue health calls for a subjective assessment of the inflammatory status of the tissue; tissue color, texture, contours, edema, and sulcular exudates are noted. The presence of specific local factors, such as plaque and calculus and their relationship to tissue inflammation, should be noted. Abnormal mucogingival architecture, such as gingival dehiscences and areas of minimal attached gingiva, should be recorded. This is especially true when these anomalies are noted in the proximity of existing or planned restorations.

During examination of the periodontium, the dentist must not only be cognizant of periodontal inflammation adjacent to existing restorations, but must estimate the location of margins for future restorations and their potential for impinging on the biologic width. Review of radiographs, especially correctly angulated bite-wing radiographs, during the periodontal examination enables the dentist to assess the relationship of existing and planned restorations to bone levels and to correlate radiographic signs with clinical findings.

When the clinical and radiographic portions of the periodontal examination have been completed, a periodontal prognosis should be established for all teeth; special attention should be given to teeth involved in the restorative dentistry treatment plan. Teeth requiring restorative treatment that have a guarded periodontal prognosis should be noted in the restorative dentistry problem list. Until the periodontal prognosis becomes predictably positive, the restorative treatment of teeth with a guarded prognosis should be as conservative as possible, and treatment planning that relies on these teeth must remain flexible.

Evaluation of Radiographs

The radiographic examination is an essential component of the comprehensive evaluation. Problems detected during evaluation of radiographs are listed under the appropriate headings on the problem list (eg, restorative, endodontic, periodontal).

Although radiographs can provide valuable information for use in diagnosis and treatment planning, exposure of patients to ionizing radiation must be minimized; therefore, discretion is required when the dentist orders radiographs. There are no inflexible rules for radiographic evaluation; rather, clinical judgment should be exercised. The goal is to minimize unnecessary exposure and cost but to avoid underutilization, which could result in inadequate diagnosis. The use of patient-specific criteria is the key. Different patients have different requirements both in terms of the radiographic views needed and the frequency with which radiographs should be repeated.

A reasonable guideline to follow is that all dentate patients should initially have a radiographic series completed that reveals the periapical areas of the entire dentition. This will permit detection of central lesions not visible on bite-wing radiographs and will serve as a baseline, allowing the clinician to assess changes over time. Although it is not common to discover pathoses by using panoramic films or complete-mouth radiograph series, it has been reported that approximately 85% of central jaw lesions are apparent in views of the apical areas of the dentition but are not visible on bite-wing radiographs.[8] For patients

who have periodontal disease, periapical radiographs are indicated. For patients who have no significant periodontal pathoses, a panoramic radiograph provides the necessary view. For all patients with approximating teeth, a series of films is indicated to show the proximal areas of posterior teeth. Bite-wing radiographs serve this purpose.

The frequency with which radiographs should be updated is determined by clinical judgment. The dentist should assess the etiologic factors present and determine whether new disease is likely to have occurred since the last radiographic examination. The dentist must weigh the risk of undetected disease against the cumulative risk of radiation exposure. A suggested guideline is to take new bite-wing radiographs of caries-active adults on an annual basis and of caries-inactive patients every 2 to 3 years.[73] Patients may be considered minimally susceptible to caries if they have had no carious lesions in recent years, demonstrate low plaque levels, have adequate salivary flow, have a noncariogenic diet, and exhibit no clinically discernible caries lesions. Periapical radiographs of the entire dentition should be repeated only as dictated by the specific needs of the treatment to be accomplished. For example, a patient under active treatment or maintenance for periodontal disease may require an updated radiographic series every 2 to 3 years to reevaluate bony contours, while another patient, because disease processes are controlled, may require subsequent periapical radiographic updates only every 4 to 5 years.

In evaluating radiographic findings for restorative purposes, the dentist should note open interproximal contacts, marginal openings, overhanging restorations, periapical radiolucencies and radiopacities, and radiolucencies within the body of the tooth. The dentist must interpret "abnormal" radiographic findings with caution. Many phenomena that are detectable radiographically can also be detected clinically and should be verified clinically before treatment is planned. This is especially true when the clinician evaluates radiolucencies that appear to represent carious tooth structure but may in fact represent nonpathologic processes. An example of this is the radiographic phenomenon commonly known as "burnout" (Fig 2-13). Burnout is a radiolucency not caused by demineralization that occurs when the x-ray beam traverses a portion of the tooth with less thickness than the surrounding areas. It is most commonly found near the cervical area of a tooth and is frequently caused by concavities in the tooth or the angulation of the beam.

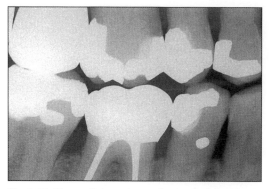

Fig 2-13 The radiolucent area beneath the restoration in the mesial surface of the maxillary first molar is radiographic burnout. No carious tooth structure is present.

The dentist must be careful not to mistakenly diagnose as demineralized tooth structure a decrease in radiopacity resulting from an abraded area. Likewise, the dentist must be cautious in diagnosing caries beneath existing restorations because certain radiolucent dental materials have a radiographic appearance similar to that of carious tooth structure. A comprehensive review of dental radiology has been provided by Goaz and White.[25]

Evaluation of Diagnostic Casts

The dentist can gain valuable information through an evaluation of diagnostic casts. By examining diagnostic casts of the dentition, the dentist can see areas that are visually inaccessible during the clinical examination. Facets and marginal openings that may be difficult to discern intraorally are readily visible on the diagnostic casts. Facets on the casts of the dentition can be aligned to provide a guide to dynamic occlusal relationships. In addition, the dentist may use gypsum casts to complete diagnostic preparations and diagnostic waxups, simulating planned treatment. Where removable partial dentures are indicated, survey and design procedures may be completed on the diagnostic casts before restorative treatment is planned. The requirements of removable partial denture design may thus be considered during the planning of restorative care.

Although not every case requires the evaluation of casts mounted on a semiadjustable articulator, some will. Cases involving multiple missing teeth or the restoration of a significant portion of the occlusion should be evaluated with mounted diagnostic casts. If multiple teeth are missing, the articulator maintains the correct interarch relationship, permitting buccal and lingual views of interarch spaces. Using a semiadjustable articulator that provides a reasonable approximation of the patient's intercondylar distance, condylar inclination, lateral guidance, and hinge axis of rotation, the dentist can simulate the patient's mandibular movements. This enables the clinician to assess the occlusal scheme and to plan restorative care accordingly.

Treatment Plan

Having completed a comprehensive examination, the dentist lists problems related to restorative dentistry on the restorative dentistry problem list (Fig 2-14). Each of the problems on the problem list is then reevaluated. After consideration, some of the problems may be deleted from the list. For example, a tooth with a defective restoration may also have a significant loss of periodontal attachment and, therefore, a poor periodontal prognosis. In such a case, the defective restoration is initially considered a problem, but, in view of the periodontal condition, the tooth would be planned for extraction rather than restoration. The defective restoration is then omitted from the restorative problem list.

Once the final problem list is formulated, the next step is to establish a plan for the treatment of each problem on the list. A problem list worksheet is a useful tool to help organize the planning of treatment for each problem. It consists of an unsequenced list of problems and their associated solutions (Fig 2-15). Later, during the sequencing process, this list of treatments will be integrated into the comprehensive treatment plan.

Planning the restoration of individual teeth is the "nuts and bolts" of restorative dentistry treatment planning. It requires the consideration of four primary factors as well as a number of modifying factors. The primary considerations are: *(1)* the amount and form of the remaining tooth structure; *(2)* the functional needs of each tooth; *(3)* the esthetic needs of each tooth; and *(4)* the final objective of the overall treatment plan.

PATIENT: Blank, Felina D.

PROBLEM LIST

Chief complaint: "My tooth hurts every time I chew, and lately iced tea has made it hurt, too."

Medical/systemic: Hypertension. Present blood pressure: 155/95.

Restorative (also see charting):

- Incomplete tooth fracture of mesiolingual cusp, #19
- Caries lesions, #20, #21, #28 (high caries risk)
- Defective restorations, #2, #12
- Facial, noncarious cervical lesion, #12
- Worn incisal edges, #6 to #11
- Fluorosis stain, #8
- Biologic width impingement, #3, distal
- Patient wishes to whiten maxillary anterior teeth

Periodontal:

- AAP Case Type I (see periodontal charting form)
- Generalized marginal gingivitis
- Generalized minimal bone loss with 3- to 4-mm pockets
- Vertical defect, #3, distolingual (5 mm)
- Biologic width problem, #3, distal
- Plaque and calculus: Generalized interproximal plaque in all posterior sextants (Modified O'Leary index: 50% plaque free), subgingival calculus revealed on bite-wing radiographs of #19 and #30; supragingival calculus present on lingual surfaces of mandibular anterior teeth.

Endodontic: None

Prosthodontic: Missing, #29

Orthodontic: None

Occlusion: Supraeruption, #4; excessive wear, #6 to #11

Temporomandibular dysfunction: None

Oral surgery: None

Fig 2-14 Example of a problem list.

PATIENT: Blank, Felina D.

PROBLEM LIST WORKSHEET

Problem	Treatment
Chief complaint: cracked #19	• Gold onlay
Hypertension	• Referral to physician for evaluation and treatment
Caries	• Educate patient: snacking, hygiene techniques, home fluoride use • Rx: neutral sodium fluoride (1.1%) gel or dentifrice • If caries continues, complete caries risk assessment (diet survey, *mutans* culture) • #20, #21: Class 5 resin-modified glass-ionomer restorations
Defective restorations	• #2: MOD amalgam • #4: Porcelain-fused-to-metal (PFM) crown (shorten to level occlusal plane) • #12: MO resin composite
Abrasion: #12	• Class 5 resin composite restoration
Wear: #6 to #11	• Protective acrylic resin occlusal splint
Fluorosis: #8	• Microabrasion
Biologic width: #3	• Surgical crown lengthening
Patient desires to lighten maxillary anterior teeth	• Home bleaching #5 to #12
Periodontal inflammation associated with local factors	• Patient education and hygiene instruction; goal: 90% plaque-free index • Prophylaxis; scaling/root planing in mandibular sextants and any areas not responding to initial care • Reevaluate; goal: eliminate bleeding on probing • Surgical crown lengthening #3: osseous recontouring and soft tissue excision
Missing: #29	• Fixed partial denture (FPD) #28 to #30; PFM retainer #28, ¾ retainer #30
Supraeruption: #4	• Shorten #4 when PFM crown is completed

Fig 2-15 Example of a problem list worksheet to accompany the problem list in Fig 2-14.

Remaining Tooth Structure

The quantity and location of remaining tooth structure determine the resistance features available for the restoration and thus greatly influence the restorative design. These factors determine not only the resistance to displacement of the restoration, but also the fracture resistance of the remaining tooth structure. The clinician should select the restoration that provides the best retention of the restoration and the optimal protection of the remaining tooth, using the least invasive design possible.

For the restoration of posterior teeth, an intracoronal restoration with amalgam or resin composite is generally the most conservative choice, and both materials have proven to be clinically successful. When the width of the intracoronal preparation of a posterior tooth reaches one third the intercuspal width, the tooth becomes significantly more susceptible to cuspal fracture and the concern becomes not only restoration failure but tooth fracture.[36]

Even more significant to the fracture resistance of the tooth than restoration width is the depth of the preparation.[9] In instances of deep and/or wide preparations, the clinician must assess the need for occlusal coverage to protect the fracture-prone portions of the tooth. Choices include cuspal-coverage amalgam, partial veneer restorations (eg, onlays, three-quarters crowns, or seven-eighths crowns), and complete crowns. The clinician should resist the temptation to progress immediately to a complete crown and, instead, should select the most conservative choice that satisfies the needs of the individual tooth and the overall treatment plan.

The quantity of remaining tooth structure has an equally important effect on the choice of restorations for anterior teeth. For conservative interproximal restorations in anterior teeth, resin composite is almost always indicated because sufficient tooth structure is generally available for effective resin-enamel and resin-dentin bonding. When extensive facial tooth structure has been esthetically compromised, but the facial enamel and the majority of the lingual aspect of the tooth remain intact, a ceramic veneer affords a conservative alternative to a complete crown. The veneer satisfies the esthetic requirement but is considerably less invasive than complete coronal coverage. When the facial enamel has been destroyed, significant lingual tooth structure has been lost, or when occlusal stress is exceptionally heavy, veneers are not a viable option, and complete crowns are required (Fig 2-16).

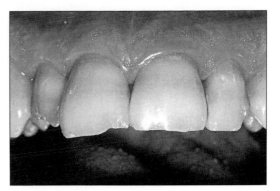

Fig 2-16 Facets and chipped incisal edges are evidence of the severe stresses placed on these anterior teeth by parafunction. Although they demonstrate tetracycline staining and possess a largely intact facial surface, these teeth would be poor candidates for veneer restorations. Complete-coverage restorations are indicated if the patient wishes to mask the tetracycline staining.

Functional Needs

The choice of restorative materials and the design of restorations must accommodate the functional needs of the individual patient. This precludes the use of a cookbook approach to treatment planning and requires that the clinician assess the circumstances peculiar to each tooth before planning restorative procedures. The functional and parafunctional stresses of the occlusion are significant considerations in this decision process. For example, a patient with average-strength musculature, an anterior-guided disocclusion of posterior teeth in excursions, and minimal tendency toward parafunction may require only an intracoronal amalgam or resin composite restoration to restore mesial and distal surfaces of a posterior tooth. In a similar circumstance, a patient with heavy musculature, signs of parafunctional activities, and no anterior-guided disclusion may require a cast-metal, occlusal restoration to minimize the chances of tooth fracture.

A useful guide in making decisions about material selection and restoration design is the evidence of functional demand provided by the existing dentition. Patients who present with a dentition exhibiting minimal destruction are good candidates for conservative, directly placed restorations. Patients whose teeth exhibit severe wear facets or considerable loss of tooth structure from occlusal attrition are best served by materials high in strength and wear resistance, such as cast-metal restorations.

Restorations placed due to noncarious cervical lesions pose little dilemma in terms of restorative choices. Any of the restorative materials suited to the restoration of Class 5 areas will serve satisfactorily. Glass-ionomer restorative materials have proven to be particularly effective in the restoration of Class 5 areas, providing longevity in excess of 10 years.[43] Resin-modified glass-ionomer restorative materials provide an alternative to conventional glass-ionomer cements and have been shown to demonstrate exceptional retention. One study[20] found a retention rate of 98% after 3 years and a second, independent study found 100% retention after 5 years.[10] Improvements in the performance of resin adhesives have made the retention of resin composites and polyacid-modified resin composite restorations predictable as well. A number of investigators have reported retention rates for resin composite restorations of over 95% after 3 years.[56,70] The glass-ionomer materials offer the anticariogenic advantage of fluoride release, while the materials containing greater amounts of resin composite generally provide better esthetics and wear resistance.

The patient's level of caries activity will influence the selection of restorative materials. Patients whose caries risk assessment indicates a high potential for caries are good candidates for treatment with anticariogenic restorative materials, as well as the use of a caries management protocol. Conventional glass-ionomer cements have been found through clinical study to provide an anticariogenic effect.[29] Resin-modified glass-ionomer materials have been found to inhibit simulated caries in vitro[64] and have been shown to possess anticariogenic properties in the clinical environment.[29] None of the anticariogenic restorative materials presently available is able to withstand the stresses of occlusal function.

Esthetic Needs

Establishing the patient's esthetic priorities is essential in planning restorative care. In most instances, the dentist will have the choice of a tooth-colored or a non–tooth-colored restoration for a given situation. Because non–tooth-colored materials (ie, metals) are generally superior in strength and durability, they are the materials of choice when strength and wear resistance are the overriding considerations. With the patient's input, the clinician must decide which requirement is more important, durability or esthetics.

For intracoronal, directly placed restorations in the anterior area of the mouth, resin composites are the obvious choice. They can be made to match most teeth in color and have been shown to provide an average service life of 43.5 to 72 months.[24,55] In stress-bearing areas in the posterior aspect of the mouth, amalgam is the material of choice for direct intracoronal restorations. Although resin composites have been steadily improving in terms of physical properties, clinical research indicates that they have not yet matched the success of amalgam for use in posterior teeth.[52] In the posterior area of the mouth, on those occasions when esthetic concerns take priority and when occlusal stresses are minimal to moderate, resin composite is the restorative material of choice.

Large resin composite restorations do not fare as well in clinical studies as do more conservative resin composite restorations.[4] In view of this, a guideline for the use of resin composites in posterior areas of esthetic concern is to restrict their use to small or medium-sized Class 2 restorations.

Where cuspal coverage is required, amalgam has been found to yield favorable results, routinely providing service in excess of 10 years[57,59]; cast-metal restorations offer even greater longevity.[6,38] When cuspal coverage is required in an area of esthetic concern, the clinician may choose between an all-ceramic and a metal-ceramic restoration. All-ceramic restorations generally provide a superior esthetic result, while the metal substructure of metal-ceramic restorations offers tremendous strength. Although long-term data are not yet available, preliminary results have shown that some all-ceramic materials may provide sufficient fracture resistance for use in the posterior areas of the mouth. Intracoronal ceramic restorations have proven quite successful, with one clinical study finding a 93% success rate over a 6-year time span for leucite-reinforced pressed ceramic inlays (Empress).[23] A study involving 232 inlays made from either a heat-pressed ceramic (Dicor, Dentsply), a leucite-reinforced ceramic material (Empress), or a conventional feldspathic porcelain found a 98% success rate over an average of 28 months.[60]

Although clinical studies have found relatively little difference in survival between the stronger and the weaker ceramics when they are used as intracoronal restorations, the same is not true in cuspal coverage situations. A clinical study involving cuspal coverage all-ceramic restorations found a 94% survival rate among leucite-reinforced ceramic onlay restorations (Empress) serving from 2 to 5 years.[74] In similar cuspal coverage situations, however, Dicor onlays demonstrated a 37% failure rate.[60] These disparate survival rates illustrate the material specificity of restoration survival and the importance of considering occlusal stresses when selecting a restorative material. Secondarily polymerized resin composites have been found to provide excellent performance in intracoronal applications but have not yet proven to be of sufficient durability to serve in cuspal coverage restorations where occlusal stress is a significant factor.[15,27]

All-ceramic materials and fiber-reinforced resin materials have been marketed for use in the fabrication of fixed partial dentures. At the present time, there are insufficient clinical data available to support their use as an alternative to metal or metal-ceramic for fixed partial denture restorations.

Final Treatment Objective

The anticipated ultimate outcome of restorative and prosthodontic rehabilitation is the final factor to consider when the design of a restoration is planned and the restorative material is selected. Teeth that may require one type of restoration to restore health and function may require a different treatment to meet the needs of the final treatment plan. For example, if implant treatment is planned or if no prosthodontic replacement is planned for teeth that are missing, the teeth adjacent to the edentulous area may require only conservative restorative care for the treatment of small carious lesions. In a different treatment plan, one calling for replacement of the missing teeth with a removable partial denture, surveyed castings may be required on the teeth adjacent to the edentulous area. In a third variation of the same case, missing teeth may be replaced with a fixed partial denture and the teeth in question may be needed as fixed partial denture abutments.

When the final treatment objective has been visualized, it is often possible to identify certain teeth as key teeth, whose retention and restoration are crucial to the success of the treatment plan. These teeth are often potential prosthodontic abutments and/or canine teeth. Because the success of the total treatment plan often hinges on these teeth, it is crucial to ascertain their periodontal and endodontic prognosis and to plan the restorative treatment that provides the best long-term prognosis. This may dictate an aggressive restorative design to achieve the most predictable success for these key teeth.

The following example serves to illustrate this principle. A hypothetical patient has a free-standing second molar that contains a defective mesio-occlusodistal (MOD) amalgam restoration. Although the facial wall of the tooth is slightly undermined, a replacement amalgam restoration appears likely to serve adequately. In the comprehensive treatment plan, the tooth will serve as a distal abutment for a removable partial denture. With mere replacement of the defective amalgam restoration, the tooth is at some risk for cuspal fracture in the future. Fracture of the tooth would necessitate fabrication of a crown beneath the removable partial denture. By planning a casting prior to fabrication of the denture, a treatment plan somewhat more aggressive than would be dictated by the needs of the individual tooth, the prognosis for the ultimate treatment objective becomes more predictable and the risk of compromising the final result is reduced. This does not mean that every removable partial denture abutment should receive a cast restoration but is intended to convey the importance of planning for predictable longevity in key teeth.

■ Treatment Sequence

When the completed treatment has been visualized and the design of the restorations required to address each problem on the restorative dentistry problem list has been established, the final step in establishing the restorative dentistry treatment plan is sequencing the treatment. Most restorative treatment will fall into the categories, discussed at the outset of the chapter, of disease control or definitive rehabilitative treatment.

Restorative treatment aimed at the control of active disease generally consists of direct restorative procedures using amalgam, resin composite, or glass-ionomer materials. The sequence of treatment within the disease-control phase is dictated by three considerations: (1) severity of the disease process (ie, the most symptomatic tooth, the tooth with the deepest lesion, or the most debilitated tooth is restored first); (2) esthetic needs; and (3) effective use of time. At each appointment, treatment is rendered in the area in most acute need of restorative treatment. When possible, the restorations should be completed quadrant by quadrant to optimize the use of time.

Treatment provided in the definitive rehabilitative phase goes beyond that needed for the stabilization of active disease and includes restorative treatment designed primarily to enhance esthetics (eg, ceramic veneers) and provide optimum function (eg, replace-

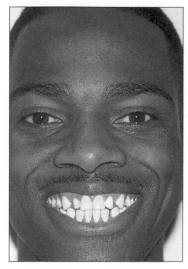

Fig 2-17a The patient wished to close the diastemata adjacent to the maxillary lateral incisors.

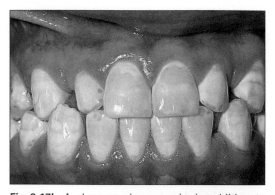

Fig 2-17b A close-up view reveals, in addition to the diastemata and discolored anterior teeth, the unesthetically short clinical crowns of teeth 7 and 10. For better space distribution prior to ceramic veneer fabrication, teeth 7 and 10 need to be repositioned distally and their crowns lengthened. Teeth 22 and 27 are obstructing movement of teeth 7 and 10 into the desired locations.

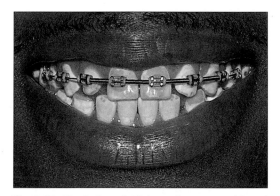

Fig 2-17c Teeth 7 and 10 have been repositioned orthodontically. Space was created by odontoplasty of teeth 22 and 27, followed by resin composite restorations. The space redistribution permits diastema closure to be completed by adding restorative material to all six anterior teeth, which avoids the problem of making any single tooth excessively wide.

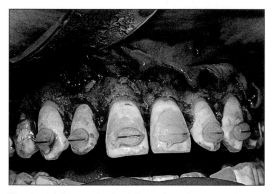

Fig 2-17d Mucogingival flap elevation reveals the osseous crest to be immediately adjacent to the cementoenamel junctions of teeth 7 and 10. This anatomic relationship is responsible for the gingiva covering a portion of the crowns of these teeth.

ment of missing teeth using fixed partial dentures) and resistance to oral stresses (eg, cast restorations).

One of the primary benefits of segregating the restorative treatment into these categories is that a formal reevaluation is completed at the end of the disease-control phase, before progressing into the definitive treatment phase. This approach incorporates into the plan the opportunity to modify or curtail restorative treatment after the control of caries and the replacement of defective restorations. There can be many

reasons for altering the original treatment plan, including the patient's desires, disease risk, finances, or the doctor-patient relationship.

The patient's financial situation or third-party payment guidelines may dictate that treatment be divided into stages and completed over a period of time. Organization of treatment in phases serves the patient's most urgent needs first, directing resources into the management of active disease and allowing less acute problems to be addressed as finances permit.

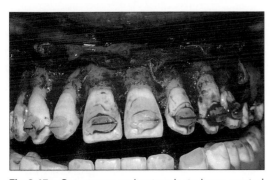

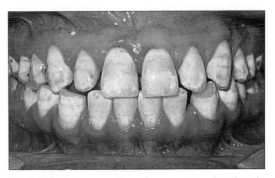

Fig 2-17e Ostectomy and osteoplasty have created approximately 3 mm of space for the combination of sulcus depth, connective tissue attachment, and epithelial attachment. This space will allow the gingival crest to reside at the level of the cervical margin of the veneers, displaying the entire crown of each tooth.

Fig 2-17f Three months after surgery, healing is complete and the teeth are ready for veneer preparation.

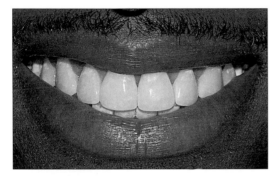

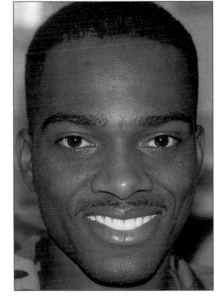

Fig 2-17g One month after veneer placement (teeth 6 to 11). The spaces have been closed, and the fluorosis-related discoloration has been eliminated.

Fig 2-17h The patient was extremely satisfied with the final results of his multidisciplinary treatment.

Treatment planning for restorative dentistry requires that the dentist recognize the sequence in which restorative care should be provided within the context of the overall plan. It also requires that the dentist be able to visualize the ultimate goal of treatment and understand the order in which restorative dental procedures must be performed to achieve this goal. It is not enough to be able to envision the final goal of treatment; one must be able to visualize each step that must be accomplished to achieve this goal. The following example and Figs 2-17a to 2-17h illustrate this.

A patient presented stating that he wished to "close the spaces" between his front teeth (Fig 2-17a). Upon evaluation, this seemingly simple request revealed a complex set of problems. The dentist recognized the problem associated with the patient's chief complaint: diastemata resulting from a tooth-size vs jaw-size discrepancy. The dentist also recognized other esthetic problems associated with the anterior teeth (Fig 2-17b): fluorosis-related discolorations of the teeth and incomplete exposure of the crowns of the anterior teeth due to altered passive eruption of teeth 6, 7, 10, and 11.

The dentist considered possible solutions to the diastema problem. The two most common solutions to this type of space-related problem are *(1)* closure of the spaces by the placement of restorations and *(2)* orthodontic retraction of the maxillary teeth, creating a smaller arch perimeter, reducing or eliminating the spaces between the teeth. An occlusal analysis revealed that the maxillary-mandibular dental relationships would not permit retraction of the maxillary anterior teeth (Fig 2-17b). Thus, complete space closure would require filling all of the open spaces with tooth-colored restorative materials. A space analysis and a diagnostic waxup revealed an important finding. Closure of all of the spaces would result in excessive (unesthetic) widening of the maxillary lateral incisors and canines. Complete space closure would be esthetically acceptable only if it were accomplished by adding a small amount of restorative material to all of the maxillary anterior teeth. The two options available were *(1)* partial closure of the diastemata with tooth-colored restorative material, leaving small spaces between teeth 6 and 7 and teeth 10 and 11, or *(2)* orthodontic redistribution of the existing spaces, followed by complete space closure using tooth-colored restorations placed on all six maxillary anterior teeth.

When presented with these possibilities, the patient stated that he would prefer complete space closure and would be willing to undergo orthodontic treatment to accomplish this. The dentist then visualized the optimal treatment goal and realized that teeth 7 and 10 would need to be moved to a more distal position to equalize the anterior spacing. This was added to the problem list. Visualizing the distal movement of teeth 7 and 10, the dentist realized that the positions of teeth 22 and 27 would interfere with this movement. This presented a new problem, which was added to the problem list. The dentist considered two options: *(1)* orthodontic movement of teeth 22 and 27, or *(2)* alteration of the contour of teeth 22 and 27 to accommodate the repositioning of teeth 7 and 10. The orthodontic movement required to reposition teeth 22 and 27 was deemed unfeasible, and so the second option was selected.

Having determined the feasibility of orthodontic space redistribution for the maxillary anterior teeth, the dentist visualized the final result. Increasing the width of the anterior teeth using tooth-colored restorations (ceramic veneers) would increase the tooth-width to tooth-height ratio, making teeth 7 and 10 appear unesthetically short and wide. Addressing this newfound problem, diagnostic periodontal probing and bone sounding procedures were completed. The

relative locations of the cementoenamel junctions and the distances from the gingival crest to the osseous crests of teeth 7 and 10 were determined. It was decided that the ideal solution for the "short tooth" problem of teeth 7 and 10 was to expose the complete crown of these teeth through surgical crown lengthening before ceramic veneer placement. This plan was presented, and was accepted by the patient.

In stepwise fashion, the entire problem complex was broken down into its individual components. Each component and its proposed solution was assessed. Any new problems that were created by proposed treatment were considered. The final chain of treatment was established and presented to the patient. By recognizing which form of treatment was required to address each component problem, the dentist was able to plan the entire sequence before initiating treatment. All of the proposed procedures were completed, and the treatment of the patient's anterior esthetic problem was realized (Figs 2-17c to 2-17h).

In the above example, discussion was limited to the management of the patient's chief complaint. Other aspects of the comprehensive problem list and treatment plan were omitted to concisely illustrate the process involved in sequencing multidisciplinary treatment.

The Dental Record

Accurate and descriptive record keeping is essential to quality dental care. The dental chart should include findings from the history and examination, the problem list, the treatment plan, and a description of the treatment accomplished. This record serves several purposes:

1. Organization and documentation of the examination findings, the problem list, the treatment plan, and the treatment rendered
2. Documentation for third-party payment, if applicable
3. Legal purposes
4. Forensic purposes

Organizing and documenting the examination findings and the problem list enable the dentist to evaluate the patient's dental problems and plan the treatment when the patient is no longer present. Once treatment has begun, documentation of the sequenced treatment plan also permits the dentist to review the anticipated treatment without the need to reconsider

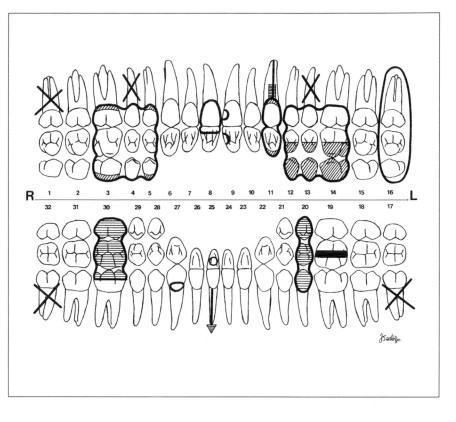

Fig 2-18 Example of a pictorial charting system used to record dental restorations. Any system that distinguishes among the various restorations is acceptable. In this example, tooth 1 is missing; tooth 4 has been replaced with a metal-ceramic fixed partial denture that extends from tooth 3 to tooth 5 with ceramic occlusal coverage; tooth 8 has a facial veneer; tooth 9 has a mesial resin composite restoration; tooth 11 has been endodontically treated and has a post and metal-ceramic crown; tooth 13 has been replaced by a metal-ceramic fixed partial denture that extends from tooth 12 to tooth 14 with metal occlusal coverage; tooth 16 is impacted; tooth 17 is missing; tooth 19 has a mesio-occlusodistal amalgam restoration; tooth 20 has been restored with a metal crown; tooth 25 has been endodontically treated, received a retrograde restoration, and has a resin composite restoration in the lingual access opening; tooth 27 has a facial tooth-colored restoration; tooth 30 has a metal three-quarter crown; and tooth 32 is missing.

the entire treatment-planning process. Dental records should include the following information:

1. Charting of examination findings, including existing restorations and dental relationships (eg, diastemata, supraeruption, tilted teeth); existing periodontal and endodontic conditions; occlusal relationships; and carious lesions and defective restorations
2. Medical history and consultations
3. Problem list
4. Treatment plan
   a. Description of treatment rendered
   b. Informed consent documentation

In addition to the usual typed or handwritten entries in a dental record, pictorial charting is an efficient means of recording a great deal of information in a small area (Figs 2-18 and 2-19). Intraoral imaging devices, either conventional cameras or videographic recording devices, provide an extremely effective means of recording findings and documenting treatment and are an ideal complement to a pictorial charting system. These offer the added advantage of simplifying communication with the patient and third-party funding agencies.

The format used to document the care provided should reflect an orderly and logical diagnostic and treatment sequence. A method commonly used in medicine that satisfies this requirement is the SOAP format. *SOAP* is an acronym for the steps involved whenever any treatment is rendered. *S* refers to subjective findings. This includes a summary of the patient's chief complaint, a description of his or her symptoms, and any other relevant information the patient provides. The patient's own words should be used as much as possible. The *O* refers to objective findings. These include examination findings and the results of consultations and diagnostic tests. *A* refers to the assessment, which is the dentist's diagnosis, based on the subjective and objective findings present. The *P* refers to the plan of treatment (when the treatment is rendered immediately, it refers to the treatment itself). An example of the use of the SOAP format is provided (see box, page 53).

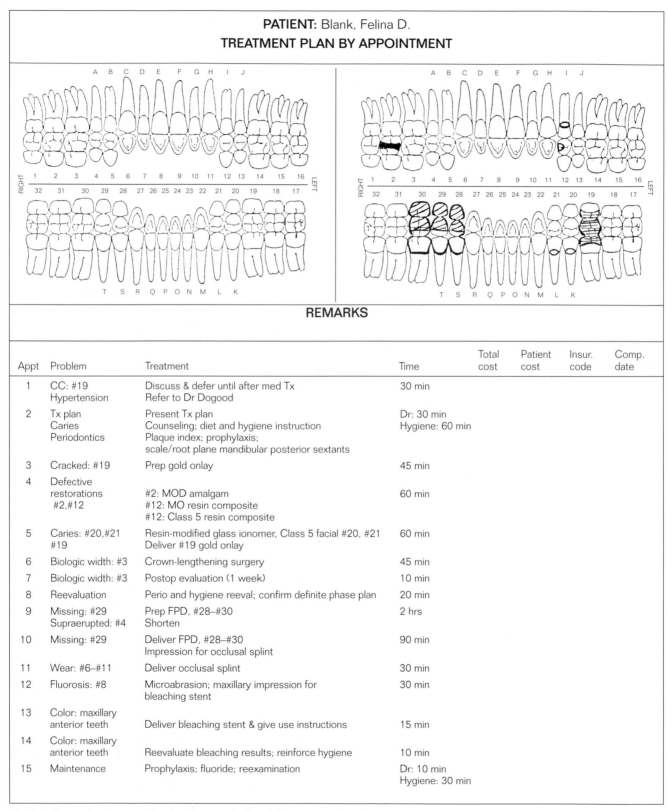

PATIENT: Blank, Felina D.
TREATMENT PLAN BY APPOINTMENT

REMARKS

Appt	Problem	Treatment	Time	Total cost	Patient cost	Insur. code	Comp. date
1	CC: #19 Hypertension	Discuss & defer until after med Tx Refer to Dr Dogood	30 min				
2	Tx plan Caries Periodontics	Present Tx plan Counseling; diet and hygiene instruction Plaque index; prophylaxis; scale/root plane mandibular posterior sextants	Dr: 30 min Hygiene: 60 min				
3	Cracked: #19	Prep gold onlay	45 min				
4	Defective restorations #2,#12	#2: MOD amalgam #12: MO resin composite #12: Class 5 resin composite	60 min				
5	Caries: #20,#21 #19	Resin-modified glass ionomer, Class 5 facial #20, #21 Deliver #19 gold onlay	60 min				
6	Biologic width: #3	Crown-lengthening surgery	45 min				
7	Biologic width: #3	Postop evaluation (1 week)	10 min				
8	Reevaluation	Perio and hygiene reeval; confirm definite phase plan	20 min				
9	Missing: #29 Supraerupted: #4	Prep FPD, #28–#30 Shorten	2 hrs				
10	Missing: #29	Deliver FPD, #28–#30 Impression for occlusal splint	90 min				
11	Wear: #6–#11	Deliver occlusal splint	30 min				
12	Fluorosis: #8	Microabrasion; maxillary impression for bleaching stent	30 min				
13	Color: maxillary anterior teeth	Deliver bleaching stent & give use instructions	15 min				
14	Color: maxillary anterior teeth	Reevaluate bleaching results; reinforce hygiene	10 min				
15	Maintenance	Prophylaxis; fluoride; reexamination	Dr: 10 min Hygiene: 30 min				

Fig 2-19 Example of a combined written and pictorial treatment planning sheet. The pictorial charts are for use in recording both completed treatment *(left)* and treatment yet to be accomplished *(right)*. Once completed, the treatment charted in pencil on the right may be erased. The remarks section is for making comments, generally made in pencil (erased and updated as needed). The area below the remarks section is for the sequenced treatment plan. A treatment planning sheet such as this allows for quick review of the overall treatment plan and provides a profile of the current status of treatment.

> S: Patient presents complaining of a "toothache that began yesterday and has hurt all night." (Patient points to tooth 30). Patient states ice water reduces the pain.
>
> O: Teeth 27 to 30 are within normal limits (WNL) to percussion, palpation, and periodontal exam, and are vital and normal to cold testing. Tooth 31 is painful to percussion and pain is alleviated with the application of cold. Radiographs of teeth 27 to 31 are unremarkable, except for a deep mesio-occlusal amalgam restoration on tooth 31.
>
> A: Tooth 31 has irreversible pulpitis.
>
> P: Patient advised of diagnosis. Patient consents to root canal treatment on tooth 31. Patient reappointed for root canal on tooth 31 at 3:00 PM today.

The SOAP format is an excellent guide in the performance and documentation of care when a challenging diagnostic problem presents itself; however, it is not suited to the routine restorative care provided based on the treatment plan. When a straightforward diagnosis is made in the absence of symptoms and patient complaint, a more concise form of documentation is appropriate (see box).

> DX: Caries in tooth 3, vital to cold and asymptomatic.
>
> TX: Tooth 3: MOD amalgam (Tytin), copal varnish, rubber dam. Local anesthesia: 36 mg lidocaine, with 0.018 mg epinephrine.
>
> Plan: Reappoint for preparation of veneers for teeth 5 to 12.

There are times when the identification of a deceased individual must be accomplished through the use of dental records. A complete record of the dentition and restorations, a radiographic survey, and photographic records are useful for identification purposes.

The dental record is a legal document. The nature and clarity of the entries made should reflect the knowledge that it may be needed in a court of law to document examination findings, informed consent, and treatment completed. The records should be accurate and should contain the elements listed above. They should not contain erasures or text that has been obliterated by any means. If errors are made, a single line should be drawn through the mistake and then the change should be initialed and dated. In the retrospective review of a legal investigation, the descriptiveness and clarity of the record is often held to be an indication of the quality of care provided.

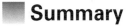

Summary

Treatment planning for restorative dentistry can be a complex undertaking. Use of a logical and orderly problem-oriented approach can simplify the process. The following principles have been offered as guidelines:

1. Be aware of pathoses that may be encountered and be able to distinguish the normal from the abnormal and stable from risk-prone situations.
2. Organize abnormal findings into a problem list.
3. Envision an overall restorative goal for the patient. This is the anticipated final state of rehabilitation. Not every patient can be restored to the ideal, but each patient has an optimum state of health that can be obtained, given the circumstances of that patient.
4. Determine a plan of treatment for each problem, so that each treatment contributes to the achievement of the anticipated ultimate treatment goal. This is the linchpin of restorative treatment planning. It requires that the dentist consider a number of factors before selecting the optimum restorative option. Chief among these considerations are: the overall goal of treatment; the functional and esthetic needs of each restorative situation (use the existing dentition and restorations as an indicator of the performance of future restorations); the strengths and weaknesses of the various restorative materials available; and the amount and location of remaining tooth structure.
5. Recognize the sequence of steps needed to achieve a specific restorative objective. The dentist must know, for example, that a tooth fractured at the level of the osseous crest and in need of a crown will require endodontic treatment, a post and core, and crown lengthening surgery before fabrication of the final restoration.
6. Sequence the treatment based on a logical model. Control active disease processes first, beginning treatment with teeth in the most acute need of care. Complete as much care as feasible in each sextant at the same appointment. Establish a restorative prognosis for key teeth early in the treatment schedule. Consider nondental factors (especially third-party payment guidelines and time-related limits) when planning the treatment schedule.

References

1. Albers HF. Treating cracked teeth. ADEPT Report 1994;4: 17–24.

2. Andreason JO. Traumatic Injuries of the Teeth, ed 2. Philadelphia: WB Saunders, 1981.

3. Bader JD, Brown JP. Dilemmas in caries diagnosis. J Am Dent Assoc 1993;124:48–50.

4. Barnes DM, Blank LW, Thompson VP, et al. A five-and eight-year clinical evaluation of a posterior resin composite. Quintessence Int 1991;22:143–154.

5. Barsh LI. Dental Treatment Planning for the Adult Patient. Philadelphia: WB Saunders, 1981.

6. Bentley C, Drake CW. Longevity of restorations in a dental school clinic. J Dent Educ 1986;50:594–600.

7. Bergman G, Linden LA. The action of the explorer on incipient caries. Sven Tandlak 1969;62:629–634.

8. Bhaskar SN. Radiographic Interpretation for the Dentist. St Louis: CV Mosby, 1986.

9. Blaser PK, Lund MR, Cochran MA, Potter RH. Effect of designs of class II preparations on the resistance of teeth to fracture. Oper Dent 1983;8:6–10.

10. Boghosian A, Ricker J, McCoy R. Clinical evaluation of a resin-modified glass ionomer restorative: 5 year results [abstract 1436]. J Dent Res 1999;78:285.

11. Cameron CE. Cracked tooth syndrome. J Am Dent Assoc 1964;68:405–411.

12. Cameron CE. The cracked tooth syndrome: additional findings. J Am Dent Assoc 1976;971–975.

13. Cavel WT, Kelsey WP, Blankenau RJ. An in vivo study of cuspal fracture. J Prosthet Dent 1985;53:38–42.

14. Chan DCN. Current methods and criteria for caries diagnosis in North America. J Dent Educ 1993;57:422–427.

15. Christensen G. Filled polymer crowns. Clinical Research Associate's Newsletter 1998;22(10):1–3.

16. Cohen SN, Silvestri AR. Complete and incomplete fractures of posterior teeth. Compend Contin Educ Dent 1984;5:652–663.

17. Cohen S, Burns RC. Pathways of the Pulp, ed 7. St Louis: Mosby–Year Book, 1998.

18. Disney JA, Graves RC, Stamm JW, et al. The University of North Carolina Caries Risk Assessment Study: future developments in caries predictors. Community Dent Oral Epidemiol 1992;20:64–75.

19. Dodds MWJ. Dilemmas in caries diagnosis—Applications to current practice and need for research. J Dent Educ 1993; 57:433–438.

20. Duke ES, Robbins JW, Summit JB, et al. Clinical evaluation of Vitremer in cervical abrasions and root caries [abstract 2578]. J Dent Res 1998;77:954.

21. Eakle WS. Effect of thermocycling on fracture strength and microleakage in teeth restored with a bonded composite resin. Dent Mater 1986;2:114–117.

22. Ekstrand K, Qvist V, Thylstrup A. Light microscope study of the effect of probing in occlusal surfaces. Caries Res 1987; 21:368–374.

23. Frankenberger R, Rumi K, Kramer N. Clinical evaluation of leucite reinforced glass ceramic inlays and onlays after six years [abstract 1623]. J Dent Res 1999;78:308.

24. Friedl K-H, Hiller K-A, Schmalz G. Placement and replacement of composite restorations in Germany. Oper Dent 1995; 20:34–38.

25. Goaz PW, White SC, eds. Oral Radiology: Principles and Interpretation, ed 3. St Louis: CV Mosby, 1994.

26. Guthrie RC, Difiore PM. Treating the cracked tooth with a full crown. J Am Dent Assoc 1991;122:71–73.

27. Hannig M. Five-year clinical evaluation of a heat- and pressure-cured composite resin inlay system [abstract 1908]. J Dent Res 1996;75:256.

28. Hansen EK. In vivo cusp fracture of endodontically treated premolars restored with MOD amalgam or MOD resin fillings. Dent Mater 1988;4:169–173.

29. Haveman C, Burgess J, Summitt J. Clinical comparison of restorative materials for caries in xerostomic patients [abstract 1441]. J Dent Res 1999;78:286.

30. Heymann HO, Sturdevant JR, Bayne S, et al. Examining tooth flexure effects. J Am Dent Assoc 1991;122:41–47.

31. Hiatt WH. Incomplete crown-root fracture in pulpal-periodontal disease. J Periodontol 1973;49:369–379.

32. Imal Y, Suzuki S, Fukushima S. In vitro enamel wear of modified porcelains [abstract 50]. J Dent Res 1999;78(SI):112.

33. Kidd EAM, O'Hara JW. The caries status of occlusal amalgam restorations with marginal defects. J Dent Res 1990;69: 1275–1277.

34. Lambrechts P, Braem M, Vanherle G. Evaluation of clinical performance for posterior composites and dentin adhesives. Oper Dent 1987;2:53–78.

35. Langouvardos P, Sourai P, Douvitsas G. Coronal fractures in posterior teeth. Oper Dent 1989;14:28–32.

36. Larson TO, Douglas WH, Geistfeld RE. Effects of prepared cavities on the strength of prepared teeth. Oper Dent 1981; 6:2–5.

37. Lee WC, Eakle WS. Possible role of tensile stress in the etiology of cervical lesions of teeth. J Prosthet Dent 1984;52: 374–380.

38. Leempoel PJB, Eschen S, DeHaan AFJ, Van't Hof MA. An evaluation of crowns and bridges in a general dental practice. J Oral Rehabil 1985;12:515–518.

39. Lindhe JA. Influence of trauma from occlusion on the progression of experimental periodontitis in beagle dogs. J Clin Periodontol 1974;1:3–14.

40. Little JW, Falace DA. Dental Management of the Medically Compromised Patient, ed 5. St Louis: Mosby–Year Book, 1997.

41. Löe H. Reaction of marginal periodontal tissue to restorative procedures. Int Dent J 1968;18:759–778.

42. Lutz F, Kreci I, Barbakow F. Chewing pressure versus wear of composites and opposing enamel cusps. J Dent Res 1992;71: 1525–1529.

43. Matis BA, Cochran M, Carlson T. Longevity of glass-ionomer restorative materials: results of a 10-year evaluation. Quintessence Int 1996;27:373–382.

44. Maynard JG, Wilson RD. Physiologic dimensions of the periodontium fundamental to successful restorative dentistry. J Periodontol 1979;50:170–174.

45. Mendoza M, Mobley CL, Hattaway K. Caries risk management and the role of dietary assessment [abstract 33]. J Dent Res 1995;74:16.

46. Mertz-Fairhurst E, Curtis JW, Ergle JW, et al. Ultraconservative and cariostatic and sealed restorations: results at year 10. J Am Dent Assoc 1998;129:55–66.

47. Mjor I. Glass-ionomer cement restorations and secondary caries: a preliminary report. Quintessence Int 1996;27: 171–174.

48. Monasky DE, Taylor DF. Studies on the wear of porcelain, enamel and gold. J Prosthet Dent 1971;25:299–306.

49. O'Leary TJ, Drake RB, Naylor JB. The plaque control record. J Periodontol 1972;43:38.

50. O'Neal SJ, Miracle RL, Leinfelder KF. Evaluating interfacial gaps for esthetic inlays. J Am Dent Assoc 1993;124:48–54.

51. Phillips RW. The Science of Dental Materials, ed 9. Philadelphia: WB Saunders, 1991.

52. Pink FE, Minder NJ, Simmonds S. Decisions of practitioners regarding placement of amalgam and composite restorations in a general practice setting. Oper Dent 1994;19:127–132.

53. Polson AM, Caton JG. Current status of bleeding in the diagnosis of periodontal disease. J Periodontol 1985;56(suppl):1.

54. Qvist V, Laurberg L, Poulsen A, Teglers PT. Longevity and cariostatic effects of everyday conventional glass-ionomer and amalgam restorations in primary teeth: three year results. J Dent Res 1997;76:1387–1396.

55. Qvist V, Qvist J, Mjör IA. Placement and longevity of tooth-colored restorations in Denmark. Acta Odontol Scand 1990; 48:305–311.

56. Robbins JW, Duke ES, Schwartz RS, Summitt JB. 3-year clinical evaluation of a dentin adhesive system in cervical abrasions [abstract 1436]. J Dent Res 1995;74:164.

57. Robbins JW, Summitt JB. Longevity of complex amalgam restorations. Oper Dent 1988;13:54–57.

58. Roberts HW, Charlton DG, Murchison DF. Effect of flowable resin on leakage at amalgam margin defects [abstract 3779]. J Dent Res 2000;79(SI):616.

59. Smales R. Longevity of cusp-covered amalgams: survival after 15 years. Oper Dent 1991;16:17–20.

60. Schmalz G, Federlin M, Hiller K-A, Felden A. Retrospective clinical investigation on ceramic inlays and partial crowns [abstract 455]. J Dent Res 1996;75:74.

61. Sorenson JA, Martinoff MD. Intracoronal reinforcement and coronal coverage: a study of endodontically treated teeth. J Prosthet Dent 1984;51:780–784.

62. Sorensen JA, Sultan E, Condon JR. Three-body in vitro wear of enamel against dental ceramics [abstract 909]. J Dent Res 1999;78(SI):219.

63. Sorensen JA, Berge HX. In vivo measurement of antagonist tooth wear opposing ceramic bridges. [abstract 2942]. J Dent Res 1999;78(SI):473.

64. Souto M, Donley KJ. Caries inhibition of glass ionomers. Am J Dent 1994;7:122–124.

65. Stanley HR. The cracked tooth syndrome. J Am Acad Gold Foil Oper 1968;11:36–47.

66. Summitt JB, Osborne JM. Initial preparations for amalgam restorations: extending the longevity of the tooth-restoration unit. J Am Dent Assoc 1993;123:67–73.

67. Svanberg M, Mjör IA, Orstavik D. Mutans streptococci in plaque from margins of amalgam, composite and glass ionomer restorations. J Dent Res 1990;69:861–864.

68. Than A, Duguid R, McKendrick AJW. Relationship between restorations and the level of periodontal attachment. J Clin Periodontol 1982;9:193–202.

69. Trabert KC, Caputo AA, Abou-Rass M. Tooth fracture: a comparison of endodontic and restorative treatments. J Endod 1978;4:341–345.

70. Trevino DF, Duke ES, Robbins JW, Summit JB. Clinical evaluation of Scotchbond Multi-Purpose adhesive system in cervical abrasions [abstract 3037]. J Dent Res 1996;75:397.

71. Trope M, Maltz DO, Tronstad L. Resistance to fracture of restored endodontically treated teeth. Endod Dent Traumatol 1985;1:108–111.

72. Tyas M. Cariostatic effect of glass ionomer cement: a five year clinical study. Aust Dent J 1991;36:236–239.

73. US Department of Health and Human Services. The Selection of Patients for X-ray Examination: Dental Radiographic Examination. US Dept of Health and Human Services Publication (FDA), 1987:87–88.

74. Van Dijken JWV, Hasselroth L, Ormin A, Olofsson A-L. Clinical evaluation of extensive dentin/enamel bonded all-ceramic onlays and onlay-crowns [abstract 2713]. J Dent Res 1999; 78:444.

75. Van Houte JH. Bacterial specificity in the etiology of dental caries. Int Dent J 1980;30:305–326.

76. Van Palenstein Helderman WH, Matee MIN, van der Hoeven JS, Mikx FHM. Cariogenicity depends more on diet than the prevailing mutans streptococcal species. J Dent Res 1996;75: 535–545.

77. Waerhaug J. Effect of rough surfaces upon the gingival tissues. J Dent Res 1956;35:323–327.

78. Waerhaug J, Hansen ER. Periodontal changes incident to prolonged occlusal overload in monkeys. Acta Odontol Scand 1966;24:91–105.

79. Wenzel A, Larsen MJ, Fejerskov O. Detection of occlusal caries without cavitation by visual inspection, film radiographs, xeroradiographs and digitized radiographs. Caries Res 1991;25:365–371.

80. Whitehead SA, Wilson NHF, Watts DC. Development of non-carious cervical notch lesions in vitro. J Esthet Dent 1999;11:332–337.

3 Esthetic Considerations in Diagnosis and Treatment Planning

J. William Robbins

Esthetic Parameters

Because beauty is primarily a matter of personal taste modified by social norms, visualizing beauty is a subjective experience. Creating a beautiful smile requires the dentist to dip into these subjective waters. This chapter provides a comprehensive, evidence-based when possible, set of guidelines that will enable dentists to provide esthetic as well as functional dentistry.

Esthetic Parameters

Face Height

The face can be divided vertically into thirds, and the length of the middle third of the face should approximately equal the lower third of the face when measured in repose[15] (Fig 3-1). The midface is measured from glabella, the most prominent point of the forehead between the eyebrows, to subnasale, the point below the base of the nose. The lower face is measured from subnasale to soft tissue menton, which is the lower border of the chin.

Variations from the norm can reflect a continuum from underdevelopment to hypertrophic development of either one or both arches. However, regarding esthetic diagnoses that impact dental treatment, exces-

sive length of the lower third of the face is most common. The long lower face is commonly the result of vertical maxillary excess and, in many cases, is accompanied by excess gingival display in the maxilla during full smile.

Lip Length

The length of the upper lip is measured from subnasale to the inferior border of the upper lip in repose (Fig 3-2a). The average length of the upper lip is 20 to 22 mm in the young adult female and 22 to 24 mm in the young adult male.[12] The upper lip tends to lengthen with age.[17] When a patient presents with excess gingival display (more than 2 mm of gingiva exposed above the maxillary central incisors during full smile), lip length may be part of the etiology (Fig 3-2b).

Lip Mobility

Mobility of the upper lip is measured from repose position to high smile position. The average lip mobility is 6 to 8 mm. In the patient with excess gingival display in full smile, hypermobility of the upper lip may be a contributing factor.

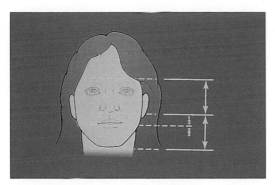

Fig 3-1 The length of the middle third of the face should equal the length of the lower third of the face.

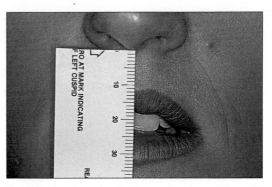

Fig 3-2a Lip length of 18 mm (average, 20 to 22 mm in females) causes gingival display in full smile.

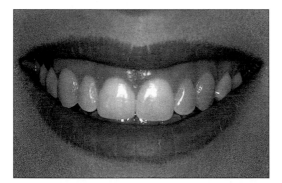

Fig 3-2b Approximately 2 mm of gingival display in full smile.

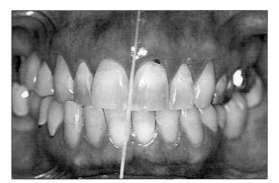

Fig 3-3 Midline canted in relation to the horizon.

Symmetry

Outline symmetry is essential at the midline[8]; the maxillary central incisors should be mirror images of each other. Additionally, a line drawn between the maxillary central incisors should be perpendicular to the horizon[10] (Fig 3-3). Finally, the maxillary dental midline should be coincident with the facial midline.[2] Asymmetry at the midline creates a visual tension in the observer resulting in an unacceptable esthetic presentation. As the eye moves peripherally from the midline, deviations from perfect symmetry (eg, notched edges or slight differences in edge lengths) become desirable.[18]

Incisal Plane

The incisal plane should be parallel to the horizon; the interpupillary line is helpful in making this determination.[18] The incisal plane is evaluated from cusp tip of the maxillary right canine to cusp tip of the maxillary left canine. Although the incisal plane must be parallel to the horizon, it is generally not flat, but has a curve that parallels the curve of the lower lip in full smile. In addition, it should not be canted up or down from right to left.

It is important not to perpetuate or create a canted incisal plane with restorations. If the interpupillary line is parallel to the horizon, the corners of the mouth should be pulled outward so that the upper lip parallels the interpupillary line (Fig 3-4). The relationship between the incisal plane and the interpupillary line, via the upper lip, can then be visualized. To transfer this information to an articulator, a facebow may be used, as long as the horizontal member of the facebow is made parallel to the horizon before attaching the bite fork. An incisal plane relationship bite may also be used. A bite registration paste is placed between the maxillary and mandibular incisors. A long cotton-tipped applicator is then embedded in the bite registration paste and set parallel to the horizon

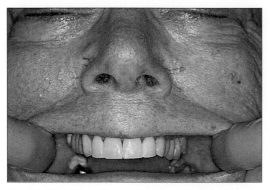

Fig 3-4 The upper lip is pulled to parallel the interpupillary line. The vermilion border of the upper lip is then used to evaluate the cant of the incisal plane and posterior occlusal plane in relation to the horizon.

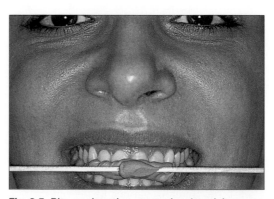

Fig 3-5 Bite registration paste is placed between maxillary and mandibular anterior teeth, and a cotton-tipped applicator is embedded in the paste. The cotton-tipped applicator is then paralleled with the interpupillary line, and the paste is allowed to set.

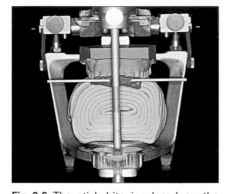

Fig 3-6 The stick bite is placed on the maxillary cast, and the stick is set parallel to the maxillary member of the articulator to orient the cast for mounting.

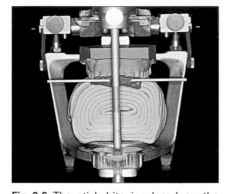

Fig 3-7 A patient with excess space in the buccal corridors.

(Fig 3-5). This relationship bite can then be used to mount the maxillary cast with an accurate incisal plane orientation to the maxillary member of the articulator (Fig 3-6).

Posterior Occlusal Plane

The buccal cusp tips of the maxillary posterior teeth should provide a visual progression from the canine cusp tips, with no step up or step down. In addition, the posterior occlusal plane should not be canted up or down from right to left.[10]

It is important not to perpetuate or create a canted posterior occlusal plane. The same techniques used to ensure an accurate mounting of the incisal plane are used for the posterior occlusal plane.

Buccal Corridor

The buccal corridor is the space between the buccal surfaces of the maxillary posterior teeth and the cheek. In full smile, the buccal corridor is almost filled with teeth. However, a minimal negative space frames the maxillary posterior teeth and is desirable.[10]

Excess buccal corridor space (Fig 3-7) is usually due to a developmental problem, ie, a constricted maxillary arch. Inadequate space in the buccal corridor is usually due to bulky posterior restorations.

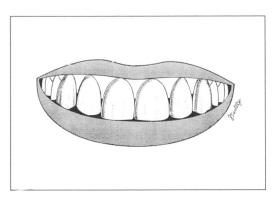

Fig 3-8a Ideal maxillary incisal edge position in relation to the lower lip.

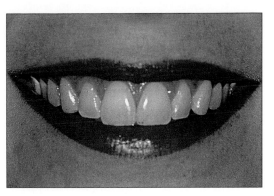

Fig 3-8b Ideal incisal edge position in relation to the lower lip. Ideal relationship between the upper lip and the gingival line.

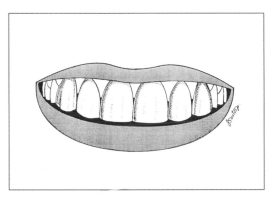

Fig 3-9 Uniform space between the maxillary incisal edges and lower lip.

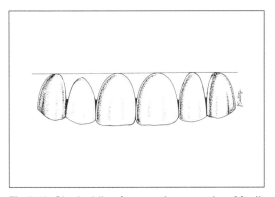

Fig 3-10 Gingival line from canine to canine. Maxillary lateral incisor can fall on this line or be up to 1.5 mm below it.

Lower Lip

In full smile, the incisal edges of the maxillary anterior teeth are ideally cradled by the lower lip[11,16] (Figs 3-8a and 3-8b). Any space between the incisal edges and the lower lip should be minimal and uniform from canine to canine (Fig 3-9). Conversely, none of the incisal edges of the maxillary anterior teeth should be concealed by the lower lip in full smile.

If there is a reverse incisal edge curve in relation to the lower lip, or a significant space between the lower lip and the maxillary incisal edges during full smile, esthetics will probably be enhanced with increased incisal edge length. Conversely, if incisal edges of maxillary anterior teeth are hidden by the lower lip during full smile, there is likely a problem with the vertical position of the maxilla. The cause may be dentoalveolar extrusion (overeruption of maxillary anterior teeth) or vertical maxillary excess, or both.

Upper Lip

In full smile, the upper lip should ideally translate up to the gingival line[11] (Fig 3-8b). This occurs in approximately 70% of the population. Approximately 10% have a high smile line, and approximately 20% have a low smile line.[16] To evaluate the gingival line, a straight line is drawn from the tooth-gingiva interface of the right maxillary canine to the tooth-gingiva interface of the left maxillary canine. The tooth-gingiva interface of both central incisors should be on this line. The tooth-gingiva interface of the lateral incisors may either fall on the gingival line or be up to 1.5 mm below it (Fig 3-10).[1]

If the upper lip does not translate up to the gingival line during full smile, some of the clinical crowns of the maxillary anterior teeth remain covered. This results in a loss of dynamism of the smile. If, in full smile, the upper lip translates above the gingival line, this results in gingival display above the clinical crowns. Gingival display of 2 mm or more above the gingival line results in compromised esthetics.

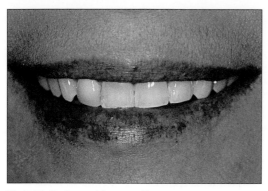

Fig 3-11 Patient with upper lip asymmetry.

Lip Asymmetry

If a patient displays an upper lip asymmetry during full smile (Fig 3-11), it does not influence treatment. However, the patient should be advised of the condition before restoration of the maxillary anterior teeth, because the brighter restored maxillary anterior teeth will draw attention to the smile and accentuate the upper lip asymmetry.

If a patient has a lower lip asymmetry during full smile, which results in a unilateral increase in negative space between the maxillary incisal edges and the lower lip, smile symmetry is lost (see Fig 3-31b). When restoring maxillary anterior teeth in this circumstance, consideration is given to subtly lengthening the incisal edges on the affected side to minimize the unilateral asymmetry. This is first accomplished in a diagnostic waxup from which provisional restorations are fabricated. The patient can then make the decision regarding the incisal edge configuration of the final restorations.

Lip asymmetries, which can play a significant role in the final restorative result, are commonly overlooked.

Incisal Edge Placement of Maxillary Central Incisors

Determining the correct position of the incisal edges of the maxillary central incisors is the first and an essential step in the provision of anterior restorative dentistry. The following five guidelines are used to determine the correct incisal edge position.

1. In full smile, the incisal edges of the maxillary anterior teeth should be cradled by the lower lip[11,16] (see Fig 3-8b).
2. In full smile, the buccal cusp tips of the posterior maxillary teeth should provide a visual progression from the canine cusp tip, with no step up or step down[10] (Figs 3-12 and 3-13).
3. In gentle repose (have the patient say "M" or "Emma"), approximately 3 to 4 mm of the incisal edges of the maxillary central incisors are displayed in the young adult female (Fig 3-14). In the young adult male, approximately 1 to 2 mm of the incisal edges are displayed. After age 40, the amount of incisal edge display decreases approximately 1 mm per decade.[17]
4. When the patient says "E," a space between the upper and lower lips is apparent (Fig 3-15a). If less than 50% of the space is occupied by the maxillary central incisors, the teeth can possibly be lengthened esthetically. If, however, more than 70% of the space is occupied by the maxillary central incisors, lengthening of the maxillary anterior teeth will probably not be esthetically pleasing (Kois J, oral communication, 1999).
5. When the patient says "F" or "V," the incisal edges of the maxillary central incisors should lightly touch the wet/dry border of the lower lip[13] (Fig 3-15b).

Steps 1 to 4 are used together to develop an approximation of the correct incisal edge position for the diagnostic waxup. At this point, incisal edge position is dictated strictly by esthetics. After tooth preparation, provisional restorations, which have been fabricated using the diagnostic waxup, are placed. The final incisal edge position is then developed dynamically, over time, in the provisional restorations to ensure suitable function and phonetics as well as esthetics. Step 5 is helpful in assessing phonetics with lengthened provisional restorations.

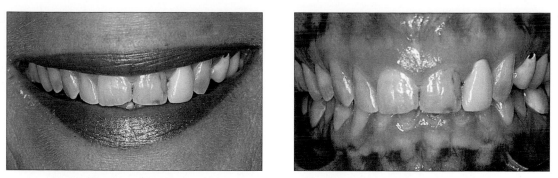

Figs 3-12a and 3-12b Note step up from maxillary left canine to maxillary left first premolar.

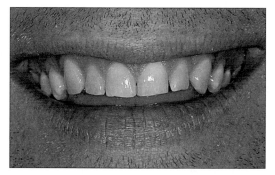

Fig 3-13 Note bilateral step down from maxillary canines to maxillary first premolars.

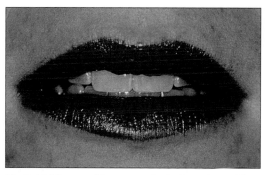

Fig 3-14 Three millimeters of display of maxillary central incisors in repose.

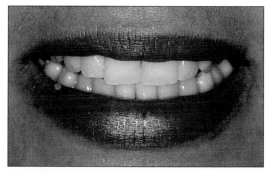

Fig 3-15a Patient in the "E" position.

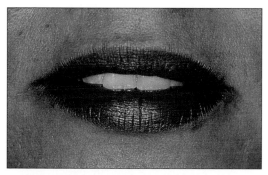

Fig 3-15b Patient in the "F" position.

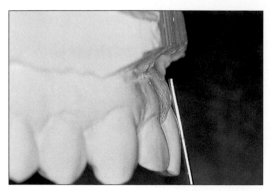

Fig 3-16 The gingival half of the maxillary central incisor is parallel to and continuous in contour with the surface of the gingival tissue overlying the alveolus.

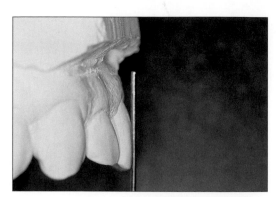

Fig 3-17 The incisal half of the central incisor is contoured to feel comfortable to the patient during lip closure and speech.

Facial Contour of Maxillary Incisors

Divide the facial surface of the maxillary central incisor into two planes. The gingival half of the tooth should be parallel to and continuous in contour with the surface of the gingival tissue overlying the alveolus[3] (Fig 3-16). The incisal half is tapered back for ease in speaking and swallowing (Fig 3-17).

Facial overcontouring of a partial- or full-coverage restoration in the gingival half can result in chronic gingival inflammation. Facial overcontouring in the incisal half may result in lip pressure, causing linguoversion of the overcontoured teeth or interference with the lip closure path.

Lingual Contour of Maxillary Incisors

Incorrect spacing between maxillary and mandibular anterior teeth may cause a lisp. A lisp can occur with too much or too little space, although, most commonly, it occurs with too little space.

If a patient develops a lisp after placement of provisional or definitive restorations, the position of the incisal edges of the mandibular incisors in relation to the maxillary central incisors when the patient makes an "S" sound must be determined. If the mandibular incisor approximates the cingulum or lingual concavity of the maxillary incisor, the lisp is most commonly corrected by increasing the lingual concavity of the maxillary incisors. If, however, the mandibular incisor approximates the incisal edge of the maxillary central incisor during the "S" sound, the lisp can most commonly be corrected by changing the length of the maxillary central incisors.

Gingival Zenith

The long axes of the maxillary anterior teeth are distally inclined. Therefore, the gingival contour adjacent to the maxillary incisors is not a symmetric rounded arch form. Rather, the marginal gingiva has a parabolic shape with the high point (gingival zenith) slightly distal to the midline of the tooth[1] (Fig 3-18).

In gingival recontouring surgery, the gingival zenith should not be overemphasized. Although a distalized zenith is more common, many patients prefer a more symmetric gingival architecture.

Interproximal Contact Areas

Maxillary interproximal contact areas become progressively more gingival from central incisor to canine (Fig 3-19). The interproximal contact between the maxillary central incisors is in the incisal third of the teeth. However, the interproximal contact between the central and lateral incisors is at the junction of the incisal and middle thirds; it is slightly more gingival between the lateral incisors and the canines.[18]

If the interproximal contact extends too far incisally, a closed and unnatural-appearing incisal embrasure results. If the interproximal contact does not extend far enough gingivally, an open gingival embrasure, or black triangle, results.

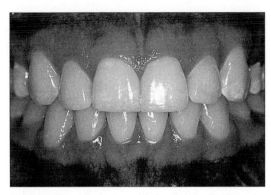

Fig 3-18 The gingival zenith is slightly distal to the midline on the maxillary central and lateral incisors.

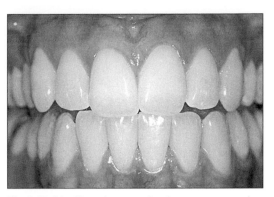

Fig 3-19 Maxillary interproximal contact areas become progressively more gingival from central incisor to canine, and incisal embrasures increase in depth from midline to canine.

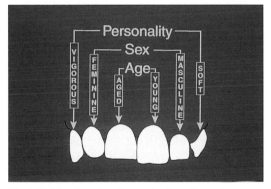

Fig 3-20 The Lombardi matrix describes characteristics associated with different incisal edge configurations.

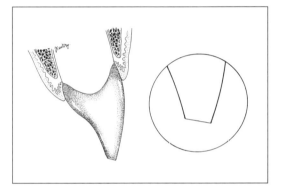

Fig 3-21 Maxillary incisal edge.

Incisal Embrasures

The incisal embrasures increase from maxillary central incisor to canine (Fig 3-19). While the incisal embrasure between the maxillary central incisors is minimal, the incisal embrasure between the maxillary central and lateral incisors is more pronounced and between the lateral incisors and canines is the most pronounced.

Uniform incisal embrasures, from maxillary canine to canine, are esthetically unnatural.

Maxillary Incisal Edge Configuration and Tooth Morphology

In nature, it is impossible to determine gender based on tooth shape or incisal edge relationships.[16] However, tooth morphology and tooth-to-tooth relationships do convey information, albeit subjective, about the individual. In 1973, based on the writings of

Frush and Fisher,[4,5] Lombardi[10] described relationships for fabricating complete dentures. His matrix is equally relevant for the dentulous patient today (Fig 3-20).

Using the Lombardi matrix, it is possible to characterize the teeth in the diagnostic waxup, the provisional restorations, and ultimately in the definitive restorations.

Maxillary Incisal Edge Shape (Buccolingual)

Natural maxillary incisal edges, in a buccolingual direction, are not rounded but rather sharp. Due to wear, the incisofacial line angle in adults is relatively sharp and blends into a 1-mm lingual facet before dropping off to the concave lingual surface (Fig 3-21).

Rounded maxillary incisal edges give the restoration an unnatural appearance due to the light reflection off a curved surface.

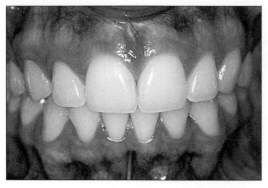

Fig 3-22 "Halo effect" in natural maxillary incisors.

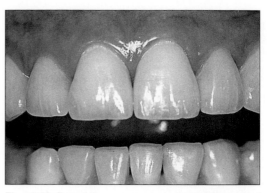

Fig 3-23 Porcelain veneers on maxillary and mandibular teeth. Note the natural appearance of the maxillary incisal edges with halo effect. (Porcelain veneers by Gilbert Young, CDT, GNS Dental Laboratory, Dallas, Texas.)

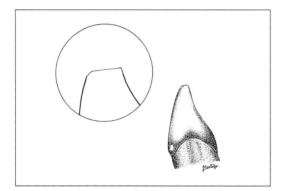

Fig 3-24 The incisal edge of a mandibular incisor. Note the pitch of the incisal table and the bevel of the incisofacial line angle.

Halo Effect

The natural incisal edge anatomy of the maxillary incisor commonly imparts a thin, white, opaque "halo effect" at the incisal edge that frames the incisal translucency (Fig 3-22). The halo effect is incorporated into porcelain restorations by building the sharp incisal edge anatomy into the crown or porcelain veneer (Fig 3-23).

Mandibular Incisal Edge Shape

The incisal edge of the mandibular incisor should have a narrow, but defined, flat incisal table. This incisal

table should be slightly canted facially. This is referred to as the *pitch* of the incisal table. The facial incisal line angle should be slightly beveled (Becker I, oral communication, 1997) (Figs 3-23 and 3-24).

This incisal edge configuration not only enhances esthetics but improves function. As the mandible moves forward, the disclusion occurs efficiently on the leading incisofacial line angle of the mandibular incisor, rather than dragging on the broader facial surface.

Outline Symmetry

The distal surfaces of the maxillary central and lateral incisors, as well as the distoincisal line angles of these teeth, should be parallel[10] (Fig 3-22).

The outline symmetry of the maxillary central and lateral incisors should be similar. A large outline discrepancy (eg, a peg-shaped lateral incisor) negatively affects the beauty of the smile.

Facial Contour of the Maxillary Incisors

The facial surfaces of the maxillary incisors should not be rounded but rather flat with resulting bold mesial and distal line angles and deep facial embrasures (Fig 3-25). Restorations with rounded facial surfaces look unnatural; facial embrasures are not well defined, resulting in a lack of visual distinction of the maxillary anterior teeth.

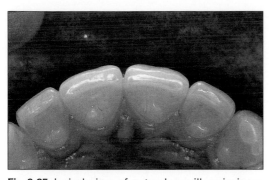

Fig 3-25 Incisal view of natural maxillary incisors. Note the flat facial surfaces, bold mesial line angles, slightly less bold distal line angles, and deep facial embrasures.

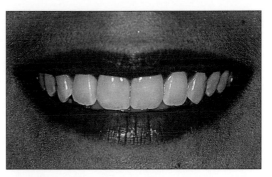

Fig 3-26 A smile that demonstrates the principle of gradation. The maxillary central incisor is visually the widest tooth, followed by the lateral incisor, the canine, and so on distally. The distal half of the canine must not be visible when viewed from the front to maintain the principle of gradation.

Outline Form of Maxillary Canines

The distal half of the maxillary canine should not be visible when viewed from the front[18] (Fig 3-26). As the eye moves laterally from the midline, each tooth should appear proportionately narrower than its mesial neighbor. This is termed the *principle of gradation*.[10] After placement of porcelain restorations on the maxillary teeth, the most common offender of this principle is the canine tooth. It appears too wide in relation to both the lateral incisor and the first premolar because the mesiodistal height of contour is too distal.

Correct placement of the mesiodistal height of contour on the facial surface of canine restorations involves the skills of both the dentist and the laboratory technician. First, the dentist must remove sufficient tooth structure on the distofacial half of the tooth to allow the technician to create the correct facial contours. Second, the technician must visualize the case from the front during final contouring of the restorations to ensure that the principle of gradation is heeded.

Color

In dentistry, color is described in four dimensions. *Hue* is the basic color of the tooth and is usually in the yellow range. *Chroma* is the saturation or intensity of the hue. *Value* is a measure of the brightness of the tooth; a high-value tooth appears bright while a low-value tooth appears darker. Finally, *maverick colors* are concentrated areas of color that are different from the overall background color.

Natural teeth are polychromatic. They generally have higher chroma in the gingival third, transition-

ing to a lower chroma and higher value in the middle third. The incisal third is characterized by the transition to incisal translucency, which is commonly framed by the halo effect (see Fig 3-22). Maverick colors can appear anywhere and individualize the tooth.

The chroma of the maxillary lateral incisor is commonly the same as the central incisor; however, the value of the lateral incisor is commonly slightly lower. In the maxillary canine, the chroma is generally higher, especially in the gingival third, and the value is lower. Incisal translucency is usually minimal in the maxillary canine, and seldom does the halo effect occur.

Polychromicity in the individual tooth and between neighboring teeth is essential in porcelain restorations if natural beauty is the goal.

Color Modifiers

It has been stated that hair color, skin color, and lipstick color all significantly affect shade selection when restorations are being placed in the esthetic zone.[13] Of these modifiers, skin color is by far the most important. A given tooth shade will look lighter and higher in value in a patient with darker skin. Conversely, the same tooth shade will appear yellower and lower in value in a patient with very light skin.

When choosing a tooth shade for a patient with variable skin color, for instance, a white patient with a deep tan, the impact of the skin color must be discussed with the patient prior to treatment. If porcelain restorations are placed while the skin is tanned, the restorations will appear to become more yellow and lower in value as the skin color lightens.

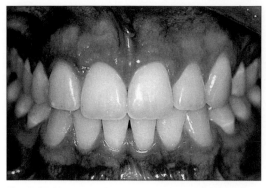

Fig 3-27 Young teeth demonstrate higher value, lower chroma, higher surface texture, and lower luster.

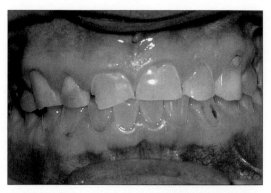

Fig 3-28 Older teeth demonstrate lower value, higher chroma, lower surface texture, and higher luster.

Image

The overall presentation of the smile can be described as the *image*. Miller[11] discusses the differences between the "natural image" and the "media image." With the media image, the teeth are generally more symmetric, monochromatic, and very high in value. The natural image incorporates asymmetries, polychromicity, and lower value with higher chroma. Dentists commonly make esthetic choices for patients based on their own notions of beauty rather than on the patient's desires.[7] When restoring maxillary anterior teeth, it is essential that the dentist understand the overall image that the patient desires.

To maximize predictability when placing anterior restorations, the issue of overall smile presentation must be developed first, to the patient's satisfaction, in the provisional restorations.

Age Characteristics of Teeth

Both tooth color and surface texture relate information about the age of the patient (Figs 3-27 and 3-28).

Chroma and Value
The value, or brightness, of a tooth is higher in young patients and decreases with age. Conversely, the chroma, or color saturation, is lower in young patients and increases with age.[8]

Surface Texture
Surface texture is higher in the young patient and decreases as the patient ages.[8] The surface luster is a function of the amount of surface texture. Therefore, the young tooth with high surface texture has a lower

luster. As the surface texture is worn away with age, the surface luster increases.

It is important to communicate with the laboratory technician about texture and luster. For example, porcelain veneers with low value, low surface texture, and high luster are not appropriate for a 25-year-old patient.

Individual Tooth Length and Proportion

The maxillary central incisor is the centerpiece of the smile. The average length of the maxillary central incisor is 10 to 11 mm[6] (Figs 3-29a to 3-29c). The ratio of height to width in the maxillary central incisor should be approximately 1.2 to 1.0. In other words, the width of the central incisor should be approximately 75% of its height.[6]

When evaluating a smile, the dentist must start with the position and size of the maxillary central incisor. It is difficult, if not impossible, to develop optimum esthetics with short maxillary anterior teeth.

Tooth-to-Tooth Proportions

The principle of gradation[10] states that as the eye moves laterally from the midline, each tooth should appear proportionately narrower than its mesial neighbor. There has been much discussion about what this mesiodistal proportion should be. The golden proportion (1.618:1.0), which was formulated as one of Euclid's elements, has been proposed.[9] Viewed from the front, the maxillary central incisor would be 1.618 times wider than the lateral incisor, the lateral incisor would be 1.618 times wider than the visual width of

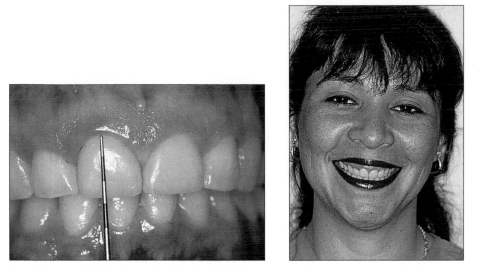

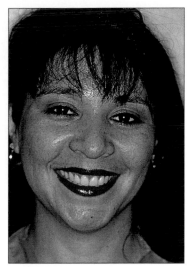

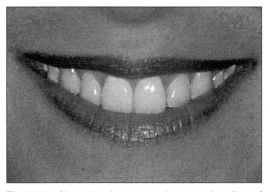

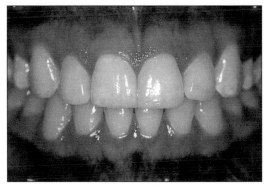

Figs 3-29a and 3-29b Short maxillary central incisor measuring 8 mm due to altered passive eruption.

Fig 3-29c After esthetic crown lengthening to treat altered passive eruption.

Fig 3-30a Note the beauty and proportionality of this natural smile.

Fig 3-30b The measurement of the visual widths of the maxillary central incisor and maxillary lateral incisor reveals a natural proportion of central incisor to lateral incisor of 1.4 to 1.0.

the canine, and so on as the eye moves distally. However, developing esthetic proportions is not that simple. In a patient with a very tapered maxillary arch, the maxillary central incisors will appear wide, and the teeth may approximate the golden proportion. However, in a patient with a very square maxillary arch form, the golden proportion would result in unesthetically wide central incisors. To some degree, the width of the central incisor, in relation to the lateral incisor, is also a matter of personal taste. The golden proportion produces very bold central incisors,[10,14] which appeals to some individuals. However, in natural teeth situated in natural arch forms, the golden proportion seldom occurs. The natural proportion of the width of the maxillary central incisor to the lateral incisor,

when measured with a caliper, is approximately 1.2 to 1.0.[7] The golden proportion is not based on actual tooth measurements, but on the tooth proportions when viewed from the front. This proportion is approximately 1.4 to 1.0 in nature (Figs 3-30a and 3-30b).

Because dental esthetics is a matter of taste, the ultimate decision on widths and proportions must be developed in provisional restorations.

Principle of Illumination

Visually, there is the perception that light objects approach the viewer and dark objects recede from the viewer.[10] This principle must be considered when high

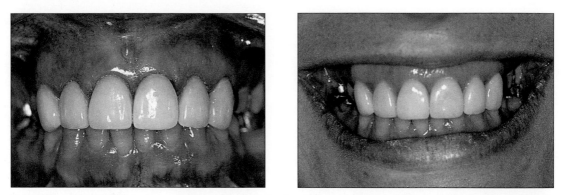

Figs 3-31a and 3-31b Porcelain veneers were placed only on the maxillary anterior teeth. Note that the maxillary first premolars are virtually invisible when viewed from the front. This results in a loss of visual coupling of the front and the back of the mouth. Note also lower lip asymmetry.

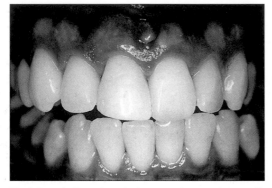

Fig 3-32a A direct bonded restoration on the maxillary right central incisor appears too wide.

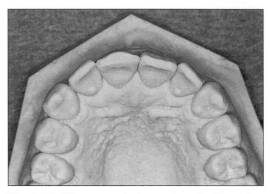

Fig 3-32b The cast of the patient in Fig 3-32a demonstrates that the mesiofacial and distofacial transitional line angles are too far into the facial embrasures, resulting in a visual widening of the tooth.

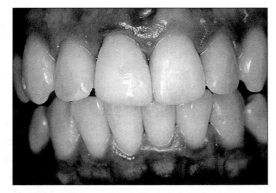

Fig 3-32c After replacement of the direct bonded restoration on the right central incisor. The tooth now appears narrower.

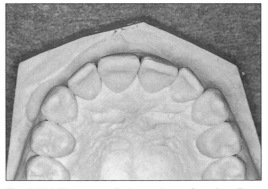

Fig 3-32d The cast of the patient after the direct bonded restoration was replaced. Note the narrower appearance of the tooth because the mesiofacial and distofacial transitional line angles are closer together.

value porcelain or composite restorations are placed only on maxillary anterior teeth, because the result may be an unesthetic visual separation of the anterior and posterior teeth. A visual coupling of the front and back of the mouth may require placement of restorations on one or more maxillary premolars (Figs 3-31a and 3-31b).

Law of the Face

The face of a tooth is that portion of the facial surface bound by transitional line angles when viewed from the front.[8] To make teeth of dissimilar widths appear similar, the apparent faces should be made equal.

To make an anterior tooth appear wider, the transitional facial line angles are moved into the interproximal facial embrasures. Conversely, to make an anterior tooth appear narrower, the transitional line angles are moved closer to the tooth midline (Figs 3-32a to 3-32d).

Conclusion

The provision of esthetic and functional restorative dentistry must be based on a set of guidelines founded on the best clinical science available. These guidelines can then be used to diagnose a patient's overall orofacial presentation and to guide the diagnostic waxup. Based on the diagnostic waxup, the provisional restorations are fabricated and placed. It is at this point that the "eye of the artist" becomes helpful for developing the final shade, shape, contour, and incisal edge configuration of the provisional restorations, which will serve as the blueprint for the final restorations.

References

1. Allen EP. Surgical crown lengthening for function and esthetics. Dent Clin North Am 1993;37:163–179.
2. Brisman AS. Esthetics: a comparison of dentists' and patients' concepts. J Am Dent Assoc 1980;100:345–352.
3. Croll BM. Emergence profiles in natural tooth contour. Part 1: photographic observations. J Prosthet Dent 1989;62:4–10.
4. Frush JP, Fisher RD. Introduction to dentogenic restorations. J Prosthet Dent 1955;5:586–595.
5. Frush JP, Fisher RD. How dentogenic restorations interpret the sex factor. J Prosthet Dent 1956;6:160–172.
6. Gillen RJ, Schwartz RS, Hilton TJ, Evans DB. An analysis of selected normative tooth proportions. Int J Prosthodont 1994;7:410–417.
7. Goldstein R. Study of need for esthetics in dentistry. J Prosthet Dent 1969;21:589–598.
8. Heymann HO. The artistry of conservative esthetic dentistry. J Am Dent Assoc (special issue) 1987:14E–22E.
9. Levin EI. Dental esthetics and the golden proportion. J Prosthet Dent 1978;40:244–252.
10. Lombardi RE. The principles of visual perception and their clinical application to denture esthetics. J Prosthet Dent 1973;29:358–382.
11. Miller CJ. The smile line as a guide to anterior esthetics. Dent Clin North Am 1989;33:157–164.
12. Peck S, Peck L, Kataja M. The gingival smile line. Angle Orthodont 1992;62:91–100.
13. Pound E. Applying harmony in selecting and arranging teeth. J Am Dent Assoc 1957;55:181–191.
14. Preston JD. The golden proportion revisited. J Esthet Dent 1993;5:247–251.
15. Proffitt WM. Contemporary Orthodontics, ed 2. St Louis: Mosby; 1992:150.
16. Tjan AHJ, Miller GD, The JGP. Some esthetic factors in a smile. J Prosthet Dent 1984;51:24–28.
17. Vig RG, Brundo GC. The kinetics of anterior tooth display. J Prosthet Dent 1978;39:502–504.
18. Williams HA, Caughman WF. Principles of esthetic dentistry: practical guidelines for the practitioner. In: Clark JW (ed). Clinical Dentistry. New York: Harper & Row, 1976;4(15):1–20.

Caries Management: Diagnosis and Treatment Strategies

J. Peter van Amerongen/Cor van Loveren/Edwina A. M. Kidd

Traditional caries management has consisted of the detection of carious lesions followed by immediate restoration. In other words, caries was managed primarily by restorative dentistry. However, when the dentist takes the bur in hand, an irreversible process begins. Placing a restoration does not guarantee a sound future for the tooth; on the contrary, it may be the start of a restorative cycle in which the restoration will be replaced several times. The decision to initiate invasive treatment should be preceded by a number of questions: Is caries present and if so, how far does it extend? Is a restoration required, or could the process be arrested by preventive treatment? Sometimes the decision to restore may be based on questionable diagnostic criteria.[22]

The introduction of adhesive restorative materials has allowed dentists to make smaller preparations, which has led to preservation of hard dental tissues and, along with declining disease prevalence, has allowed elimination of G. V. Black's principle of "extension for prevention." Maximum tooth structure is preserved. However, this approach, sometimes described as a "dynamic treatment concept," cannot prevent repeated treatment procedures and the occurrence of iatrogenic damage (Fig 4-1). Lussi and Gygax showed that during the preparation of a proximal surface, the neighboring surface was damaged 100% of the time, despite very careful operating procedures.[61]

A different treatment strategy is recommended, based on a proper diagnosis of caries, taking into account the dynamics of the caries process. The activity of caries should be determined, and causative factors should be evaluated. Caries risk should be assessed before treatment is considered, and treatment should include preventive regimens to arrest the caries process by redressing the imbalance between demineralization and remineralization.[56]

The treatment goal in caries management should be to prevent new lesions from forming and to detect lesions sufficiently early in the process so that they can be treated and arrested by nonoperative means.[56] Such management requires skill and is time-consuming and worthy of appropriate payment. If these attempts have failed, high-quality restorative dentistry will be required to restore the integrity of the tooth surface.

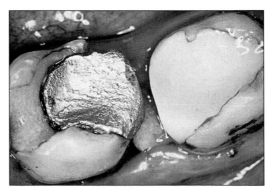

Fig 4-1 Iatrogenic damage caused by repeated treatment procedures.

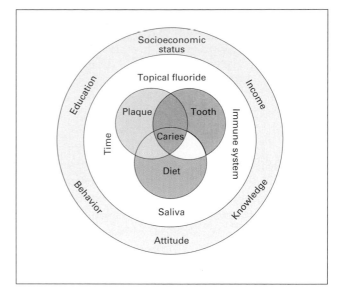

Fig 4-2 Factors influencing the equilibrium between the three prerequisites for the caries process as first described by Keyes and Jordan.[48]

Etiology

The factors involved in the caries process, which include the tooth, dental plaque, and diet, were presented in the 1960s in a model of overlapping circles.[48] Since then, the model has been supplemented with the factors of time, fluoride, saliva, and social and demographic factors (Fig 4-2). At first sight, these circles constitute a simple model to explain caries risk, which is represented by the overlap of the three inner circles. When one of the risk factors increases, the respective circle becomes larger, as does the overlap of the circles, indicating increased caries risk. If there is, for instance, hyposalivation, the saliva circle will tighten the three inner circles, enlarging the overlap, again indicating a greater risk. Inversely, the model explains why reduction in any risk factor decreases caries risk.

Dental Plaque

The prevalence of mutans streptococci and lactobacilli is associated with dental caries.[12,47,58] *Streptococcus mutans* is involved in caries formation from its initiation, while lactobacilli are so-called secondary organisms that flourish in a carious environment and contribute to caries progression. Dental plaque may be more cariogenic locally where mutans streptococci and lactobacilli are concentrated, but in everyday practice it is difficult for the dentist to identify cariogenic plaque to make this knowledge useful in treating individual patients. Plaque can be sampled and

mutans streptococci and lactobacilli can be quantified, but the procedure is quite complicated and requires the support of a microbiologic laboratory. It is easier to count mutans streptococci and lactobacilli in saliva, and kits are commercially available for this purpose. These counts, however, do not give site-specific information and are poor predictors for high caries activity in general, although low counts or absence of mutans streptococci are good predictors of low caries activity.[88]

High numbers of mutans streptococci and lactobacilli are probably the consequence of a high sugar intake and the resulting periods of low pH levels in dental plaque.[18,66] Inversely, it has been shown that restriction of sugar intake reduces the numbers of mutans streptococci and lactobacilli.[18,55] In one study of individuals complying with a Weight Watchers diet, the numbers of mutans streptococci and lactobacilli were reduced by half.[1] A comparable reduction was found in subjects who reduced their sugar intake frequency from 7.2 to 1.8 times a day.[117] Interestingly, after a period of sugar restriction, the pH response to glucose was reduced in buccal[100] but not in interdental plaque.[117] Apparently, the reductions in numbers of mutans streptococci and lactobacilli are insufficient to reduce the acidogenicity of interdental plaque.[117]

The oral flora colonizes on teeth continuously, but it takes up to several days before the dental plaque contains enough acidogenic bacteria to lower plaque pH to the level that causes demineralization.[43] Theoretically, plaque removal every second day would be sufficient. If the dentition is professionally cleaned, an even lower frequency of cleaning has been demonstrated to prevent caries.[3,4] But we have only to consider the caries prevalence in the prefluoride era to realize that few people are capable of cleaning their teeth to a level adequate to prevent caries.

Teeth

Teeth consist of a calcium phosphate mineral that demineralizes when the environmental pH lowers. As the environmental pH recovers, dissolved calcium and phosphate can reprecipitate on remaining mineral crystals. This process is called *remineralization*. Remineralization is a slower process than demineralization. When remineralization is given enough time, it can eliminate the damage done during demineralization, but in the absence of this the caries process will progress and a lesion will develop. Dentin is more vulnerable than enamel because of structural differences and impurities in the lattice. For many years, much emphasis was given to the pre-eruptive effect of fluoride improving the quality of the dental hard tissues. However, it is now clear that posteruptively used fluoride is more protective against caries.[80,96,105]

Diet

Dietary carbohydrates are necessary for the bacteria to produce the acids that initiate demineralization. In general, dietary advice for caries prevention is based on three principles: *(1)* the drop in pH lasts for approximately 30 minutes; *(2)* the frequency of intake is more important than the quantity; and *(3)* the stickiness is an important factor in the cariogenicity of foods. It has become obvious, however, from many epidemiologic studies that where fluoride is used daily, sugar consumption and caries prevalence have become independent for many individuals. Even when there was a significant correlation between sugar consumption and caries prevalence, the caries-preventive effect of sugar restriction was small. For instance, in Basel, Switzerland, wartime restriction had reduced sugar supply from about 40 to 16 kg/person/year, but the number of caries-free children rose only from approximately 3% to 15%.[36,54] At that time, the improvement seemed impressive, but it was dwarfed by the effect of nationwide use of fluoride. With this evidence, the role of dietary counseling in caries prevention should be re-examined. This does not negate the value of diet analysis and advice for patients presenting with

multiple carious lesions, but the importance of the proper use of fluoride should also be emphasized.

Information gathered with the reliable pH-telemetry method has revealed that a pH drop induced by eating may last for hours if there is no stimulation of the salivary flow.[43–45] Even the consumption of an apple can depress the pH for 2 hours or longer.[43] Long pH depressions will be most prevalent in areas where saliva has little or no access, and these are the most caries-prone areas. It is unknown how much additional harm is caused by a second sugar intake during such a period of low pH or how beneficial it is to omit a second sugar intake during that period. These considerations emphasize that at sites where caries lesions develop, advice based on a 30-minute duration of the pH drop is not necessarily effective for caries prevention. In addition, foods believed to be "good" for teeth may not be better than foods that are supposedly "bad." A chocolate and caramel bar might be considered bad because it feels sticky. In reality, the caramel dissolves and leaves the mouth relatively quickly, whereas potato chips, generally considered less harmful, take a longer time to clear the mouth.[46] During this retention, the carbohydrate fraction may be hydrolyzed to simple sugars, providing a substrate for the acidogenic bacteria.[57]

All the uncertainties about the determinants of the cariogenicity of foods make it impossible to provide strict dietary guidelines. To snack in moderation, limited to 3 or 4 snacks a day, is the only wise recommendation.

Time

Time affects the caries process in several ways. When caries was commonly considered to be a chronic disease, time was introduced to indicate that the substrate (dietary sugars) must be present for a sufficient length of time to cause demineralization.[75] Now we know that caries is not a chronic disease and that its effects can be arrested or completely repaired should enough time be given for remineralization. Finally, it is clear that caries lesions do not develop overnight, but take time; in fact, it may take years for cavitation to occur. This potentially gives the dentist and the patient ample time for preventive treatment strategies.

Fluoride

Experiments have shown that fluoride protects enamel more effectively when it is present in the ambient solution during acid challenges than when it is incorporated into the enamel lattice.[80] The mechanism by which fluoride inhibits demineralization is by reprecipitation of dissolved calcium and phosphate, thereby preventing these constituents from being leached out of the enamel into the plaque and saliva.[105] Part of the reprecipitation takes place at the surface of the tooth. This narrows the pores in the enamel surface that provide diffusion pathways for the acids produced in the dental plaque to penetrate into the enamel. Acid penetration is thus hampered. In addition, during periods where the ambient pH is above 5.5, fluoride will facilitate remineralization, promoting lesion arrest and repair. A lack of fluoride constitutes a caries risk.

The retention of fluoride in the mouth is site-specific. In plaque and saliva and in dentin samples fixed in dental splints, most fluoride was found on the labial surfaces of maxillary incisors and buccal surfaces in the mandibular molar region after rinsing with a fluoride solution.[16,114] In addition, it was observed that fluoride from passively dissolving fluoride tablets remained highly concentrated only at the site of tablet dissolution. There was very little or no transport of fluoride between the right and the left sides of the mouth and between the maxillary and mandibular arches.[16] Because of this, localized caries lesions in the mouth may be related to an insufficient spread of fluoride when subjects use fluoride toothpaste. Certainly when patients use fluoride toothpaste they should be encouraged to spit out any excess rather than to rinse vigorously with water.

Saliva

The important role of saliva is clearly demonstrated by the rampant caries that may occur in subjects with compromised salivary flow. These subjects lack the protective qualities of saliva of which the flow rate and buffering capacity may be the most important. Both help to neutralize and clear the acids and carbohydrates from dental plaque. Clearance, however, is not uniform throughout the mouth and may be slowest at the labial aspects of the maxillary incisors and buccal aspects of the mandibular molars. Other sites in the dentition may not be easily accessible to saliva as a result of an individual's anatomy, including inter-

proximal spaces and fissures. Dental plaque in a cavity may also be protected from salivary clearance.

The sites that are difficult for saliva to reach may also be difficult to reach with mechanical cleaning devices, such as a toothbrush or dental floss. Plaque and food may adhere for long times in these areas, making these sites more caries prone. Furthermore, this caries risk factor may be easily overlooked in children, whose teeth appear to be clean as judged from the sites that are easily cleaned. These children may even brush their teeth twice daily and have only a moderate number of sugar intake episodes per day. The most feasible way to prevent caries at these sites is by thorough oral hygiene measures and use of a fluoride-containing toothpaste so that plaque is removed and fluoride is applied.

Social and Demographic Factors

Many studies have shown that, at least in the western world, dental caries is more prevalent in the lower socioeconomic categories, in the less affluent areas, and among some ethnic minorities (Table 4-1).[108] Differences related to the socioeconomic status are very clear for the primary dentition and less clear for the permanent dentition, although this pattern may differ in other parts of the world. Studies have shown that for the prediction of caries development, social and demographic factors may be successful in very young children without a long dental history, but for older children, clinical parameters are more predictive.[17,33] In the elderly population, however, root caries again seems to be more prevalent in people from lower socioeconomic backgrounds.

Caries Prediction

To make the most appropriate treatment decisions, a good estimate of the caries risk is necessary. Indicators of past caries experience are the strongest predictors, and the status of the most recently erupted or exposed surfaces is a strong predictor for the newly emerging surfaces. One very elegant review plots the strongest clinical predictors against age and dentition (Table 4-2).[88] The sensitivity and specificity of the predictors varied from 0.60 to 0.80, indicating that 20% to 40% of the children who developed caries during the study were not identified and that 20% to 40% of the children who were not caries active were, in contrast, predicted to develop caries. In addition, it is impor-

Table 4-1 Percentages of 6- and 12-year-old caries-free children and mean dmfs and DMFS scores in children who were not caries free in 1989, 1993, and 1996 according to socioeconomic level[108]

Socioeconomic status	6-year-old children					12-year-old children				
	%	d	m	f	dmf ± SD	%	D	M	F	DMF ± SD
Low										
1989	43	4.7	0.6	2.8	8.2 ± 8.5	46	0.2	0.0	3.4	3.6 ± 2.2
1993	39	4.8	0.3	2.7	7.8 ± 9.0	67	0.1	0.0	3.9	4.0 ± 3.1
1996	49	5.0	1.1	3.5	9.6 ± 9.8	50	0.1	0.0	3.1	3.2 ± 2.4
Medium										
1989	60	3.4	0.8	1.3	5.5 ± 6.9	49	0.2	0.1	3.5	3.9 ± 2.7
1993	69	4.0	0.3	1.4	5.8 ± 7.5	61	0.3	0.0	2.5	2.8 ± 1.9
1996	79	3.7	0.9	0.4	4.9 ± 5.3	89	0.0	0.0	3.6	3.6 ± 2.6
High										
1989	77	1.5	0.0	0.6	2.1 ± 1.3	59	0.9	0.2	1.8	2.9 ± 2.0
1993	77	2.5	0.2	1.7	4.4 ± 3.5	63	0.3	0.0	1.7	2.1 ± 1.6
1996	84	1.6	0.9	2.2	4.7 ± 5.1	86	0.3	0.0	2.0	2.3 ± 2.1

dmfs = decayed, missing, or filled surfaces in primary teeth; DMFS = decayed, missing, or filled surfaces in permanent teeth.

Table 4-2 Time line of strongest clinical predictors of caries incidence[88]

	Age (y)						
	0 and 1	2–5	6–9	10–13	14–21	22–45	>45
Dentition	Primary	Primary	Mixed dentition	Mixed dentition	Early permanent	Mature permanent	Mature permanent and gingival recession
Predictor*	Mutans streptococci	**dmfs, especially primary incisors;** mutans streptococci and lactobacilli	**dmfs, especially primary molars;** 1st molar occlusal morphology; DMFS	**DMFS, especially 1st permanent molars;** 1st molar occlusal morphology; incipient smooth surface lesions	**Incipient smooth surface lesions;** DMFS	Not studied	Coronal and root DMFS; number of teeth; periodontal disease

dmfs = decayed, missing, or filled surfaces in primary teeth; DMFS = decayed, missing, or filled surfaces in permanent teeth.
*The strongest predictors are in bold.

tant to recognize that none of the studies in the review were designed to predict the progression rate of caries at a specific site. So, even if it could be predicted that an individual would develop caries, the lesion that is going to progress cannot be confidently identified.

Rate of Caries Progression

The decline in caries prevalence has been accompanied by a change in lesion behavior. Caries lesions progress more slowly than they did several decades ago, probably due to increased use of fluoride, which delays lesion progression. It is clear that the progression rate is not the same for each site. Little is known about the progression rate of fissure caries. Longitudinal epidemiologic data from the 1950s, when fluoride was not yet widely used, showed that it took approxi-

mately 1 year for an enamel fissure lesion to develop into a dentinal lesion.[5] More recent data from the same geographic area, after the introduction of fluoride toothpaste, showed that 50% of the enamel fissure lesions had progressed to involve dentin within 2 years while 75% had become dentinal lesions after 4 years.[112] Data from Switzerland showed that, for first permanent molars, approximately 10%, 20%, and 45%, respectively, of sound fissures, fissures with a yellowish discoloration, and fissures with a dark discoloration progressed to dentinal caries or tooth restoration in 4 years.[65] These progression rates were slightly lower than those found by the same investigators 10 years earlier. It is the experience of many clinicians that not all initial fissure lesions will develop to involve the dentin but that a number of them may become arrested. In populations where not all fissure lesions develop into open cavities, the dentist will be confronted with clinically undetected occlusal dentinal caries. This is not a new phenomenon; it was discussed as early as 1931.[42] Today, reported prevalence rates vary greatly.[15,116]

Based on epidemiologic data from the 1950s, the progression rates of proximal caries lesions from initial enamel caries to dentinal caries in the permanent dentition was estimated to be 2 years at age 7 and approximately 4 years at age 12.[5] Data collected after fluoride supplementation became available showed a progression rate of 3 to 4 years for proximal caries lesions to reach the dentin in 12 year olds.[9] Shwartz et al[103] concluded from data collected in Sweden and the United States that it takes an average of 4 years for caries lesions to progress through the proximal enamel of permanent teeth. The progression rate seemed to be independent of the number of DMFS (decayed, missing, or filled surfaces) of the individuals.

Not all caries lesions progress, however. In one study, over 50% of initial proximal caries lesions had not advanced in a 3-year period in 13-year-old children.[35] The majority of the lesions that progressed were found in the children who had the highest number of lesions at the start of the study, which probably reflects the difference between caries-active and caries-inactive children. Recently, Mejàre et al[67] published data on the caries prevalence on the proximal surfaces of the posterior teeth at various ages (Fig 4-3). The caries prevalence was low, with the distal surfaces of the first molars being the most caries prone.

Caries on free smooth surfaces seems to progress more slowly than on proximal surfaces or in fissures. Many lesions do not progress into the dentin and even show regression to sound enamel.[5,34,51,99] In one study, dentists were asked at what point they would treat small noncavitated lesions on the buccal surfaces of teeth. Approximately 40% indicated that they would use a preventive rather than an operative strategy.[76] This indicates that many dentists believe that they are well able to judge the severity of buccal lesions and to monitor lesion development.

Altogether, the evidence indicates that along with the decline in caries prevalence has come a decline in caries progression rate. Between the initiation of caries and the involvement of dentin in the caries process, there is ample time for a preventive management strategy. This implies that the early lesion should be detected so that preventive treatment can arrest its progress and bring about remineralization. If this strategy is successful, operative intervention will not be required.

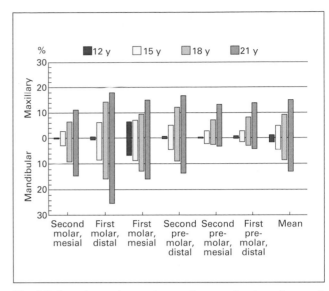

Fig 4-3 Prevalence (percentage of approximal surfaces affected) of dentinal lesions in the respective approximal surfaces in different age groups (Mejàre et al[67]).

Detection and Diagnosis

When a dentist identifies a carious lesion, it is a change in mineral content that is detected. The dentist must also determine whether a lesion is active or arrested before a logical management plan can be proposed; the dynamics of the caries process must be recognized.[56]

Detection

Teeth must be clean for the clinical detection of carious lesions. Otherwise, reliable detection may be obstructed by the presence of plaque (Figs 4-4a and 4-4b). The teeth are cleaned and an air/water syringe used so that the tooth surface may be dried. This drying has two functions: the first is to remove saliva, which can obscure a lesion; the second is to dry a white spot lesion. Removing water from the porous tissue in this way enables the dentist to gauge how far through the enamel a lesion has progressed. A white spot lesion visible on a wet tooth surface indicates that demineralization is over halfway through the enamel, possibly extending into dentin. A white spot lesion that becomes visible only after thorough air-drying will be less than halfway through enamel.

The dentist also requires bite-wing radiographs to assist in the detection of proximal caries lesions, occlusal caries lesions, and recurrent caries. The radio-

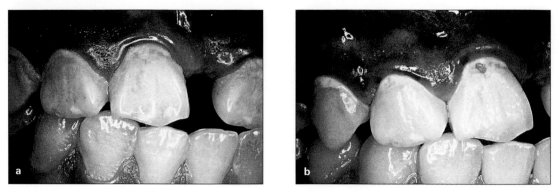

Figs 4-4a and 4-4b Reliable detection of caries lesions can be obstructed by plaque. (a) Plaque covers labial surfaces and conceals a cavity in tooth 8. (b) Same surface, cleaned, reveals the cavity. (Courtesy K. R. Ekstrand.)

Table 4-3	Criteria for visual examination of caries[47,58]
Score	**Criteria**
0	No or slight change in enamel translucency after prolonged air drying (> 5 s)
1	Opacity or discoloration hardly visible on the wet surface, but distinctly visible after air drying
2	Opacity or discoloration distinctly visible without air drying
3	Localized enamel breakdown in opaque or discolored enamel and/or grayish discoloration from the underlying dentin
4	Cavitation in opaque or discolored enamel, exposing the dentin

Table 4-4	Criteria for the histologic examination of fissure caries[47,58]
Score	**Criteria**
0	No enamel demineralization or a narrow surface zone of opacity (edge phenomenon)
1	Enamel demineralization limited to the outer half of the enamel layer
2	Demineralization involving between half of the enamel and outer third of the dentin
3	Demineralization involving the middle third of the dentin
4	Demineralization involving the pulpal third of the dentin

graphs should be taken using a film holder and beam-aiming device to take the guesswork out of tube alignment and allow comparable views to be taken on subsequent occasions. Because lesions confined to enamel on radiographs should be managed by preventive treatment, monitoring them is important. Magnification is a great adjunct to caries detection.

Pit and Fissure Lesions

Detection of caries in fissures and pits is most often done by visual inspection. Good lighting and dry, clean teeth are prerequisites. It appears that any sign of visible cavitation in the occlusal surface corresponds to progression of the lesion into the dentin.[24,109] Interpretation of the occlusal surface that appears caries free can be difficult, but it is possible if all plaque is removed and the teeth are dried, as shown by Ekstrand et al.[25,26] When occlusal surface caries was recorded visually using a caries score ranking system (Table 4-3), a high correlation with the histologic depth of the lesions into enamel and dentin was found (Table 4-4).[25,26]

A clear ranked caries scoring system is useful for subsequent assessment and monitoring. Careful examination of bite-wing radiographs is also important, although enamel lesions will not be visible. Caries in dentin, however, can usually be detected, and such lesions are often large (Fig 4-5). Bite-wing radiographs can be considered to provide a safety net function for large occlusal lesions.[25,28,110] For assessment and monitoring, a ranked scoring system can be used (Table 4-5).

Tactile examination of fissures with a dental explorer has been advocated for many decades (even centuries) as an important method to detect caries, but research has shown this to be an unwise practice. The method is inaccurate,[84] and, worse, the explorer can damage a white spot lesion by breaking through the relatively intact surface zone (Fig 4-6).[23] Vigorous use of a sharp explorer can cause a cavity, which will subsequently trap dental plaque and encourage lesion progression. Detection of fissure caries lesions should rely on sharp eyes, not sharp explorers.

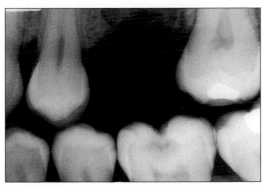

Fig 4-5 The radiograph as "safety net": occlusal caries in dentin is well detected (tooth 19).

Table 4-5	Criteria for the radiographic examination of fissure caries[47,58]
Score	Criteria
0	No radiolucency visible
1	Radiolucency visible in the enamel
2	Radiolucency visible in the dentin but restricted to the outer third of the dentin
3	Radiolucency extending to the middle third of the dentin
4	Radiolucency in the pulpal third of the dentin

Lesions Involving Proximal Surfaces

When there is contact between proximal surfaces, the radiograph is the most accurate method for detecting demineralization. In the premolar and molar regions, lesion progression or arrest can be monitored, provided that appropriate film holders and beam-aiming devices have been used to ensure that subsequent bitewing radiographs are taken at approximately the same angulation.[85] The radiograph should be examined carefully to determine whether carious lesions are present in the outer enamel, at the dentinoenamel junction, in the outer half of dentin, or in the inner half of dentin (Figs 4-7a and 4-7b).

Fiberoptic transillumination techniques have proven useful. With these techniques, a fine light, coned down to a 0.5-mm diameter, is transmitted through a contact point. Lesions appear as a dark shadow. It is difficult, however, to discriminate between demineralization extending just into enamel and that progressing further into dentin, especially in the posterior areas. For detection of proximal lesions in anterior teeth, however, the fiberoptic transillumination technique is particularly appropriate and convenient.[71]

Finally, use of an orthodontic separator has been advocated in some cases to allow the dentist to see more clearly and to *gently* feel for a break in the enamel surface.[92]

Lesions in Smooth, Free Surfaces

Lesions in smooth, free surfaces, whether in the enamel of the crown or the dentin of the root, can be detected easily with visual inspection. The surface to be examined must be cleaned, dried, and well illuminated. Again, drying with an air syringe can be used to assess the depth of penetration of a white spot lesion through the enamel.

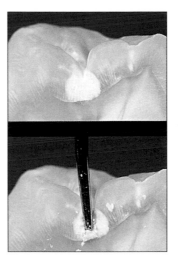

Fig 4-6 The explorer tip can easily damage white spot lesions.

New Detection Devices

The development of several new devices and detection methods is promising. Electronic caries monitors are based on the principle that porous carious lesions have lower conductive values than intact tooth structures.[91] Various optical methods, including several laser systems, are promising,[2,59,62,63,89] as are the new ultrasonic devices.[119] Experimental results, however, show that further development and research are required before application in general practice can be recommended.

Diagnosis

What is the difference between lesion detection and diagnosis?

Caries is a ubiquitous, natural process that does not have to progress.[31] Detecting mineral loss resulting from the carious process is only the first step.

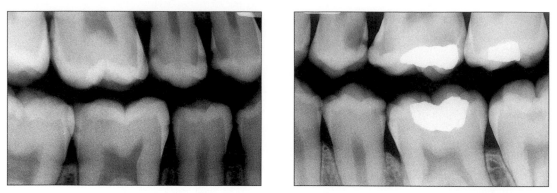

Figs 4-7a and 4-7b Radiographs showing approximal demineralizations in the outer enamel, to the dentino-enamel junction, and in the outer and inner half of dentin. (Occlusal lesions are visible on teeth 18, 30, and 31, and recurrent caries under the restoration on tooth 14).

Table 4-6	Parameters concerning caries activity
Immediate past caries experience	Development of new lesions within a certain period of time
Progression of the lesions	Progression or arrest of previously registered lesions
Appearance of the lesions/cavities	Structure: shiny, matte, smooth, cavitated Consistency: hard, soft Moistness: wet, dry Color: white, yellow, brown, black
Location of the lesions/cavities	Lesions only on sites of predilection or on sites not normally affected by caries
Presence of plaque/gingivitis	Lesion covered or not covered by plaque; gingival inflammation near the lesion or not

If this information is to be useful, whether the detected lesion is arrested or active must be determined. If the lesion is arrested, no treatment is required unless for esthetic or functional reasons; if the lesion is active, preventive treatment, which may include operative dentistry, is needed to arrest lesion progression. Thus diagnosis adds the dimension of lesion activity to detection.[29]

Assessing Caries Activity

There are some features of individual lesions that indicate whether a lesion is active or arrested. Some of these features will be obvious the first time a dentist and patient meet. However, most patients see their dentist at regular intervals. Thus the initial diagnosis can and should be refined at recall, and these visits provide the opportunity to assess the effects of preventive treatment. Has a lesion, previously diagnosed as active, apparently arrested? Table 4-6 lists some of the parameters relevant in the assessment of caries activity.

Following are discussions of the individual sites where caries may occur with definitions of the features of active and arrested lesions.[79] Difficulties in making this distinction are highlighted.

Occlusal lesions. The visual and radiographic features of occlusal caries have been presented (see Tables 4-3 and 4-5). The following features indicate lesion activity:

- White spot lesions that have a matte or visibly frosted surface or are plaque-covered after drying or application of a disclosing solution[13]
- Cavitated lesions, including microcavities as well as cavities exposing dentin (Fig 4-8)
- Lesions visible in dentin on bite-wing radiographs[90]

The following feature indicates that the lesion may be arrested:

- White or brown spot lesions with a shiny surface (Fig 4-9)[13]

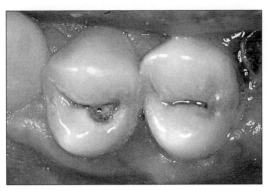

Fig 4-8 Active occlusal caries.

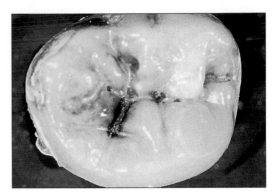

Fig 4-9 Arrested lesions.

Proximal lesions. Diagnosis of lesion activity is more difficult when the adjacent tooth precludes a direct visual assessment. (The radiographic features are presented in Chapter 2 and in preceding paragraphs.) The presence or absence of a cavity is relevant to lesion activity, but unfortunately this cannot be judged from the radiograph. The reason a cavity is important is that for an active carious lesion to be arrested, plaque must be regularly removed from it. But on a proximal surface, there is no access for the toothbrush, and even the most fastidious of flossers will only skate over the surface.

The following tend to indicate lesion activity:

- A patient with proximal lesions on the radiograph who is judged to be at high caries risk[60] (described later in this chapter)
- A proximal lesion present radiographically and persistent gingival inflammation despite the patient's attempts to remove plaque with dental floss[27]
- A lesion not present at previous examination

The following features indicate that the lesion may be arrested:

- Successive, reproducible, bite-wing radiographs showing no lesion progression
- A patient who is now judged to be at low risk for caries following preventive treatment

Smooth-surface lesions. These are probably the most straightforward lesions for assessing activity because they are the most visible. Of all lesions, these are the ones most likely to be arrested by preventive treatment alone. Indeed, they are a barometer that a patient can and should watch in the quest for dental health.

The following indicate lesion activity:

- White spot lesions close to the gingival margin that have a matte or visibly frosted surface; these are often plaque-covered (Fig 4-10).
- Cavitated, plaque-covered lesions with or without exposed dentin; if dentin is exposed and soft, the dentin is heavily infected and the lesion is active (Figs 4-11a and 4-11b).

The following indicate that the lesion is arrested:

- Shiny white or brown lesions, often well exposed due to recession; the lesions are not plaque-covered (Fig 4-12).
- Cavitated lesions, often dark brown, with hard dentin at their bases; the lesions are not plaque-covered and are often remote from the gingival margin (Fig 4-13).

Root caries. Active lesions are:

- Close to the gingival margin and plaque-covered
- Soft or leathery in consistency

Arrested lesions are:

- Often some distance from the gingival margin and not covered with plaque (Fig 4-14)
- As hard as the surrounding healthy root surface[39]

Color is unreliable in differentiating active from inactive lesions. While arrested lesions may be dark, so may the soft dentin in some active lesions. The research community has yet to fully explain why demineralized dentin is brown.

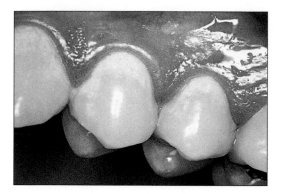

Fig 4-10 Matte, white, active cervical lesions.

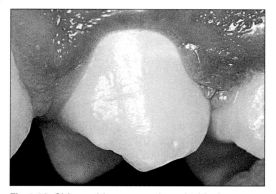
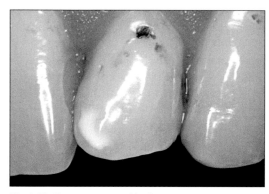

Figs 4-11a and 4-11b Cavitated, active cervical lesions.

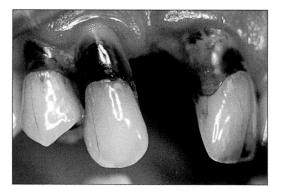

Fig 4-12 Shiny, white, arrested cervical lesion.

Fig 4-13 Brown, arrested lesion.

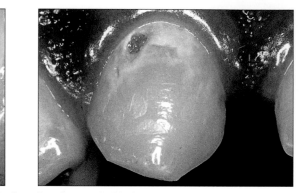

Fig 4-14 Arrested root caries.

Recurrent caries. Caries at the margin of or beneath a restoration is called *recurrent caries*, and its diagnosis on various tooth surfaces is as described previously. The bite-wing radiograph is very important in the diagnosis of recurrent caries since lesions often form cervical to an existing proximal restoration, in the area of plaque stagnation. Lesions that are obviously in dentin as seen radiographically tend to be cavitated and active. However, research has shown that the following are not reliable indicators of active caries beneath a restoration: ditching and staining around an amalgam restoration[49]; staining around a tooth-colored restoration.[50]

Assessment of Caries Risk

In addition to differentiating active from inactive lesions, determining the overall caries risk for the patient is an important factor. If a patient presents with many cavitated lesions and a dentist skillfully restores the teeth, is the patient still at risk of caries? The answer is "yes" unless the biologic environment that caused the caries to occur has been changed. Preventive treatment is needed, in addition to operative care, to help the patient to remove plaque more effectively, to modify the diet if appropriate, to use fluoride to delay lesion progression, and to attempt to stimulate saliva if the mouth is dry. The role of operative procedures in caries control is to facilitate plaque control, but restorations alone cannot be relied on to change the patient's caries risk status, particularly if the risk status is high.

Patients should be made aware of their caries risk status to encourage them to become involved in their own preventive care, to keep appropriate recall appointments, and perhaps to help them budget for dental costs. It is also important for patients to realize that caries risk status can change and their dentist can detect this change. Examples of a change in risk status may be the onset of a dry mouth or a change in ability to remove plaque.

Assessment of caries risk is an important part of contemporary dental practice, and it is something that general practitioners do rather well.[19] Indeed, research has shown that a dentist's best guess of a patient's caries risk may be as accurate as any combination of more objective factors.[52] These factors include:

- Clinical evidence
- Plaque control
- Use of fluoride
- Dietary habits
- Saliva
- Medical history
- Social history

An experienced practitioner will be able to assess caries risk in less time than it takes the reader to read these descriptions. Risk assessment is an intellectual process demanding both clinical skill and experience.[56]

Dentists should define the caries risk status of each patient, and, whether the risk is high or low, they should identify the reasons. Interestingly, it can be more difficult to explain low risk than high risk. However, it is with the high-risk patient that the definition becomes critical to patient management. It is important to determine whether or not the risk factors can be modified and if so, how this can best be done.

Clinical Evidence

Clinical evidence has been shown to be the best predictor of caries risk.[19,111] The findings of many initial lesions or many restorations requiring frequent replacement provide evidence of high risk for caries. There may also be a history of teeth being extracted because "they were too carious to be restored."

Clinical and radiographic examinations, described earlier in this section, are very important. If the dentist can review earlier radiographs, perhaps taken over years, the caries status of the patient may be graphically displayed.

It should also be remembered that adding a dental appliance to the environment, such as an orthodontic appliance[118] or a partial denture,[20] may tip the balance toward high risk.

Because appliances favor plaque retention, they should be avoided in high-risk patients when possible.

Plaque Control

Dental plaque is the primary risk factor for dental caries.[30] Not all patients with poor plaque control will inevitably develop caries, but oral hygiene is the bedrock of a caries control program in a high-risk patient. If for any reason plaque control becomes difficult, perhaps because of age or long-term illness, caries risk can change.

Use of Fluoride

Fluoride delays the progression of the carious process, and patients living where the water is fluoridated will benefit, particularly in areas of social deprivation.[74] Today most patients use a toothpaste containing fluoride, but it is wise to ascertain this in those with multiple, active lesions.

Dietary Habits

High sugar intake is considered an important factor in caries risk,[97] but not all patients with high sugar intake will develop caries. It is, however, unusual to find a patient with multiple active carious lesions who does not have a high sugar intake. It is also important to remember that dietary habits can change. Changes in lifestyle such as unemployment, retirement, or bereavement can have profound implications, and a vigilant dentist will take such changes into consideration.

Saliva

A dry mouth is one of the most important factors predisposing to high caries risk.[106] The four most common causes are:

- Many medications, such as antidepressants, antipsychotics, tranquilizers, antihypertensives, and diuretics, can cause dry mouth.
- Patients with rheumatoid arthritis may also have Sjögren's syndrome, which affects the salivary and lacrimal glands, leading to a dry mouth and dry eyes.
- People with eating disorders may suffer from hyposalivation, which, combined with a poor diet, can lead to extensive caries.[72]
- Patients who have received radiation therapy in the region of the salivary glands for a head and neck malignancy will often suffer from xerostomia.

Numerous research studies have also shown that salivary counts of mutans streptococci and lactobacilli help predict caries risk.[111] This huge volume of work appears to show that in individual patients, low counts often predict low risk well, but the opposite is not necessarily true. The routine use of salivary counts for prediction of risk status is, therefore, not recommended.

Medical History

Medically compromised and handicapped people may be at high risk for developing caries.[102] For these patients, oral hygiene may be difficult, and long-term use of medicines can be a problem if the medicines are sugar-based[40] or cause reduced salivary flow.[51]

The most important caries risk factor in a medical history is the complaint of dry mouth,[51] discussed previously. It is important to realize that the medical history is one factor in a caries risk assessment that can change. A vigilant dentist will detect such changes and help the patient with the potential dental consequences.

Social History

Many studies have shown that social deprivation[7,41] can be an indicator of caries risk. Other diseases, such as coronary heart disease and some cancers, are also prevalent in socially deprived people. The dentist may notice high caries in siblings, and the patient or parent may possess little knowledge of dental disease. Concern about dental health may be low and dental visits irregular.

Identifying Relevant Risk Factors

While it is relatively easy for an experienced dentist to classify patients into a high- or low-risk category, determining the cause of the risk may take longer. However, this is time well spent and an essential part of diagnosis.[111] An appropriate plan of action cannot be formulated until the factors that require modification have been defined. Identifying the reasons that the patient is at high risk is also relevant to prognosis. Can the patient modify the risk factor? Some causes of dry mouth are impossible to alter and the patient may always be at high risk. Another individual may be able to change his or her risk status by modifying plaque control and/or diet, but these changes demand behavioral modification. The patient must take responsibility for the problem rather than transferring responsibility to the dentist.[6] Unless the high-risk patient accepts responsibility for modifying behavior and improving his or her dental health, no restorative services, no matter how well executed, will prevent the caries recurrence.

Treatment Strategy

Traditionally, radiographic evidence of demineralization in enamel or to the dentinoenamel junction led to the immediate decision to place a restoration. Such management is still an accepted part of some state board examinations. However, contemporary research has shown that this is not the optimal approach. Radiographs may reveal demineralization, but the caries activity of the lesion must be assessed. If the lesion is arrested, it requires no treatment. The management of an active lesion should be directed to redressing the imbalance of demineralization and remineralization. This management may arrest the lesion so that a restoration is never required.

Caries is often presented as a one-way process; sugar in the presence of plaque causes demineralization that presents as a white dull lesion. As the process progresses, a hole or cavity results (Fig 4-15). In fact, caries is a dynamic process in which periods of demineralization and remineralization alternate depending on the oral environment. It may be possible to cure or arrest an early lesion on a free smooth surface (Fig 4-16). On a smooth surface, even cavitated lesions can be arrested because plaque may be removed with a toothbrush.

Caries is caused by a multifactorial process, and its management should reflect this.[8] The general ap-

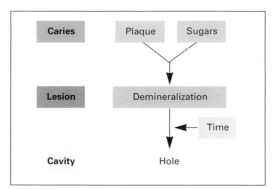

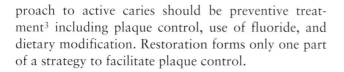

Fig 4-15 Caries presented as a one-way process.

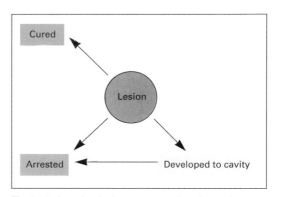

Fig 4-16 A caries lesion presented as dynamic.

proach to active caries should be preventive treatment[3] including plaque control, use of fluoride, and dietary modification. Restoration forms only one part of a strategy to facilitate plaque control.

Preventive Management Strategies

The most plausible explanation for the decline of caries prevalence is the steady improvement in oral hygiene, which results in regular (at least partial) removal of dental plaque, combined with a regular daily administration of fluoride, provided via toothpaste.[10,96] A recently published analysis of data derived from a sample of 1,450 preschool children studied in the British National Diet and Nutrition Survey confirmed the significant caries-inhibiting effect of toothbrushing with a fluoride dentifrice twice daily. On a population basis, sugar-containing foods and drinks were not associated with caries experience, unless children brushed once a day or less.[32] Thus, the cornerstone of any preventive strategy for the management of caries is oral self-care: twice daily careful cleaning of the teeth with a toothbrush and an effective fluoride toothpaste. Additionally, dental floss should be used, but patients should be instructed carefully and the frequency should be individually recommended. In areas where the water is fluoridated to optimal levels, twice daily careful cleaning of the teeth is a safe and effective preventive treatment and caries management strategy.[73,81,83]

If caries or caries progression is not prevented, the reasons should be carefully examined (Fig 4-17). A first step in this procedure is to carefully assess the quality of the oral hygiene. If hygiene is adequate, it is appropriate to evaluate whether additional risk fac-

tors such as multiple intake episodes of sugar-containing foods and drinks are present. If so, these risks must be reduced as much as possible. In the meantime, the patient can be helped with professionally applied preventive measures such as topical application of concentrated fluoride solutions, gels, or varnishes, or chlorhexidine gels or varnishes. Salivary flow can be stimulated by daily use of sugar-free chewing gum. When no additional risks can be identified, the fluoride supply must be intensified, perhaps by adding a third daily fluoride application in the form of additional brushing, mouthwash, or tablet.

If the daily oral hygiene procedures are inadequate, an attempt should be made to determine whether the problem is due to an inability to use a toothbrush or whether the patient simply is noncompliant. The dentist should apply disclosing solution to the teeth and watch as the patient demonstrates the oral hygiene procedures. If he or she is not able to remove the plaque, the patient should be taught alternative methods. Sometimes a patient can be helped by professionally applied preventive measures. If a patient is able to remove plaque but is not motivated to do so, the dentist must try to determine the reasons. The patient may not be convinced of the necessity for thorough plaque removal. This puts the dentist in the realm of behavior modification, a subject not in the scope of this textbook but an important part of dental practice.

Professionally Applied Preventive Measures

Professionally applied topical fluorides in solutions, gels, or varnishes have been shown to be effective in many clinical trials.[64,94] The effectiveness seems not to depend on the method of application, the use of addi-

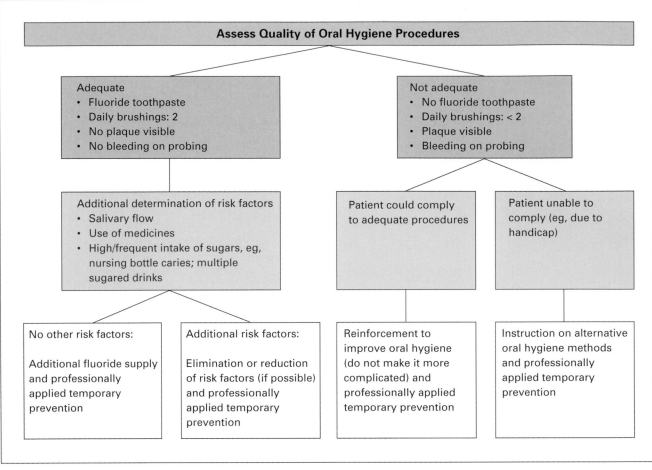

Fig 4-17 Assessment of oral hygiene procedures when caries or caries progression is not prevented.

tional fluoride supplements, or baseline caries prevalence. A recent meta-analysis revealed a 22% to 26% overall caries-inhibiting effect for fluoride gel treatments.[14,94,113] Chlorhexidine, as a 1% gel or a 40% varnish, has also been successfully applied to prevent caries.[113] Applications of the chlorhexidine products are more laborious than fluoride applications and must be performed every 3 to 4 months. In addition, they have been shown to reduce caries only in those who harbor 10^6 mutans streptococci or more per milliliter of saliva. To select these patients, the number of mutans streptococci should be quantified in saliva.

With the decline in caries prevalence, the professionally applied preventive treatments do not seem appropriate on a population basis. In a population with, for example, a mean caries incidence of 0.25 DMFS/year, a preventive treatment with 22% effect would theoretically save 0.055 DMFS/year/individual. In the total population, 36 treatments would be needed to prevent 1 DMFS/year. With a low caries activity, the cost-effectiveness ratio is unfavorable. Based on cost-effectiveness calculations, an individual can decide whether he or she is willing to pay for professionally applied treatments to prevent tooth decay.

Treatment of the Lesion or Cavity

Carious lesions are detected at a relatively late point of development. This may be due to difficulties in detecting the early lesion or it may be because the patient did not visit the dentist early in the lesion process. Although this may suggest the value of a rigorous, invasive approach, it is preferable, because of the iatrogenic damage that may occur during preparation, to select a treatment option that is as conservative as possible. The treatment should be based on the interpretation of the activity of the lesion and on fu-

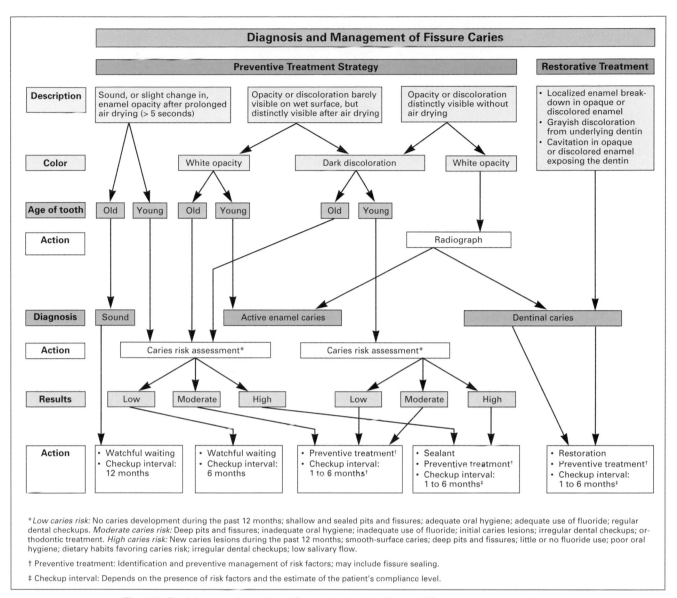

Diagnosis and Management of Fissure Caries

| | **Preventive Treatment Strategy** | | | **Restorative Treatment** |

Description: Sound, or slight change in, enamel opacity after prolonged air drying (> 5 seconds) | Opacity or discoloration barely visible on wet surface, but distinctly visible after air drying | Opacity or discoloration distinctly visible without air drying | • Localized enamel breakdown in opaque or discolored enamel • Grayish discoloration from underlying dentin • Cavitation in opaque or discolored enamel exposing the dentin

Color: White opacity — Dark discoloration — White opacity

Age of tooth: Old | Young — Old | Young — Old | Young

Action: Radiograph

Diagnosis: Sound — Active enamel caries — Dentinal caries

Action: Caries risk assessment* — Caries risk assessment*

Results: Low | Moderate | High — Low | Moderate | High

Action:
• Watchful waiting
• Checkup interval: 12 months

• Watchful waiting
• Checkup interval: 6 months

• Preventive treatment†
• Checkup interval: 1 to 6 months†

• Sealant
• Preventive treatment†
• Checkup interval: 1 to 6 months‡

• Restoration
• Preventive treatment†
• Checkup interval: 1 to 6 months‡

*Low caries risk: No caries development during the past 12 months; shallow and sealed pits and fissures; adequate oral hygiene; adequate use of fluoride; regular dental checkups. Moderate caries risk: Deep pits and fissures; inadequate oral hygiene; inadequate use of fluoride; initial caries lesions; irregular dental checkups; orthodontic treatment. High caries risk: New caries lesions during the past 12 months; smooth-surface caries; deep pits and fissures; little or no fluoride use; poor oral hygiene; dietary habits favoring caries risk; irregular dental checkups; low salivary flow.

† Preventive treatment: Identification and preventive management of risk factors; may include fissure sealing.

‡ Checkup interval: Depends on the presence of risk factors and the estimate of the patient's compliance level.

Fig 4-18 Decision tree for occlusal fissure lesions leading to different treatment options.

ture caries risk. Figure 4-18 demonstrates a decision-making tree for occlusal fissure lesions with different features leading to different treatment options dependent on lesion activity and risk assessment.

Although lesions that are cavitated are treated traditionally by preparation and restoration, a preventive treatment approach is often successful, especially when the lesion is in a free smooth surface. When a lesion is present in an occlusal or proximal surface, it will often be difficult to arrest lesion progression because of the difficulty of removing plaque. However, when lesions are in buccal or lingual surfaces, or in

the roots of teeth, it is often possible for the patient to tip the balance of demineralization and remineralization in the right direction and stop further progression of the lesion.

Causal, Noninvasive, or Preventive Treatment

Where individual lesions or cavities are concerned, the treatment options are to restore or not to restore. If the decision is made not to restore, the question arises, can the lesion or cavity be cured, or at least prevented from

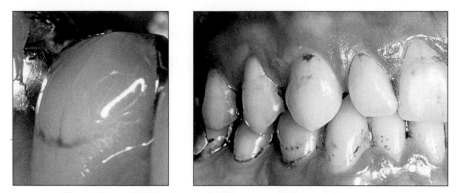

Figs 4-19a and 4-19b Arrested lesions seen as brownish scar tissue.

further extension; in other words, can it be arrested? When considering caries, factors such as plaque, fluoride, and diet are of paramount importance. Management of the lesion should be directed such that optimal plaque removal, sufficient fluoride application, and a healthy diet prevent further deterioration. It is still relevant to ask what effects preventive treatment has on initial demineralized lesions and on cavities: Can they be cured (healed) or merely arrested?

Initial Lesions

Von der Fehr et al[115] and Koch[53] have shown that normal individuals can be turned into individuals with high caries risk. Within a short period of time, numerous initial carious lesions can develop when oral hygiene is withdrawn and a sugar-rich diet is offered.[53,115] However, when effective oral hygiene and application of topical fluoride are instituted, and a normal, less sugar-rich diet is consumed, reversal of the situation seems possible; after a period of time, the initial lesions are no longer visible. But are they healed or controlled? Thylstrup et al[107] demonstrated that in the very early lesion, only the external microsurface is dissolved by plaque. When the plaque is removed mechanically at this stage, the eroded area will change from the chalky white appearance of the earlier active lesion into a hard and shiny surface. It has been suggested that this phenomenon is caused by wear and polishing and not by recovery of the carious surface.[107]

Further progression of the lesion leads to deeper surface and subsurface dissolution. Intervening in the process with plaque removal, fluoride application, and a better diet leads again to wear and a polished surface, and a slowly remineralizing subsurface lesion.[107] Although these lesions decrease in depth and width in course of time, they may remain visible as shiny white lesions, commonly seen on facial sur-

faces. In this case, the lesion cannot be considered completely recovered, but it can be concluded that the caries process has ceased. These arrested lesions may be seen throughout life as whitish or brownish "scar tissue" (Figs 4-19a and 4-19b). Research has shown that these areas are more resistant to a subsequent caries attack than sound enamel.

The average speed of progression of carious lesions on different surfaces has been determined.[86,87] On proximal and free smooth areas, caries proceeds slowly. It is thus reasonable to postpone restorative intervention. A procedure whereby the patient is examined regularly ("watchful waiting") creates the opportunity for arrest and remineralization. "Watchful waiting" implies that nothing is done, but in fact it is based on the intellectual decision not to restore because of knowledge of the caries process. The dentist is performing active preventive treatment by helping the patient to improve oral hygiene, by applying fluoride, and by encouraging the patient to modify his or her diet. These measures should always be carried out when active noncavitated lesions exist. But what should be done when further progression has led to a cavity?

Cavitated Lesions

Several authors have shown that when an occlusal lesion has cavitated, the dentin is always involved in the process.[24,109] Moreover, these lesions, mostly detectable on radiographs, contain many microorganisms and are therefore considered active.[2,25,26,28,110]

It is not difficult to imagine that measures directed to a thorough removal of plaque are ineffective on the occlusal surface because the bristles of the toothbrush cannot get into the undermined cavity. Proximal cavitations are also difficult to reach. Dental floss will skim the surface but will not have access to the cavi-

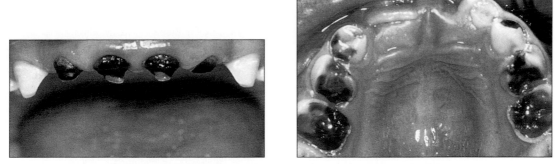

Figs 4-20a and 4-20b Arrested carious lesions in the primary dentition.

tated area. However, where there are cavitated areas on free smooth surfaces, the situation is different. Those areas are easily reached by the toothbrush but may be difficult to clean due to undermining of the enamel. Removal of the overhanging enamel margins must be considered to aid in keeping the whole area free of plaque. Cavities in these surfaces, cleaned twice daily with a fluoride toothpaste, can be arrested and converted into leathery or hard lesions[77,79] (see Figs 4-13 and 4-14). When the activity of highly infected caries lesions is decreased and finally arrested, the carious layers contain few bacteria that can be cultivated.[78,82,98,101] Though occlusal or proximal caries lesions cannot be approached by preventive measures alone, in primary molars this method can be successful. Therefore, undermined enamel margins should be eliminated, so that when plaque is removed, fluoride can be applied easily to the carious dentin. Under ideal conditions, carious dentitions can be managed so that caries is arrested and demineralization and remineralization are in equilibrium (Figs 4-20a and 4-20b).

Sealants

Fissures are more susceptible to caries than smooth surfaces because fissure anatomy favors plaque maturation and retention.[95] When active fissure caries has been diagnosed or if a high risk has been established and fissures have susceptible morphologic characteristics, sealants may be indicated (see Fig 4-18). After acid etching, a lightly filled resin fissure sealant or a flowable resin composite is used to penetrate the fissures and prevent plaque accumulation. This is especially important during the period of tooth eruption, although the application of sealants in suspect fissures is also advisable in older patients with high caries risk.[93] Advantages of fissure sealants are that no irreversible interventions are necessary, active dentin lesions inadvertently covered by the resin do not progress

further, and the possible development of new lesions in other sites of the fissure is prevented. Sealants have been used successfully for many years.[104] Concern has been expressed about placement of sealants over undiagnosed dentin caries lesions. However, there is ample evidence that caries does not progress as long as the fissure remains sealed.[37,38,68,69] Sealed, radiographically evident caries has been shown in one study not to progress over a 10-year period.[11,70] Also, sealed restorations placed directly over frankly cavitated lesions arrested the progress of these lesions. Sealing of restorations, therefore, appears to be very effective in conserving sound tooth structure, protecting the margins of restorations, and preventing recurrent caries.[70]

Symptomatic (Invasive or Restorative) Treatment

It is necessary to have well-defined criteria for the decision to restore due to caries. The most important reason for placing a restoration is to aid plaque control. Elderton and Mjör formulated the following indications for restorative treatment[21]:

• The tooth is sensitive to hot, cold, sweetness, etc.
• Occlusal and proximal lesions extend into dentin.
• The pulp is endangered.
• Previous attempts to arrest the lesion have failed and there is evidence that the lesion is progressing (such evidence usually requires an observation period of months or years).
• The patient's ability to provide effective home care is impaired.
• Drifting is likely to occur through loss of proximal contact.
• Esthetic reasons.

Treatment will be directed in such a way that infected dental tissue is removed and the remaining cavity is adapted so that the restorative material can be optimally placed. The particular preparation methods and restorative procedures are discussed in the following chapters.

Most dentists enjoy the technical, esthetic, and intellectual challenges of restorative dentistry. However, before invasive procedures are initiated, noninvasive options must be explored and preventive measures taken. Restorative dentistry is one part of preventive treatment. Above all, it must be remembered that caries is a dynamic process and the diagnosis requires the determination of caries activity and risk assessment.

References

1. Andréen I, Köhler B. Effects of Weight Watchers' diet on salivary secretion rate, buffer effect and number of mutans streptococci and lactobacilli. Scand J Dent Res 1992;100:93–97.

2. Angmar-Månsson B, Al-Khateeb S, Tranaeus S. Monitoring the caries process. Optical methods for clinical diagnosis and quantification of enamel caries. Eur J Oral Sci 1996;104:480–485.

3. Axelsson P, Lindhe J. Effect of controlled oral hygiene procedures in caries and periodontal diseases in adults. J Clin Periodontol 1978;5:133–151.

4. Axelsson P, Lindhe J, Nyström B. On the prevention of caries and periodontal disease. Results of a 15 year longitudinal study in adults. J Clin Periodontol 1991;18:182–189.

5. Backer Dirks O. Posteruptive changes in dental enamel. J Dent Res 1966;45(suppl):503–511.

6. Barker T. Patient motivation. In: Kidd EAM, Joyston-Bechal S (eds). Essentials of Dental Caries. Oxford: Oxford University Press, 1997:146–162.

7. Beal JF. Social factors and preventive dentistry. In: Murray JJ (ed). Prevention of Oral Disease. Oxford: Oxford University Press, 1996:216–233.

8. Benn DK. Practical evidence-based management of the initial caries lesion. J Dent Educ 1997;61:853–854.

9. Bjarnason S, Kingman A. Caries progression in populations with different caries prevalence. Caries Res 1991;25:215.

10. Brathall D, Hänsel-Petersson G, Sundberg H. Reasons for the caries decline: what do the experts believe? Eur J Oral Sci 1996;104:416–422.

11. Briley JB, Dove SB, Mertz-Fairhurst EJ. Radiographic analysis of previously sealed carious teeth [abstract 2514]. J Dent Res 1994;73:416.

12. Carlsson J, Grahnen H, Jonsson G. Lactobacilli and streptococci in the mouth of children. Caries Res 1975;9:333–339.

13. Carvalho JC, Thylstrup A, Ekstrand K. Results after 3 years non-operative occlusal caries treatment of erupting permanent first molars. Community Dent Oral Epidemiol 1992;20:187–192.

14. Clark DC, Hanley JA, Stamm JW, Weinstein PL. An empirically based system to estimate the effectiveness of caries-preventive agents. Caries Res 1985;19:83–95.

15. Creanor SL, Russell JI, Strang DM, et al. The prevalence of clinically undetected occlusal dentin caries in Scottish adolescents. Br Dent J 1990;169:126–129.

16. Dawes C, Weatherell JA. Kinetics of fluoride in the oral fluids. J Dent Res 1990;69(special issue):638–644.

17. Demers M, Broduer J-M, Mouton C, et al. A multivariate model to predict caries increment in Montreal children aged 5 years. Community Dent Health 1992;9:273–281.

18. De Stoppelaar JD, Van Houte J, Backer Dirks O. The effect of carbohydrate restriction on the presence of Streptococcus mutans, Streptococcus sanguis and iodophylic polysaccharide-producing bacteria in human dental plaque. Caries Res 1970;4:114–123.

19. Disney JA, Graves RC, Stamm JW, et al. The University of North Carolina Risk Assessment Study: further developments in caries risk prediction. Community Dent Oral Epidemiol 1992;20:64–75.

20. Drake CW, Beck JD. The oral status of elderly removable partial denture wearers. J Oral Rehabil 1993;20:53–60.

21. Elderton RJ, Mjör IA. Treatment planning. In: Hörsted-Bindslev P, Mjör IA (eds). Modern Concepts in Operative Dentistry. Copenhagen: Munksgaard, 1988.

22. Elderton RJ. Principles in the management of dental caries. In: Elderton R (ed). The Dentition and Dental Care. Oxford: Heinemann Medical Books, 1990.

23. Ekstrand KR, Qvist V, Thylstrup A. Light microscope study of the effect of probing in occlusal surfaces. Caries Res 1987;21:368–374.

24. Ekstrand KR, Kuzmina I, Bjørndal L, Thylstrup A. Relationship between external and histologic features of progressive stages of caries in the occlusal fossa. Caries Res 1995;29:243–250.

25. Ekstrand KR, Ricketts DNJ, Kidd EAM. Reproducibility and accuracy of three methods for assessment of demineralization depth on the occlusal surface: an in vitro examination. Caries Res 1997;31:224–231.

26. Ekstrand KR, Ricketts DNJ, Kidd EAM, et al. Detection, diagnosing, monitoring and logical treatment of occlusal caries in relation to lesion activity and severity: an in vivo examination with histological validation. Caries Res 1998;32:247–254.

27. Ekstrand KR, Brunn C, Brunn M. Plaque and gingival status as indicators for caries progression on proximal surfaces. Caries Res 1998;32:41–45.

28. Espelid I, Tveit AB, Fjelltveit A. Variations among dentists in radiographic detection of occlusal caries. Caries Res 1994;28:169–175.

29. Featherstone JDB. Clinical implications: New strategies for caries prevention. In: Stookey GK (ed). Early Detection of Dental Caries. Indianapolis: Indiana University, 1996:287–295.

30. Fejerskov O, Manji F. Reactor paper: risk assessment in dental caries. In: Bader JD (ed). Risk Assessment in Dentistry. Chapel Hill, NC: University of North Carolina Dental Ecology, 1990:215–217.

31. Fejerskov O. Concepts of dental caries and their consequences for understanding the disease. Community Dent Oral Epidemiol 1997;25:5–12.

32. Gibson S, Williams S. Dental caries in preschool children: associations with social class, toothbrushing habit and the consumption of sugars and sugar containing foods. Caries Res 1999;33:101–113.

33. Grindefjord M, Dahlöf G, Nilsson D, Modéer T. Prediction of dental caries development in 1-year-old children. Caries Res 1995;29:343–348.

34. Groeneveld A. Longitudinal study of prevalence of enamel lesions in a fluoridated and non-fluoridated area. Community Dent Oral Epidemiol 1985;13:159–163.

35. Gröndhal H-G, Hollender L, Malmcrona E, Sundquist B. Dental caries and restorations in teenagers. II. A longitudinal radiographic study of the caries increment of proximal surfaces among urban teenagers in Sweden. Swed Dent J 1977;1: 51–57.

36. Gülzow H-J, Maeglin B, Mühlemann R, et al. Kariesbefall und Kariesfrequenz bei 7-15 jährigen Basler Schulkindern im Jahre 1977, nach 15 jähriger Trinkwasserfluoridierung. Schweiz Monatsschr Zahnheilk 1982;92:255–266.

37. Handelman S, Washburn F, Wopperer P. Two-year report of sealant effect on bacteria in dental caries. J Am Dent Assoc 1976;93:967–970.

38. Handelman S. Effect of sealant placement on occlusal caries progression. Clin Prev Dent 1982;4:11–16.

39. Hellyer PH, Beighton D, Heath MR, Lynch E. Root caries in older people attending a general dental practice in East Sussex. Br Dent J 1990;169:201–206.

40. Hobson P. Sugar-based medicines and dental disease. Community Dent Health 1985;2:57–62.

41. Hunt RJ. Behavioural and sociodemographic risk factors for caries. In: Bader JD (ed). Risk Assessment in Dentistry. Chapel Hill, NC: University of North Carolina Dental Ecology 1990;29–34.

42. Hyatt TP. Observable and unobservable pits and fissures. Dent Cosmos 1931;73:586–592.

43. Imfeld T. Identification of Low Risk Dietary Components. Basel: Karger, 1983.

44. Jensen ME, Schachtele CF. Plaque pH measurements by different methods on the buccal and proximal surfaces of human teeth after a sucrose rinse. J Dent Res 1983;62:1058–1061.

45. Jensen ME, Wefel JS. Human plaque pH responses to meals and the effects of chewing gum. Br Dent J 1989;167:204–208.

46. Kashket S, Van Houte J, Lopez LR, Stocks S. Lack of correlation between food retention on the human dentition and consumer perception of food stickiness. J Dent Res 1991;70: 1314–1319.

47. Keene H, Shklair I. Relationship of Streptococcus mutans carrier status to the development of caries lesions in initially caries free recruits. J Dent Res 1974;53:1295–1299.

48. Keyes PH, Jordan HV. Factors influencing the initiation, transmission and inhibition of dental caries. In: Harris RJ (ed). Mechanisms of Hard Tissue Destruction. New York: Academic Press, 1963:261–283.

49. Kidd EAM, Joyston-Bechal S, Beighton D. Marginal ditching and staining as a predictor of secondary caries around amalgam restorations: a clinical and microbiological study. J Dent Res 1995;74:1206–1211.

50. Kidd EAM, Beighton D. Prediction of secondary caries around tooth-colored restorations: a clinical and microbiological study. J Dent Res 1996;75:1942–1946.

51. Kidd EAM, Joyston-Bechal S (eds). Saliva and caries. In: Essentials of Dental Caries. Oxford: Oxford University Press, 1997:66–78.

52. Kidd EAM. Assessment of caries risk. Dent Update 1998;25: 385–390.

53. Koch G. Importance of early determination of caries risk. Int Dent J 1988;38:203–210.

54. König KG. Changes in the prevalence of dental caries: how much can be attributed to changes in diet? Caries Res 1990:24 (suppl 1):16–18.

55. Krasse B. The effect of the diet on the implantation of caries inducing streptococci in hamsters. Arch Oral Biol 1967;10: 215–226.

56. Lagerlöf F, Oliveby A. Clinical implications: new strategies for caries treatment. In Stookey GK (ed). Early detection of dental caries. Indianapolis: Indiana University, 1996:297–321.

57. Lingstrom P, Birkhed D. Plaque pH and oral retention after consumption of starchy snack products at normal and low salivary secretion rate. Acta Odontol Scand 1993;51:379–388.

58. Loesche W. Dental Caries: A Treatable Infection. Springfield, IL: Thomas, 1982.

59. Longbottom C, Pitts NB, Reich E, Lussi A. Comparison of visual and electrical methods with a new device for occlusal caries detection. Caries Res 1998;32:297.

60. Lunder N, von der Fehr FR. Proximal cavitation related to bitewing image and caries activity in adolescents. Caries Res 1996;30:143–147.

61. Lussi A, Gygax M. Iatrogenic damage to adjacent teeth during classical proximal box preparation. J Dent 1998;26:435–441.

62. Lussi A, Imwinkelried S, Longbottom C, Reich E. Performance of a laser fluorescence system for detection of occlusal caries. Caries Res 1998;32:297.

63. Lussi A, Pitts N, Hotz P, Reich E. Reproducibility of a laser fluorescence system for detection of occlusal caries. Caries Res 1998;32:297.

64. Marthaler T. Clinical cariostatic effects of various fluoride methods and programs. In: Ekstrand J, Fejerskov O, Silverstone LM (eds). Fluoride in Dentistry, ed 1. Copenhagen: Munksgaard, 1988:252–275.

65. Marthaler TM, Stener M, Bandi A. Werden verfärbte Molarenfissuren innerhalb van vier Jahren häufiger kariös als Nichtverfärbte? Schweiz Monatsschr Zahnmed 1990;100: 841–849.

66. McDermid AS, McKee AS, Ellwood DC, Marsh PD. The effect of lowering the pH on the composition and metabolism of a community of nine oral bacteria grown in a chemostat. J Gen Microbiol 1986;132:1205–1214.

67. Mejàre I, Källestål C, Stenlund H, Johansson H. Caries development from 11 to 22 years of age: a prospective radiographic study. Prevalence and distribution. Caries Res 1998;32:10–16.

68. Mertz-Fairhurst E, Schuster G, Fairhurst C. Arresting caries by sealants: results of a clinical study. J Am Dent Assoc 1986; 112:194–197.

69. Mertz-Fairhurst EJ, Adair SM, Sams DR, et al. Cariostatic and ultraconservative sealed restorations: nine-year results among children and adults. J Dent Child 1995;62:97–107.

70. Mertz-Fairhurst EJ, Curtis JW, Ergle JW, et al. Ultraconservative and cariostatic sealed restorations: results at year 10. J Am Dent Assoc 1998;129:55–66.

71. Mitropoulos CM. The use of fibre-optic transillumination in the diagnosis of posterior-proximal caries in clinical trials. Caries Res 1985;19:379–384.

72. Montgomery MT, Ritvo J, Ritvo J, Weiner K. Eating disorders; phenomenology, identification and dental intervention. Gen Dent 1988;36:485–488.

73. Murray JJ, Breckon JA, Reynolds PJ, et al. The effect of residence and social class on dental caries experience in 15-16-year-old children living in three towns (natural fluoride, adjusted fluoride and low fluoride) in the north east of England. In: Murray JJ (ed). The Prevention of Dental Disease, ed 2. Oxford: Oxford Medical, 1989.

74. Murray JJ, Breckon JA, Reynolds PJ, et al. The effect of residence and social class on dental caries experience in 15-16-year-old children living in three towns (natural fluoride, adjusted fluoride and low fluoride) in the north east of England. Br Dent J 1991;171:319–322.

75. Newbrun E. Cariology. Baltimore, MD: Williams & Wilkins, 1978.

76. Nuttal NM, Fyffe HE, Pitts NB. Caries management strategies used by a group of Scottish dentists. Br Dent J 1994;176: 373–378.

77. Nyvad B, Fejerskov O. Active root surface caries converted into inactive caries as a response to oral hygiene. Scand J Dent Res 1986;94:281–284.

78. Nyvad B, Fejerskov O. An ultrastructural study of bacterial invasion and tissue breakdown in human experimental root surface caries. J Dent Res 1990;69:2218–2225.

79. Nyvad B, Fejerskov O. Assessing the stage of caries lesion activity on the basis of clinical and microbiological examination. Community Dent Oral Epidemiol 1997;25:69–75.

80. Øgaard B, Rølla G, Ruben J, et al. Microradiographic study of demineralization of shark enamel in a human caries model. Scand J Dent Res 1988;96:209–211.

81. O'Mullane D, Whelton H. Caries prevalence in the Republic of Ireland. Int Dent J 1994;44:387–391.

82. Parikh SR, Massler M, Bahn A. Microorganisms in active and arrested carious lesions of dentin. NY State Dent J 1963;29: 347–355.

83. Pendrys GP, Katz RV, Morse DE. Risk factors for enamel fluorosis in a fluoridated population. Am J Epidemiol 1994;140: 461–471.

84. Penning C, Van Amerongen JP, Seef RE, Ten Cate JM. Validity of probing for fissure caries diagnosis. Caries Res 1992;26: 445–449.

85. Pitts NB, Kidd EAM. Some of the factors to be considered in the prescription and timing of bitewing radiography in the diagnosis and management of dental caries. J Dent 1992; 20:74–84.

86. Pitts NB, Kidd EAM. The prescription and timing of bitewing radiography in the diagnosis and management of dental caries: contemporary recommendations. Br Dent J 1992;172: 225–227.

87. Pitts NB, Kidd EAM. Some of the factors to be considered in the prescription and timing of bitewing radiography in the diagnosis and management of dental caries. J Dent 1992; 20:74–84.

88. Powell LV. Caries prediction: a review of the literature. Community Dent Oral Epidemiol 1998;26:361–371.

89. Reich E, Al Marrawi F, Pitts N, Lussi A. Clinical validation of a laser caries diagnosis system. Caries Res 1998;32:297.

90. Ricketts DNJ, Kidd EAM, Beighton D. Operative and microbiological validation of visual, radiographic and electronic diagnosis of occlusal caries in non-cavitated teeth judged to be in need of operative care. Br Dent J 1995;79:214–220.

91. Ricketts DNJ, Kidd EAM, Liepins PJ, Wilson RF. Histological validation of electrical resistance measurements in the diagnosis of occlusal caries. Caries Res 1996;30:148–155.

92. Rimmer PA, Pitts NB. Temporary elective tooth separation as a diagnostic aid in general practice. Br Dent J 1990;169:87–92.

93. Ripa LW, Leske GS, Varma OA. Longitudinal study of the caries susceptibility of occlusal and proximal surfaces of first permanent molars. J Public Health Dent 1988;48:8–13.

94. Ripa LW. Review of the anticaries effectiveness of professionally applied and self-applied topical fluoride gels. J Public Health Dent 1989;49(special issue):297–309.

95. Ripa LW. Sealants revisited: an update of the effectiveness of pit and fissure sealants. Caries Res 1993;27:77–82.

96. Rølla G, Øgaard B, de Almeida Cruz R. Clinical effect and mechanism of cariostatic action of fluoride-containing toothpastes: a review. Int Dent J 1991;41:171–174.

97. Rugg-Gunn AJ. Diet and dental caries. In: Murray JJ (ed). Prevention of Oral Disease. Oxford: Oxford University Press, 1996:3–31.

98. Sarnat H, Massler M. Microstructure of active and arrested dentinal caries. J Dent Res 1965;44:1389–1401.

99. Saxer UP, Marthaler TM. Karieszuwachs über 10 Jahre bei jungen Erwachsenen mit und ohne Prophylaxe-Program im Pflichtschulalter (II). Quintessenz 1982;4:833–840.

100. Scheie AA, Arneberg P, Orstavik D, Afseth J. Microbial composition, pH-depressing capacity and acidogenicity of 3-week smooth surface plaque developed on sucrose-regulated diets in man. Caries Res 1984;18:74–86.

101. Schüpbach P, Guggenheim B, Lutz F. Human root caries: histopathology of arrested lesions. Caries Res 1992;26: 153–164.

102. Shou L. Social and behavioural aspects of caries prediction. In: Johnson NW (ed). Dental Caries: Markers of High and Low Risk Groups and Individuals. Cambridge: Cambridge University Press, 1991:172–197.

103. Shwartz M, Gröndhal H-G, Pliskin JS, Boffa J. A longitudinal analysis from bitewing radiographs of the rate of progression of proximal carious lesions through human dental enamel. Arch Oral Biol 1984;29:529–536.

104. Simonsen R. Retention and effectiveness of dental sealant after 15 years. J Am Dent Assoc 1991;122:34–42.

105. Ten Cate JM, Duijsters PPE. The influence of fluoride in solution on tooth enamel demineralization I. Chemical data. Caries Res 1983;17:193–196.

106. Tenovuo J. Salivary parameters of relevance for assessing caries activity in individuals or populations. Community Dent Oral Epidemiol 1997;25:82–86.

107. Thylstrup A, Bruun C, Holman L. In vivo caries models-Mechanisms for caries initiation and arrestment. Adv Dent Res 1993;8:144–157.

108. Truin GJ, König KG, Bronkhorst EM, et al. Time trends in caries experience of 6- and 12-year-old children of different socioeconomic status in The Hague. Caries Res 1998;32:1–4.

109. Van Amerongen JP, Penning C, Kidd EAM, Ten Cate JM. An in vitro assessment of the extent of caries under small occlusal cavities. Caries Res 1992;26:89–93.

110. Van Amerongen JP, Van Amerongen-Pieko A, Penning C. Validity of caries diagnosis in molars with discolored fissures by radiography. J Dent Res 1993;72:344.

111. Van Houte J. Microbiological predictors of caries risk. Adv Dent Res 1993;7:87–96.

112. Van Palenstein Helderman WH, Ter Pelkwijk L, Van Dijk JW. Caries in fissures of permanent first molars as a predictor for caries increment. Community Dent Oral Epidemiol 1989;17: 282–284.

113. Van Rijkom HM, Truin GJ, van't Hof MA. A meta-analysis of clinical studies on the caries-inhibiting effect of chlorhexidine treatment. J Dent Res 1996;75:790–795.

114. Vogel GL, Carey CM, Ekstrand J. Distribution of fluoride in saliva and plaque fluid after a 0.2% NaF rinse: short term kinetics and distribution. J Dent Res 1992;71:1553–1557.

115. Von der Fehr FR, Löe H, Theilade E. Experimental caries in man. Caries Res 1970;4:131–136.

116. Weerheijm KL, Kidd EA, Groen HJ. The effect of fluoridation on the occurrence of hidden caries in clinically sound occlusal surfaces. Caries Res 1997;31:30–34.

117. Wennerholm K, Birkhed D, Emilson CG. Effects of sugar restriction on Streptococcus mutans and Streptococcus sobrinus in saliva and dental plaque. Caries Res 1995;29:54–61

118. Zachrisson BK, Zachrisson S. Caries incidence and orthodontic treatment with fixed appliances. Scand J Dent Res 1971; 79:183–192.

119. Ziv A, Gazit D, Beris D, et al. Correlative ultrasonic histologic and roentgenographic assessment of proximal caries. Caries Res 1998;32:294.

chapter 5

Pulpal Considerations

Thomas J. Hilton/James B. Summitt

Because caries is a bacterial infection, it has a deleterious effect on the pulp, ranging from mild inflammation to pulpal death. In addition, virtually all restorative procedures cause pulpal irritation. As discussed in Chapter 1, the pulp has inherent defense mechanisms to limit damage caused by irritants. There are also a number of dental procedures performed with the goal of preserving pulpal health. Most of these procedures attempt to provide a barrier to external irritants by placing a protective sealer or liner on the cavity walls.

Before placing or cementing a restoration into a cavity preparation, the clinician must decide if a cavity base or a protective cavity sealer or liner should be placed. While seemingly simple, this decision has been complicated by an ever-increasing number of products for sealing and lining. The purpose of this chapter is to review pulpal considerations relevant to operative dentistry, including the effects of cavity preparation, caries, and restorative materials on the pulp. In addition, this chapter defines the various protective materials, describes the ways they interact with and provide protection for the pulp, reviews the properties of current materials, and discusses the changes that have occurred in this area of operative dentistry in recent years.

Physiologic Considerations

The physiology of the pulp is influenced by several factors that form the basis for the decision to use a sealer, liner, and/or base.

Remaining Dentin Thickness

No material that can be placed in a tooth provides better protection for the pulp than dentin. Dentin has excellent buffering capability to neutralize the effects of cariogenic acids.[195] The remaining dentinal thickness, from the depth of the cavity preparation to the pulp, is the single most important factor in protecting the pulp from insult.[194] In vitro studies have shown that a 0.5-mm thickness of dentin reduces the effect of toxic substances on the pulp by 75%; a 1.0-mm thickness of dentin reduces the effect of toxins by 90%.[130] Little if any pulpal reaction occurs when there is a remaining dentinal thickness of 2 mm or more.[194] Conservation of remaining tooth structure is more important to pulpal health than is replacement of lost tooth structure with a cavity liner or base.

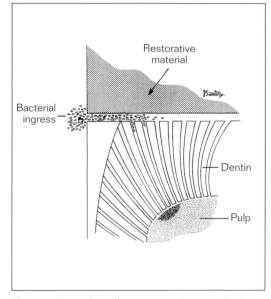

Fig 5-1a Bacteria will penetrate the marginal gap and dentinal tubules from the saliva, which may cause pulpal irritation, pulpal necrosis, or recurrent caries.

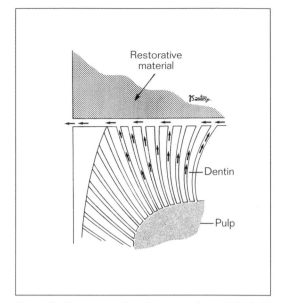

Fig 5-1b If a restoration is not well sealed, fluid flows out of the dentinal tubules and into the space between the restorative material and the tooth surface *(arrows)*. A stimulus such as hot or cold causes a change in the flow rate, which is interpreted by mechanoreceptors as painful.

Causes of Pulpal Inflammation

Like other soft tissues, the pulp reacts to an irritant with an inflammatory response.[235] It was previously believed that pulpal inflammation was the result of toxic effects of dental materials.[198,199] More recent evidence, however, demonstrates that pulpal inflammatory reactions to dental materials are mild and transitory; significant adverse pulpal responses occur more as the result of pulpal invasion by bacteria or their toxins (Figs 5-1a and 5-1b).[12,19,38,234] Even early enamel caries lesions that extend less than one fourth of the way to the dentinoenamel junction (DEJ) have been shown to induce a pulpal reaction, particularly when the caries lesion has advanced rapidly. This is probably due to an increase in the permeability of enamel, allowing the transmission of stimuli along enamel rods.[14,18]

As a lesion progresses deeper into the tooth, pulpal reaction increases.[14] When actual pulpal encroachment by bacteria and/or their toxins occurs, severe inflammation or pulpal necrosis frequently occurs.[234] The outward flow of fluid through dentinal tubules does not prevent bacteria or their toxins from reaching the pulp and initiating pulpal inflammation.[229] The caries process also induces the formation of reparative dentin and reactive dentin sclerosis, which increases the protective effects of the remaining dentin.[201]

When bacterial contamination is prevented, favorable responses in pulpal tissue adjacent to many restorative materials have been found. Those materials include amalgam, light-activated resin composite, autocured resin composite,[144] zinc phosphate cement, silicate cement,[38] glass-ionomer cement, and acrylic resin.[20] Acid etching of dentin has long been considered detrimental to the pulp, but the pulp can readily tolerate the effects of low pH if bacterial invasion is prevented.[19,107,144]

A number of instrumentation techniques elicit pulpal responses as well. The most common are rotary instruments used in high- and low-speed handpieces for tooth preparation. Tooth preparation can be traumatic to the pulp, and a number of factors affect pulpal reaction. The degree of pulpal reaction is dependent on the amount of friction and desiccation.[77,108] The key to controlling both is water spray at the site of contact between the bur and tooth structure. This is more important than the amount of water that is used on a rotating bur.[108] Frictional heat generated by tooth preparation can result in burn lesions in the pulp and abscess formation.[202] While it is often advantageous to refine aspects of a cavity preparation without water spray to aid visibility, this must be done conservatively. The pulp can tolerate dry preparation in a limited area, but the severity of the pulpal reaction increases as the area of dentin subjected to preparation without water spray increases.[108] Another adverse consequence of desiccating dentin in a preparation is that the dentinal fluid is lost from the tubules. The lost fluid may be replaced with chemicals that can elicit a harmful pulpal reaction.[108]

The temperature rise is considerably greater when enamel or a combination of enamel and dentin is prepared versus preparation of dentin alone.[164] Additionally, research has shown that pressure applied during rotary instrumentation has a greater effect on temperature rise than does rotational speed,[164] which is probably why preparation using low-speed rotary instrumentation has been shown to be more traumatic to the pulp than high-speed preparation.[202] Diamonds tend to produce more temperature increase than do carbide burs,[202] and the reaction of the pulp tends to increase as the depth of the cavity preparation increases. Considering these latter two findings, it should not be surprising that an occasional consequence of full-coverage restorations is pulpal necrosis. One study found that 13.3% of teeth with full-coverage crowns required endodontic therapy.[57] Key to controlling temperature rise and minimizing adverse pulpal reaction from rotary instrumentation are adequate air/water spray coolant and light pressure during preparation.[109,164,202]

Two new methods for tooth preparation are available—lasers and kinetic cavity preparation, also known as air abrasion. Animal studies have shown that air-abrasion cavity preparation is no more traumatic to the pulp than rotary instrumentation.[95,109] Likewise, the use of a variety of lasers, including CO_2, Er:YAG, and free electron lasers (FEL) on tooth structure has demonstrated minimal pulpal response, comparable to that of high-speed rotary instrumentation.[48,171,191]

One other modality commonly used in conjunction with operative dentistry—electrosurgery to remove gingival tissue for enhanced access during tooth preparation and impression making—may affect the dental pulp. Several animal studies have shown that as long as the contact of the electrosurgery probe is with intact enamel, little or no pulpal reaction ensues. However, if the probe contacts a metallic restoration, adverse and often severe pulpal reaction results.[45,106,180,193] This adverse reaction occurs regardless of whether a cavity base is present or not.[193] The pulpal response is more severe with increased contact time (> 0.4 sec)[106] and decreased dentin thickness between the metallic restoration and the pulp.[45,193]

Causes of Pulpal Pain

The causes of pulpal pain and sensitivity, while not fully explained, are becoming better understood. Increased intrapulpal pressure on nerve endings, secondary to an inflammatory response, is one mechanism that may explain pain as a result of bacterial invasion.[196] However, this interpretation fails to explain sensitivity that occurs in the absence of inflammation. The explanation for pulpal pain in the absence of inflammation that is most accepted is the hydrodynamic theory.[17] In a vital tooth with exposed dentin, there is a constant slow movement of fluid outward through the dentinal tubules. The hydrodynamic theory proposes that when a stimulus causes the slow fluid movement to become more rapid, nerve endings in the pulp are deformed, a response that is interpreted as pain. Stimuli such as tooth preparation, air drying, and application of cold have been suggested as causes of this sudden, rapid movement of fluid.[17]

Causes of Thermal Sensitivity

Prevention of postoperative thermal sensitivity has long been a rationale for the placement of cavity bases beneath metallic restorations. Initial in vivo research documenting the alleged problem was sparse and poorly controlled. Although one study showed reduced postoperative sensitivity in patients when thick cement bases were used,[132] another demonstrated that, by 6 months postoperatively, few patients had thermal sensitivity regardless of whether a cavity base had been placed.[168] In one survey, 50% of patients questioned 24 hours after restoration placement reported some discomfort, but 78% of these patients described the discomfort as mild and fleeting.[186] Several more recent studies have demonstrated that a significant majority of patients receiving amalgam restorations do not experience postoperative thermal sensitivity, regardless of lesion depth or the absence or presence of a particular cavity sealer or liner. Of those patients with postoperative thermal discomfort, almost all describe it as minor, and it has almost always disappeared within 30 days.[8,24,75,76,100,116] Any discussion of the need for protection against postoperative thermal sensitivity must be tempered by the understanding that the prevalence and magnitude of this problem have likely been overestimated.

Theory of Thermal Shock

There are two theories about the cause of thermal sensitivity (usually to cold) following restoration placement, and consequently two philosophies as to how to best address the problem. The first theory states that sensitivity is the result of direct thermal shock to the pulp via temperature changes transferred from the oral cavity through the restorative material,[74,163] especially when remaining dentin is thin. Protection from this insult would then be provided by an adequate thickness of an insulating material with low thermal diffusivity.[83,163] It has been noted that resin composite exhibits such low thermal diffusivity that a thermal insulating base would be unnecessary in conjunction with resin composite restorations.[49,83] Use of an insulating base for thermal protection would, therefore, be limited to metallic restorative materials that exhibit higher rates of temperature transfer.

When a base is used to provide insulation to counter thermal sensitivity in amalgam restorations, the thickness of the material must be minimized in areas subject to occlusal loading. Research has shown that, as the thickness of the base increases, the fracture resistance of the overlying amalgam decreases.[56,92] Because temperature diffusion through amalgam to the floor of the cavity preparation is effectively reduced by 0.50 to 0.75 mm of basing material, if a base is used, its thickness should be restricted to that dimension.[83] Modulus of elasticity (high modulus of elasticity indicates stiffness; low modulus of elasticity indicates flexibility) is the key property that determines how effectively a base or liner will support an amalgam restoration. As the modulus of elasticity of a basing material decreases, the resistance to fracture of overlying amalgam decreases.[56,92,166]

Theory of Pulpal Hydrodynamics

The more widely accepted theory of thermal sensitivity holds that temperature sensitivity is based on pulpal hydrodynamics. Most restorations have a gap between the wall of the preparation and the restorative material that allows the slow outward movement of dentinal fluid (see Fig 5-1b). Cold temperatures cause a sudden contraction of this fluid, resulting in a rapid increase in the flow, which is perceived by the patient as pain.[17] As dentin nears the pulp, tubule density and diameter increase,[197] as does permeability,[155] thus increasing both the volume and flow of pulpal fluid susceptible to the hydrodynamic effects of cold temperatures. This may explain why deeper restorations are sometimes associated with more problems of sensitivity.

According to this theory, if the tubules can be occluded, fluid flow is prevented and a cold temperature does not induce pain. The operative factor in reducing sensitivity to thermal change thus becomes effective sealing of dentinal tubules rather than placement of an insulating material of certain thickness.[17] Scanning electron microscopic observations have revealed significantly higher numbers of open tubule orifices in hypersensitive dentin, lending credence to this theory.[50,242]

The theory of pulpal hydrodynamics has gained general acceptance in recent years and has changed the direction of restorative procedures away from thermal insulation and toward dentinal sealing. Thus there is increasing emphasis on the integrity of the interface between restorative material and cavity preparation.

Cavity Sealers, Liners, and Bases

The terms *varnish*, *sealer*, *liner*, and *base*, used to describe a variety of materials, have been a source of confusion in dental literature. In 1995, McCoy[124] provided the following definitions for these terms.

1. Cavity sealers: Materials in this category provide a protective coating to the walls of the prepared cavity and a barrier to leakage at the interface of the restorative material and the walls. The term *sealer* implies total prevention of leakage, but, in fact, the barrier provides various degrees of seal. Sealers usually coat all walls of a cavity preparation. Commonly used sealers fall into two categories:
   a. Varnish: A natural rosin or gum (such as copal), or a synthetic resin, dissolved in an organic solvent such as acetone, chloroform, or ether.[5]
   b. Resin bonding systems: The adhesive systems designed to provide sealing as well as bonding at the interface between restoration and cavity preparation walls.
2. Cavity liners: Cement or resin coating of minimal thickness (usually less than 0.5 mm) to achieve a physical barrier to bacteria and their products and/or to provide a therapeutic effect, such as an antibacterial or pulpal anodyne effect. Liners are usually applied only to dentin cavity walls that are near the pulp.
3. Cavity bases: Materials to replace missing dentin, used for bulk buildup and/or for blocking out undercuts in preparations for indirect restorations.

Table 5-1	Tooth-Restoration Interface: Materials and Clinical Failures						
	Composite			Amalgam	Glass ionomer		
Study	Secondary caries	Marginal gap/fracture	Marginal discoloration	Secondary caries	Secondary caries	Marginal gap/fracture	Marginal discoloration
Friedl et al, 1995[64] (Germany)	40%	18%	—	—	—	—	—
Browning and Dennison, 1996[22] (US)	28.6%	14.1%	21.7%	—	—	—	—
Mjör and Qvist, 1997[137] (Denmark)	62%	—	—	70%	—	—	—
Mjör and Toffenetti,[138] 1992 (Italy)	44%	6%	9%	—	—	—	—
Mjör, 1996[136] (Sweden)	33%	—	—	—	50%	5%	3%

Knowledge of the properties and indications for the materials in each category will aid the practitioner faced with an array of choices.

Cavity Sealers

Cavity sealers provide a protective coating for freshly cut tooth structure of the prepared cavity. The tooth-restoration interface has always been considered critical in dentistry, a fact apparent in the profession's emphasis on marginal adaptation of dental restorations. The concern is that any interfacial gap, even one not readily apparent under magnification, will allow microleakage. Kidd[101] defined microleakage as the passage of bacteria, fluids, molecules, or ions along the interface of a dental restoration and the wall of the cavity preparation. This process is theorized to cause marginal discoloration, secondary caries, and pulpal pathosis. A summary of some retrospective studies on the causes of clinical failure of existing restorations is provided in Table 5-1.

Clearly, the junction between the restorative material and tooth structure is the source of a considerable number of restoration failures; providing a seamless transition from restoration to tooth structure has long been a goal in dentistry. Cavity sealers, used to fulfill this function, take two forms.

Varnishes

A varnish is a natural gum (such as copal), a rosin, or a synthetic resin dissolved in an organic solvent, such as acetone, chloroform, or ether, that evaporates, leaving behind a protective film.[5] It is used as a barrier against the passage of bacteria and their by-products into dentinal tubules, and it reduces the penetration of oral fluid at the restoration-tooth interface. This film is very thin, usually 2 to 5 μm, and provides no thermal insulation.[44,165,206]

Copal varnishes have been used for many years to fill the gap at the amalgam-tooth interface until corrosion products form to reduce it.[3,44,113] Varnishes have also been used as barriers against the passage of irritants from cements and bacteria into dentinal tubules.[44] Two applications have been shown to be more effective than a single coat, but a third application does not significantly improve the coating of the cavity walls.[159] Copal varnish is capable of reducing dentin permeability by 69%[158] and significantly reducing microleakage for 4 to 6 months.[61,123,139] Varnish is commonly used under amalgam restorations and before cementation of indirect restorations with zinc phosphate cement. Placement of copal varnish before crown cementation with zinc phosphate does not have a detrimental effect on retention.[58]

Adhesive Sealers

The most recent materials to be used as cavity sealers have a demonstrated multisubstrate bonding ability that allows the restorative material to adhere to tooth structure. Examples include adhesive bonding systems, resin luting cements, and glass-ionomer luting cements. The benefits of using adhesive bonding systems (described in Chapter 8) to attach resin composite materials to tooth structure are well documented and accepted. It is well established that acid etching will promote a reliable, durable bond to enamel.[19] Its mechanism of action (ie, the diffusion of polymerizable monomers into porosities and channels established in enamel and dentin as a result of the demineralizing action of acid) is well accepted. Bonding systems also provide a chemical bond between the unfilled resin of the adhesive system and the resin composite. Enamel's more consistent and highly mineralized structure provides a more reliable bond than that achieved to dentin.

Researchers and clinicians have worked to develop cavity sealers that can improve the seal provided by cavity varnishes for amalgam restorations. Some studies have demonstrated that varnishes reduce, but do not eliminate, microleakage around amalgam restorations,[61,157,190] while other studies have shown no benefit or even increased microleakage when a varnish is used.[118,122,239] Because of postplacement amalgam marginal leakage, the duration of which is prolonged when the slower-corroding high-copper alloys are used, more effective and longer lasting sealers have been sought. This has led to the frequent use of adhesive resins in conjunction with amalgam restorations.[32] At least one study has shown an adhesive to be inferior to varnish in the seal it provides;[115] others have shown adhesives and varnishes to exhibit similar degrees of microleakage,[53,204] while still others have shown the adhesive resin to impart no greater seal than when no sealer at all is used.[118,146] However, numerous studies have shown resin adhesives to provide a significant reduction in leakage.[10,27,30,91,123,127,139,181,214,220,227]

While not unanimous, the evidence is compelling that adhesive resins, used as sealers, reduce interfacial microleakage compared to either unsealed or varnish-sealed amalgam restorations when evaluated short term (24 hours to 14 days). Superior sealing of dentinal tubules by bonding resins compared to varnish has also been demonstrated.[10,139,181,227] Animal research has demonstrated that dentin primers alone or in conjunction with dentin adhesives can significantly reduce dentin sensitivity[233] and that they have good pulpal compatibility when used in cavity prepara-

tions.[207,238] However, modern adhesives continue to exhibit significant leakage when cavity margins are on dentin or cementum.[89,152,205,217] Most in vitro research on the use of bonding systems with amalgam restorations is of short duration, and uncertainty exists concerning the durability of the bonded interface between amalgam and tooth structure. Studies have found that both interfacial and dentinal tubule leakage increase significantly over periods of 1 month to 1 year after placement of the resin bonding/sealing resin and amalgam.[10,127,139,181]

Most important, numerous controlled clinical trials have failed to demonstrate a decrease in postoperative sensitivity with the use of adhesive agents under amalgam restorations compared with the use of either traditional sealers and liners or no cavity sealer at all.[8,23,75,76,100,114,116,121] These results are consistently found regardless of cavity depth and remaining dentin thickness.[75,76]

Given these facts, there are some concerns about the use of adhesive resins under amalgam restorations. The insoluble adhesive layer may act as a barrier to prevent amalgam corrosion products from ultimately sealing the tooth-restoration interface. As a result, the dentin bonding resins may potentially put the patient at greater risk in the long term for marginal leakage and recurrent caries. In addition, bonding resins are much more technique sensitive than varnishes,[88,217] and bonding systems are more expensive and time-consuming.[33] Time and additional research should provide an answer to this dilemma.

Cavity Liners

Cavity liners placed with minimal thickness, usually less than 0.5 mm, provide not only seal, but fluoride release, adhesion to tooth structure, and/or antibacterial action that promotes pulpal health.[124]

Calcium Hydroxide

Calcium hydroxide [$Ca(OH)_2$] has long been used as a liner because of its pulpal compatibility and purported ability to stimulate reparative dentin formation with direct pulpal contact.[195] However, research has shown that not all formulations of $Ca(OH)_2$ have a stimulatory effect on human pulpoblasts.[78] There is a growing belief that reparative dentin formation is assisted, rather than stimulated, and that this is due to the antibacterial action of calcium hydroxide that reduces or eliminates the inflammatory effects of bacteria and their by-products on the pulp.[17,36,234]

Conventional formulations of calcium hydroxide liners have demonstrated poor physical properties.[43,56] High solubility of some calcium hydroxide liners may lead to contamination of bonding resins and result in increased marginal leakage.[105] High solubility may also result in softening of the liner and in material loss under poorly sealed restorations.[17,161] Visible light–activated calcium hydroxide products have overcome most of these deficiencies. They exhibit improved physical properties[213] and significantly reduced solubility.[43] While modulus of elasticity of the light-activated products has been shown to be increased relative to conventional $Ca(OH)_2$ in one study,[112] in another it was lower,[213] with a resulting reduced ability to support an overlying amalgam restoration.[167] These unfavorable physical properties restrict $Ca(OH)_2$ use to application over the smallest area that would suffice to aid in the formation of reparative dentin when a known or suspected pulp exposure exists.

Glass Ionomer

Glass ionomer has been used as a cavity liner in an attempt to take advantage of two highly desirable properties: chemical bond to tooth structure and fluoride release.[41] Although fluoride release from glass ionomer decreases with time,[148] sustained release has been demonstrated[135] with corresponding uptake into adjacent tooth structure.[69] This is thought to aid in anticariogenic activity.[68] Like zinc phosphate, glass ionomer is quite acidic on initial mixing but tends to neutralize within 24 hours.[31] Pulpal response to both visible light–activated and conventional glass-ionomer formulations has been shown to be favorable,[66,87,93,144] probably because glass ionomer decreases interfacial bacterial penetration.[87] The exact mechanism by which this is achieved is uncertain, but it may be due to one or more of the following: fluoride release, initial low pH,[46] chemical bond to tooth structure (physically excluding bacteria),[87] or release of a metal cation.[131,184] Both visible light–activated and conventional glass-ionomer liners exhibit good physical properties, with the conventional version exhibiting reduced interfacial gap formation,[94] a higher modulus of elasticity,[26] and subsequently improved support for amalgam restorations.[167] Glass ionomer has been shown to reduce microleakage under amalgam restorations.[6,118] Conventional glass ionomers are relatively soluble in an acidic environment and are susceptible to rapid surface deterioration when subjected to acid etching.[189] Visible light–activated glass ionomers show improved resistance to acid solubil-

ity[213] while maintaining fluoride release and bond to tooth structure.[26] Therefore, the visible light–activated formulations are more desirable for use with resin composite restorations.

Glass-ionomer cements (GIC) have been recommended as liners under resin composite restorations to reduce microleakage. The use of GIC as an intermediate layer between dentin and resin composite, particularly in Class 5 restorations, is often referred to as the "sandwich technique." Glass ionomer use, most often in conjunction with Class 2 resin composite restorations, is sometimes called the "bonded-base" technique. Either the sandwich or bonded-base techniques can be "open," in which the GIC at the gingival margin is exposed, or "closed," in which the GIC is completely covered by resin composite. Glass-ionomer liners, both visible light–cured and autocured, have been studied extensively for their ability to seal the interface between resin composite and the cavity preparation. The preponderance of in vitro evidence indicates that GIC liners perform at least as well as, and in most cases significantly better than, bonding resins used alone to seal the restoration-tooth interface. This is probably due to the delayed set and increased strain capacity provided by the GIC. In addition, the open sandwich or bonded-base restoration appears to be superior to the closed technique in achieving this superior seal.[1,34,65,99,133,174,185,226,237,240]

Cavity Bases

As previously stated, cavity bases are used as dentin replacement materials, allowing for less bulk of restorative material or blocking out undercuts for indirect restorations[124] (Figs 5-2a and 5-2b). Although cavity bases generally are not used for pulpal protection or health, they are briefly described here.

Zinc Oxide–Eugenol and Zinc Phosphate Cements

Zinc oxide–eugenol and zinc phosphate cements have been used for a number of years as bases for a variety of restorative materials. Although both provide excellent thermal insulation,[38,83] and zinc phosphate cement exhibits superior physical properties,[42] their use has diminished in recent years with the growing question of their benefit to pulpal health and with the advent of materials that are adhesive to dentin and release fluoride.[117]

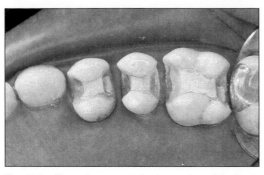

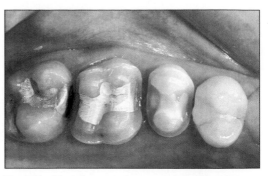

Figs 5-2a The primary use for bases is to block out undercuts in divergent preparations. Glass-ionomer bases are used here to block out undercuts in inlay preparations.

Fig 5-2b Glass-ionomer bases are used in this case to block out undercuts in porcelain onlay preparations.

Glass Ionomer

As previously mentioned, glass-ionomer materials have excellent physical properties, with the conventional versions offering excellent modulus of elasticity and restoration support. As a result, glass ionomers can be used as cavity bases as well as cavity liners.

Guidelines for Basing, Lining, and Sealing

Clinicians must always consider the limitations of currently available materials. The best possible base for any restoration is sound tooth structure. The following are guidelines for placement of bases, liners, and sealers:

1. Do not remove sound tooth structure to provide space for a base. Maintaining sound dentin will enhance restoration support and provide maximum dentin thickness for pulpal protection.
2. Use bases as indicated for build-up materials and block-out materials for cemented indirect restorations. If used for direct amalgam restorations or bonded restorations, minimize the extent of the base. Basing a preparation to "ideal" depth and internal form is contraindicated.[179] Bases in cavity preparations for amalgam restorations and bonded resin or ceramic restorations lead to decreased bulk of restorative material and increased potential for restoration fracture.
3. Use the minimum thickness of liner necessary to achieve the desired result. For liners under amalgam restorations, this should not exceed 0.5 mm.[54]
4. Currently, there is no convincing evidence for the routine use of adhesive sealers (dentin bonding resins) under metallic restorations.

Direct and Indirect Pulp Capping

Pulp capping is defined as "endodontic treatment designed to maintain the vitality of the endodontium."[7] Several favorable conditions must be present before considering direct or indirect pulp capping:

1. The tooth must be vital and have no history of spontaneous pain.[7]
2. Pain elicited during pulp testing with a hot or cold stimulus should not linger after stimulus removal.
3. A periapical radiograph should show no evidence of a periradicular lesion of endodontic origin.
4. Bacteria must be excluded from the site by the permanent restoration.

If these conditions can be met, an indirect pulp capping procedure is much preferable to a direct pulp capping procedure. Because of the uncertainty for success with either procedure, pulpal health should be monitored for several months in teeth that are to receive castings or serve as abutments for fixed or removable partial dentures. If the pulpal status of a tooth is uncertain, the clinician should consider endodontic therapy before initiating restorative treatment.

Direct Pulp Capping

Animal studies have demonstrated that direct pulpal exposures can heal normally, but a bacteria-free environment is required.[160] The adverse consequences of bacterial contamination of the pulp have been well documented.[19,20,38,144,234] Therefore, the only reason-

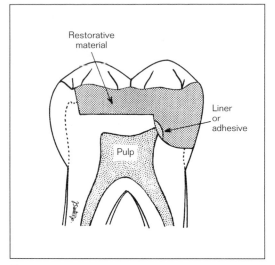

Fig 5-3 For a direct pulp capping procedure, a calcium hydroxide lining material is placed on the exposed pulpal tissue and a small amount of surrounding dentin. A sealing liner and/or a sealing restoration is then placed to seal out bacteria and their by-products.

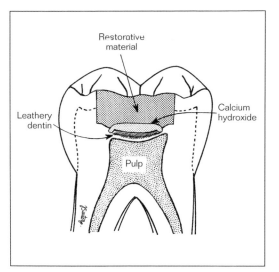

Fig 5-4 In an indirect pulp capping procedure, all carious, demineralized dentin is removed in the periphery of the preparation, but a small amount of demineralized dentin is left immediately over the area of the pulp. A calcium hydroxide lining material is placed to cover the remaining demineralized dentin. A sealing liner and/or a sealing restoration is then placed to seal out bacteria and their by-products.

able chance that a direct pulp cap has to permit formation of a dentin bridge and to maintain pulp vitality is under the most ideal conditions. If a large number of bacteria from a caries lesion or exposure to the oral flora have contaminated the pulp, the likelihood of regaining or maintaining a healthy pulp is slight. In addition, aged pulps have increased fibrosis and a decreased blood supply,[13] and thus a decreased ability to mount an effective response to invading microorganisms.

In one clinical study of direct pulp capping of 38 patients over 3 years, no relationship between success and factors such as patient age, tooth type, or size of exposure was found.[120] However, in a larger study of both direct and indirect pulp capping involving 592 patients over a 24-year period, age, tooth type, and extent of exposure did have a bearing on success.[178] The degree of bleeding affects the success of direct pulp capping; increased bleeding is associated with increased likelihood of failure.[37,120,151]

Direct pulp capping should be attempted only when a small mechanical exposure of an otherwise healthy pulp occurs. The tooth must be isolated with a rubber dam, and adequate hemostasis must be achieved. The exposure should be covered with calcium hydroxide because of its documented ability to

provide the highest percentage of success[7,62,120,236] (Fig 5-3). It must be possible to restore the tooth with a well-sealed restoration that will prevent subsequent bacterial contamination.

Indirect Pulp Capping

An indirect pulp capping procedure (Fig 5-4) should be considered when there is a radiographically evident, deep carious lesion encroaching on the pulp and the tooth has no history of spontaneous pain and responds normally to vitality tests. Pulp exposure must be avoided; if it occurs, it should be regarded as an iatrogenic event. A direct pulp capping procedure should be necessary only if the operator inadvertently exposes the pulp in attempting an indirect pulp capping procedure. With a deep carious lesion, the indirect pulp capping procedure is always preferred to a direct pulp capping procedure.

In the procedure (Figs 5-5 and 5-6), after the initial entry into the carious dentin (Fig 5-5c), a spoon excavator or large round bur, rotating very slowly in a low-speed handpiece, should be used to excavate the caries-softened dentin (Fig 5-6e). Demineralized dentin not near the pulp should be completely removed, leav-

Fig 5-5 Indirect pulp capping procedure, mandibular left first molar.

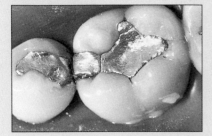

Fig 5-5a Mandibular first molar with deep recurrent carious involvement. Preoperative evaluation indicated vital pulpal tissue and no history of spontaneous pain.

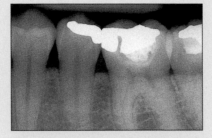

Fig 5-5b Preoperative radiograph shows demineralized dentin around the base, under the amalgam, with carious demineralization advancing toward the pulp chamber.

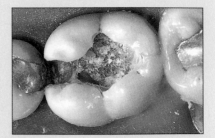

Fig 5-5c The old restoration and base are removed, revealing soft, carious dentin.

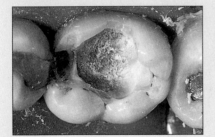

Fig 5-5d The preparation is widened to enable removal of a large amount of carious dentin and some undermined enamel.

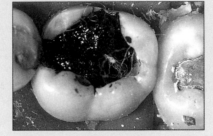

Fig 5-5e A cotton pellet, saturated with a blue caries-disclosing dye solution (Cari-D-Tect, Gresco Products), is placed so that the dye coats all areas of the preparation. The cotton pellet is left in place for 10 seconds and removed. The area is then washed with air/water spray.

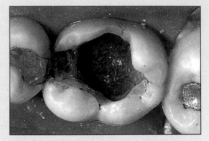

Fig 5-5f The preparation after being washed. Note the remaining large amount of demineralized dentin, as revealed by the blue dye. The stained dentin is checked for softness, and softened dentin is removed with a large round bur rotating very slowly. The dye is then reapplied, rinsed, and additional softened dentin, as disclosed by the dye, is removed.

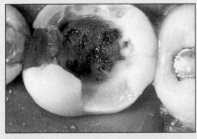

Fig 5-5g Most of the demineralized dentin has been removed. Only a small amount of dye-stained dentin is left; this dentin is believed to immediately overlie the pulp.

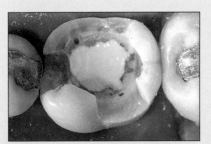

Fig 5-5h A calcium hydroxide liner (Dycal, Caulk/Dentsply) is placed over the remaining demineralized dentin.

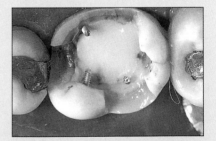

Fig 5-5i A glass-ionomer liner (Vitrebond, 3M) is placed over the calcium hydroxide liner. The glass-ionomer liner provides some seal and improved strength for amalgam condensation.

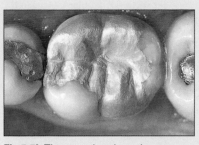

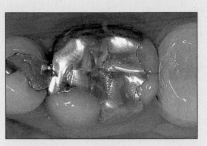

Fig 5-5j The completed amalgam restoration immediately after placement.

Fig 5-5k The restoration after 7 years of service.

Fig 5-6 Indirect pulp capping procedure, mandibular right second molar.

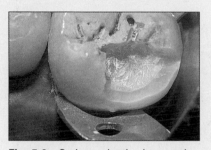

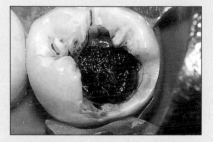

Fig 5-6a Carious dentin has undermined the distolingual cusp of the mandibular second molar. Overlying enamel and some carious dentin have been removed.

Fig 5-6b Caries-disclosing dye is applied.

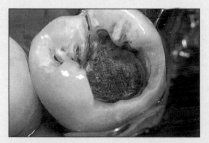

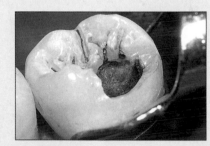

Figs 5-6c and 5-6d Dye-stained dentin.

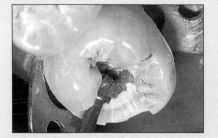

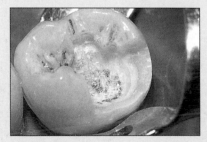

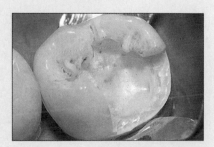

Fig 5-6e A large round bur (No. 8, Midwest), rotating very slowly, is used to remove the soft, dye-stained, carious dentin.

Fig 5-6f After several applications of caries-disclosing dye and removal of caries-softened dentin, only a small amount of dye-stained dentin remains, adjacent to the pulp chamber.

Fig 5-6g Calcium hydroxide and glass-ionomer liners are applied over the remaining demineralized dentin.

Protocol for Indirect Capping Procedures

Diagnosis

The preoperative status of the pulp and periradicular tissues should be carefully evaluated. The tooth is a candidate for indirect pulp capping only if the following conditions exist:

1. There is no history of spontaneous pulpal pain.
2. Pulpal vitality has been confirmed with thermal or electric pulp testing.
3. There is no history of pain that lingers after the tooth has returned to mouth temperature following the application of a hot or cold stimulus.
4. Pain elicited during pulp testing with a hot or cold stimulus does not linger after the tooth returns to mouth temperature.
5. A periapical radiograph shows no evidence of a periradicular lesion of endodontic origin.

Treatment

1. Isolation: After administering anesthesia, isolate the tooth with a rubber dam.
2. Preparation: Prepare the tooth for the final restoration, leaving demineralized dentin only in the area immediately adjacent to the pulp. Use a caries-disclosing dye if necessary to ensure complete carious dentin removal (other than that immediately adjacent to the pulp). After this is accomplished, use a spoon excavator or a large round bur in a low-speed handpiece using a very low speed. Use very gentle, featherweight strokes over the area of the demineralized dentin to remove only the wet (soft, amorphous) carious dentin. Leave the dry, fibrous, demineralized dentin that gives some moderate resistance to gentle scraping with a spoon excavator.

3. Lining: Place a calcium hydroxide liner over the remaining demineralized dentin. If additional sealing is indicated, use a glass-ionomer liner.
4. Restoration:
   a. Direct restorations: For direct restorations (bonded amalgam, composite, ionomer), place the final restoration. If time does not allow for placement of a final restoration at the first appointment, an ionomer or reinforced zinc oxide–eugenol provisional restoration should be placed and the patient reappointed for the final restoration as soon as possible. The indirect pulp capping liner should not be disturbed during the subsequent restoration process.
   b. Indirect restorations: For indirect restorations (cast metal restorations, ceramic onlays, or crowns), place a definitive buildup if time allows (bonded amalgam, composite, ionomer) at the appointment in which the indirect pulp capping procedure was performed. Delay placement of the final restoration for 4 to 8 months. Before proceeding with the definitive restoration, ensure normal pulp vitality.

Precautions

1. Use care in removing carious dentin near the pulp to prevent accidental pulp exposure.
2. If a temporary restoration has been previously placed over an indirect pulp capping liner and the tooth is re-entered for a restorative procedure, do not remove the indirect pulp capping material.
3. Prior to excavation, use tactile exploration to confirm that dye-stained dentin lacks hardness.

---

ing hard, sound dentin. As the caries excavation nears the pulp, caution must be exercised to avoid pulpal exposure. If a bur has been used to excavate softened dentin, a spoon excavator may be used to aid in tactile detection of softened dentin. The wet (soft, amorphous) carious dentin should be removed; as the pulp is approached, the dry, fibrous, demineralized dentin that gives some moderate resistance to gentle scraping with a spoon excavator should be allowed to remain.

Caries-disclosing dyes may be used to assist in caries excavation (Figs 5-5e to 5-5g and 5-6b to 5-6f). Studies have demonstrated the benefit of these dyes to aid in identification and removal of demineralized dentin[203] and to greatly reduce remaining viable bacteria.[15] It must be recognized that the dyes stain not only demineralized dentin, but anything porous, such as debris that may have been left in the cavity preparation. In addition, noncarious deep dentin will absorb the dye[4,102,241] because of the increased number and size of dentinal tubules in deep dentin; if this dye-stained sound dentin is removed, pulp exposure will result. If the operator uses a caries-disclosing dye, he or she must be aware of this characteristic of dye use in deep dentin. Any residual dye left on dentin before use of a dentin bonding system will cause a significant reduction in bond strength.[245] This dye-stained dentin should be covered with a liner before placement of a bonding resin.

In the procedure, carious dentin is removed except for the last portion of firm, leathery dentin immediately overlying the pulp; this layer is left because its removal would likely expose the pulp. At this point, a calcium hydroxide liner is placed over the demineralized area of dentin (Fig 5-5h). Placement of calcium hydroxide over this layer of leathery dentin has been shown to virtually eliminate all remaining bacteria and render the residual carious dentin operationally sterile.[52,55,111] If any vital bacteria remain, a well-sealed restoration should isolate them from life-sustaining substrate and prevent further acid production, thereby arresting the caries process.[128,129] These facts argue against a two-step procedure in which the tooth is re-entered for the purpose of excavating the remaining acid-affected dentin to confirm reparative dentin formation. This procedure risks creating a pulp exposure and causing further traumatic insult to the pulp.[51] If desired, a glass-ionomer liner may be placed over the calcium hydroxide liner to improve strength during amalgam condensation and to enhance the seal (Figs 5-5i and 5-6g). The definitive restoration should then be placed (Fig 5-5j). This restoration should be placed to minimize microleakage at the interface of the restoration with the cavity preparation walls.

Calcium Hydroxide vs Dentin Bonding Agents

It has been suggested that dentin bonding agents may be used for direct and indirect pulp capping.[97,172] The rationale is based on the belief that an effective, permanent seal against bacterial invasion is provided and will promote pulpal healing. This theory is supported by a number of studies. Animal research has shown good compatibility of mechanically exposed pulps to visible light–activated resin composites when bacteria are excluded.[36] In addition, adhesive resins and pulpal tissues were shown to be compatible for up to 90 days when the smear layer was removed from cavity walls before the application of a dentin adhesive, confirming the ability of the bonding agents to minimize bacterial invasion for this period of time.[40,207,238] Several animal studies have shown that while calcium hydroxide may result in faster dentin bridge formation, adhesives can be successfully associated with dentin bridge formation, and this can occur without long-term pulpal inflammation.[37,70,103,104,147] Many components of dentin bonding agents are directly toxic to pulp cells,[79,96,177] but their release is rapid and slows dramatically with time, so these materials are not

thought to be deterrents to the regeneration of pulp tissues.[59]

Clinical success of direct pulp capping with adhesive resins following traumatic pulp exposure[97] and exposure during excavation of carious dentin have been described.[172] In a clinical study of 64 cases of direct pulp capping with a dentin bonding agent following exposure during removal of carious dentin, it was reported that 60 of the teeth were vital 1 year later. In this same study, the pulps of six caries-free third molars were intentionally exposed with a bur, capped with a dentin bonding agent, and the teeth extracted up to 1 year later for histologic evaluation. All cases revealed dentin bridge formation and no inflammatory changes in the pulp.[98]

A number of in vivo studies counter the claims of success of direct pulp capping with adhesive sealers. The animal studies showing successful direct pulp capping with dentin bonding agents are invariably accomplished in an environment not contaminated by bacteria.[37,70,103,104,147,200,207,216,238] When the exposed pulps of experimental animals were intentionally contaminated to simulate the clinical setting, the majority of direct pulp caps accomplished with adhesive sealers failed (75%), with resulting pulpal death or failure to form dentin bridges; most of the contaminated pulps capped with calcium hydroxide succeeded (77%).[151] Several human studies have confirmed the superiority of calcium hydroxide to adhesive resin sealers for direct pulp capping. One study showed mixed results with pulp capping using a dentin bonding agent.[218] Two other studies showed no evidence of dentin bridge formation in the exposures capped with adhesive resin, while all of the calcium hydroxide–capped pulps demonstrated repair and dentin bridge formation.[86,162]

Although clinical success has been reported for direct pulp capping with dentin bonding agents,[98] most of these recommendations are empirical and are based on case reports.[97,172] In an animal study comparing direct pulp capping with a conventional and a visible light–activated calcium hydroxide to direct pulp capping with a dentin bonding agent, dentin bridges formed in almost all pulps capped with $Ca(OH)_2$, whereas dentin bridges formed in less than 25% of the pulps capped with dentin bonding agents.[169] Several other in vivo studies have shown very high failure rates using adhesive sealers for pulp capping, especially compared to calcium hydroxide.[86,162,200,218]

Additional concerns regarding pulp capping with dentin bonding agents is provided by laboratory studies. In vitro microleakage tests showing imperfect seals with dentin bonding agents have been criticized as being invalid because many dye tracer molecules are orders of magnitude smaller than the oral bacteria that cause pulpal inflammation.[238] These tests, therefore, may not be reliable indicators of the ability of bacteria to penetrate dentin toward the pulp. In addition, the outward flow of dentinal fluid in vivo partially opposes the diffusion of toxins into dentin,[230] and those toxins that ultimately reach the pulp are diluted and removed by the circulation.[154] However, while pathogenic intraoral bacteria may be larger than the initial interfacial gaps associated with dentin bonding agents, key components of pulpal inflammation are bacterial by-products,[11] the molecules of which are much smaller than the bacteria.

Interconnecting microporosities within the hybrid layer, created by dentin bonding resins in the demineralized dentin surface, have been shown to be permeable to very small molecules via "nanoleakage."[182,183] This demonstrates the potential for diffusion of even smaller water molecules, which could then lead to the hydrolysis of exposed collagen fibers within the hybrid layer.[232] Likewise, nearly all dye molecules are at least as large as, if not larger than, glucose, which allows for the possibility that bacteria present in the smear layer or in caries-affected dentin could be sustained by the diffusion of this nutrient source. Finally, gap formation seen at the tooth-restoration interface in a number of studies indicates the presence of openings considerably larger than bacteria, viruses, and endotoxins.[34,35,60,173,192,211,219] It would seem reasonable to assume that dye penetration between dentin and the bonding resin would indicate an imperfect seal, ultimately leading to bacterial penetration, especially as the size of the interfacial gap and subsequent leakage is increased by thermal stress.[25]

There are additional concerns regarding indirect and/or direct pulp capping using dentin bonding resins. Numerous studies have found a significant loss of bond strength of adhesive resins to human carious dentin vs sound dentin,[63,142,143,242] leading to further questioning of the integrity of the bond and subsequent ability to prevent bacterial invasion of a carious substrate. Proponents of the use of dentin bonding agents for direct pulp capping point to the shortcomings of calcium hydroxide in this role, including breakdown when acid etchants are used, dissolution under leaky restorations, interfacial failure during amalgam condensation, and the presence of tunnel defects in reparative dentin that remain open from the pulp to the medicament interface, allowing recurring microleakage of bacteria to the pulp.[39] The ultimate failure of $Ca(OH)_2$ is thought to be its inability to provide a long-term seal against microleakage.[40] These are all valid concerns; methods for gaining maximum benefit from calcium hydroxide in direct pulp capping, while compensating for its shortcomings, are described at the end of this chapter.

The success of dentin bonding agents for pulp capping depends on the quality and durability of the bond and requires that their placement has no deleterious effects on the pulp.

Quality and Durability of the Bond

Improvements in dentin bonding agents have been dramatic. However, in vitro research has demonstrated that modern dentin bonding resins leak almost immediately when bonded to superficial dentin.[89,152,205,217] The anatomy of dentin near the pulp can have an even greater adverse impact on bond formation. As dentin nears the pulp, more area of a cut surface is taken up by tubules and less by intertubular dentin.[67] The collagen of intertubular dentin is required for the formation of a hybrid layer or hybrid zone, which is thought to be the primary means by which modern bonding resins adhere to dentin.[141] In addition, the bond immediately adjacent to dentinal tubules is often loose, allowing fluid shift and leakage of substrates due to a cuff of collagen-poor peritubular dentin.[156] Bond strengths of dentin bonding agents to surfaces of cut dentin are directly related to the area of sound dentin minus the area of the tubules,[208] since resin tags in the dentin tubules contribute little to the bond strength.[215] It is, therefore, not surprising that dentin bonding agents show a significant loss of bond strength to deep dentin compared to superficial dentin.[134,153,208,212,215] In addition, the bond degrades with time.[181,232] This is significant because animal studies of pulpal compatibility are short term (21 to 90 days)[38,40,207,238]; studies have not provided long-term in vivo evaluation of the effectiveness of bonding systems as barriers to bacterial penetration.

Effect of Dentin Bonding Agent Application on Pulp

Modern dentin bonding systems require conditioning that removes the dentinal smear layer, usually through acid etching.[141,207,217,238] Acid etching of dentin has been demonstrated in multiple animal studies not to cause pulpal damage.[21,107,144,207,238] However, removal of the smear layer before placement of a dentin bonding resin and composite restoration significantly increased dentin fluid flow and pulpal nerve firing in dogs.[90] The increased dentin fluid flow that can result from opening the dentinal tubules can also cause fluid contamination, poor bonding, and fluid-filled gaps, which can allow bacterial penetration into dentin tubules if the restorative material provides an imperfect seal.[156] These bacteria and their toxins can progress to the pulp despite the outward flow of dentinal tubular fluid.[229] Dentin tubules opened by acid etching have been shown to allow the passage of adhesive sealer particulates into the human dental pulp, eliciting foreign body responses that inhibit dentin bridge formation.[218] Finally, applying acid to exposed pulps tends to increase bleeding, which inhibits good adhesion to dentin adjacent to the exposure.[104,200]

Many components of modern dentin bonding resins, primarily unpolymerized monomers, are toxic to cells[79,110,176,177] and capable of diffusing into the dental pulp.[72] Cellular toxicity decreases with improved degree of cure of the resin, since fewer unpolymerized monomers are available to leach from the adhesive resin.[29] Greater remaining dentin thickness and dentin fluid flow significantly reduce diffusion to the dental pulp and help to decrease the toxic effects of these components.[16] Although the concentration at which they reach the pulp is difficult to determine with certainty,[79] research has indicated that reducing remaining dentin thickness to 0.5 mm allows reactions to range from mild biologic responses[80] to mild toxic reactions after 12 hours to significant toxicity after 24 hours.[16] The presence of pulpal inflammation and direct placement of adhesives on pulp tissue, such as would occur with direct pulp capping, will exacerbate these responses.[16,80] The inward diffusion of these components is not prevented by intrapulpal pressure, even at a level of intrapulpal pressure that would simulate that of an inflamed pulp.[71] More important, at certain concentrations, most resin components in dentin bonding agents inhibit pulp T lymphocytes, leading to speculation that immunosuppression of pulpal immunocompetent cells may enhance potential for bacterial injury to pulpal tissues.[96]

Another issue in placing bonding resins directly on pulpal tissue is heat generation from the curing light. An intrapulpal temperature increase of more than 20°F (11.2°C) has been shown to cause irreversible damage in vivo.[243] A recent study investigated the temperature rise in a bonding resin during light polymerization. An increase of 18.2°C was found with a 10-second cure, and a 25.2°C increase was detected with a 20-second cure.[175] Because most bonding resins require a 20-second cure, there is potential for the pulp to be exposed to dangerous heat levels.

The Future of Direct Pulp Capping Materials

A number of materials are being investigated for future use as direct pulp capping agents. Hydroxyapatite elicited a better pulpal response than calcium hydroxide in one animal study, because the hydroxyapatite acted as a scaffold for dentin formation.[85] Another material that has shown promise is mineral trioxide aggregate (MTA), a combination of tricalcium silicate, tricalcium aluminate, tricalcium oxide, and silicate oxide. This material demonstrates a high pH similar to calcium hydroxide, exhibits compressive strength comparable to reinforced zinc oxide–eugenol, and is radiopaque.[223] It also displays some antibacterial activity and has shown significantly decreased microleakage compared to amalgam and two temporary restorative materials (Super-EBA [Harry J. Bosworth] and IRM [Caulk/Dentsply]).[224,225] Most important, MTA has been shown to stimulate dentin bridge formation in primate animal studies.[170,221] The primary disadvantage demonstrated to date with MTA is its extended setting time of 2 hours, 45 minutes.[222]

Antibacterial Efficacy of Restorative Materials

One of the keys to any successful restoration, but particularly for a tooth that has undergone a pulp capping procedure, is the ability to exclude bacteria and their by-products from entry into the pulp.[7,38] Of concern are the cariogenic bacteria, since they tend to invade the interface between the restoration and the cavity preparation. Ultimately, these bacteria may lead to recurrent caries, and, if they reach the pulp in sufficient quantities, they will cause inflammatory and ultimately pathologic responses.[38] In particular, *Streptococcus mutans* is often used in in vitro studies evaluating the efficacy of restorative materials against bacteria, since this organism is associated with recurrent caries[231] (see Chapter 4).

The discussion so far has focused on the materials placed immediately adjacent to the site of near or actual pulp exposure. However, the seal provided by the restorative material will also affect the ultimate success of the procedure. Restorative materials can effectively prevent bacterial contamination by one of two means: by providing an impermeable seal with the cavity walls to physically exclude bacteria and the toxins they produce, or by possessing antibacterial properties to destroy bacteria entering the restoration-tooth interface. No material yet provides an impermeable seal that can ensure the physical exclusion of bacteria.

Amalgam

Although typically not considered a material possessing antibacterial properties, dental amalgam has demonstrated varying levels of antibacterial activity.[140,145,150,228] This activity has been attributed to a variety of elements released from amalgam, including copper, mercury, zinc, silver, and chloride compounds. A number of studies have shown that amalgam is effective against cariogenic bacteria, including *S mutans*, *Actinomyces viscosus*, and *Lactobacillus spp*.[140,145,150,228]

S mutans thrive and produce lactic acid in an acidic environment.[82] The tooth-amalgam interface has a decreased pH,[119] which results in demineralization of tooth structure.[125] In vivo studies have shown that metallic solutions of copper, silver, and zinc are all capable of reducing acid production in plaque.[2] In one case, ions of these metals reduced acid production more than did fluoride in a comparable concentration.[149] All of these ions are released by amalgam and would, therefore, be present at the tooth-restoration interface.[140,145,150,228]

In addition to its antibacterial properties, amalgam is the only restorative material in which the marginal seal improves with time. This is due to the acidic environment and low oxygen concentration that exists in the amalgam–to–cavity wall gap, which promotes corrosion. In conventional amalgam, the gamma-2 phase forms SnO_2, $SnCl_2$, and $Sn(OH)_2Cl$, which slowly fill the interfacial gap. In high-copper alloys, in which there is no gamma 2, the eta phase (Cu_6Sn_5) corrodes to form CuO_2 and $CuCl_2$, but this occurs much more slowly. Corrosion in high-copper alloys may take twice as long as in conventional alloys to produce the same level of seal.[9]

Glass Ionomer

Glass ionomer has the ability to decrease bacterial penetration,[87] possibly through its fluoride release,[87] initial low pH,[46] physical exclusion of bacteria,[87] or release of a metal cation.[131,184] Whatever the mechanism, glass-ionomer restorative and liner/base materials inhibit cariogenic bacteria[126] and demineralization at tooth-restoration interfaces.[47,73] In vivo plaque studies assessing the level of cariogenic bacteria in-

variably show significantly lower levels of these organisms adjacent to glass ionomer compared to either resin composite or amalgam.[209,210,244]

Resin Composite

In contrast to amalgam and glass ionomer, resin composite is most dependent on the formation of an impermeable seal to exclude bacterial penetration. This is because, as shown in in vitro bacterial inhibition studies, there is little, if any, inhibitory effect demonstrated by resin composite against cariogenic bacteria,[184] and, therefore, there is little resistance to secondary caries activity.[73] This is true even if a resin composite contains fluoride.[73] In fact, research has indicated that certain monomers released from resin composite actually stimulate cariogenic bacteria growth.[81] In vivo plaque studies have demonstrated that levels of cariogenic bacteria in the plaque present on surfaces of resin composite restorations are significantly higher than on either amalgam or glass ionomer.[187,188,210,244] While certain adhesive systems are similar to resin composite in that they demonstrate no bacterial inhibition,[28] some glutaraldehyde-containing bonding systems have shown an inhibitory effect on cariogenic organisms.[28,126] As previously stated, the quality and durability of adhesive bonding to dentin is questionable, and an impermeable seal is not achieved. Because resin composite does not have the ability to inhibit cariogenic bacteria, placement of a resin composite restoration with a dentin margin in a tooth that has been treated with pulp capping may decrease the chances of successful treatment.

Summary

1. Most operative procedures are traumatic to the pulp, and the effects are at least somewhat cumulative. Excessive heat and dehydration should be avoided. Questionable teeth should receive pulp vitality testing before undergoing clinical procedures.
2. Because, in direct pulp capping, no dentin remains between the capping material and the pulp, the problem of exposure of pulpal tissues and surrounding vital dentin to caustic or toxic materials is significant. The effects of thermal and chemical insults are magnified with an exposed vital pulp. Of the current materials available, calcium hydroxide remains the material of choice for direct pulp

capping, and it should be used with very specific clinical procedures and excellent isolation. Indirect pulp capping is preferred to direct pulp capping; with proper diagnosis and good clinical procedure, direct pulp capping should rarely be required.

3. Calcium hydroxide is also the material of choice for indirect pulp capping. If the restoration–to–cavity wall interface is well sealed, calcium hydroxide eliminates or greatly reduces the numbers of vital bacteria in the remaining demineralized dentin. Dentin bonding resins adhere poorly to carious dentin, provide a poor seal, and impart little to no antimicrobial activity.

4. Drawbacks attributed to the use of calcium hydroxide as a pulp capping agent include dissolution with acid etching, degradation under leaky restorations, and interfacial failure during amalgam condensation. While the most significant drawback of calcium hydroxide is its inability to provide a permanent seal against bacterial invasion, the integrity and durability of the bond achieved with dentin adhesives is questionable as well. Although there is potential as a possible future treatment modality, the lack of long-term documentation of clinical success for pulp capping with dentin bonding resins in controlled clinical trials should be weighed against literature that demonstrates 75% to 90% success for up to 12 years when calcium hydroxide is used.[7,84,87,120]

5. When $Ca(OH)_2$ is used as a pulp capping material, it should be limited to as small an area as possible, and some method of protecting it should be considered during subsequent restorative procedures. Most of the drawbacks to its use can be overcome by the use of a light-activated form of calcium hydroxide. This eliminates most problems, except microleakage. Another approach is to place a glass-ionomer lining material over the $Ca(OH)_2$. This provides a combination of clinically proven materials associated with clinical success in pulp capping. Calcium hydroxide provides antibacterial properties; glass ionomer provides resistance to acids, condensation pressures, and dissolution, as well as fluoride release and adhesion to tooth structure. A well-sealed restoration should then be placed to further reduce the potential for microleakage and enhance the success of the pulp cap.

References

1. Aboushala A, Kugel G, Hurley E. Class II composite resin restorations using glass-ionomer liners: microleakage studies. J Clin Pediatr Dent 1996;21(1):67–71.
2. Afseth J, Oppermann RV, Rolla G. The in vivo effect of glucose solutions containing Cu++ and Zn++ on the acidogenicity of dental plaque. Acta Odontol Scand 1980;38(4):229–233.
3. Andrews JT, Hembree JH. Marginal leakage of amalgam alloys with high content of copper: a laboratory study. Oper Dent 1980;5:7.
4. Ansari G, Beeley JA, Reid JS, Foye RH. Caries detector dyes—an in vitro assessment of some new compounds. J Oral Rehabil 1999;26:453–458.
5. Anusavice KJ. Phillips' Science of Dental Materials, ed 10. Philadelphia: Saunders; 1996:545.
6. Arcoria CJ, Fisher MA, Wagner MJ. Microleakage in alloy-glass ionomer lined amalgam restorations after thermocycling. J Oral Rehabil 1991;18:9–14.
7. Baume LJ, Holz J. Long term clinical assessment of direct pulp capping. Int Dent J 1981;31(4):251–260.
8. Belcher MA, Stewart GP. Two-year clinical evaluation of an amalgam adhesive. J Am Dent Assoc 1997;128:309–314.
9. Ben-Amar A, Cardash HS, Judes H. The sealing of the tooth/amalgam interface by corrosion products. J Oral Rehabil 1995;22:101–104.
10. Ben-Amar A, Liberman R, Rothkoff Z, Cardash HS. Long term sealing properties of amalgambond under amalgam restorations. Am J Dent 1994;7:141–143.
11. Bergenholtz G, Cox CF, Loesche WJ, Syed SA. Bacterial leakage around dental restorations: its effect on the dental pulp. J Oral Pathol 1982;11:439–450.
12. Bergenholtz G, Lindhe J. Effect of soluble plaque factors on inflammatory reactions in the dental pulp. Scand J Dent Res 1975;83(3):153–158.
13. Bernick S, Nedelman C. Effect of aging on the human pulp. J Endod 1975;1(3):88–94.
14. Bjorndal L, Darvann T, Thylstrup A. A quantitative light microscopic study of the odontoblast and subodontoblastic reactions to active and arrested enamel caries without cavitation. Caries Res 1998;32(1):59–69.
15. Boston DW, Graver HT. Histological study of an acid red caries-disclosing dye. Oper Dent 1989;14:186–192.
16. Bouillaguet S, Wataha JC, Hanks CT, Ciucchi B, Holz J. In vitro cytotoxicity and dentin permeability of HEMA. J Endod 1996;22:244–248.
17. Brannstrom M. Communication between the oral cavity and the dental pulp associated with restorative treatment. Oper Dent 1984;9(2):57–68.
18. Brannstrom M, Lind PO. Pulpal response to early dental caries. J Dent Res 1965;44:1045–1050.
19. Brannstrom M, Nordenvall KJ. Bacterial penetration, pulpal reaction and the inner surface of Concise enamel bond. Composite fillings in etched and unetched cavities. J Dent Res 1978;57:3–10.
20. Brannstrom M, Vojinovic O. Response of the dental pulp to invasion of bacteria around three filling materials. ASDC J Dent Child 1976;43(2):83–89.
21. Brannstrom M, Vojinovic O, Nordenvall KJ. Bacteria and pulpal reactions under silicate cement restorations. J Prosthet Dent 1979;41:290–295.
22. Browning WD, Dennison JB. A survey of failure modes in composite resin restoration. Oper Dent 1996;21(4):160–166.

23. Browning WD, Johnson WW, Gregory PN. Clinical performance of bonded amalgam restorations at eighteen months [abstract 427]. J Dent Res 1997;76(special issue):67.

24. Browning WD, Johnson WW, Gregory PN. Postoperative pain following bonded amalgam restorations. Oper Dent 1997;22(2):66–71.

25. Bullard RH, Leinfelder KF, Russell CM. Effect of coefficient of thermal expansion on microleakage. J Am Dent Assoc 1988;116:871–874.

26. Burgess JO, Barghi N, Chan DCN, Hummert T. A comparative study of three glass ionomer base materials. Am J Dent 1993;6:137–141.

27. Cao DS, Hollis RA, Christensen RP, et al. Shear strength and microleakage of 23 adhesives for amalgam bonding [abstract 1760]. J Dent Res 1995;74(special issue):231.

28. Carvalhaes Fraga R, Freitas Siqueira JJ, de Uzeda M. In vitro evaluation of antibacterial effects of photo-cured glass ionomer liners and dentin bonding agents during setting. J Prosthet Dent 1996;76:483–486.

29. Caughman WF, Caughman GB, Shiflett RA, et al. Correlation of cytotoxicity, filler loading and curing time of dental composites. Biomaterials 1991;12:737–740.

30. Chang JC, Chan JT, Chheda HN, Iglesias A. Microleakage of a 4-methacryloxyethyl trimellitate anhydride bonding agent with amalgams. J Prosthet Dent 1996;75:495–498.

31. Charlton DG, Moore BK, Swartz ML. Direct surface pH determinations of setting cements. Oper Dent 1991;16:231–238.

32. Christensen G. Product use survey—1995. Clin Res Assoc Newsletter 1995;19(10):1–4.

33. Christensen GJ. Should you and can you afford to bond amalgams? J Am Dent Assoc 1994;125:1381–1382.

34. Ciucchi B, Bouillaguet S, Delaloye M, Holz J. Volume of the internal gap formed under composite restorations in vitro. J Dent 1997;25:305–312.

35. Coli P, Brannstrom M. The marginal adaptation of four different bonding agents in Class II composite resin restorations applied in bulk or in two increments. Quintessence Int 1993;24:583–591.

36. Cox CF. Biocompatibility of dental materials in the absence of bacterial infection. Oper Dent 1987;12:146–152.

37. Cox CF, Hafex AA, Akimoto N, et al. Biocompatibility of primer, adhesive and resin composite systems on non-exposed and exposed pulps of non-human primate teeth. Am J Dent 1998;11(special issue):S55–S63.

38. Cox CF, Keall CL, Keall HJ, et al. Biocompatibility of surface-sealed dental materials against exposed pulps. J Prosthet Dent 1987;57:1–8.

39. Cox CF, Subay RK, Ostro E, et al. Tunnel defects in dentin bridges: their formation following direct pulp capping. Oper Dent 1996;21:4–11.

40. Cox CF, Suzuki S. Re-evaluating pulp protection: calcium hydroxide liners vs. cohesive hybridization [review]. J Am Dent Assoc 1994;125:823–831.

41. Craig RG. Restorative Dental Materials, ed 8. St. Louis: Mosby, 1989:284.

42. Craig RG. Restorative Dental Materials, ed 8. St. Louis: Mosby, 1989:200.

43. Craig RG. Restorative Dental Materials, ed 8. St. Louis: Mosby, 1989:218.

44. Craig RG. Restorative Dental Materials, ed 9. St. Louis: Mosby-Year Book; 1993:203–207.

45. D'Souza R. Pulpal and periapical immune response to electro-surgical contact of cervical metallic restorations in monkeys. Quintessence Int 1986;17:803–808.

46. DeSchepper EJ, Thrasher MR, Thurmond BA. Antibacterial effects of light-cured liners. Am J Dent 1989;2(3):74–76.

47. Donly KJ, Gomez C. In vitro demineralization-remineralization of enamel caries at restoration margins utilizing fluoride-releasing composite resin. Quintessence Int 1994;25:355–358.

48. Dostalova T, Jelinkova H, Krejsa O, et al. Dentin and pulp response to Erbium:YAG laser ablation: a preliminary evaluation of human teeth. J Clin Laser Med Surg 1997;15(3):117–121.

49. Drummond JL, Robledo J, Garcia L, Toepke TRS. Thermal conductivity of cement base materials. Dent Mater 1993;9:68–71.

50. Duke ES, Lindemuth JS. Variability of clinical dentin substrates. Am J Dent 1991;4:241–246.

51. Dumsha T, Hovland E. Considerations and treatment of direct and indirect pulp-capping. Dent Clin North Am 1985;29:251–259.

52. Dumsha T, Hovland EJ. Evaluation of long-term calcium hydroxide treatment in avulsed teeth—an in vivo study. Int Endod J 1995;28:7–11.

53. Dutton FB, Summitt JB, Garcia-Godoy F. Effect of a resin lining and rebonding on the marginal leakage of amalgam restorations. J Dent 1993;21:52–56.

54. Eames WB, Scrabeck JG. Bases, liners and varnishes: interviews with contemporary authorities. Gen Dent 1980;33:201–207.

55. Fairbourn DR, Charbeneau GT, Loesche WJ. Effect of improved Dycal and IRM on bacteria in deep carious lesions. J Am Dent Assoc 1980;100:547–552.

56. Farah JW, Clark AE, Mohsein M, Thomas PA. Effect of cement base thicknesses on MOD amalgam restorations. J Dent Res 1983;62:109–111.

57. Felton D, Madison S, Kanoy E, Kantor M, Maryniuk G. Long term effects of crown preparation on pulp vitality [abstract 1139]. J Dent Res 1989;68(special issue):1009.

58. Felton DA, Kanoy BE, White JT. Effect of cavity varnish on retention of cemented cast crowns. J Prosthet Dent 1987;57:411–416.

59. Ferracane JL, Condon JR. Rate of elution of leachable components from composite. Dent Mater 1990;6:282–287.

60. Finger WJ, Fritz U. Laboratory evaluation of one-component enamel/dentin bonding agents. Am J Dent 1996;9:206–210.

61. Fitchie JG, Reeves GW, Scarbrough AR, Hembree JH. Microleakage of a new cavity varnish with a high-copper spherical amalgam alloy. Oper Dent 1990;15:136–140.

62. Fitzgerald M, Heys RJ. A clinical and histological evaluation of conservative pulpal therapy in human teeth. Oper Dent 1991;16:101–112.

63. Frankenberger R, Sindel J, Kramer N, Petschelt A. Dentin bond strength and marginal adaptation: direct composite resins vs ceramic inlays. Oper Dent 1999;24:147–155.

64. Friedl K-H, Hiller K-A, Schmalz G. Placement and replacement of composite restorations in Germany. Oper Dent 1995;20:34–38.

65. Friedl K-H, Schmalz G, Hiller K-A, Mortazavi F. Marginal adaptation of composite restorations versus hybrid ionomer/composite sandwich restorations. Oper Dent 1997;22:21–29.

66. Gaintantzopoulou MD, Willis GP, Kafrawy AH. Pulp reactions to light-cured glass ionomer cements. Am J Dent 1994;7:39–42.

67. Garberoglio R, Brannstrom M. Scanning electron microscopic investigation of human dentinal tubules. Arch Oral Biol 1976;21:355–362.

68. Garcia-Godoy F, Jensen ME. Artificial recurrent caries in glass ionomer-lined amalgam restorations. Am J Dent 1990; 3:89–93.

69. Geiger SB, Weiner S. Fluoridated carbonatoapatite in the intermediate layer between glass ionomer and dentin. Dent Mater 1993;9:33–36.

70. Gerbo L, Cox CF, Suzuki S, Suzuki SH. Histologic pulp response of a dentin bonding system [abstract 937]. J Dent Res 1993;72(special issue):220.

71. Gerzina TM, Hume WR. Effect of hydrostatic pressure on the diffusion of monomers through dentin in vitro. J Dent Res 1995;74:369–373.

72. Gerzina TM, Hume WR. Diffusion of monomers from bonding resin-resin composite combinations through dentine in vitro. J Dent 1996;24:125–128.

73. Gilmour ASM, Edmunds DH, Newcombe RG. Prevalence and depth of artificial caries-like lesions adjacent to cavities prepared in roots and restored with a glass ionomer or a dentin-bonded composite material. J Dent Res 1997;76:1854–1861.

74. Going RE. Cavity liners and dentin treatment. J Am Dent Assoc 1964;69:415–422.

75. Gordan VV, Mjor IA, Hucke RD, Smith GE. Effect of different liner treatments on postoperative sensitivity of amalgam restorations. Quintessence Int 1999;30:55–59.

76. Gordan VV, Mjor IA, Moorhead JE. Amalgam restorations: postoperative sensitivity as a function of liner treatment and cavity depth. Oper Dent 1999;24:377–383.

77. Hamilton AI, Kramer IR. Cavity preparation with and without waterspray. Effects on the human dental pulp and additional effects of further dehydration of the dentine. Br Dent J 1967;123:281–285.

78. Hanks CT, Bergenholtz G, Kim JS. Protein synthesis in vitro, in the presence of Ca(OH)$_2$-containing pulp-capping medicaments. J Oral Pathol 1983;12:356–365.

79. Hanks CT, Strawn SE, Wataha JC, Craig RG. Cytotoxic effects of resin components on cultured mammalian fibroblasts. J Dent Res 1991;70:1450–1455.

80. Hanks CT, Wataha JC, Parsell RR, et al. Permeability of biological and synthetic molecules through dentine. J Oral Rehabil 1994;21:475–487.

81. Hansel C, Leyhausen G, Mai UEH, Geurtsen W. Effects of various resin composite (co)monomers and extracts on two caries-associated micro-organisms in vitro. J Dent Res 1998; 77:60–67.

82. Harper DS, Loesche WJ. Growth and acid tolerance of human dental plaque bacteria. Arch Oral Biol 1984;29: 843–848.

83. Harper RH, Schnell RJ, Swartz ML, Phillips RW. In vivo measurements of thermal diffusion through restorations of various materials. J Prosthet Dent 1980;43:180–185.

84. Haskell EW, Stanley HR, Chellemi J, Stringfellow H. Direct pulp capping treatment: a long-term follow-up. J Am Dent Assoc 1978;97:607–612.

85. Hayashi Y, Imai M, Yanagiguchi K, et al. Hydroxyapatite applied as direct pulp capping medicine substitutes for osteodentin. J Endod 1999;25:225–229.

86. Hebling J, Aparecida Giro EM, de Souza Costa CA. Biocompatibility of an adhesive system applied to exposed human dental pulp. J Endod 1999;25:676–682.

87. Heys RJ, Fitzgerald M. Microleakage of three cement bases. J Dent Res 1991;70:55–58.

88. Hilton TJ, Schwartz RS. The effect of air thinning on dentin adhesive bond strength. Oper Dent 1995;20:133–137.

89. Hilton TJ, Schwartz RS, Ferracane JL. Microleakage of four Class II resin composite insertion techniques at intraoral temperature. Quintessence Int 1997;28:135–144.

90. Hirata K, Nakashima M, Sekine I, et al. Dentinal fluid movement associated with loading of restorations. J Dent Res 1991;70:975–978.

91. Hollis RA, Hein DK, Rasmussen TE, et al. Shear strength and microleakage of 14 amalgam bonding adhesives [abstract 2958]. J Dent Res 1996;75(special issue):387.

92. Hormati AA, Fuller JL. The fracture strength of amalgam overlying base materials. J Prosthet Dent 1980;43:52–57.

93. Hosoda H, Inokoshi S, Shimada Y, et al. Pulpal response to a new light-cured composite placed in etched glass-ionomer lined cavities. Oper Dent 1991;16:122–129.

94. Irie M, Suzuki K. Marginal gap formation of light-activated base/liner materials: effect of setting shrinkage and bond strength. Dent Mater 1999;15:403–407.

95. James VE, Schour I. Early dentinal and pulpal changes following cavity preparations and filling materials in dogs. Oral Surg Oral Med Oral Pathol 1955;8:1305–1314.

96. Jontell M, Hanks CT, Bratel J, Bergenholtz G. Effects of unpolymerized resin components on the function of accessory cells derived from the rat incisor pulp. J Dent Res 1995;74: 1162–1167.

97. Kanca JI. Replacement of a fractured incisor fragment over pulpal exposure: a case report. Quintessence Int 1993;24: 81–84.

98. Kashiwada T, Takagi M. New restoration and direct pulp capping systems using adhesive composite resin. Bull Tokyo Med Dent Univ 1991;38(4):45–52.

99. Kemp-Scholte CM, Davidson CL. Complete marginal seal of Class V resin composite restorations effected by increased flexibility. J Dent Res 1990;69:1240–1243.

100. Kennington LB, Davis R, Murchison DF, Langenderfer WR. Short-term clinical evaluation of post-operative sensitivity with bonded amalgams. Am J Dent 1998;11:177–180.

101. Kidd EA. Microleakage: a review. J Dent 1976;4:199–206.

102. Kidd EAM, Joyston-Bechal S, Beighton D. The use of a caries detector dye during cavity preparation: a microbiological assessment. Br Dent J 1993;174:245–248.

103. Kitasako Y, Inokoshi S, Fujitani M, et al. Short-term reaction of exposed monkey pulp beneath adhesive resins. Oper Dent 1998;23:308–317.

104. Kitasako Y, Inokoshi S, Tagami J. Effects of direct resin pulp capping techniques on short-term response of mechanically exposed pulps. J Dent 1999;27:257–263.

105. Krejci I, Lutz F. Mixed Class V restorations: the potential of a dentine bonding agent. J Dent 1990;18:263–270.

106. Krejci RF, Reinhardt RA, Wentz FM, et al. Effects of electrosurgery on dog pulps under cervical metallic restorations. Oral Surg Oral Med Oral Pathol 1982;54:575–582.

107. Kurosaki N, Kubota M, Yamamoto Y, Fusayama T. The effect of etching on the dentin of the clinical cavity floor. Quintessence Int 1990;21:87–92.

108. Langeland K, Langeland LK. Indirect capping and the treatment of deep carious lesions. Int Dent J 1968;18:326–380.

109. Laurell KA, Carpenter W, Daugherty D, Beck M. Histopathologic effects of kinetic cavity preparation for the removal of enamel and dentin. An in vivo animal study. Oral Surg Oral Med Oral Pathol 1995;80:214–225.

110. Lefebvre CA, Schuster GS, Rueggeberg FA, et al. Responses of oral epithelial cells to dental resin components. J Biomater Sci Polym Ed 1996;7:965–976.

111. Leung RL, Loesche WJ, Charbeneau GT. Effect of Dycal on bacteria in deep carious lesions. J Am Dent Assoc 1980;100: 193–197.

112. Lewis BA, Burgess JO, Gray SE. Mechanical properties of dental base materials. Am J Dent 1992;5:69–72.

113. Lin JHC, Marshall GW, Marshall SJ. Microstructures of Cu-rich amalgams after corrosion. J Dent Res 1983;62:112–115.

114. Mahler DB, Engle JH. Clinical evaluation of bonding amalgam in traditional Class I and Class II restorations. J Am Dent Assoc 2000;131:43–49.

115. Mahler DB, Engle JH, Adey JD. Bond strength and microleakage of amalgam adhesives [abstract 42]. J Dent Res 1992;71(special issue):111.

116. Mahler DB, Engle JH, Simms LE, Terkla LG. One-year clinical evaluation of bonded amalgam restorations. J Am Dent Assoc 1996;127:345–349.

117. Manders CA, Garcia-Godoy F, Barnwell GM. Effect of a copal varnish, ZOE or glass ionomer cement base on microleakage of amalgam restorations. Am J Dent 1990;3:63–66.

118. Marchiori S, Baratieri LN, Andrade e Silva F, et al. The use of liners under amalgam restorations: an in vitro study on marginal leakage. Quintessence Int 1998;29:637–642.

119. Marek M, Hochman RF. Mechanism of crevice corrosion of dental amalgam [abstract 166]. J Dent Res 1975;54(SI):242.

120. Matsuo T, Nakanishi T, Shimizu H, Ebisu S. A clinical study of direct pulp capping applied to carious-exposed pulps. J Endod 1996;22:551–556.

121. Mazer RB, Leinfelder KF, Barnette JH. Post-operative sensitivity and margin adaptation of amalgam and composite restorations treated with ProBond adhesive [abstract 748]. J Dent Res 1995;74(special issue):105.

122. Mazer RB, Rehfeld R, Leinfelder KF. Effect of cavity varnishes on microleakage of amalgam restorations. Am J Dent 1988;1(5):205–208.

123. McComb D, Ben-Amar A, Brown J. Sealing efficacy of therapeutic varnishes used with silver amalgam restorations. Oper Dent 1990;15:122–128.

124. McCoy RB. Bases, liners and varnishes update. Oper Dent 1995;20(5):216.

125. McTigue D, Brice C, Nanda CR, Sarkar NK. The in vivo corrosion of Dispersalloy. J Oral Rehabil 1984;11:351–359.

126. Meiers JC, Miller GA. Antibacterial activity of dentin bonding systems, resin-modified glass ionomers, and polyacid-modified composite resins. Oper Dent 1996;21(6):257–264.

127. Meiers JC, Turner EW. Microleakage of dentin/amalgam alloy bonding agents: results after 1 year. Oper Dent 1998;23(1):30–35.

128. Mertz-Fairhurst EJ, Curtis JW Jr, Ergle JW, et al. Ultraconservative and cariostatic sealed restorations: results at year 10. J Am Dent Assoc 1998;129:55–66.

129. Mertz-Fairhurst EJ, Schuster GS, Williams JE, Fairhurst CW. Clinical progress of sealed and unsealed caries. Part I: depth changes and bacterial counts. J Prosthet Dent 1979;42:521–526.

130. Meryon SD. The model cavity method incorporating dentine. Int Endod J 1988;21(2):79–84.

131. Meryon SD, Jakeman KJ. Zinc release from dental restorative materials in vitro. J Biomed Mater Res 1986;20(3):285–291.

132. Miller BC, Charbeneau GT. Sensitivity of teeth with and without cement bases under amalgam restorations: a clinical study. Oper Dent 1984;9:130–135.

133. Miller MB, Castellanos ER, Vargas MA, Denehy GE. Effect of restorative materials on microleakage of Class II composites. J Esthet Dent 1996;8(3):107–113.

134. Mitchem JC, Gronas DG. Effect of time after extraction and depth of dentin on resin dentin adhesives. J Am Dent Assoc 1986;113:285.

135. Mitra SB. In vitro fluoride release from a light-cured glass-ionomer liner/base. J Dent Res 1991;70:75–78.

136. Mjör IA. Glass-ionomer cement restorations and secondary caries: a preliminary report. Quintessence Int 1996;27:171–174.

137. Mjör IA, Qvist V. Marginal failures of amalgam and composite restorations. J Dent 1997;25(1):25–30.

138. Mjör IA, Toffenetti F. Placement and replacement of resin-based composite restorations in Italy. Oper Dent 1992;17(3):82–85.

139. Moore DS, Johnson WW, Kaplan I. A comparison of amalgam microleakage with a 4-META liner and Copal varnish. Int J Prosthodont 1995;8:461–466.

140. Morrier JJ, Suchett-Kaye G, Nguyen D, et al. Antimicrobial activity of amalgams, alloys and their elements and phases. Dent Mater 1998;14(2):150–157.

141. Nakabayashi N, Ashizawa M, Nakamura M. Identification of a resin-dentin hybrid layer in vital human dentin created in vivo: durable bonding to vital dentin. Quintessence Int 1992;23:135–141.

142. Nakajima M, Sano H, Burrow MF, et al. Tensile bond strength and SEM evaluation of caries-affected dentin using dentin adhesives. J Dent Res 1995;74:1679–1688.

143. Nakajima M, Sano H, Zheng L, et al. Effect of moist vs. dry bonding to normal vs. caries-affected dentin with Scotchbond Multi-Purpose Plus. J Dent Res 1999;78:1298–1303.

144. Nordenvall KJ, Brannstrom M, Torstensson B. Pulp reactions and microorganisms under ASPA and Concise composite fillings. ASDC J Dent Child 1979;46:449–453.

145. Nunez LJ, Schmalz G, Hembree J. Influence of amalgam, alloy, and mercury on the in vitro growth of Streptococcus mutans: I. Biological test system. J Dent Res 1976;55:257–261.

146. Oliveira HP, Araujo MAJ, Figueiredo MOG. Adhesive amalgam: a microleakage study [abstract 69, Brazilian Div]. J Dent Res 1996;75(5):1086.

147. Olmez A, Oztas N, Basak F, Sabuncuoglu B. A histopathologic study of direct pulp-capping with adhesive resins. Oral Surg Oral Med Oral Pathol Oral Radiol Endod 1998;86(1):98–103.

148. Olsen BT, Garcia-Godoy F, Marshall TD, Barnwell GM. Fluoride release from glass ionomer-lined amalgam restorations. Am J Dent 1989;2:89.

149. Oppermann RV, Johansen JR. Effect of fluoride and non-fluoride salts of copper, silver and tin on the acidogenicity of dental plaque in vivo. Scand J Dent Res 1980;88:476–480.

150. Orstavik D. Antibacterial properties of and element release from some dental amalgams. Acta Odontol Scand 1985;43:231.

151. Pameijer CH, Stanley HR. The disastrous effects of the "Total Etch" technique in vital pulp capping in primates. Am J Dent 1998;11(special issue):S45–S54.

152. Pameijer CH, Wendt SL Jr. Microleakage of "surface-sealing" materials. Am J Dent 1995;8:43–46.

153. Panighi MM, Allart D, Jacquot BM, et al. Influence of human tooth cryopreservation on dentin bond strength. Dent Mater 1997;13(1):56–61.

154. Pashley DH. The influence of dentin permeability and pulpal blood flow on pulpal solute concentrations. J Endod 1979;5:355–361.

155. Pashley DH. Clinical considerations of microleakage. J Endod 1990;16:70–77.

156. Pashley DH. Clinical correlations of dentin structure and function. J Prosthet Dent 1991;66:777–781.

157. Pashley DH, Depew DD. Effects of the smear layer, copalite, and oxalate on microleakage. Oper Dent 1986;11:95–102.

158. Pashley DH, Livingston MJ, Outhwaite WC. Rate of permeation of isotopes through human dentin, in vitro. J Dent Res 1977;56:83–88.

159. Pashley DH, O'Meara JA, Williams EC, Kepler EE. Dentin permeability: effects of cavity varnishes and bases. J Prosthet Dent 1985;53:511–516.

160. Paterson RC. Bacterial contamination and the exposed pulp. Br Dent J 1976;140(7):231–236.

161. Pereira JC, Manfio AP, Franco EB, Lopes ES. Clinical evaluation of Dycal under amalgam restorations. Am J Dent 1990;3:67–70.

162. Pereira JC, Segala AD, Costa CAS. Human pulp response to direct capping with an adhesive system-histologic study [abstract 1329]. J Dent Res 1997;76(special issue):180.

163. Peters DD, Augsburger RA. In vitro cold transference of bases and restorations. J Am Dent Assoc 1981;102:642–646.

164. Peyton FA, Henry EE. The effect of high speed burs, diamond instruments and air abrasive in cutting tooth tissue. J Am Dent Assoc 1954;49:426–435.

165. Phillips RW. Skinner's Science of Dental Materials, ed 9. Philadelphia: WB Saunders, 1991.

166. Pierpont W, Gray S, Hermesch C, Hilton T. Effect of various bases on the fracture resistance of amalgam [abstract 981]. J Dent Res 1993;72:226.

167. Pierpont WF, Gray SE, Hermesch CB, Hilton TJ. The effect of various bases on the fracture resistance of amalgam. Oper Dent 1994;19(6):211–216.

168. Piperno S, Barouch E, Hirsch SM, Kaim JM. Thermal discomfort of teeth related to presence or absence of cement bases under amalgam restorations. Oper Dent 1982;7(3):92–96.

169. Pitt Ford TR, Roberts GJ. Immediate and delayed direct pulp capping with the use of a new visible light-cured calcium hydroxide preparation. Oral Surg Oral Med Oral Pathol 1991;71:338–342.

170. Pitt Ford TR, Torabinejad M, Abedi HR, et al. Using mineral trioxide aggregate as a pulp-capping material. J Am Dent Assoc 1996;127:1491–1494.

171. Powell GL, Morton TH, Larsen AE. Pulpal response to irradiation of enamel with continuous wave CO2 laser. J Endod 1989;15:581–583.

172. Prager M. Pulp capping with the total-etch technique. Dent Econ 1994;84(1):78–79.

173. Prati C, Nucci C. Marginal gap, microleakage and shear bond strength of adhesive restorative systems [abstract 1036]. J Dent Res 1989;68(special issue):996.

174. Prati C, Nucci C, Davidson CL, Montanari G. Early marginal leakage and shear bond strength of adhesive restorative systems. Dent Mater 1990;6:195–200.

175. Puckett A, Thompson N, Phillips S, Reeves G. Heat generation during curing of a dentin adhesive and composite [abstract 1380]. J Dent Res 1965;74(special issue):184.

176. Ratanasathien S, Wataha JC, Hanks CT, Dennison JB. Cytotoxic interactive effects of dentin bonding components on mouse fibroblasts. J Dent Res 1995;74:1602–1606.

177. Rathbun MA, Craig RG, Hanks CT, Filisko FE. Cytotoxicity of a BIS-GMA dental composite before and after leaching in organic solvents. J Biomed Mater Res 1991;25:443–457.

178. Reuver J. 592 Pulp cappings in a dental office—a clinical study (1966-1990). Dtsch Zahnärztl Zeitschr 1992;47:29–32.

179. Robbins JW. The placement of bases beneath amalgam restorations: review of literature and recommendations for use. J Am Dent Assoc 1986;113:910–912.

180. Robertson PB, Luscher B, Spangberg LS, Levy BM. Pulpal and periodontal effects of electrosurgery involving cervical metallic restorations. Oral Surg Oral Med Oral Pathol 1978;46:702–710.

181. Saiku JM, St Germain HA Jr, Meiers JC. Microleakage of a dental amalgam alloy bonding agent. Oper Dent 1993;18:172–178.

182. Sano H, Takatsu T, Ciucchi B, et al. Nanoleakage: leakage within the hybrid layer. Oper Dent 1995;20:18–25.

183. Sano H, Yoshiyama M, Ebisu S, et al. Comparative SEM and TEM observations of nanoleakage within the hybrid layer. Oper Dent 1995;30:160–167.

184. Scherer W, Lippman N, Kaim J. Antimicrobial properties of glass-ionomer cements and other restorative materials. Oper Dent 1989;14(2):77–81.

185. Sidhu SK, Henderson LJ. In vitro marginal leakage of cervical composite restorations lined with a light-cured glass ionomer. Oper Dent 1992;17:7–12.

186. Silvestri AR Jr, Cohen SH, Wetz JH. Character and frequency of discomfort immediately following restorative procedures. J Am Dent Assoc 1977;95:85–89.

187. Skjorland KK. Plaque accumulation on different dental filling materials. Scand J Dent Res 1973;81:538–542.

188. Skjorland KK, Sonju T. Effect of sucrose rinses on bacterial colonization on amalgam and composite. Acta Odontol Scand 1982;40(4):193–196.

189. Smith GE. Surface deterioration of glass-ionomer cement during acid etching: an SEM evaluation. Oper Dent 1988;13(1):3–7.

190. Sneed WD, Hembree JH Jr, Welsh EL. Effectiveness of three cavity varnishes in reducing leakage of a high-copper amalgam. Oper Dent 1984;9(1):32–34.

191. Sonntag KD, Klitzman B, Burkes EJ, et al. Pulpal response to cavity preparation with the Er:YAG and Mark III free electron lasers. Oral Surg Oral Med Oral Pathol 1996;81:695–702.

192. Sorensen JA, Munksgaard EC. Relative gap formation adjacent to ceramic inlays with combinations of resin cements and dentin bonding agents. J Prosthet Dent 1996;76:472–476.

193. Spangberg LS, Hellden L, Robertson PB, Levy BM. Pulpal effects of electrosurgery involving based and unbased cervical amalgam restorations. Oral Surg Oral Med Oral Pathol 1982;54:678–685.

194. Stanley HR. Human Pulp Response to Restorative Dental Procedures. Gainesville, FL: Storter, 1981:41.

195. Stanley HR. Human Pulp Response to Restorative Dental Procedures. Gainesville, FL: Storter, 1981:42–43.

196. Stanley HR. Human Pulp Response to Restorative Dental Procedures. Gainesville, FL: Storter, 1981:9.

197. Stanley HR. Human Pulp Response to Restorative Dental Procedures. Gainesville, FL: Storter, 1981:38.

198. Stanley HR. Pulpal responses to ionomer cements—biological characteristics. J Am Dent Assoc 1990;120:25–29.

199. Stanley HR, Going RE, Chauncey HH. Human pulp response to acid pretreatment of dentin and to composite restoration. J Am Dent Assoc 1975;91:817–825.

200. Stanley HR, Pameijer CH. Dentistry's Friend: calcium hydroxide. Oper Dent 1997;22(1):1–3.

201. Stanley HR, Pereira JC, Spiegel E, et al. The detection and prevalence of reactive and physiologic sclerotic dentin, reparative dentin and dead tracts beneath various types of dental lesions according to tooth surface and age. J Oral Pathol 1983;12:257–289.

202. Stanley HR Jr, Swerdlow H. Reaction of the human pulp to cavity preparation: results produced by eight different operative grinding techniques. J Am Dent Assoc 1959;58(5):49–59.

203. Starr CB, Langenderfer WR. Use of a caries-disclosing agent to improve dental residents' ability to detect caries. Oper Dent 1993;18:110–114.

204. Stefanoni JI, Abate PF, Polack MA, Macchi RL. In vitro marginal leakage in amalgam restorations [abstract 37, Argentine Div]. J Dent Res 1996;75:1063.

205. Strydom C, Retief DH, Russell CM, Denys FR. Laboratory evaluation of the gluma 3-step bonding system. Am J Dent 1995;8:93–98.

206. Summitt JB. On bases, liners, and varnishes [letter]. Oper Dent 1994;19:35.

207. Suzuki S, Cox CF, White KC. Pulpal response after complete crown preparation, dentinal sealing, and provisional restoration. Quintessence Int 1994;25:477–485.

208. Suzuki T, Finger WJ. Dentin adhesives: site of dentin vs bonding of composite resins. Dent Mater 1988;4:379.

209. Svanberg M, Krasse B, Ornerfeldt HO. Mutans streptococci in interproximal plaque from amalgam and glass ionomer restorations. Caries Res 1990;24(2):133–136.

210. Svanberg M, Mjor IA, Orstavik D. Mutans streptococci in plaque from margins of amalgam, composite, and glass-ionomer restorations. J Dent Res 1990;69:861–864.

211. Symons AL, Wing G, Hewitt GH. Adaptation of eight modern dental amalgams to walls of Class I cavity preparations. J Oral Rehabil 1987;14:55.

212. Tagami J, Tao L, Pashley DH, et al. Effects of high-speed cutting on dentin permeability and bonding. Dent Mater 1991;7:234–239.

213. Tam LE, Pulver E, McComb D, Smith DC. Physical properties of calcium hydroxide and glass-ionomer base and lining materials. Dent Mater 1989;5(3):145–149.

214. Tangsgoolwatana J, Chochran MA, Moore BK, Li Y. Microleakage evaluation of bonded amalgam restorations: Confocal microscopy versus radioisotope. Quintessence Int 1997;28:467–477.

215. Tao L, Pashley DH. Shear bond strengths to dentin: effects of surface treatments, depth and position. Dent Mater 1988;4:371.

216. Tarim B, Hafez AA, Suzuki SH, et al. Biocompatibility of compomer restorative systems on nonexposed dental pulps of primate teeth. Oper Dent 1997;22(4):149–158.

217. Tay FR, Gwinnett AJ, Pang KM, Wei SHY. Variability in microleakage observed in a total-etch wet-bonding technique under different handling conditions. J Dent Res 1995;74:1168–1178.

218. Tay FR, Gwinnett AJ, Wei SHY. Ultrastructure of the resin-dentin interface following reversible and irreversible rewetting. Am J Dent 1997;10(2):77–82.

219. Tjan AHL, Bergh BH, Lidner C. Effect of various incremental techniques on the marginal adaptation of Class II composite resin restorations. J Prosthet Dent 1992;67:62–66.

220. Tjan AHL, Tan DE, Sun JC, Tjan AH. Marginal leakage of amalgam restorations pretreated with various liners. Am J Dent 1997;10(6):284–286.

221. Torabinejad M, Chivian N. Clinical applications of mineral trioxide aggregate. J Endod 1999;25:197–205.

222. Torabinejad M, Hong CU, McDonald F, Pitt Ford TR. Physical and chemical properties of a new root-end filling material. J Endod 1995;21:349–353.

223. Torabinejad M, Hong CU, Pitt Ford TR, Kettering JD. Cytotoxicity of four root end filling materials. J Endod 1995;21:489–492.

224. Torabinejad M, Rastegar AF, Kettering JD, Pitt Ford TR. Bacterial leakage of mineral trioxide aggregate as a root-end filling material. J Endod 1995;21:109–112.

225. Torabinejad M, Watson TF, Pitt Ford TR. Sealing ability of a mineral trioxide aggregate when used as a root end filling material. J Endod 1993;19:591–595.

226. Trushkowsky RD, Gwinnett AJ. Microleakage of Class V composite, resin sandwich, and resin-modified glass ionomers. Am J Dent 1996;9(3):96–99.

227. Turner EW, St Germain HA, Meiers JC. Microleakage of dentin-amalgam bonding agents. Am J Dent 1995;8:191–196.

228. Updegraff DM, Chang RW, Joos RW. Antibacterial activity of dental restorative materials. J Dent Res 1971;50:382–387.

229. Vojinovic O, Nyborg H, Brannstrom M. Acid treatment of cavities under resin fillings: bacterial growth in dentinal tubules and pulpal reactions. J Dent Res 1973;52:1189–1193.

230. Vongsavan N, Matthews B. The permeability of cat dentine in vivo and in vitro. Arch Oral Biol 1991;36:641–646.

231. Wallman-Bjorklund C, Svanberg M, Emilson CG. Streptococcus mutans in plaque from conventional and from non-gamma-2 amalgam restorations. Scand J Dent Res 1987;95(3):266–269.

232. Watanabe I, Nakabayashi N. Bonding durability of photocured Penyl-P in TEGDMA to smear layer-retained bovine dentin. Quintessence Int 1993;24:335–342.

233. Watanabe T, Sano M, Itoh K, Wakumoto S. The effects of primers on the sensitivity of dentin. Dent Mater 1991;7:148–150.

234. Watts A, Paterson RC. Bacterial contamination as a factor influencing the toxicity of materials to the exposed dental pulp. Oral Surg Oral Med Oral Pathol 1987;64:466–474.

235. Weine FS. Endodontic Therapy, ed 3. St Louis: Mosby, 1982:118.

236. Weine FS. A preview of the canal-filling materials of the 21st century. Compend Contin Educ Dent 1992;13:688–698.

237. Wells DL, Davis RD, Osborne PB. Effect of dentin treatment on the cervical marginal integrity of Class II composite restorations [abstract 199]. J Dent Res 1998;77(special issue):130.

238. White KC, Cox CF, Kanca JI, et al. Pulpal response to adhesive resin systems applied to acid-etched vital dentin: damp versus dry primer application. Quintessence Int 1994;25:259–268.

239. Wright W, Mazer RB, Teixeira LC, Leinfelder KR. Clinical microleakage evaluation of a cavity varnish. Am J Dent 1992;5(5):263–265.

240. Yap AUJ, Mok BYY, Pearson G. An in vitro microleakage study of the "bonded-base" restorative technique. J Oral Rehabil 1997;24:230–236.

241. Yip HK, Stevenson AG, Beeley JA. The specificity of caries detector dyes in cavity preparation. Br Dent J 1994;176:417–421.

242. Yoshiyama M, Masada J, Uchida A, Ishida H. Scanning electron microscopic characterization of sensitive vs. insensitive human radicular dentin. J Dent Res 1989;68:1498–1502.

243. Zach L, Cohen G. Pulp response to externally applied heat. Oral Surg Oral Med Oral Pathol 1965;19:515–530.

244. Zalkind M, Keisar O, Ever-Hadani P, Sela M. Accumulation of Streptococcus mutans on light-cured composites and amalgam: an in vitro study. J Esthet Dent 1998;10(4):187–190.

245. Zanata RL, Palma RG, Navarro L. Two years clinical assessment of Permite C and Dispersalloy amalgam restorations [abstract 1490]. J Dent Res 1997;76(special issue):200.

Nomenclature and Instrumentation

James B. Summitt

Basic to any science is a language understood by the members of the community of the discipline. This chapter is devoted to a review of the language of operative dentistry and to the basic instrumentation of that discipline. *Operative dentistry* today may be defined as that part of restorative dentistry involving assessment, prevention, and treatment of diseases and defects of the hard tissues of individual teeth to maintain or restore functional, physiologic, and esthetic integrity and health.

Nomenclature and Classification of Caries and Cavity Preparations

Systems for Naming and Numbering Teeth

Each tooth may be identified by its location in the mouth and by its individual name. Examples include the *maxillary right central incisor* and the *mandibular left second premolar*. Areas of the mouth are referred to by arch (*maxillary* or *upper* and *mandibular* or *lower*) and by the side of the patient's midline (left and right) (Fig 6-1). Each arch is divided in half at the midline, forming four *quadrants* (maxillary right and left quadrants and mandibular right and left quadrants). In addition, each tooth is identified as *primary* or *permanent*. Finally, the individual name of the tooth, eg, *molar* or *central incisor,* completes the iden-

tification of the tooth. Examples of complete tooth names are *mandibular left permanent first molar* and *maxillary right primary canine.*

Because their names are cumbersome, teeth are frequently referred to by number. The tooth-numbering systems primarily used today are the Universal system and the Fédération Dentaire Internationale (FDI) system (Fig 6-2). In the Universal system, the numbering begins with the maxillary (upper) right third molar (tooth 1), proceeds around the arch to the maxillary left third molar (tooth 16), then to the mandibular (lower) left third molar (tooth 17) and around the mandibular arch to the mandibular right third molar (tooth 32).

In the FDI system, the first digit of the tooth number represents a quadrant (1, maxillary right; 2, maxillary left; 3, mandibular left; and 4, mandibular right). The second digit represents the tooth (1, a central incisor, regardless of the arch or quadrant; 2, lateral incisor; 3, canine; and so on to 8, third molar). The maxillary left first premolar would be identified as tooth 24; the mandibular right second molar would be identified as tooth 47.

Incisors and canines are referred to as *anterior teeth*, regardless of the arch; premolars and molars are *posterior teeth*.

In addition to quadrants, the mouth may also be divided into *sextants*, or sixths. There are three sextants in each arch, with divisions between the canines and first premolars—the maxillary right, anterior, and left sextants and the mandibular right, anterior, and left sextants.

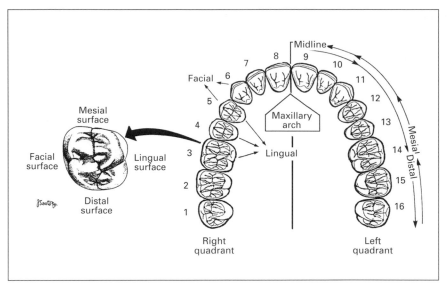

Fig 6-1 Nomenclature of directions and tooth surfaces.

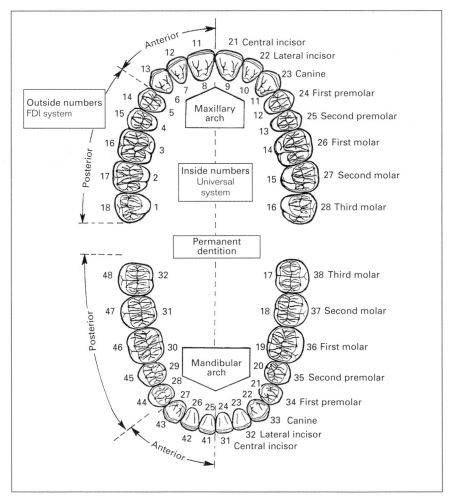

Fig 6-2 Tooth-numbering systems and nomenclature.

Figs 6-3a and 6-3b Directions, features, and tooth surfaces of anterior teeth.

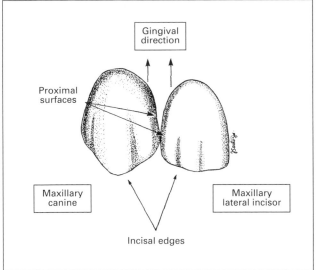

Fig 6-3a Facial view.

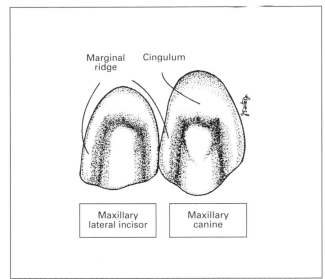

Fig 6-3b Lingual view.

Figs 6-4a and 6-4b Directions, features, and tooth surfaces of posterior teeth.

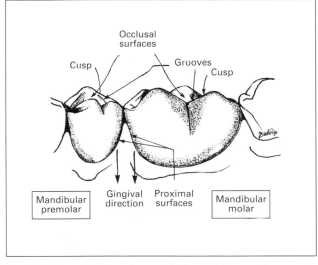

Fig 6-4a Lingual view of mandibular right second premolar and first molar.

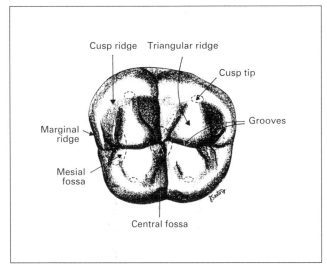

Fig 6-4b Occlusal view of mandibular right first molar.

Nomenclature of Tooth Surfaces and Cavity Preparations

The surfaces of the teeth are identified by their locations. Any surface or movement toward the midline of the arch is referred to as *mesial* (see Fig 6-1). A surface or movement away from the midline is *distal*. Surfaces and movements toward the tongue are termed *lingual*; those that are in the direction of the cheek or lips are termed *facial*. For the anterior teeth, facial may be referred to as *labial* (toward the lips); for posterior teeth, facial may be referred to as *buccal* (toward the cheek).[7]

On any tooth, *gingival* refers to a surface or movement toward the gingiva (Figs 6-3 and 6-4). A distinction is made, however, between the chewing surfaces of posterior teeth, which are called *occlusal* (Figs 6-4a and 6-4b) and the biting edges of anterior teeth, which are called *incisal* (Figs 6-3a and 6-3b). A *proximal* surface is one that faces an adjacent tooth; it may be further identified as mesial or distal.[7]

115

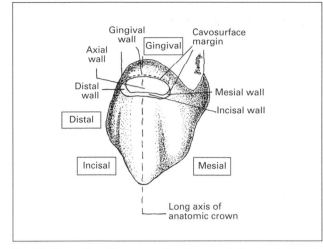

Fig 6-5 Class 5 cavity preparation in an anterior tooth (maxillary canine, facial view). In posterior teeth, there would be an occlusal wall instead of an incisal wall.

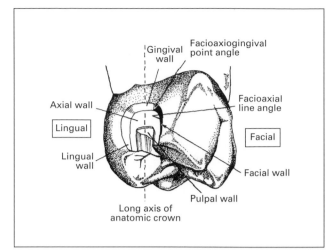

Fig 6-6 Class 2 cavity preparation (maxillary molar, proximal view).

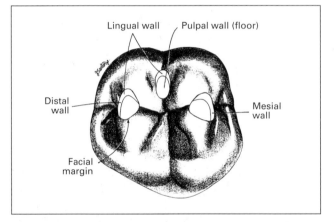

Fig 6-7 Class 1 cavity preparations in a posterior tooth. The occlusal surface of this mandibular left molar is viewed slightly from the facial aspect (occlusofacial), so the facial wall is hidden from view.

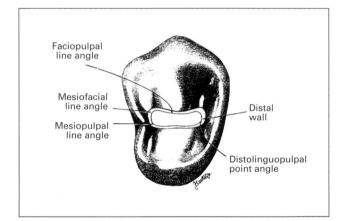

Fig 6-8 Class 1 cavity preparation in a posterior tooth (maxillary premolar, occlusal view). In a direct restoration (such as for amalgam), the facial and lingual walls would be parallel or convergent for retention of the amalgam. The walls of a preparation for bonded resin composite could diverge as shown here or by considerably more, because the restoration would be bonded to the enamel and dentin.

The anatomic contour of anterior teeth is less complicated than that of posterior teeth, in which the occlusal surfaces are characterized by grooves, cusp tips and ridges, marginal ridges, and fossae. *Marginal ridges* (both mesial and distal) border the lingual surfaces of anterior teeth (see Fig 6-3b) and the occlusal surfaces of posterior teeth (see Fig 6-4b). A *groove* is a linear channel between enamel elevations, such as cusps and/or ridges. A *fissure* is a developmental linear cleft usually found at the base of a groove; it is commonly the result of the lack of fusion of the enamel of adjoining dental cusps or lobes. A *pit* is a small depression in enamel, usually located in a groove and often at the junction of two or more fissures. A *fossa* is a hollow, rounded, or depressed area in the enamel surface of a tooth. For example, a mesial fossa lies just distal to a mesial marginal ridge (see Fig 6-4b).[7]

With the advent of bonding restorative materials to teeth, walls of cavity preparations are less distinct than they are in preparations for restorations that are retained by mechanical undercuts in the preparation walls or by nonadhesive cements. The walls of cavity preparations, however, are generally referred to by the same terms as the surface features of the teeth, for

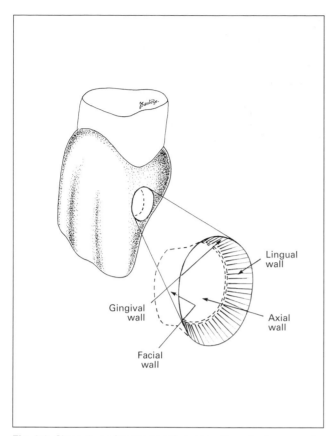

Fig 6-9 Class 3 cavity preparation (maxillary incisor, mesiofacial view). The preparation is for a bonded, tooth-colored restoration.

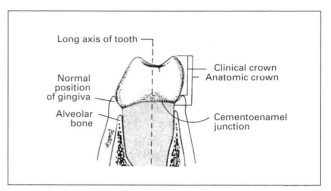

Fig 6-10 Anatomic and clinical crowns of a mandibular molar with the periodontal attachment at the normal, healthy level.

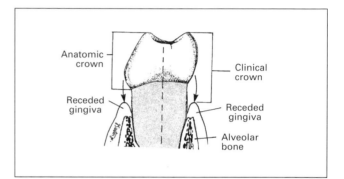

Fig 6-11 Anatomic and clinical crowns of a mandibular molar with the periodontal attachment at a more apical level (periodontal recession). With loss of gingival height comes an increase in the length of the clinical crown, but the anatomic crown, which is defined by the cementoenamel junction (or cervical line), stays constant. The occlusogingival dimension of the anatomic crown can be reduced by loss of occlusal tooth structure from wear or erosion.

example, the gingival and distal walls (Figs 6-5 to 6-9). Exceptions are the *pulpal wall* (or floor), which is only in the occlusal portion of a preparation and is the wall adjacent or nearest to the pulp chamber of the tooth (Figs 6-6 and 6-7), and the *axial wall*, which, in all other areas of a preparation, is the wall adjacent or nearest to the pulp chamber or pulp canal(s) and is approximately parallel to the long axis of the tooth (Figs 6-5, 6-6, and 6-9).[7]

The junction of two walls in a cavity preparation is called a *line angle*.[7] Again, in preparations for bonded restorations, line angles may not be well defined, but the names for line angles may be used to refer to general areas of the preparation. For example, the meeting of the facial and axial walls forms the facioaxial (or axiofacial) line angle (Fig 6-6). Similarly, the junction of three walls is referred to as a *point angle*. For example, the junction of the facial, axial, and gingival walls

creates the facioaxiogingival (or axiofaciogingival or gingivofacioaxial) point angle. Again, the junction of two walls is often rounded, so it does not actually form a line, but it is still referred to as a line angle; likewise, a point angle is usually not a sharp point.

The *margins* (or *cavosurface angles*[7]) of a preparation, which are formed by the junction of a cavity wall and an external tooth surface, are identified by the names of the adjacent walls (eg, incisal margin, mesial margin, or gingival margin).

The *anatomic crown* of a tooth is the portion that extends from the cementoenamel junction, or cervical line, to the occlusal surface or incisal edge; it is covered by enamel (Figs 6-10 and 6-11). The *clinical crown* is the portion that is visible in the oral cavity.[7] Depending on the tooth, the clinical crown may include only part of the anatomic crown (Fig 6-10) or it may include all of the anatomic crown and part of the root (Fig 6-11).

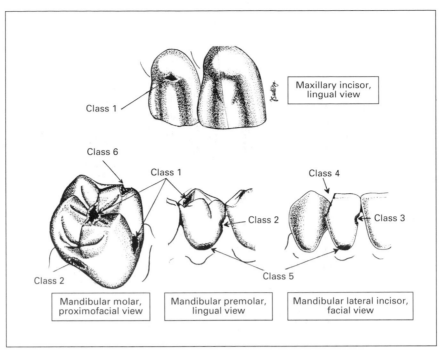

Fig 6-12 Classification of cavity preparations.

Classification of Carious Lesions and Tooth Preparations

Near the beginning of the 20th century, G. V. Black,[2] who is known as the father of operative dentistry, classified carious lesions into groups according to their locations in permanent teeth. The same classification is used to refer to cavity preparations, because the location of carious tooth structure is a major factor in the design of the cavity preparation and the selection of instruments (Fig 6-12).

Class 1 (I) lesions occur in pits and fissures on the facial, lingual, and occlusal surfaces of molars and premolars and, less often, the lingual surfaces of maxillary anterior teeth (most frequently lateral incisors, less frequently central incisors, rarely canines) (see Figs 6-7 and 6-8).

Class 2 (II) lesions occur on the proximal surfaces of the posterior teeth (molars and premolars). If a proximal surface of a posterior tooth is involved in a restoration, it is a Class 2 restoration (see Fig 6-6).

Class 3 (III) lesions occur on the proximal surfaces of anterior teeth (central and lateral incisors and canines). Class 3 cavities do not involve an incisal angle (see Fig 6-9).

Class 4 (IV) lesions occur on the proximal surfaces of anterior teeth when the incisal angle requires restoration. The angle may have to be removed because of its fragility or for proper placement of the restoration, or it may have been fractured by trauma (Fig 6-13).

Class 5 (V) lesions occur on smooth facial and lingual surfaces in the gingival third of teeth. Class 5 cavities begin close to the gingiva and may involve a cementum or dentinal surface as well as enamel (see Fig 6-5).

Class 6 (VI) lesions are pit or wear defects on the incisal edges of anterior teeth or the cusp tips of posterior teeth (Fig 6-14).

In addition to being named for their classifications, cavity preparations and restorations are named for the tooth surfaces involved. For example, a restoration involving the mesial and occlusal surfaces of a posterior tooth is called a *mesio-occlusal Class 2 restoration*; simply saying *mesio-occlusal restoration* identifies it as a Class 2 restoration because the proximal surface of a posterior tooth is involved. A preparation or restoration involving the mesial, occlusal, distal, and facial surfaces of a posterior tooth is called a *mesio-occlusodistofacial preparation* or *restoration*.

For brevity's sake, the names of the surfaces are often abbreviated (distal, *D*; lingual, *L*; facial, *F*; mesial, *M*; incisal, *I*; occlusal, *O*). A mesio-occlusal restoration in a posterior tooth would be abbreviated *MO*, and a distolingual restoration in an anterior tooth is abbreviated *DL*.

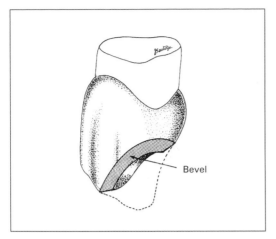

Fig 6-13 Class 4 preparation for a bonded, tooth-colored restoration. Maxillary incisor, facial view.

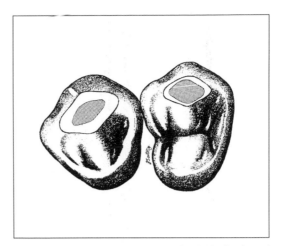

Fig 6-14 Class 6 preparations in the incisal edge of a maxillary canine and the cusp tip of a premolar (incisal/occlusal view). The dotted area of the preparation represents dentin; the clear area of the preparation represents enamel. The preparations have no mechanical, or undercut, retention; they are for bonded, tooth-colored restorations.

Black's Steps in Cavity Preparation

Treatment modalities for dental caries other than surgical removal are discussed in Chapter 4. When it has been determined that nonsurgical means of treating caries will not suffice, however, restorative therapy is indicated. This involves the surgical removal of carious tooth structure and restoration of the tooth to its original anatomic form with a suitable restorative material. The design of the cavity preparation is determined first by the location of the caries lesion(s) in the tooth. The shape or outline of the cavity preparation, as it meets the external surface of the tooth, is referred to as *outline form*. Other factors influencing the design include the need to obtain access for the instruments as the operator is preparing the cavity or placing the restoration *(convenience form)* and the need to provide retention for the restorative material *(retention form)*. Also required is resistance to stress on the restoration and the tooth to the forces of biting and chewing *(resistance form)*. Because cavity preparation is a surgical procedure in which a mistake can mean injury to living tissue, it is essential that the operator be knowledgeable and highly skilled.

The sequential steps of cavity preparation were established by Black.[2] Black's steps represent a systematic, scientific procedure for efficiency in cavity preparation. Although the technology of bonding restorative materials to enamel and dentin was not available to Black,

his steps of cavity preparation are generally as appropriate today as they were when he formulated them:

1. *Establish outline form.* Outline form is based primarily on the location and extent of the carious lesion, tooth fracture, or erosion. In carious teeth, the outline form is established after penetration into carious dentin and removal of the enamel overlying the carious dentin. The extent of carious dentin should be a primary determinant of the outline form of the preparation; the final outline is not established until the carious dentin and its overlying enamel have been removed.

2. *Obtain resistance form.* Resistance for the remaining tooth structure and for the restoration must be designed in the preparation, so that the restoration is resistant to displacement and both the tooth and the restoration are resistant to fracture during function.

3. *Obtain retention form.* Retention may be obtained through mechanical shaping of the preparation to retain the restoration and/or via bonding procedures that attach the restorative material to tooth structure.

4. *Obtain convenience form.* Convenience form allows adequate observation, accessibility, and ease of operation during preparation and restoration of the tooth. Convenience form that involves the removal of sound, strong tooth structure should be limited to that which is necessary.

5. *Remove remaining carious dentin.* Removal of remaining carious dentin applies primarily to that in the deepest part (pulpally) of the preparation. Other carious tooth structure was removed when the outline form was established.

6. *Finish enamel walls and cavosurface margins.* For indirect restorations (those requiring the making of an impression and fabrication of a stone duplicate of the preparation), finishing involves making the walls relatively smooth. For direct and indirect restorations not utilizing bonding, finishing involves removing any unsupported, weak, or fragile enamel and making the cavosurface margin smooth and continuous to facilitate finishing of restoration margins. For bonded resin composite restorations, enamel that is not supported by dentin and is not going to be exposed to significant occlusal loading is frequently allowed to remain in place and is reinforced by bonding to its internal surface.

7. *Clean the preparation.* Black referred to this step as "performing the toilet of the cavity." It includes washing or scrubbing away any debris in the preparation and drying the preparation. Afterward, the cavity is inspected for any remaining debris, fragile enamel, and demineralized tooth structure.

Instrumentation

Hand Instruments

Black[2] organized not only the classification of cavity preparations and their parts, but the naming and numbering of hand instruments. *Cutting instruments*, which he also called *excavators*, were to be used in shaping the tooth preparation. All other hand instruments are grouped into the noncutting category.

Metals

For many years, carbon steel was the primary material used in hand instruments for operative dentistry because carbon steels were harder and maintained sharpness better than stainless steels. Stainless steels are now the preferred materials for hand instruments, because all instruments must be sterilized with steam or dry heat between patients and because the properties of stainless steels have improved. There are literally hundreds of formulas for stainless steels,[10] all incorporating a significant amount of chromium, some carbon, and iron. Chromium imparts corrosion resistance and brightness to the metal; carbon imparts hardness.

Cutting Instruments

Before rotating instruments were available, dentists could cut well-shaped cavity preparations using sharp hand instruments alone. The process was slow. The advent of the dental handpiece in 1871,[11] first attached to a foot-operated engine, allowed increased speed of tooth preparation. Most tooth preparation today is accomplished with rotary instruments, but hand cutting instruments are still important for finishing many tooth preparations. Few preparations involving a proximal surface can be properly completed without the use of hand cutting instruments. It is crucial that hand instruments used for cutting tooth structure or carving restorative materials be sharp.

Design. Hand cutting instruments are composed of three parts: *handle* (or *shaft*), *shank*, and *blade*[2] (Fig 6-15). The primary cutting edge of a cutting instrument is at the end of the blade (called the *working end*), but the sides of the blade are usually beveled and also may be used for cutting tooth structure (Fig 6-16). The shank joins the blade to the handle of the instrument and is angled to keep the working end of the blade within 2.0 to 3.0 mm of the axis of the handle (Fig 6-17). This angulation is intended to provide balance, so that when force is exerted on the instrument it is not as likely to rotate, decreasing the effectiveness of the blade and possibly causing damage to the tooth. Figure 6-17a illustrates an instrument that has a single angle at the junction of the blade and the shank. Because the working end of the blade is not aligned with the handle, the instrument is said to be out of balance. Such an instrument may still be useful in tooth preparation. Its blade will usually be relatively short, and it will usually be used with minimal force. Figure 6-17b shows a shank that has two angles to bring the cutting edge into near alignment with the long axis of the handle to provide balance.

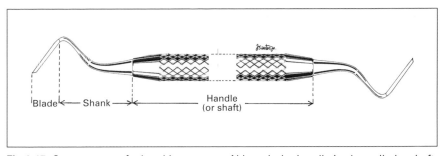

Fig 6-15 Components of a hand instrument. Although the handle is also called a shaft, that designation is little used.

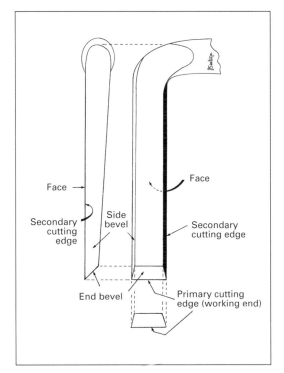

Fig 6-16 Blade bevels. Most hand cutting instruments not only have a bevel on the end of the blade but also have bevels on the sides. Although most of the work of a hand cutting instrument is accomplished with the end of the blade, the sides may also be used to plane walls and margins. (In the drawing on the right, the blade is lying face down.)

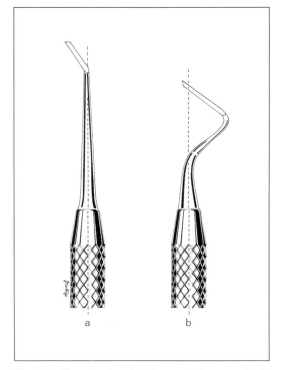

Fig 6-17 The shanks of instruments have multiple angles to keep the working end of the instrument within 2.0 to 3.0 mm of the long axis of the handle. (a) The working end of this instrument is not close to the long axis of the handle, and the instrument is, therefore, not balanced. (b) The shank of this instrument has two angles in it so that the working end is brought near to (within 2.0 mm) the long axis of the handle; this provides balance for the instrument to facilitate control of the instrument during the application of force. The instrument is said to be contra-angled.

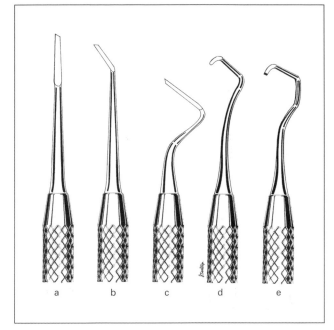

Fig 6-18 Instruments classified by the number of angles in the shank: (a) straight; (b) monangle; (c) binangle; (d) triple-angle; (e) quadrangle.

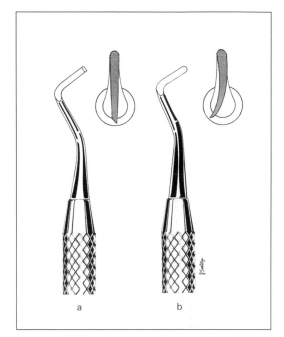

Fig 6-19 (a) Binangle hatchet. (b) Binangle spoon. A double-ended hatchet or spoon would have a left-cutting end and a right-cutting end (see Fig 6-20).

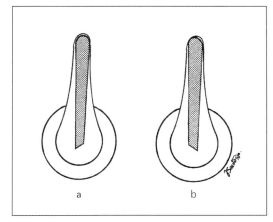

Fig 6-20 End view of binangle hatchets, paired: (a) right-cutting; (b) left-cutting. A double-ended binangle hatchet has left-cutting and right-cutting ends.

Fig 6-21 Monangle hatchets (left-cutting).

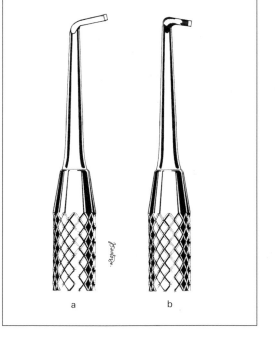

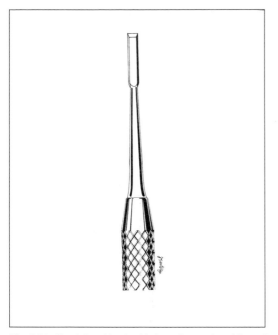

Fig 6-22 Straight chisel with bevels on the sides of the blade, to give secondary cutting edges, as well as on the end (primary cutting edge).

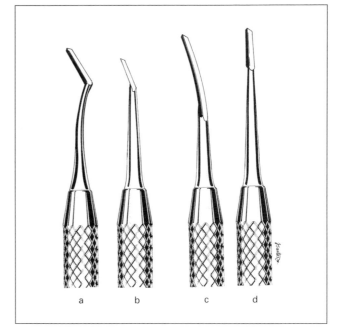

a   b   c   d

Fig 6-23 Chisels: (a) binangle; (b) monangle; (c) Wedelstaedt; (d) straight. The blades for a, c, and d are slightly rotated to visualize the face, as well as the side bevel.

Nomenclature. The terminology organized by Black[2] in the early part of the last century is still used today with minor modifications. Most names Black assigned to cutting instruments were based on the appearance of the instrument, such as *hatchet, hoe, spoon,* and *chisel.* For an instrument that did not have the appearance of a commonly used item, Black based the name on the intended use, for example, *gingival margin trimmer.* Black called all cutting instruments used for tooth preparation *excavators,* and he referred to instruments as *hatchet excavators, spoon excavators,* etc. The term *excavator* is still applicable, but, in the day-to-day language of operative dentistry, it is little used. In catalogs of instruments, however, cutting instruments are often indexed as excavators.

Black combined the name of each instrument with a designation of the number of angles in the shank of the instrument. Shanks may be *straight, monangle* (one angle), *binangle* (two angles), *triple-angle* (three angles), or *quadrangle* (four angles) (Fig 6-18). The term *contra-angled* refers to a shank in which two or more angles are necessary to bring the working end into near alignment with (within 2.0 to 3.0 mm) the axis of the handle (see Fig 6-17b).

Hatchet. In a *hatchet* (also called an *enamel hatchet*), the blade and cutting edge are on a plane with the long axis of the handle; the shank has one or more angles (Figs 6-18e, 6-19a, 6-20, and 6-21). The

face (see Fig 6-16) of the blade of the hatchet will be directed either to the left or the right in relation to the handle, and the instrument is usually supplied in a double-ended form. Therefore, there are left-cutting and right-cutting ends of the double-ended hatchet.

Chisel. A *chisel* has a blade that is either aligned with the handle (Figs 6-18a, 6-22, and 6-23d), slightly angled (Figs 6-18b, 6-23a, and 6-23b), or curved (Fig 6-23c) from the long axis of the handle, with the working end at a right angle to the handle.

Hoe. A *hoe* has a cutting edge that is at a right angle to the handle, like that of a chisel. However, its blade has a greater angle from the long axis of the handle than does that of the chisel; its shank also has one or more angles (Figs 6-15, 6-18c, and 6-24). A general guideline for distinguishing between a hoe and a chisel will be given later in the chapter.

Spoon. The blade of a *spoon* is curved, and the cutting edge at the end of the blade is in the form of a semicircle (Figs 6-19b and 6-25b); this gives the instrument an outer convexity and an inner concavity that make it look somewhat like a spoon. Like the hatchet, the spoon has a cutting edge at the end of its blade that is parallel to the handle of the instrument; therefore, there are left-cutting and right-cutting spoons. The shank of some spoons holds a small circular, or disk-shaped, blade at its end, and the cutting

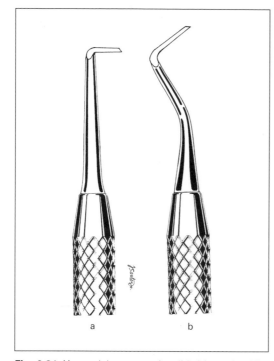

Fig 6-24 Hoes: (a) monangle; (b) binangle. The blade of a hoe has an angle from the long axis of the handle of greater than 12.5 centigrades; in contrast, the blade of a chisel will have an angle from the long axis of the handle of 12.5 centigrades or less.

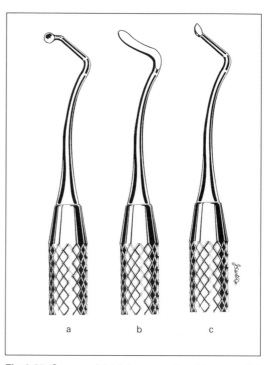

Fig 6-25 Spoons: (a) triple-angle discoid spoon; (b) binangle spoon (or regular spoon or banana spoon); (c) binangle discoid spoon. Spoons are used in tooth preparation for removing (or "spooning out") carious dentin.

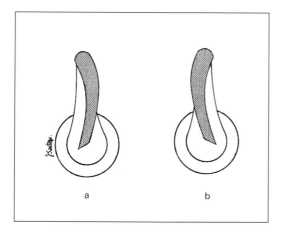

Fig 6-26 End view of gingival margin trimmers, paired: (a) right-cutting, (b) left-cutting. A double-ended gingival margin trimmer has both left-cutting and right-cutting ends, but there must be two double-ended gingival margin trimmers to complete a set, one double-ended mesial gingival margin trimmer and one double-ended distal gingival margin trimmer.

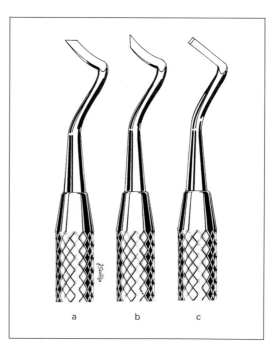

Fig 6-27 (a) Left-cutting mesial gingival margin trimmer. (b) Left-cutting distal gingival margin trimmer. (c) Right-cutting binangle hatchet.

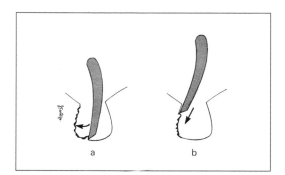

Fig 6-28 (a) Gingival margin trimmer being used in a proximal box of a Class 2 preparation with a horizontal (left or right) stroke to scrape (plane) a gingival wall and margin. (b) Gingival margin trimmer being used with a vertical, or chopping, stroke to plane a facial or lingual wall and margin. A hatchet could be used in a similar way.

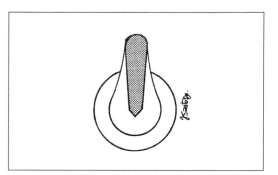

Fig 6-29 Bi-beveled cutting edge, useful in placing retention points in some direct gold (gold foil) preparations, has little use in any of the preparations described in this book.

edge extends around the disk except for its junction with the shank; these are called *discoid spoons* (Figs 6-25a and 6-25c).

Gingival margin trimmer. A *gingival margin trimmer* is similar to an enamel hatchet, except that the blade is curved, and the bevel for the cutting edge at the end of the blade is always on the outside of the curve; the face of the instrument is on the inside of the curve (Figs 6-26 and 6-27). Gingival margin trimmers, like hatchets and spoons, come in pairs (left cutting and right cutting) (Fig 6-26), but there are also mesial gingival margin trimmers and distal gingival margin trimmers (Fig 6-27). Thus, a set of gingival margin trimmers is composed of four instruments: left-cutting and right-cutting mesial gingival margin trimmers, and left-cutting and right-cutting distal gingival margin trimmers. Because these are usually double-ended instruments, one instrument is a mesial gingival margin trimmer (with left- and right-cutting ends), and the other is a distal gingival margin trimmer (with left- and right-cutting ends). Figure 6-27a illustrates a mesial left-cutting gingival margin trimmer. Figure 6-27b illustrates a distal left-cutting gingival margin trimmer. Contrasted with these is a right-cutting hatchet (Fig 6-27c). Gingival margin trimmers have many uses in addition to trimming gingival margins (Fig 6-28).

Off-angle hatchet. Black's instrument names apply to instruments that have cutting edges that are either parallel or at a right angle to the handle. Instruments have been developed that have blades rotated 45 degrees from the plane of the long axis of the handle; these are called *off-angle hatchets*.

Usage. Hand cutting instruments are, for the most part, made in pairs, and, as with the gingival margin trimmers, most instruments used today are double-ended and will have one of the pair on each end (see Figs 6-15, 6-20, and 6-26). A cutting instrument may be used with horizontal strokes, in which the long axis of the blade is directed at between 45 and 90 degrees to the surface being planed or scraped (Fig 6-28a), or with vertical or chopping strokes, in which the blade is nearly parallel to the wall or margin being planed (Fig 6-28b). For horizontal (scraping) or vertical (chopping) strokes, the acute angle of the cutting edge is intended to be used. The acute angle is the junction of the face of the blade with the bevel; in other words, the bevel is on the back of the blade, not the face of the blade. A double-ended hatchet, gingival margin trimmer, or spoon will have one end that is designated as right-cutting and one that is designated as left-cutting. In a double-ended hoe, in addition to allowing vertical or chopping strokes, one end is intended for pushing strokes (beveled end) and the other is intended for pulling strokes (contrabeveled end).

The cutting edges of most hand cutting instruments used today are single beveled, as are all of those described here (see Fig 6-16). Double-beveled, or bi-beveled, cutting edges are also available but have limited application in contemporary operative dentistry (Fig 6-29). These instruments usually have narrow blades and are used for tasks such as adding mechanical retention points in areas of preparations that cannot be reached by a bur.

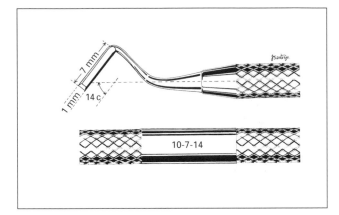

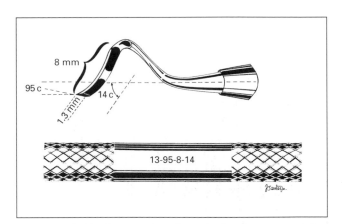

Fig 6-30 Black's three-number formula for instruments that have a primary cutting edge (working end) that is at a right angle (90 degrees) to the long axis of the blade: The first number is the width of the blade in tenths of a millimeter; the second number is the length of the blade in millimeters; and the third number is the blade angle, the angle the blade makes with the long axis of the handle, in centigrades. The complete name of the instrument illustrated would be binangle hatchet, 10-7-14. The formula would be the same if the blade were rotated 90 degrees on the shank to form a hoe, but the name would be different. Assuming the instrument illustrated is double-ended, the right-cutting end is shown.

Fig 6-31 Black's four-number formula for instruments that have a primary cutting edge (working end) that is not at a right angle to the long axis of the blade: The first number is the width of the blade in tenths of a millimeter; the second number is the cutting edge angle, the angle the primary cutting edge makes with the long axis of the handle, in centigrades; the third number is the length of the blade in millimeters; and the fourth number is the blade angle, the angle the blade makes with the long axis of the handle, in centigrades. Illustrated is the right-cutting end of a distal gingival margin trimmer, 13-95-8-14.

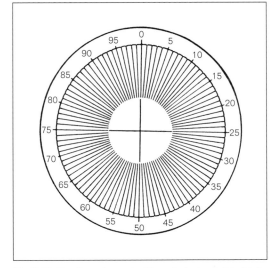

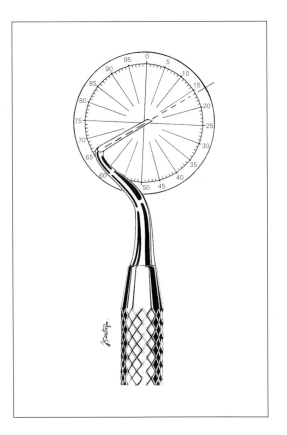

Fig 6-32 Centigrade scale. The circle is divided into 100 units.

Fig 6-33 Centigrade scale inset to show angulation indicator of 16.0 centigrades for the blade angle of this hoe (three-number formula). The vertical axis (0.0 centigrades) is the axis of the instrument's handle. If the blade of the instrument were 1.4 mm wide and 10.0 mm long, the formula for the instrument would be 14-10-16.

Numeric formulas. The configuration of the shanks combined with the appearance of the blade or the use of the instrument produces names such as *straight chisel, monangle chisel, binangle hoe,* and *triple-angle hatchet.* These are descriptive terms, but they are imprecise because they do not indicate sizes or angles. For more complete identification of hand cutting instruments, Black[2] developed a system of assigning numeric formulas to instruments (Figs 6-30 and 6-31). The formulas make use of the metric system. For designating the degree of angulation, centigrades are used. Centigrades are based on a circle divided into 100 units (Fig 6-32), as opposed to the 360-degree circle ordinarily used to designate angles. In a centigrade circle, a right angle has 25.0 centigrades.

Three-number formula. For instruments in which the primary cutting edge (at the end of the blade) is at a right angle to the long axis of the blade, Black developed a formula that has three numbers (Fig 6-30). The first number is the width of the blade in tenths of a millimeter; the second is the length of the blade in millimeters, and the third is the angle (in centigrades) made by the long axis of the blade and the long axis of the handle (Fig 6-33).

Four-number formula. For instruments in which the cutting edge at the end of the blade is not at a right angle to the long axis of the blade, such as the gingival margin trimmers, Black designed a four number formula (Fig 6-31). The first number is the width of the blade in tenths of a millimeter; the second number is the angle (in centigrades) that the primary cutting edge (working end) makes with the axis of the handle (Fig 6-34); the third number is the length of the blade in millimeters; and the fourth number is the angle (in centigrades) that the long axis of the blade makes with the handle. In margin trimmers, a cutting edge angle of greater than 90 centigrades is intended for distal gingival margins (Fig 6-31); an angle of 85 centigrades or less is intended for mesial gingival margins.

Chisel versus hoe. Although Black defined a chisel as having a blade that is aligned with the handle or slightly curved from it, terminology has evolved so that a chisel may also have a blade that is angled from the handle up to 12.5 centigrades.[5] A chisel with a blade angled more than 3 or 4 centigrades from the axis of the handle must be binangle for the instrument to be balanced.

If the blade is angled more than 12.5 centigrades, the instrument is defined as a hoe. In a curved or angled chisel or a hoe, a blade with its primary cutting edge (and its face) on the side of the blade toward the

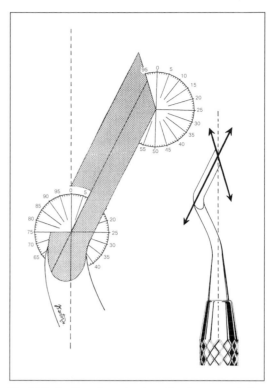

Fig 6-34 Centigrade scales inset to show angulation indicators of 7.0 centigrades for the blade angle and 95.0 centigrades for the cutting edge angle of this gingival margin trimmer (four-number formula). The vertical axis (0.0 centigrades) is the axis of the instrument's handle. If the blade were 1.5 mm wide and 10.0 mm long, the formula for the instrument would be 15-95-10-7.

handle is said to be *beveled* (see Figs 6-23a to 6-23c); a blade with its primary cutting edge (and its face) on the side of the blade away from the handle is said to be *contrabeveled* (see Fig 6-18c).

Recommended instrument kit. Black recommended a long set of 96 cutting instruments, a university set of 44 cutting instruments, or a short set of 25 cutting instruments. Because bonding technology and high-speed handpieces were not available, the dental materials of the time were more limited, and a primary restorative material was direct gold; the longevity of restorations depended on the retention and resistance form developed with hand cutting instruments.

With access to advanced materials and technology, current use of hand cutting instruments is greatly diminished. The kit recommended in this chapter has only 12 hand cutting instruments (six double-ended instruments). Because it is now recognized that there is no need to plane walls and floors of cavity prepara-

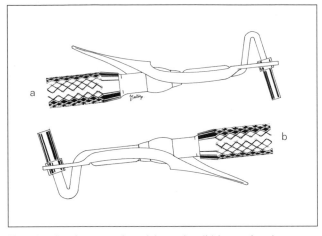

Fig 6-35 Amalgam carriers: (a) regular; (b) large. Amalgam carriers are usually supplied as double-ended instruments. They are available in several different diameters; for example, mini is 1.5 mm; regular (medium) is 2.0 mm; large is 2.5 mm; and jumbo is 3.0 to 3.5 mm. These are the approximate inside diameters of the cylinders of amalgam carriers and may vary slightly from manufacturer to manufacturer.

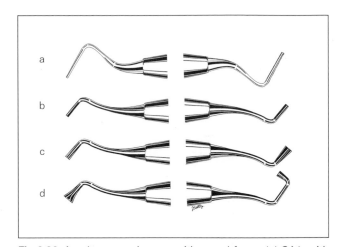

Fig 6-36 Amalgam condensers with round faces: (a) SA1, with 0.5- and 0.6-mm diameter faces; (b) SA2 with 0.7- and 1.0-mm faces; (c) SA3 with 1.5- and 2.0-mm faces; (d) SA4, with a 2.5-mm face on the binangle end and a 1.5-mm face on the triple-angle or back-action end.

tions to smoothness with hand instruments for a restoration to perform well, hand cutting instruments play only a small, albeit important, part in cavity preparation. If burs alone were used for shaping proximal preparations, excessive sound tooth structure would have to be removed from the tooth being restored or the bur would damage the adjacent tooth. Hand cutting instruments enable the dentist to shape and refine small proximal boxes without damaging adjacent teeth.

Hatchets, hoes, chisels, and gingival margin trimmers have straight cutting edges and are designed to plane enamel and dentinal walls and margins in shaping cavity preparations, especially in areas of the preparation that cannot be reached with a bur. Spoons, on the other hand, have rounded cutting edges; their intended use is the removal of carious dentin. Although slowly rotating round burs are most useful in removing carious dentin, a spoon gives more tactile sensation and is preferred by many operators.

Noncutting Instruments

Non–tooth-cutting hand instruments are similar in appearance to cutting instruments, except that the blade used for tooth preparation is replaced with a part that has a totally different use. In noncutting instruments such as burnishers and amalgam condensers, the blade is replaced by a *nib* or *point*.[2] The flat end of the nib of a condenser is called the *face*.

Amalgam carvers have carving blades instead of tooth-cutting blades.

Condensers, carvers, and burnishers are used to place dental amalgam and, to a certain extent, resin composite restorative materials. Plastic filling instruments are used to place resin composite materials, provisional restorative materials, and sometimes cavity-basing materials into tooth preparations. Spatulas are necessary for mixing cavity-lining and cavity-basing materials, provisional restorative materials, and cements for luting inlays, onlays, and crowns.

Amalgam carriers. For silver amalgam restorations, amalgam is placed into the preparation with an *amalgam carrier*, an instrument with a hollow cylinder that is filled with amalgam (Fig 6-35). A plunger operated with a finger lever pushes the amalgam out of the carrier into the preparation. For some of the more viscous resin composite materials, carriers have been fitted with plastic cylinders to reduce sticking of the resin material to the internal walls of the cylinder.

Condensers. *Amalgam condensers* are used to compress the amalgam into all areas of the preparation. The working ends, or nibs, of condensers may be any shape, but usually they are round with flat ends (faces). Figure 6-36 shows four round condensers of different sizes and configurations. Other commonly used condenser nibs are triangular, rectangular, or

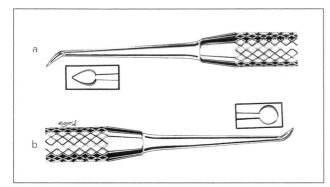

Fig 6-37a Cleoid-discoid carver: (a) cleoid end; (b) discoid end. This type of carver is a double-ended instrument. *Cleoid* means claw shaped. Both shapes are useful in carving occlusal surfaces of amalgam restorations. The point of the cleoid carver is used to carve the bases of grooves in the occlusal amalgam, and the tip is usually very slightly rounded so that grooves are not sharp.

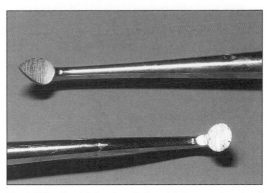

Fig 6-37b Cleoid *(top)* and discoid *(bottom)* ends of the cleoid-discoid carver.

diamond shaped. Amalgam is condensed by pushing the condenser directly into the preparation and confining the amalgam between the condenser face and the preparation floor through vertical pressure (vertical condensation). The amalgam is condensed against the vertical walls of the preparation (lateral condensation) by angling the nib and using the end for condensation, or by lateral, or side-to-side, movements of the condenser, using the sides of the nib to condense the amalgam.

The condensation pressure applied to the amalgam with a condenser depends on the size of the face and the amount of force used by the operator. For small condensers, such as the SA1 condenser (Fig 6-36a), little force is needed. The nibs of the SA1 condenser are 0.5 and 0.6 mm in diameter. For larger condensers, such as the SA3 (Fig 6-36c), with nib diameters of 1.5 and 2.0 mm, a significant amount of force (6 to 8 lbs) gives optimum condensation.

Amalgam condensers may also be used to place resin composite materials. The resin material is not actually condensed, however, but pushed or patted into all areas of the preparation with the largest condenser face that will fit into the area.

Carvers. Carvers are used to shape amalgam and resin composite (tooth-colored) materials after they have been placed in tooth preparations. Figures 6-37a and 6-37b show the shapes of the blades of a cleoid-dis-

coid carver. Figure 6-38 illustrates six commonly used carvers. In general, when a convex amalgam contour is being carved, a concave-shaped carver facilitates the shaping or carving. Likewise, a convex carver facilitates carving of a concave shape. A convex carver may be used to carve a convex surface; the surface is carved tangentially, with multiple strokes. Whether a carver is used to carve amalgam or resin composite, it is important that the blade be sharp.

The cleoid-discoid (or discoid-cleoid) carvers shown in Figs 6-38a and 6-38b are used primarily for occlusal carving in amalgam restorations. The Walls No. 3 carver (Fig 6-38c) is useful for carving occlusal surfaces; the end that is shaped like a hoe is also useful for shaping cusps and for carving facial and lingual surfaces of large amalgam restorations. The Hollenback No. ½ carver (Fig 6-38d) is useful for occlusal, proximal, and axial (facial and lingual) surfaces; several larger Hollenback carvers, with the same general shape, are also available. The interproximal carver (IPC) (Fig 6-38e) has very thin blades and is extremely valuable for carving proximal amalgam surfaces near the interproximal contact area. The No. 14L carver (Fig 6-38f) can be used for interproximal areas, or it may be used for carving convex facial and lingual surfaces of very large amalgam restorations. The No. 14L carver has a very strong, hollow-ground triangular blade, so it can be used to remove amalgam overhangs from completely set amalgam.

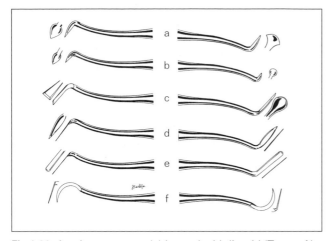

Fig 6-38 Amalgam carvers: (a) large cleoid-discoid (Tanner No. 5 [5T]) carver; (b) small cleoid-discoid (UWD5) carver; (c) Walls No. 3 carver; (d) Hollenback No. ½ carver; (e) interproximal carver (IPC); (f) No. 14L sickle-shaped carver.

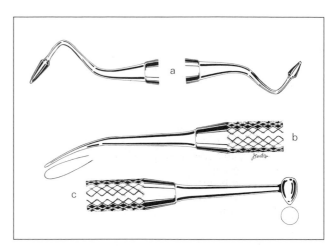

Fig 6-39 Burnishers: (a) PKT3 (rounded cone-shaped) burnisher, designed by Peter K. Thomas as a waxing instrument but useful in placing direct restorations as well; its rounded end and cone shape allow it to serve most functions that a small ball-shaped burnisher would serve, plus others; (b) beavertail (No. 2) burnisher; (c) football or ovoid (No. 30) burnisher. The ovoid burnisher, available in various sizes (eg, 28, 29, and 31), can be used for final condensation of amalgam and the initial shaping of the occlusal anatomy in amalgam. The beavertail and ovoid burnishers are useful for burnishing margins of cast-gold restorations.

Although most of the shaping of resin composite restorations should be completed before the material is polymerized, several amalgam carvers are also useful for carving resin composite. The discoid carvers are especially useful for lingual concavities of anterior teeth; cleoid and discoid carvers and the hoe-shaped end of the Walls No. 3 carver are useful for occlusal surfaces of posterior resin composite restorations. Another carver very useful for resin composite restorations is a disposable scalpel blade (No. 12 or No. 12b blade) mounted in a scalpel handle.

Burnishers. Burnishers are used for several functions. The word *burnish* is defined as "to make shiny or lustrous, especially by rubbing; to polish"; and "to rub (a material) with a tool for compacting or smoothing or for turning an edge."[13] Burnishing is probably used in all of those ways in dentistry. Two frequently used double-ended burnishers are illustrated in Fig 6-39.

One use of burnishers is to shape metal matrix bands so that they impart more desirable contours to restorations. Large burnishers are used with considerable force to pinch off freshly condensed amalgam at the margins, or, in other words, to impart some condensation and to begin shaping the occlusal surfaces of amalgam restorations. After the amalgam has been

carved, a burnisher may be used with a gentle rubbing motion to smooth the surface. The PKT3 (P. K. Thomas No. 3) burnisher (Fig 6-39a) is also useful for sculpting occlusal anatomy in posterior resin composite restorations prior to polymerization of the resin.

Burnishers are used to "bend" cast gold near the margin to narrow the gap between the gold and the tooth. This closing of a marginal gap is best accomplished with a narrow burnisher, such as the side of a beavertail burnisher, used with heavy force in strokes parallel to the margin but about 1.0 or 1.5 mm away from it. If burnishing is accomplished directly on a thin gold margin, the gold can be bent severely and may break.

Plastic instruments. Plastic instruments (or plastic filling instruments) are so named because they were originally designed to use with plastic restorative materials, such as the silicates and acrylic resins used in the middle of the 20th century. They are currently used to carry and shape tooth-colored restorative materials such as resin composites and glass-ionomer restorative materials.

A commonly used plastic instrument is the No. 1-2 (Fig 6-40a). The double-ended instrument has a nib or blade on each end, one at a 90-degree angle to the other. Other double-ended plastic instruments have a blade-type nib on one end and a condenser nib on the

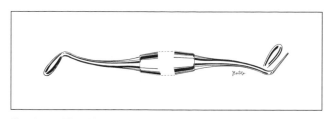

Fig 6-40a The No. 1-2 plastic instrument, made of stainless steel, is useful for placing a rubber dam, placing and shaping resin composite and other tooth-colored restorative materials, and packing gingival retraction cord around a crown or abutment preparation before an impression is made. Some cord-packing instruments are similar to the No. 1-2 plastic instrument but have serrated ends to provide better control of the cord.

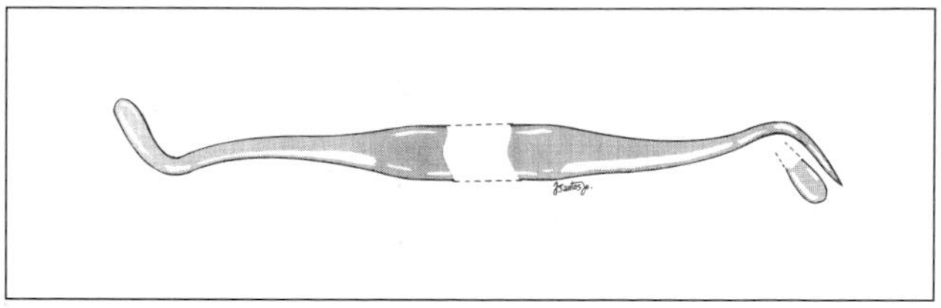

Fig 6-40b A plastic instrument made of hard plastic, rather than metal, is preferred by some operators for placing resin composites.

other. The bladed plastic instruments have many uses in operative dentistry in addition to carrying and contouring restorative materials. The interproximal carver (Fig 6-38e), for instance, is preferred by some operators for packing knitted cord and placing and shaping resin composite.

These instruments are now available in both hard plastic and metal; the original rationale for using an instrument made of plastic (Fig 6-40b) was to eliminate abrasion of metal by the quartz in resin composites, which caused grayness in the tooth-colored material. Because of changes in the inorganic fillers used in today's resin composites, the problem of metal abrasion and graying has been eliminated; thus, a metal instrument functions well to carry and shape resin composite.

Cement spatulas. A variety of materials in operative dentistry require mixing, some on a glass slab, others on a paper pad. Several spatulas are available, and they vary in size and thickness (Fig 6-41). The larger cement spatulas were originally designed for mixing luting cements and the smaller spatulas for cavity liners, but with the advent of resin luting cements, the smaller spatulas are frequently used for mixing small amounts of those materials. The thinner spatulas are flexible; the thicker ones are rigid. Selection of a rigid or flexible cement spatula is dependent on the desired viscosity of the cement and personal preference.

Sharpening of Hand Instruments

To assess sharpness, the user of the instrument should look at the cutting edge in bright light; the presence of a "glint" indicates that the edge is dull or rounded

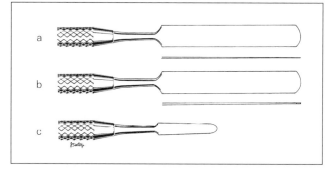

Fig 6-41 Spatulas. (a) No. 24, a flexible spatula, is used for luting cements such as zinc phosphate and glass ionomer. (b) No. 24A is thicker, for more rigidity. (c) No. 313 is used for cavity liners, such as the calcium hydroxide liners.

(Figs 6-42a and 6-42b). Alternatively, the dentist can pull the instrument across hard plastic, such as the handle of a plastic mouth mirror or an evacuator tip. A dull blade will slide across the plastic; a sharp blade will cut into the surface, stopping movement. A specially made, sterilizable, sharpness-testing stick is also available (Figs 6-43a and 6-43b) (Dalron Test Stick, Thompson Dental).

Sharpening is performed in different ways for different hand instruments. When chisels, hatchets, hoes, and margin trimmers are sharpened, the cutting-edge bevel is placed flat against a flat stone, which is on a stable surface, and the instrument is pushed or pulled so that the acute cutting angle is moved forward, with fairly heavy force on the forward stroke, and with little or no force on the back stroke (Figs 6-44 and 6-45). Usually, unless the instrument has been

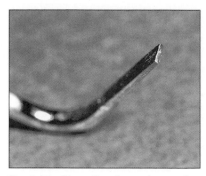

Fig 6-42a The glint from the cutting edge of this hoe indicates that the blade is quite dull.

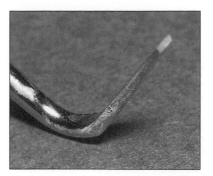

Fig 6-42b After sharpening, no glint is noticeable.

Figs 6-43a and 6-43b The sharpness-testing stick is a hard plastic stick used for testing the sharpness of instruments. For testing sharpness, the blade should be applied to the stick at an angle that is similar to that applied during use and pulled or pushed in a direction that is similar to the direction of its intended use.

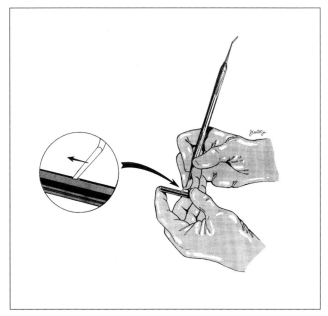

Fig 6-43a Testing the sharpness of a monangle chisel.

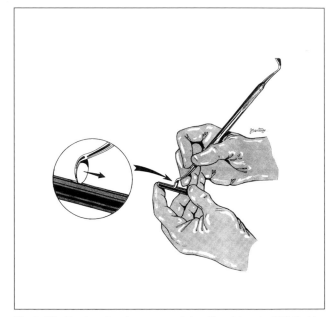

Fig 6-43b Testing the sharpness of the discoid end of Walls No. 3 carver.

badly neglected, only two or three forward strokes are required. Because the bevels of these instruments should usually make a 45-degree angle with the face of the blade, the blade should make a 45-degree angle with the surface of the sharpening stone (Figs 6-45 and 6-46).

When spoons, discoid carvers, and cleoid carvers are sharpened, the instrument is rotated as the blade is advanced on the flat stone (Fig 6-47). The bevel is

at 45 degrees, or slightly more or less, to the face, and the instrument is advanced on the stone with the bevel against the surface of the stone and the cutting edge of the instrument perpendicular to the path of advancement. When a blade with a rounded edge is being sharpened, the handle cannot be simply twirled to achieve the desired rotation, but must actually be swung in an arc to keep the cutting edge of the blade perpendicular to the direction of the stroke.

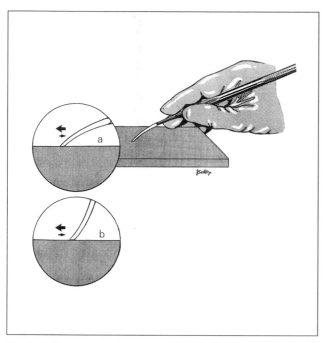

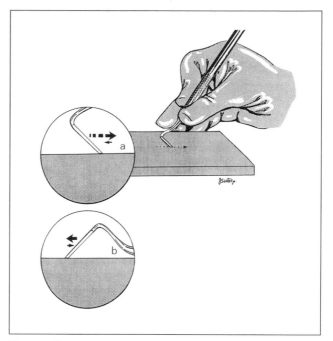

Fig 6-44 Sharpening the two ends of a double-ended Wedel-staedt chisel: (a) sharpening the contrabevel end (inside bevel); (b) sharpening the bevel end (outside bevel). The end bevel (for the primary cutting edge or working end) of each blade is placed flat on the stone; the blade will make a 45-degree angle with the stone. In the primary sharpening stroke, the cutting edge is moved forward. Unless the instrument is very dull, only two or three fairly heavy forward strokes will be necessary to sharpen the cutting edge.

Fig 6-45 Sharpening the two ends of a double-ended binangle hoe: (a) sharpening the bevel end (outside bevel); (b) sharpening the contrabevel end (inside bevel). The primary bevel is always flat against the stone; the face of the blade is up.

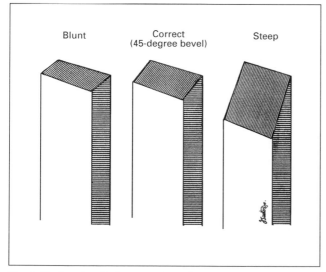

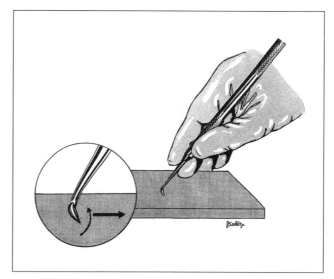

Fig 6-46 Bevels of sharpened cutting instruments. Working end bevels of chisels, hatchets, and hoes, as well as the bevels of amalgam carvers, should be at approximately 45 degrees to the face of the blade. The cutting edge at the left is too blunt, the center blade has a correctly angled cutting edge, and the cutting edge at the right is too acute and will dull rapidly.

Fig 6-47 Sharpening a cleoid carver. The handle is swung in an arc to rotate the blade as the bevel is pulled forward on the stone. This movement is used to keep the cutting edge perpendicular to the direction of the stroke.

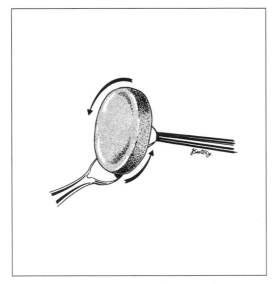

Fig 6-48 Sharpening a discoid spoon with a rotating sharpening stone. A discoid spoon may also be sharpened on a flat stone; the blade is rotated as it is pulled with the cutting edge forward. If the face is ground with a rotating stone, the blade will be thinned.

The discoid carver and spoon may be sharpened with a continuous rotation of the blade; the shank moves clockwise from the 9 o'clock position to the 3 o'clock position in one motion. For the cleoid carver, however, the rotation begins with the shank in the 9 o'clock position and continues clockwise only until the bevel just next to the point is ground (see Fig 6-47); to sharpen the other side of the cleoid, the rotation begins with the shank at the 3 o'clock position and continues counterclockwise to the point.

The blade of a discoid spoon may be sharpened by grinding the face of the blade with a rotating stone (Fig 6-48). This method of sharpening also thins the blade, and care must be taken to avoid rendering the blade so thin that it could easily break.

Sharpening machines are available. A slowly rotating sharpening wheel is employed by one type of machine; an oscillating flat stone, or hone, is used by another. These machines are useful for sharpening instruments between patients and before sterilization.

When instruments are sharpened during an operative procedure, they should be sharpened with a sterile stone. When a stone is sterilized, it should not have oil in or on it, because the oil may thicken during sterilization and form a shellaclike coating that will prevent the abrasion needed for sharpening. A good

substitute for oil is water. Stones lubricated with water should be washed well or cleaned in an ultrasonic cleaner after use to remove the metal filings prior to sterilization. A flat, white Arkansas stone or fine synthetic sharpening stone should be made a part of the operative dentistry instrument kit so that it is available during each procedure.

Mirrors, Explorers, Periodontal Probes, and Forceps

Mirrors, explorers, periodontal probes, and forceps are basic instruments that will be needed during each appointment for diagnosis or treatment.

Mirrors. For every procedure performed in the mouth, the dentist must have clear and distinct vision of the field. Wherever possible, the field should be viewed with direct vision. When needed, the mouth mirror allows the operator to visualize areas of the mouth that he or she would not otherwise be able to see. It also allows the operator to maintain a body position that will reduce health problems associated with poor posture.

Almost as important as its allowing indirect visualization of obscure areas of the mouth is the mirror's function as a reflector of light into the area being examined or treated. A mirror that is positioned properly allows the operator to visualize the field of operation in the mirror and, at the same time, reflects the operating light into that area. To accomplish this, the light should be positioned behind and just to the side of the operator's head.

The mouth mirror can also serve as a retractor of soft tissue (tongue, cheeks, or lips) to aid access and visualization.

For clarity of vision, the reflective surface of the mirror should be on the surface of the glass. This type of mirror is called a front-surface mirror (Fig 6-49a). Mouth mirrors are usually round and come in a variety of sizes (Fig 6-49b). The most widely used sizes for adults are the No. 4 and No. 5. For constricted areas in posterior regions of the mouth, when a rubber dam is in place, a smaller mirror, such as a No. 2, is helpful.

Explorers. Explorers are pointed instruments used to feel tooth surfaces for irregularities and to determine the hardness of exposed dentin. The explorer that is used most often is the shepherd's hook, or No. 23, explorer (Fig 6-50a). Another useful shape is a cowhorn explorer, which provides improved access for exploring proximal surfaces (Fig 6-50b). The No. 17 explorer is also useful in proximal areas (Fig 6-50c).

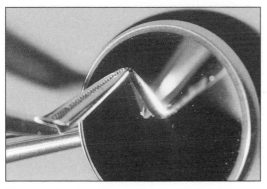

Fig 6-49a Front-surface mirror. Any object touching the mirror, such as the tips of the cotton forceps, will appear to be touching itself.

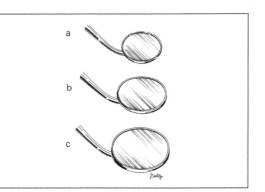

Fig 6-49b Mouth mirrors: (a) No. 2 (⅞-inch diameter); (b) No. 4 (⅞-inch diameter); (c) No. 5 (¹⁵⁄₁₆-inch diameter).

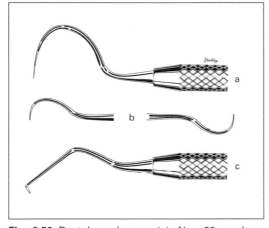

Fig 6-50 Dental explorers: (a) No. 23 explorer (shepherd's hook); (b) 3CH explorer (cowhorn or pigtail); (c) No. 17 explorer.

Fig 6-51 Periodontal probes: (a) QOW probe (Michigan O probe with Williams markings); (b) PCP12 probe (Marquis markings); (c) PSR (periodontal screening and recording) probe.

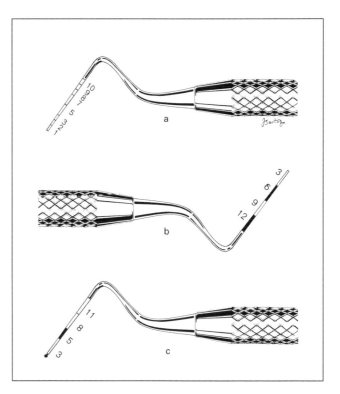

Periodontal probes. Periodontal probes are designed to detect and measure the depth of periodontal pockets. In operative dentistry, they are also used to determine dimensions of instruments and of various features of preparations or restorations. There are many periodontal probe designs; the differences are in the diameters, the position of the millimeter markings, the configuration of the markings (eg, whether they are notched or painted), and the design of the tip. Three commonly used probes are illustrated in Fig 6-51.

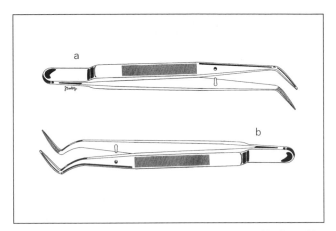

Fig 6-52 Cotton forceps: (a) College (No. 17); (b) Meriam (No. 18).

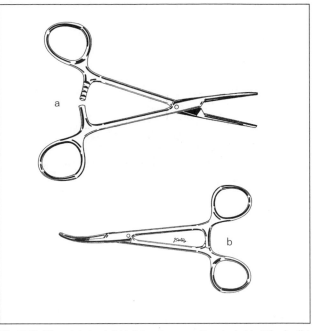

Fig 6-53 Hemostats: (a) Halstead mosquito straight, 6-inch; (b) Halstead mosquito curved, 5-inch.

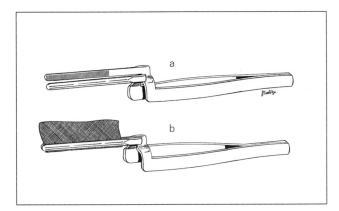

Fig 6-54 Articulating paper forceps: (a) Forceps handles provide a spring that keeps the jaws closed together; they are opened (as shown) by squeezing the handle. (b) The entire length of the piece of articulating paper or tape is supported by the jaws of the forceps.

Forceps. Forceps of various kinds are useful in operative dentistry. Cotton forceps are used for picking up small items, such as cotton pellets (small cotton balls), and carrying them to the mouth (Fig 6-52). Other forceps useful in operative dentistry are hemostats (Fig 6-53). A hemostat locks tightly, so it is often helpful in placing or removing items used to confine amalgam for condensation. Articulating paper forceps are designed to carry an inked tape to the mouth to mark the contacts of teeth in opposing arches during closure (Fig 6-54).

Instrument Grasps

The operator should master two basic instrument grasps, the pen grasp, which provides more flexibility of movement, and the palm or palm-thumb grasp, which provides limited movement but controlled power. Usually only one-handed grasps are used, but occasionally two-handed instrumentation is needed to make refinement of a preparation more precise (Fig 6-55).

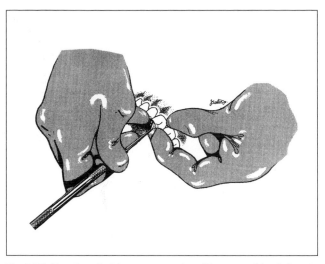

Fig 6-55 Two-handed instrumentation. The use of both hands can make refinement of a preparation more precise. The right hand is thrusting and rotating the instrument while the index finger of the left hand guides and assists the motion of the working end to refine a proximal margin of a Class 2 preparation. A similar dual-handed action is useful for condensing amalgam; it allows increased condensation force to be controlled.

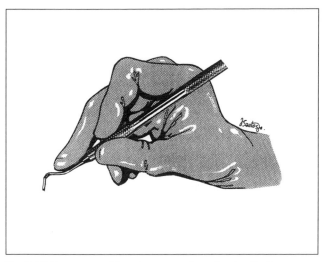

Fig 6-56 Pen grasp. The pen grasp is not actually the way a pen is held for writing. The instrument is held between the index finger and thumb, and the middle finger is placed atop the handle or shank, nearer the working end of the instrument, to provide more force, or thrust, directed toward the working end of the instrument.

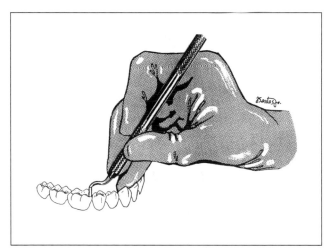

Fig 6-57a Pen grasp used in a chopping (downward) motion. The ring finger is resting on the incisal edges of the anterior teeth. During the use of any instrument in the mouth (with the exception of the mirror), a firm rest must be achieved on teeth or attached gingival tissue.

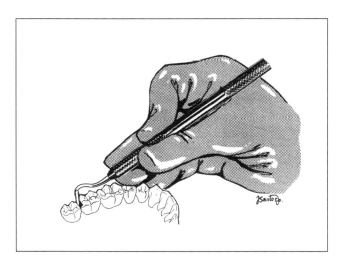

Fig 6-57b Pen grasp as the instrument is used more posteriorly and with a side-to-side or scraping motion. The small finger and ring finger are resting on the facial and occlusal surfaces, respectively.

Pen grasp. This is the most frequently used instrument grasp in operative dentistry. The pen grasp is actually different from the way one would grasp a pen (Fig 6-56); the shaft of the instrument is engaged by the end, not the side, of the middle finger; this provides more finger power. The pen grasp is initiated by placement of the instrument between the thumb and index finger; the middle finger engages the handle or shank of the instrument. The ring finger is braced against the teeth to stabilize instrument movement (Figs 6-57a and 6-57b).

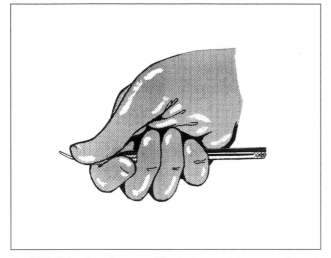

Fig 6-58 Palm-thumb grasp. The instrument is grasped much nearer to its end than in the pen grasp, so that the thumb can be braced against the teeth to provide control during movement of the instrument.

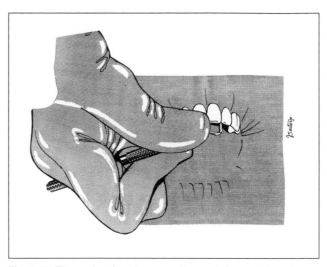

Fig 6-59 The palm-thumb grasp is used frequently when a hand cutting instrument, such as a gingival margin trimmer, is used in Class 3 preparations that have lingual access. The thumb is resting on the incisal edges of the teeth. The palm-thumb grasp is also used frequently with the Wedelstaedt chisel, usually for facial access in posterior and anterior operations, and occasionally for lingual access.

Palm or palm-thumb grasp. In this grasp, the thumb serves as a brace (Fig 6-58). Side-to-side, rotation, or thrusting movements of the instrument by the wrist and fingers are controlled by the thumb, which is firmly in contact with the teeth (Fig 6-59).

Instrument Motions

The following are some of the many motions used with hand instruments:

- *Chopping* (in the direction of the working end of the instrument, or parallel to the long axis of the blade)
- *Pulling* (toward the operator's hand)
- *Pushing* (away from the hand)
- *Rotating*
- *Scraping* (with the blade directed at an angle between 45 and 90 degrees to the surface being scraped and moved side to side or back and forth on the surface)
- *Thrusting* (forcibly pushing against a surface)

Rotating Instruments

Handpieces

In dentistry, two basic types of handpiece, the straight handpiece (Fig 6-60) and the contra-angle handpiece (Fig 6-61), are used. In the straight handpiece, the long axis of the bur is the same as the long axis of the handpiece. The straight handpiece is used more frequently for laboratory work but is occasionally useful clinically.

The primary handpiece used in the mouth is the contra-angle handpiece. As with hand instruments, *contra-angle* indicates that the head of the handpiece is angled first away from, and then back toward, the long axis of the handle. Also as with hand instruments, this contra-angle design is intended to bring the working point (the head of the bur) to within a few millimeters of the long axis of the handle of the contra-angle handpiece to provide balance. Without balance, the handpiece would be unstable and could rotate in the hand with any application of pressure at the working point.

There are two types of contra-angle handpieces, which are classified by their speed potential. Low-speed contra-angle handpieces have a typical free-running speed range of 500 to 15,000 rpm; some are able

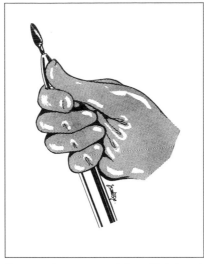

Fig 6-60 Straight handpiece. This handpiece is used occasionally in the mouth, but it is more frequently used extraorally, for tasks such as making adjustments to removable prostheses or adjusting and repolishing a cast-gold or ceramic restoration prior to insertion. The bur installed in this handpiece is a tree-shaped denture bur.

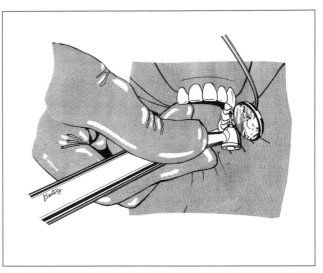

Fig 6-61 Contra-angle handpiece. This is a high-speed contra-angle handpiece, which is used with small-diameter burs for rapid cutting of tooth structure or restorations. A low-speed contra-angle is also useful for removal of carious dentin, with a slowly rotating round bur, and for shaping and polishing with abrasive disks and impregnated rubber polishers. Some operators also prefer the low-speed contra-angle for refining tooth preparations.

to slow to 200 rpm, and others are able to achieve speeds of 35,000 rpm. High-speed handpieces have a free-running speed range greater than 160,000 rpm, and some handpieces attain free-running speeds up to 500,000.[14] In the United States, dentists are accustomed to air-turbine high-speed handpieces; their speeds during tooth preparation are significantly less than their free-running speeds. In Europe, some handpieces powered by an electric motor can achieve free-running speeds of only around 165,000 rpm, but these handpieces are electronically regulated to maintain speed during tooth preparation.[9]

High-speed techniques are generally preferred for cutting enamel and dentin. Penetration through enamel and extension of the cavity outline are more efficient at high speed. Small-diameter burs should be used in the high-speed handpiece. High speed generates considerable heat, even with small-diameter burs, and should be used with water coolants[9] and high-efficiency evacuation. For refining preparations, a high-speed handpiece may be slowed considerably and used with only air coolant and a gentle brushing or painting motion in which each application of the bur to the tooth is brief. This technique allows visualization and prevents overheating.[4]

Low-speed contra-angle handpieces, with round burs rotating very slowly, are used for removal of carious dentin.

There are two types of contra-angle heads for the low-speed handpiece, a friction-grip head and a latch-type head. The shanks of the burs that fit into each of these types of contra-angle head are shown in Fig 6-62. The high-speed handpiece will receive only the friction-grip bur.

Burs

Hand-rotated dental instruments are known to have been used since the early 1700s. The foot engine came into use in dentistry in 1871 and the electric engine in 1872.[11] The most significant advance, which has made present-day high-speed cutting possible, is the tungsten carbide bur, which became available in 1947.[12]

Burs have three major parts, the head, the neck, and the shank (Fig 6-63). For the different types of handpieces or handpiece heads, there are burs with different designs and dimensions (Fig 6-62).

The head of a bur is the portion of the bur that cuts. The cutting action is produced by blades on the head, and the blades are produced by cuts made into the head. The blades of a bur are usually obtuse to

Table 6-1	Shapes and diameters of regular carbide burs used for tooth preparation (US designations*)

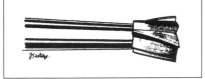

Round

Bur size	1/16	1/8	1/4	1/2	1	2	3	4	5
Diameter (mm)	.30	.40	.50	.60	.80	1.0	1.2	1.4	1.6

Bur size	6	7	8	9	11
Diameter (mm)	1.8	2.1	2.3	2.5	3.1

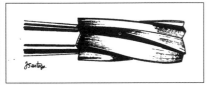

Inverted cone

Bur size	33½	34	35	36	37	39	40
Diameter (mm)	.60	.80	1.0	1.2	1.4	1.8	2.1

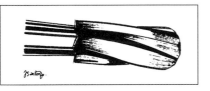

Straight fissure†

Bur size	55½	56	57	58	59	60
Diameter (mm)	.60	.80	1.0	1.2	1.4	1.6

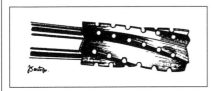

Straight fissure, rounded end (straight dome)†

Bur size	1156	1157	1158
Diameter (mm)	.80	1.0	1.2

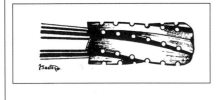

Straight fissure, crosscut†

Bur size	556	557	558	559	560
Diameter (mm)	.80	1.0	1.2	1.4	1.6

Straight fissure, rounded end, crosscut (straight dome crosscut)

Bur size	1556	1557	1558
Diameter (mm)	.80	1.0	1.2

Table 6-1   *continued*

Tapered fissure[†]

Bur size	168	169	170	171
Diameter (mm)	.80	.90	1.0	1.2

Tapered fissure, rounded end (tapered dome)[†]

Bur size	1169	1170	1171
Diameter (mm)	.90	1.0	1.2

Tapered fissure, crosscut[†]

Bur size	699	700	701	702	703
Diameter (mm)	.90	1.0	1.2	1.6	2.1

Pear[†]

Bur size	329	330	331	332
Diameter (mm)	.60	.80	1.0	1.2

Long inverted cone, rounded corners (amalgam preparation)

Bur size	245	246
Diameter (mm)	.80	1.2

End-cutting

Bur size	956	957
Diameter (mm)	.80	1.0

*Adapted from American National Standards Institute/American Dental Association Specification 23 and catalogs of Midwest Dental Products and Brasseler.
[†]Some sizes available with a long head (L).

| Table 6-2 | Shapes and diameters of some of the available 12-bladed carbide finishing burs used for smooth cuts in tooth preparation and for finishing restorations (US designations)* |

Egg

Bur size	7404	7406	7408
Diameter (mm)	1.4	1.8	2.3

Bullet

Bur size	7801	7802	7803
Diameter (mm)	.90	1.0	1.2

Needle

Bur size	7901	7902	7903
Diameter (mm)	.90	1.0	1.2

Round

Bur size	7002	7003	7004	7006
Diameter (mm)	1.0	1.2	1.4	1.8
Bur size	7008	7009	7010	
Diameter (mm)	2.3	2.7	3.1	

Flame

Bur size	7102	7104	7106	7108
Diameter (mm)	1.2	1.4	1.8	2.3

Cone

Bur size	7202	7204	7205	7206
Diameter (mm)	1.0	1.4	1.6	1.8

Table 6-2	*continued*

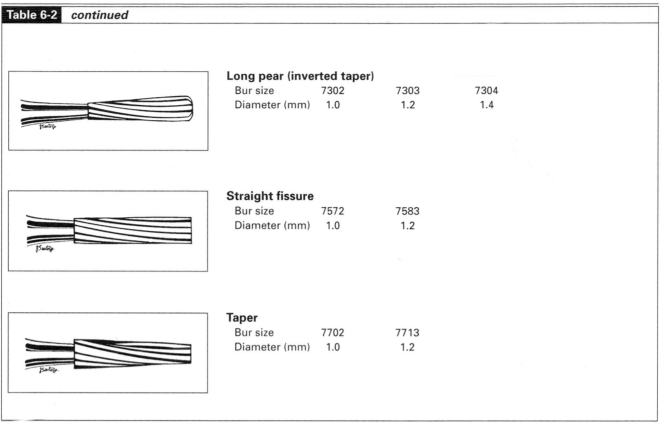

Long pear (inverted taper)

Bur size	7302	7303	7304
Diameter (mm)	1.0	1.2	1.4

Straight fissure

Bur size	7572	7583
Diameter (mm)	1.0	1.2

Taper

Bur size	7702	7713
Diameter (mm)	1.0	1.2

*Adapted from catalogs of Midwest Dental Products and Brasseler.

Air-Abrasion Technology

In the 1940s, an instrument called the Airdent (SS White) was introduced as a means of cavity preparation.[3] Because all restorations placed at that time depended on cavity preparation shape for retention, and as the Airdent did not prepare undercuts in preparations, the technology soon lost favor. When it was reintroduced in the 1980s, it received a greater degree of acceptance because bonded restorations had become routine.[8] Etched enamel and dentin, rather than the shape of the cavity preparation, give retention to many restorations. A large number of air-abrasion units are being marketed for opening of fissures, for some cavity preparations, and to facilitate repair of existing restorations with bonding technology (Figs 6-66a to 66c).

Magnifiers

The quality, and therefore the serviceability and longevity of dental restorations, is dependent on the ability of the operator to see what he or she is doing. One of the primary advantages of the rubber dam in operative dentistry is improvement of the visualization of the operating field (see Chapter 7). Most current contra-angle handpieces have fiberoptic systems by which lights are placed in the contra-angle heads to improve visualization of the operating field.

Magnification devices are extremely helpful in restorative procedures, and some form of magnification is recommended for every dentist providing restorative dentistry services.[6] Available magnification devices run the gamut of effectiveness and expense. Among the finest magnifiers are the telescopes (Figs 6-67a to 6-67c), which are the most expensive. Less expensive loupes are available from several manufacturers (Figs 6-68a to 6-68c).

In choosing a magnification device, the operator is wise to select one that gives a focal distance in the range of 10 to 14 inches. The 2.0- to 4.0-diopter range is recommended.

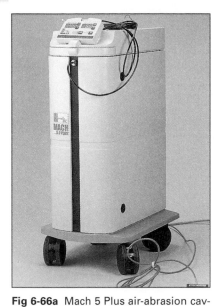

Fig 6-66a Mach 5 Plus air-abrasion cavity preparation unit from Welch Allyn/ Kreativ.

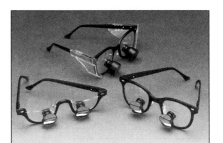

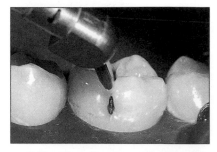

Figs 6-66b and 6-66c Handpiece in use for a small Class 1 cavity preparation for resin composite.

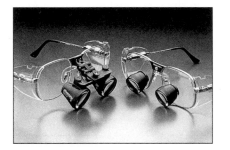

Fig 6-67a Binocular telescopes manufactured by Designs for Vision.

Fig 6-67b Binocular telescopes manufactured by Orascoptic Research.

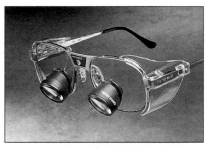

Fig 6-67c Binocular telescope manufactured by SurgiTel Systems, General Scientific Corp.

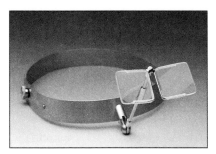

Fig 6-68a Binocular loupes manufactured by Almore International.

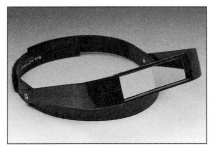

Fig 6-68b Binocular loupes manufactured by Lactona.

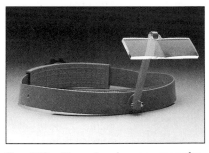

Fig 6-68c Binocular loupes manufactured by Edroy Products.

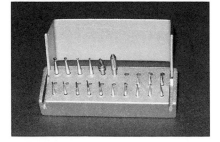

Fig 6-69 Bur block (No. A600, Brasseler), containing the burs listed in the instrument kit recommended in this chapter.

Suggested Operative Dentistry Instrument Kit

A compact assembly of hand instruments that will satisfy most operators' needs during any amalgam, resin composite, glass ionomer, ceramic, or cast-gold restorative procedure is presented here. Dental students, residents, and practitioners have used the kit, and, although another instrument may have to be added for a specific situation from time to time, the kit will more than suffice for most procedures. The kit was designed with the sequence of most operative procedures in mind. Therefore, instrument sequence in the kit proceeds from the mirror and explorer for examination, to the plastic instrument used to facilitate dam placement as well as for placement of materials, to tooth preparation instruments, to restoration placement instruments. The kit uses a 23-slot tray with a small well (open, boxlike section) from Thompson Dental. Thompson Dental has this tray and others available with customizable color-coded tabs to facilitate replacement of similarly color-coded instruments into the correct positions in the tray.

In slots (in this order, from left to right, with the open well to the rear):
- Mirror (No. 5 with handle)
- Explorer–periodontal probe (XP23/QOW)
- Cotton forceps (college, with serrations)
- Plastic instrument, No. 1-2
- Spoon, discoid, 11½-7-14
- Hatchet, 10-7-14
- Hoe, 12-10-16
- Gingival margin trimmer, 10-80-7-14
- Gingival margin trimmer, 10-95-7-14
- Wedelstaedt chisel, 10-15-3
- TD applicator/No. 313 spatula (Thompson Dental)
- Condenser, SA1 (Thompson Dental)
- Condenser, SA2 (Thompson Dental)
- Condenser, SA3 (Thompson Dental)
- Burnisher, beavertail-ovoid, 2/30
- Burnisher, PKT3
- Carver, cleoid-discoid, UWD5
- Carver, Walls No. 3
- Carver, Hollenback No. ½
- Carver, interproximal (IPC)
- Carver, No. 14L
- Articulating paper forceps
- Carrier, amalgam, medium/large

In well of tray:
- Scalpel handle, No. 3, flat
- Sharpening stone, flat, Arkansas or ceramic
- Tofflemire retainer, straight
- Tofflemire retainer, contra-angle
- Amalgam well, stainless steel, small (Thompson Dental)

Clipped to lid of tray:
- Hemostat, mosquito, 5-inch curved
- Scissors, Quimby

Sterilized separately and available for each operative procedure:
- Anesthetic syringe
- Rubber dam kit (forceps; punch; frame; 1 each of clamps W2A, 27, 212SA and 2 W8ASA clamps [Hu-Friedy])
- Brasseler bur block (No. A600) with burs arranged in the following order (Fig 6-69):
- Friction-grip burs, No. ⅛, ¼, 1, 2, 33½, 56, 169L, 170, 329, 330, 7404, 7803, 7901
- Latch burs, No. 2, 4, 6, 8
- Mandrel for pop-on disks

Sterilized separately and available for occasional use:
- Chisel, monangle, 10-4-8
- Condenser, SA4
- Hemostat, mosquito, 5-inch straight
- Mirror, No. 2 (on handle)
- Proximal contact disks (Thierman Products or Centrex) (see Chapter 7)
- Rubber dam clamps, 00, W1A, W8A
- Scaler, McCalls, SM13s-14s
- Spatula, No. 24 (or 324)
- Spoon, discoid, 15-8-14
- Spoon, discoid, 25-9-15
- Triple angle hoe, 8-3-23

References

1. American National Standards Institute/American Dental Association Specification No. 23 (Revised) for Dental Excavating Burs. Chicago: American Dental Association, 1982.

2. Black GV. A Work on Operative Dentistry. Chicago: Medico-Dental Publishing, 1908.

3. Black RB. Technique for nonmechanical preparation of cavities and prophylaxis. J Am Dent Assoc 1945;32:955–965.

4. Bouschor CR, Matthews JL. A four-year clinical study of teeth restored after preparation with an air turbine handpiece with an air coolant. J Prosthet Dent 1966;16:306–309.

5. Charbeneau GT. Principles and Practice of Operative Dentistry, ed 3. Philadelphia: Lea & Febiger, 1988.

6. Christensen GJ. Magnification. Clin Res Assoc Newsletter 1990;14(10):1.

7. Glossary of Operative Dentistry Terms, ed 1. Washington, DC: Academy of Operative Dentistry, 1983.

8. Goldstein RE, Parkins FM. Air-abrasive technology: its new role in restorative dentistry. J Am Dent Assoc 1994;125:551–557.

9. Lauer H, Kraft E, Rothlauf W, Zwingers T. Effects of the temperature of cooling water during high-speed and ultrahigh-speed tooth preparation. J Prosthet Dent 1990;63:407–414.

10. Metals Handbook, ed 10, vol 1. Materials Park, OH: American Society of Metals International, 1990:841–842, 908–909.

11. Ring ME. Dentistry, an Illustrated History. New York: Abrams, 1985:251.

12. Sturdevant CM, Roberson TM, Heymann HO, Sturdevant JR. The Art and Science of Operative Dentistry, ed 3. St Louis: Mosby, 1995.

13. Webster's Ninth New Collegiate Dictionary. Springfield, MA: Merriam-Webster, 1988.

14. Young JM. Dental air-powered handpieces: selection, use, and sterilization. Compend Contin Educ Dent 1993;14:358–366.

Field Isolation

James B. Summitt

There are many ways to isolate an area of the mouth or a tooth so that restorative services can be performed without interference from soft tissue, the tongue, saliva, or other fluids. Various tongue- and cheek-retracting devices and suction methods may be used; some of these are discussed later in this chapter. By far the most complete method of obtaining field isolation is the rubber dam, the primary subject of this chapter.

Rubber Dam

Sanford C. Barnum is credited with introducing the rubber dam to the profession in 1864.[5] For many years, the rubber dam has been recognized as an effective method of obtaining field isolation, improving visualization, protecting the patient, and improving the quality of operative dentistry services. It has been demonstrated that most patients prefer the use of the rubber dam for restorative procedures.[9,16] In recent years, the dam has been acknowledged as an important barrier for prevention of microbial transmission from patients to members of the dental care team. In addition, it is medicolegally prudent to use a dam for procedures in which small objects, such as dental burs or endodontic files, could be aspirated by the patient.

Christensen[6] has emphatically stated that the use of the rubber dam not only boosts the quality of restorations but also increases quantity of restorative services because patients are unable to talk or expectorate when the dam is in place. He has further stated that the operating field can only be maintained free of saliva and other contaminants with the dam in place, and the field is more accessible, airborne debris is reduced, and the patient feels more comfortable.

There is convincing evidence of the importance of rubber dam use during resin bonding procedures. Barghi et al[1] used cotton roll isolation or rubber dam isolation in bonding resin composite buttons to facial enamel surfaces of teeth that were to be extracted. They found shear bond strengths to be significantly greater when rubber dam isolation was used. The same group, using similar techniques, showed that rubber dam isolation significantly reduced microleakage of resin composite buttons bonded to etched enamel[10] and that salivary contamination may affect the bond strength provided by some dentin bonding systems.[11]

Most dentists are taught the use of the rubber dam in dental school, and many suffer tremendous frustrations during rubber dam applications. For the dam to be used and to actually save chair time, the practitioner must be able to apply it quickly and easily. This chapter is designed to describe methods that facilitate use of the rubber dam.

Table 7-1	Available rubber dam thicknesses (gauges)*	
Gauge	**Thickness (range)***	
Thin	0.006 (0.005–0.007) inch	
Medium	0.008 (0.007–0.009) inch	
Heavy	0.010 (0.009–0.015) inch	
Extra heavy	0.012 (0.0115–0.0135) inch	
Special heavy	0.014 (0.0135–0.0155) inch	

*Thickness ranges listed by Hygenic.

Instruments and Materials

Rubber Dam Material

Rubber dam materials are currently available in an array of colors, ranging from green to lavender to gray to ivory. It is important in operative dentistry to use a dam color that contrasts with the color of teeth; ivory-colored dam is therefore not recommended for operative dentistry procedures. The original gray dam is still the most used, but the bright colors are gaining popularity. Some operators use the gray dam because they believe that it is better for matching shades in tooth-colored restorations. Because shades of restorative materials are selected prior to rubber dam placement and tooth color changes with the enamel desiccation that accompanies rubber dam use, the restorative shade is probably not affected by the use of a brightly colored rubber dam.

Rubber dam material is available in rolls, either 5 or 6 inches wide, from which squares may be cut. It is also available in sheets that are 5 inches square, usually used for children, and 6 inches square.

Rubber dam material is available in several thicknesses, or gauges (Table 7-1). The heavy and extra heavy gauges are recommended for isolation in operative dentistry. If the rubber of the heavier gauges is passed through the interproximal tooth contacts in a single thickness and not bunched in the contacts, the heavy dams are no more difficult to apply than are the thinner materials, and heavier dams are less likely to tear. The heavier materials provide a better seal to teeth and retract tissues more effectively than the thinner materials.

Rubber dam material has a shelf life of more than a year, but aging is accelerated by heat. Extra boxes of dam material can be stored in a refrigerator to extend the shelf life. Dam material that has exceeded its shelf life becomes brittle and tears easily; unfortunately, this is usually noticed during dam application. A simple test for the resistance of rubber dam material to tearing is to attempt to tear a sheet grasped with thumbs and index fingers; a strong dam will be very difficult to tear. Brittle dam material should be discarded. If the material was recently purchased, it should be returned to the supplier for replacement.

Napkin

The rubber dam napkin is a piece of strong, absorbent cloth or paper placed between the rubber dam and the patient's face. The napkin provides greater comfort for the patient, especially during unusually long procedures. Napkins are available in two shapes (Fig 7-1). The smaller napkin is usually used with rubber dam frames; the larger provides padding for the side of the face when retracting straps are used.

Punch

At least two types of rubber dam punches are available (Figs 7-2a and 7-2b). The Ainsworth-type punch, which is made by several manufacturers, is excellent if it is well made. The Ivory punch (Heraeus Kulzer) is also excellent and has a self-centering coned piston, or punch point, that helps to prevent partially punched holes (Fig 7-3). Punches should have hardened steel cutting tables (or anvils) with a range of hole sizes so that the dam will seal against teeth of various cervical diameters (Fig 7-4).

Occasionally, the rim of a hole may be damaged because the rotating cutting table was not snapped completely into position before an attempt was made to punch a dam. Holes must be cleanly cut; incompletely punched holes (Fig 7-3) will allow tearing of the dam during application or will affect the ability of the dam to seal.

A damaged hole rim in the cutting table will cause incomplete cutting. The damaged or dull rim can sometimes be sharpened with a mounted flat, coarse sandpaper disk or separating disk used in a low-speed handpiece or a finishing bur used in a high-speed handpiece. The level of the rim of the hole is evenly lowered to an area of the wall of the hole that is beyond the damage. The metal around that hole may then be polished with finer disks. A damaged cutting wheel should usually be replaced; a replacement wheel can be ordered from the manufacturer.

Hole-Positioning Guides

Although many operators punch the holes without a positioning aid, most find it helpful to have some form of guide to determine where the holes should be punched. There are several ways to mark a rubber dam so that holes can be located optimally.

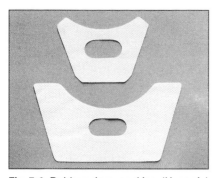

Fig 7-1 Rubber dam napkins (Hygenic) for longer procedures. Napkins provide padding between the rubber dam and the face and lips, making the dam more comfortable for the patient. The small napkin is for use with rubber dam frames. The larger napkin is for use with strap- or harness-type rubber dam holders.

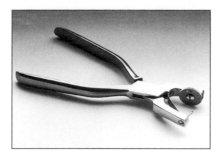

Fig 7-2a Ainsworth-design (Hygenic) rubber dam punch.

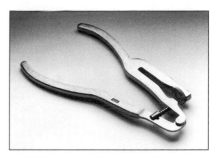

Fig 7-2b Ivory-design rubber dam punch.

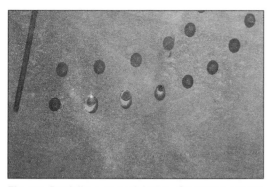

Fig 7-3 Partially punched holes. Stretched rubber dam shows the flaps of dam material left when holes are incompletely punched. The flaps will prevent proper seal. If the flaps are torn off, ragged edges can lead to tearing of the dam during application.

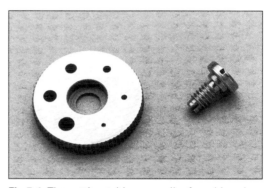

Fig 7-4 The cutting table, or anvil, of a rubber dam punch should have a range of sizes. Pictured is the cutting table from an Ivory punch.

Teeth as a guide. The teeth themselves, or a stone cast of the teeth, can be used in marking the dam. To use the teeth, the dam is held in the desired position in the mouth over the teeth to be included in the isolation. The cusp tips of posterior teeth and incisal edges of anterior teeth can be visualized through the dam, and the centers of the teeth are marked on the dam with a pen. An advantage of this method is precise positioning of the marks even when teeth are malaligned. Its disadvantages include the time-consuming nature of the procedure and the inability to punch a dam before the patient is seated.

Template. Templates are available to guide the marking of the dam (Fig 7-5). These templates are approximately the same size and shape as the unstretched rubber dam itself. Holes in each template correspond to tooth positions. The template is laid over the dam, and a pen is used to mark through selected holes onto the dam. With the template, the dam can be marked and punched before the patient is seated.

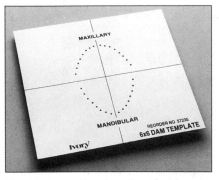

Fig 7-5 Ivory template for marking the dam. Marks corresponding to the teeth to be isolated are made on a 6.0-inch rubber dam through the holes with a felt-tipped or ballpoint pen.

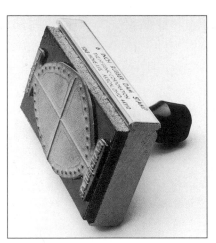

Fig 7-6a Rubber dam stamp for the adult dentition (Hygenic).

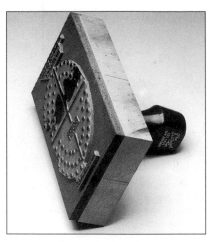

Fig 7-6b Stamp made by a rubber stamp–manufacturing company.

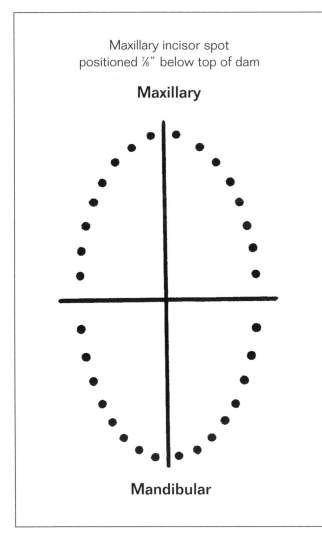

Maxillary incisor spot positioned ⅞" below top of dam

Maxillary

Mandibular

Fig 7-7 Pattern for a rubber dam stamp. This may be duplicated and taken to a rubber stamp manufacturer.

Rubber dam stamp. Rubber stamps provide a very convenient and efficient way of marking the dam for punching (Figs 7-6a and 7-6b). There are commercially available stamps, or stamps can be made by any rubber stamp manufacturer from a pattern such as the one shown in Fig 7-7 or any custom design. Dams should be prestamped by an assistant so that the marks for the maxillary central incisors are positioned approximately 0.9 inch from the top of the dam. Exceptions to normal tooth position are easily accommodated.

Rubber Dam Holders

Strap holders. Strap holders such as the Woodbury holder or retractor (Fig 7-8) provide the most cheek and lip retraction, access, and stability, but may cause the most discomfort to the patient. A rubber dam napkin is a necessity for patient comfort when a strap holder is used. The Woodbury retractor grasps the dam material with spring-loaded clips. When posterior teeth are isolated with a Woodbury-type holder, a tuck or fold in the dam may be needed (Fig 7-9).

Frame holders. Frame holders are exemplified by the Young frame (Young Dental) and the Nygaard-Ostby frame (Figs 7-10a to 7-10d). A U-shaped Young frame is made by several manufacturers in both metal and plastic. The Young-type frames are available in both adult and child sizes. A plastic frame is advantageous when radiographs will be a part of the procedure because it is radiolucent. The plastic frames do not,

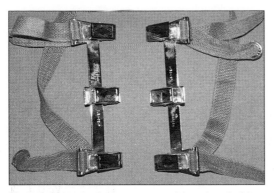

Fig 7-8 Strap- or harness-type rubber dam holders provide excellent lip and cheek retraction. Pictured is a Woodbury retractor.

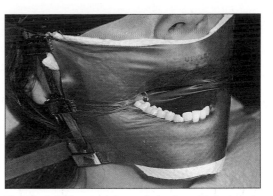

Fig 7-9 A fold or tuck is made in the rubber dam to provide an uncluttered operating field.

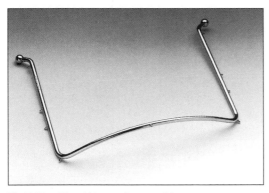

Fig 7-10a Metal Young frame with eye protectors.

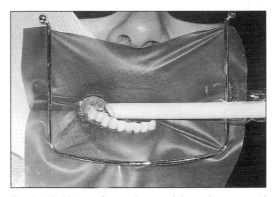

Fig 7-10b Young frame inserted into the external surface of the dam.

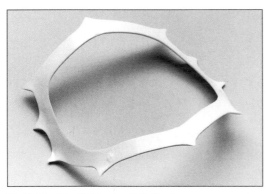

Fig 7-10c Plastic Nygaard-Ostby frame.

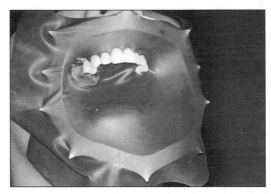

Fig 7-10d Nygaard-Ostby frame inserted into the internal surface of the dam.

however, stand up to heat sterilization as well as metal frames, and they have a shorter life span. Metal frames are less bulky and last for years.[15] They are available with balls on the ends to protect the patient in the event that the frame is inadvertently pushed toward the eyes.

The Young frame is usually positioned on the outside surface of the dam so that it is not in contact with the patient's face. The Nygaard-Ostby frame is normally positioned on the tissue surface or inside surface of the dam and touches the patient's face (or the rubber dam napkin). All frames have points or pegs over which the dam material is stretched to provide a clear operating field and to hold the frame in position.

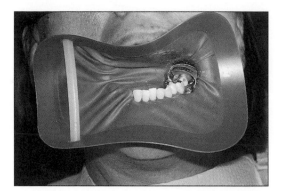

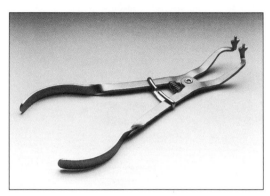

Fig 7-11 In the HandiDam, the frame is an integral part of the dam.

Fig 7-12a Ivory forceps.

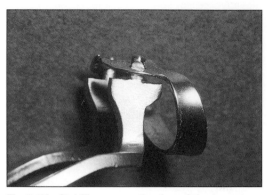

Fig 7-12b Stabilizers near the tips of the Ivory-type forceps limit rotation of the clamp when it is held by the forceps.

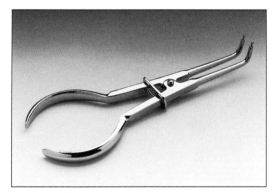

Fig 7-12c Stokes-type forceps.

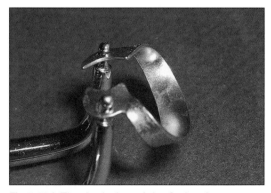

Fig 7-12d The tip design of the Stokes forceps provides more freedom for rotation of the clamp while it is held by the forceps.

Preattached frames. One commercially available rubber dam (HandiDam, Aseptico) comes with a built-in frame and a rod for insertion to keep the dam open (Fig 7-11).

Clamp Forceps

Ivory-type clamp forceps are available from several manufacturers and with differently angled beaks (Fig 7-12a). Ivory forceps (Ivory, Heraeus Kulzer) have stabilizers that prevent the clamp from rotating on the beaks (Fig 7-12b). This is usually advantageous, but it limits the use of these forceps to teeth that are within a range of normal angulation.

Stokes-type clamp forceps (Fig 7-12c), which have notches near the tips of their beaks in which to locate the holes of a rubber dam clamp (Fig 7-12d), allow a range of rotation for the clamp so that it may be positioned on teeth that are mesially or distally angled.

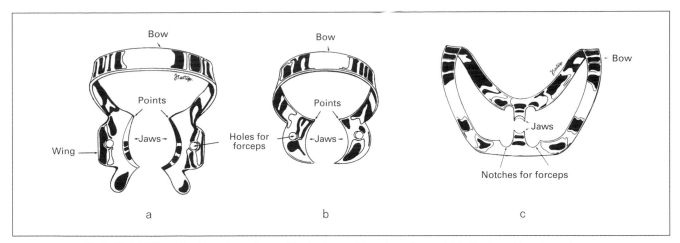

Fig 7-13 (a) Winged rubber dam clamp; (b) wingless rubber dam clamp; (c) butterfly rubber dam clamp.

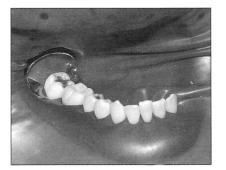

Fig 7-14 Isolated mandibular right quadrant. The clamp is positioned on the distal-most exposed tooth.

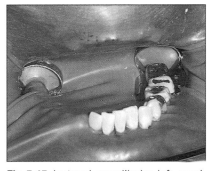

Fig 7-15 Isolated mandibular left quadrant with a second clamp placed on an unexposed molar on the right side of the mouth to give additional access to the lingual surfaces of the teeth in the left quadrant. The dam has been loosely stretched over the unexposed tooth to prevent the clamp from initiating a tear. The mirror and other instruments will now be unimpeded when the defective lingual margin of the crown on the first molar is treated.

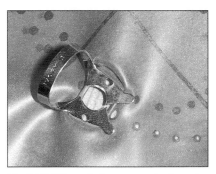

Fig 7-16 Winged clamp attached to the rubber dam. The edges of the hole are stretched over the wings of the clamp.

Either of these types of clamp forceps will serve the practitioner well, and selection should be based on personal preference. The Ivory-type forceps are probably the most popular because of cost.

Clamps

Rubber dam clamps are the usual means of retaining the rubber dam. The three basic types of clamps and their parts are shown in Fig 7-13. When a posterior segment is isolated, the clamp is usually placed on the distal-most exposed tooth (Fig 7-14). The clamp may also be placed on an unexposed tooth (one for which a hole has not been punched) (Fig 7-15).

There are clamps with jaw sizes to fit every tooth. Some clamps simply have a number designation; others have a W in front of the number. The W indicates that the clamp is wingless (Fig 7-13b); those clamps that do not bear a W have wings (Fig 7-13a) so that the dam may be attached to the wings before the clamp is placed on the tooth (Fig 7-16).

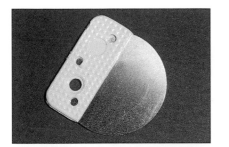

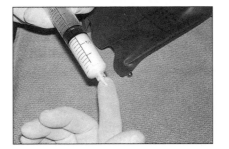

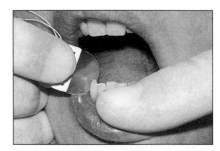

Figs 7-27a and 7-27b Proximal contact disk or plane with handle.

Fig 7-27c The proximal contact disk is used to plane rough contact.

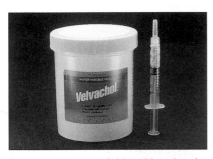

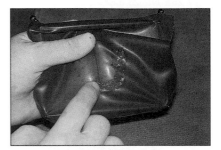

Fig 7-28 A water-soluble rubber dam lubricant, such as Velvachol, can be loaded into a syringe, such as a 3.0-mL disposable syringe. The lubricant can be dispensed from the syringe onto the tissue surface (underside) of the rubber dam or onto a glove for coating of the dam adjacent to the holes.

Fig 7-29a Water-soluble lubricant can be carried to the dam with a finger.

Fig 7-29b The dam lubricant is layered on the tissue surface of the dam in the area of the holes.

before it is taken to the mouth (Figs 7-29a and 7-29b). The lubricant makes passage of the dam through the interproximal contacts much easier, and the dam will often pass through the contacts, in a single layer, without the use of floss. If additional lubrication is desired, lubricant may be applied to the teeth prior to placement of the dam.

A lubricant for the lips will make the patient more comfortable during the procedure. A petroleum-based lubricant, such as Vaseline, cocoa butter, silicate lubricant, or lip balm, functions well as a lip lubricant.

Application and Removal

Preparation of the Mouth

Teeth should be cleaned, if necessary, and contacts should be checked with floss. The rapid passage of dental floss through each contact that will be involved in the isolation is very important and, if accomplished as a part of the routine, will save chair time. Any

rough contact should be smoothed with the proximal contact disk (Fig 7-27), not only to facilitate dam placement, but to enable the patient to clean each interproximal area during routine flossing.

If a restorative procedure that involves an occlusal surface is planned, centric occlusion (maximum intercuspation) contacts should be marked with articulating paper or tape prior to application of the dam. Centric occlusion markings may be coated with a cavity varnish or light-cured resin to protect them from being rubbed off. If a cavity varnish containing a solvent is used, the cotton pellet or brush used to apply it to the centric occlusion markings should not touch the markings, or it may dissolve them and wipe them away. Instead, the pellet or brush containing the varnish is touched to the enamel adjacent to the markings, and the material is allowed to flow across the markings and dry (Fig 7-30).

If lips are to be lubricated, this should be accomplished prior to application of the dam (Fig 7-31).

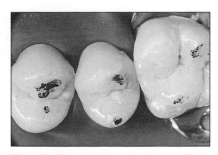

Fig 7-30 The centric occlusion markings were protected by cavity varnish during dam placement; had the markings not been protected with varnish, the placement procedure would likely have erased them.

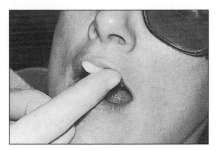

Fig 7-31 Lips are lubricated with petroleum-based lubricant prior to placement of the rubber dam.

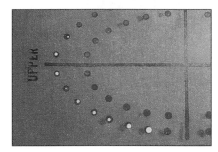

Fig 7-32 Varying hole sizes are used to seal against various sizes of teeth.

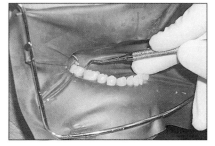

Fig 7-33 The incisal edges of the anterior teeth are used as a finger rest.

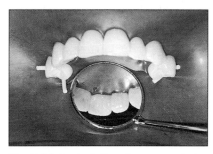

Fig 7-34 In isolation for an anterior restoration, the anterior teeth and first premolars are exposed to provide anchorage of the dam and to leave adequate working room on the lingual aspect of the anterior teeth.

Preparation of the Dam

Use of a prestamped dark (gray or green), heavy (or extra heavy) gauge dam material is recommended. Various hole sizes should be used to ensure a seal around the variety of tooth sizes (Fig 7-32). For example, an Ivory punch has six hole sizes, numbered 1 through 6 from smallest to largest (see Fig 7-4). Hole sizes recommended are 5 for clamped molars; 4 for other molars; 3 for premolars, canines, and maxillary central incisors; and 2 for lateral incisors and mandibular central incisors.

Slight variation from the recommended hole sizes may be needed, depending on the size of individual teeth, operator preference, and gauge of the dam, but a range of hole sizes should be used to prevent leakage between the dam and the teeth.

For operative procedures involving posterior teeth, the tooth or teeth to be restored should be exposed, as well as at least one tooth posterior to the most distal tooth to be restored, if possible. In addition, all teeth around to the central or lateral incisor on the opposite side of the same arch should be exposed. This extension of the area of isolation to the opposite side will hold the dam flat in the arch to give room for fingers and instruments in the area of the teeth to be restored. It will also expose teeth in the anterior area for finger rests during the operation (Fig 7-33).

For anterior restorations, exposure of the first premolar through the first premolar on the opposite side is recommended (Fig 7-34). This will provide room for the mirror and for hand instruments on the lingual aspect of the anterior teeth.

When a prestamped dam or a template is used, holes should be punched away from the spots to accommodate atypical alignment of teeth. In addition, when the dam is being prepared to provide isolation for Class 5 restorations, the hole for the tooth to receive a facial Class 5 restoration should be punched approximately 1.0 mm facial to the spot to allow retraction with the No. 212SA clamp. No holes should be punched for missing teeth.

After the dam is punched, the tissue side of the dam should be lubricated with a water-soluble lubricant. A small dollop of lubricant is applied to the tissue surface and smeared over the surface of the dam in the area of the holes (see Fig 7-29). The rubber dam frame can then be attached loosely to the dam to hold the edges of the dam away from the holes during application (see Fig 7-35b).

Placement of the Dam

If a local anesthetic agent has been administered to provide pulpal anesthesia for the tooth or teeth being restored, at least a portion of the gingival tissue will have also been anesthetized. If an inferior alveolar block has been given, the lingual nerve will almost always have been anesthetized as well, so the gingival tissue lingual to the mandibular posterior teeth will also have been anesthetized. If infiltration anesthesia has been administered to maxillary teeth, the facial gingival tissue will have been anesthetized. For application of a rubber dam clamp, the portions of the gingival tissue that have not been anesthetized along with the delivery of pulpal anesthesia will not normally need to be anesthetized. When the clamp is applied, as long as the points of the clamp's jaw are firmly on the tooth and have not penetrated gingival tissue, the patient may feel some discomfort for a few seconds where the jaws are pressing against tissue. This pressure discomfort will usually disappear within 1 minute due to "pressure anesthesia," and injection anesthesia for the gingival tissue is usually unnecessary. If additional gingival anesthesia is necessary, topical anesthetic solutions or gels may suffice.

When the clamp is applied to the tooth with the clamp forceps, the clamp should be expanded only enough to allow it to pass over the crown of the tooth. Overexpansion of the clamp will permanently distort it so that it will be weak, unstable, and more likely to dislodge from the tooth.

There are several methods of dam placement:

Dam over clamp. A wingless clamp is placed on the tooth. It is recommended that a finger be maintained over the inserted clamp to prevent its dislodgment until its stability on the tooth has been confirmed. The operator checks stability by engaging the bow of the clamp with an instrument and firmly attempting to pull it occlusally (Fig 7-35a). If the clamp rotates on the tooth, it is not stable and should be repositioned or replaced.

The top and bottom attachment points of the Young frame are engaged at the top and bottom of the dam to give a slackness or pouching of the dam (Fig 7-35b). The tissue side of the dam is lubricated in the area of the holes. Then, with a finger on each side of the distal hole in the dam, the dentist (or assistant) stretches the dam so that the hole is enlarged and appears to be an open slit; the hole is then carried over the bow and jaws of the clamp (Fig 7-35c). The hole at the opposite end of the row (usually for the lateral or central incisor on the opposite side) is then passed over the appropriate tooth, and the septa are worked through the interproximal contacts.

A gloved fingernail used to slightly separate the anterior teeth is very helpful, and floss is rarely needed to carry the dam through anterior interproximal contacts (Fig 7-35d). Good lubrication of the dam is necessary for easy and quick application. The dam should be passed through each contact in a single layer. This may be accomplished by stretching a septum over one of the teeth adjacent to the contact and sliding the edge of the rubber to the contact so that a leading edge of dam is touching the contact (Fig 7-35e).

In posterior areas, the leading edge should be touching the occlusal portion of the contact in the occlusal embrasure. Waxed tape (ribbon floss) or waxed floss is then used to move the dam progressively through the contact (Figs 7-35e to 7-35g). Tape will carry more of the rubber through the contact in a single pass than will floss. If tape is used, like the rubber, it should be taken through the contact in a single layer, not twisted or bunched up.

If the dam goes through with one pass of the floss, the floss may be removed from the contact without pulling the rubber back out. To accomplish this, the tail of the floss that is on the lingual side of the teeth is doubled back across the occlusal embrasure of the contact so that both ends are on the facial aspect; then the tape is pulled facially through the contact. If only a portion of the septum goes through the contact with the first pass of the floss or tape, the floss should be doubled back and passed through the contact again; it is then pulled facially out of the gingival embrasure (Fig 7-35h). The tape should be passed through repeatedly until the entire septum has been carried through the contact.

Fig 7-35 Dam over clamp method of dam application.

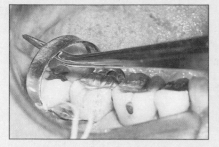

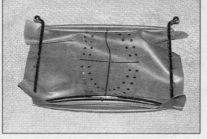

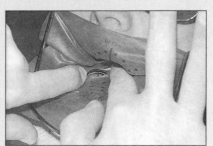

Fig 7-35a The clamp (modified No. W8A) is tested for stability. To do so, the operator attempts to pull the bow occlusally.

Fig 7-35b The dam is fitted loosely on the frame.

Fig 7-35c The distal hole of the dam is carried over the bow of the clamp.

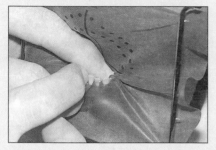

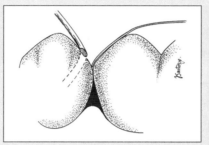

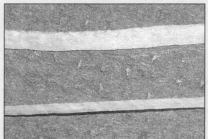

Fig 7-35d The septa are worked through anterior contacts as a gloved fingernail is used to slightly separate teeth.

Fig 7-35e The leading edge of the dam is touching the occlusal aspect of the interproximal contact; floss is on the adjacent tooth.

Fig 7-35f Waxed dental tape, or ribbon floss *(top)*, if it is not folded or bunched, will carry more of the dam septum through the contact in a single pass than will waxed floss *(bottom)*, but either type will serve the purpose.

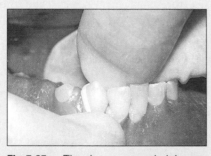

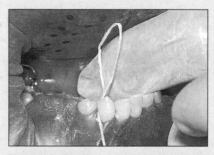

Fig 7-35g The dam septum is lying on the mesial aspect of the mandibular first premolar, with its leading edge at the mesial contact; the floss is lying on the distal aspect of the canine, ready to move to the contact, meeting the dam there. The floss will then carry at least a portion of the septum through the contact.

Fig 7-35h The floss has been doubled back to the facial aspect and passed through the contact again, carrying another portion of the septum through the contact. The floss is then removed from the contact; one or both of the tails of the floss are pulled facially away from the teeth.

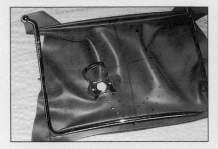

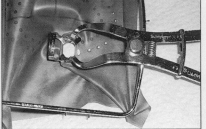

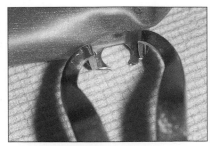

Fig 7-36 *Winged clamp in dam method of dam application.*

Fig 7-36a A winged clamp (No. 27) is inserted into the distal hole of the dam.

Fig 7-36b The clamp-dam-frame assembly is carried to the mouth as a unit.

Fig 7-37a Wingless clamp in dam method of dam application. Shown is the clamp in the dam.

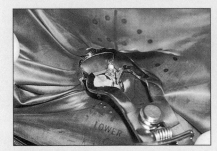

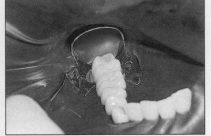

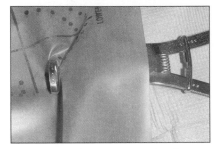

Fig 7-36c The clamp is placed on the mandibular second molar.

Fig 7-36d The dam has been applied to the quadrant, and a No. 1-2 plastic instrument is used to pull the edges of rubber off the wings of the clamp.

Fig 7-37b Dam and clamp with forceps in place.

Winged clamp in dam. Prior to lubrication of the dam, the clamp is placed into the distal hole so that the hole is stretched over the wings of the clamp from its tissue side (Fig 7-36a). The dam is then lubricated, and the frame is attached. The forceps are inserted into the holes of the clamp, and the clamp, dam, and frame are carried as a unit into place (Figs 7-36b and 7-36c). After the stability of the clamp is confirmed, the dam material on the wings of the clamp is pulled off the wings with finger tension or with a bladed instrument such as a plastic instrument (Fig 7-36d). The remainder of the dam is placed as previously described.

Wingless clamp in dam. The distal hole of the lubricated dam is passed over the bow of a wingless clamp, such as the No. W8A, so that the hole comes to rest at the junction of the bow and the jaw arms (Fig 7-37a). The frame is not attached to the dam at this point. The dam is gathered up and elevated to expose the jaw arms of the clamp, and the forceps are then inserted into the forceps holes (Figs 7-37a and 7-37b). The gathered dam is carried to the mouth with one hand and the forceps with the other. After the clamp is ap-

plied to the distal tooth and the dam has been pulled over the jaws of the clamp, the frame is attached and the other teeth are isolated as previously described.

Clamp after dam. The dam is applied to the teeth and then the clamp is placed. This technique, occasionally necessary, is the most difficult.

Completion of Application

Application of the napkin. For longer procedures, the use of a rubber dam napkin is recommended. The napkin may be positioned before or after the dam is in place on the teeth. For placement of the napkin after the dam has been applied, the frame is removed, the napkin is placed so that the edges of the napkin remain on the skin and not in the mouth, and the frame is replaced.

Adjustment of the dam in the frame. The frame and dam are adjusted so that there is a minimum of folds and wrinkles and so that the dam does not obstruct the nostrils.

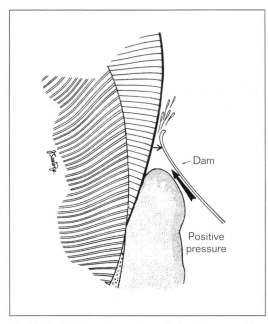

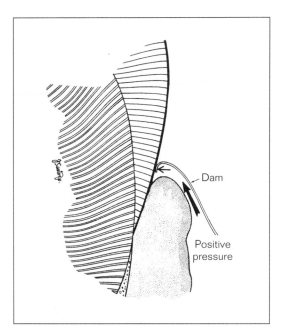

Fig 7-38a Without inversion of the dam, positive pressure under the dam, created by tongue movement, swallowing, etc, will cause leakage of saliva into the operating field.

Fig 7-38b With inversion of the dam, positive pressure under the dam only causes the dam to seal more tightly against the tooth, preventing leakage.

Washing of the dam. The dam and isolated teeth are washed with an air/water spray to remove the lubricant. After they are washed, the dam and teeth should be dried with air from the air syringe.

Inversion of the dam. The dam should be inverted around the necks of the teeth, at least in the area of the tooth or teeth to be restored. The edge of the dam that is against the tooth acts as a valve. If the edge is directed occlusally (Fig 7-38a), when a positive pressure is created by the tongue and cheeks under the dam, the valve opens, and saliva and other liquids under the dam are pushed between the tooth and dam to flood the operating field; then when a negative pressure is created under the dam, the valve closes and the saliva is trapped in the field. When the dam is inverted, a positive pressure under the dam simply serves to push the valve more tightly against the tooth (Fig 7-38b) so that no flooding of the field occurs.

Almost any instrument may be used to tuck the edge of the dam gingivally (see Figs 7-25a to 7-25c). A steady, high-volume stream of air should be directed at the tip of the instrument used to invert the dam, and the instrument should be moved along the margin of the dam so that the inversion is progressive.

Floss may be used to invert the dam in interproximal areas (Fig 7-39a). When it is used to carry the edge of the dam gingivally, the floss should not then be pulled occlusally for removal because it will frequently pull the edge of the dam with it, eliminating the inversion. Instead, the floss can be doubled over on itself on the lingual aspect and passed again through the contact. Then one end is pulled in a facial direction so that it rolls from the sulcus, leaving the dam inverted (Fig 7-39b). In this floss-facilitated inversion, a steady stream of air is as helpful as it is when inversion is accomplished with an instrument. The dam inverts more easily when the surfaces of the tooth and adjacent dam are dry.

Protection of the Dam

Torn dams provide poor isolation, so expenditure of a little effort to prevent tearing is worthwhile. An example of protection would be the use of a wedge interproximally when rotary instruments are used in the proximity of the dam. Another example is the use of a second clamp to retract the dam below a margin that is near, or below, the level of the gingival crest (see Fig 7-46).

Fig 7-44 *Rubber dam isolation around a fixed partial denture (cyanoacrylate method).*

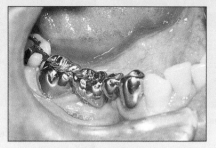

Fig 7-44a A four-unit fixed partial denture extends from the mandibular first premolar to the second molar.

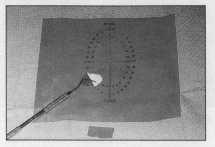

Fig 7-44b The holes for the abutment teeth are connected with an arched cut. Note small piece of dam material at bottom that will be used as shown in Figs 7-44c and 7-44d.

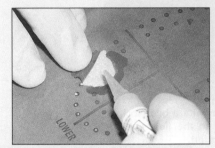

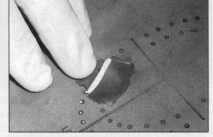

Figs 7-44c and 7-44d A small piece of dam is glued in place.

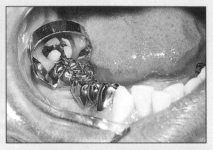

Fig 7-44e A No. W8A clamp is positioned on the second molar.

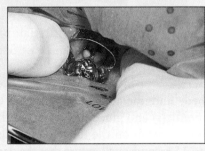

Fig 7-44f The dam is carried to place.

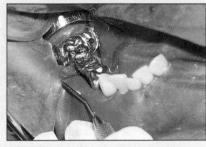

Fig 7-44g The tongue of dam material is tucked under the pontics with a periodontal probe.

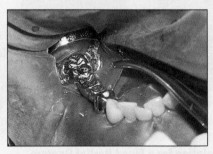

Fig 7-44h The tongue of material is grasped and pulled lingually with a hemostat.

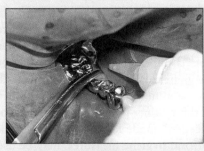

Fig 7-44i Glue is applied for attachment of the rubber dam tongue.

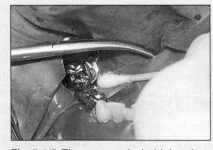

Fig 7-44j The tongue is held in place with a hemostat and a cotton-tipped applicator while the glue sets.

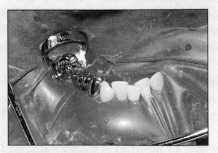

Fig 7-44k Isolation is complete.

Fig 7-45 Isolation around a three-unit fixed partial denture or splinted teeth (ligation method).

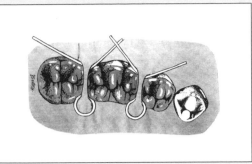

Fig 7-45a Holes are punched for the abutment teeth and pontic, and the dam is positioned. The septa on the mesial aspect of the mesial abutment and the distal aspect of the distal abutment are flossed to place, and then the holes are stretched over the abutments and the pontic.

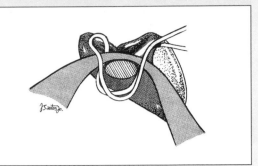

Fig 7-45b A ligature is threaded through an abutment hole on the facial aspect, under the retainer-pontic connector, through the same hole again on the lingual aspect, around the septum, through the pontic hole on the lingual aspect, back under the connector to the facial aspect, and back through the pontic hole.

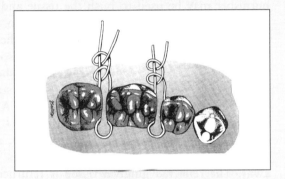

Figs 7-45c to 7-45e The ends of the ligature are tied together to pull the rubber septum tightly around the connector.

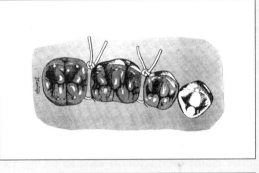

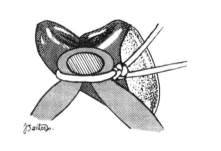

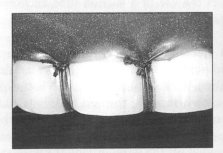

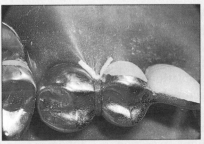

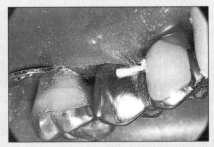

Figs 7-45f Sutures have been used for field isolation involving an anterior three-unit fixed partial denture.

Figs 7-45g and 7-45h Floss has been used for isolation involving a cantilevered canine pontic attached to splinted premolars.

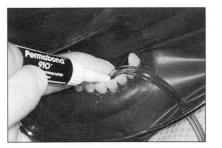

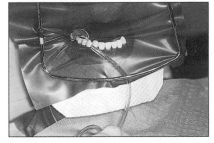

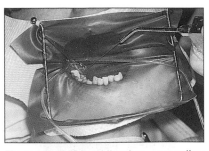

Figs 7-49a and 7-49b The washed field apparatus[2,4] is used for evacuation of fluids from the dam when no assistant is available. A small tube is attached to the dam with cyanoacrylate. (Courtesy of Dr James M. Childers and Dr Thomas D. Marshall.)

Fig 7-49c Two small tubes, extending from a Y connector, are tucked under the frame and behind the bow of the clamp to provide evacuation. (Courtesy of Dr James M. Childers and Dr Thomas D. Marshall.)

tioned fluids. A similar apparatus, described by Benavides and Herrera,[2] involves a Y-type connector (DCI International) to which two small-diameter plastic tubes are attached (Fig 7-49c).

Sealing a Root Concavity

The rubber dam seals well on convex tooth surfaces. If the dam is retracted so that its edge goes across a root concavity, however, saliva will leak into the operating field. A solution is to seal the gap between the edge of the dam and the concave root surface. This may be accomplished with a provisional restorative material, such as Cavit (ESPE Premier), which hardens with moisture (Fig 7-50).

Repair of a Torn Rubber Dam

A small tear in a dam may often be patched. A piece of dam material is cut to cover the tear and extend 1.0 cm or so beyond the tear on all sides. The piece is attached over the tear with cyanoacrylate.

Placement of a Second Dam Over the First

If a dam is torn beyond repair during a procedure, the dentist might choose to remove the dam and replace it. Alternatively, another dam may be placed over the top of the first. Brownbill[3] recommended that this technique be used when there is leakage around teeth through incorrectly sized holes and when strong chemicals are to be used.

Latex Allergies

There is an increasing awareness of latex sensitivity.[8,13,14] One survey[14] reported 3.7% of patients to have a latex allergy; the investigators recommended

careful questioning of patients regarding a history of sensitivity to latex-based products, so that the use of latex products, such as gloves and the rubber dam, may be avoided with these patients.

For latex-sensitive patients, use of the latex dam should be avoided, as should other latex products. Nonlatex rubber dam material is available and should be on hand for latex-allergic patients. One such product from Hygenic has elastic properties very similar to latex (Fig 7-51).

Summary of Recommendations

Following are some of the procedures that facilitate rubber dam use:

1. Use a heavy-gauge, prestamped dam.
2. Floss through contacts prior to dam placement, planing any contact that shreds or tears the floss.
3. Use a good water-soluble lubricant, such as Velvachol.
4. Use a clamp designed for four-point contact on the tooth, and avoid overexpansion of the clamp so that the clamp will maintain its strength and will be stable as a retainer.
5. Isolate enough teeth to hold the dam on the lingual aspect of the teeth away from the operating field and to provide exposed teeth for finger rests.
6. With waxed floss, floss the dam through interproximal contacts in a single layer and avoid doubling or bunching the dam in the contact.
7. Master the use of modeling compound to stabilize rubber dam retainers.

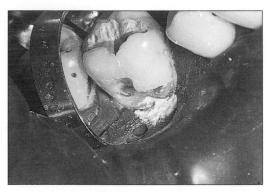

Fig 7-50 Sealing of the root concavity. The dam is retracted by the clamp to allow isolation for a large Class 5 restoration; the retraction is apical to the beginning of the root concavity of the furcation. The gap between the dam and the concave root surface is sealed with Cavit, a provisional restorative material that hardens when it comes into contact with moisture.

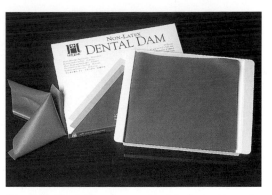

Fig 7-51 Nonlatex dam material from Hygenic. Nonlatex dams should be used for patients with a latex allergy.

Other Methods of Isolation

Svedopter

The Svedopter (EC Moore) is probably the most commonly used tongue retraction device (Figs 7-52a and 7-52b). It is designed so that the vacuum evacuator tube passes anterior to the chin and mandibular anterior teeth, over the incisal edges of the mandibular anterior teeth, and down to the floor of the mouth, to either the left or the right of the tongue. A mirrorlike vertical blade is attached to the evacuator tube so that it holds the tongue away from the field of operation. Several sizes of vertical blades are supplied by the manufacturer. An adjustable horizontal chin blade is attached to the evacuation tube so that it will clamp under the chin to hold the apparatus in place.

Absorbent cotton rolls are placed adjacent to the Svedopter in the floor of the mouth and in the maxillary buccal vestibule adjacent to the opening of the parotid gland (Stinson's) duct. The Svedopter is especially useful for preparation and cementation of fixed prostheses. It is less effective than the rubber dam for procedures in which total isolation from the fluids and vapors of the oral cavity is desired.

Hygoformic Saliva Ejector

The Hygoformic (Pulpdent) coiled saliva ejector is used in the same way as the Svedopter, but it does not have a reflective blade (Figs 7-53a to 7-53c). It is, however, usually more comfortable and less traumatic to lingual tissues than is the Svedopter. For use, the saliva ejector must be re-formed (rebent) so that the evacuator tube passes under the chin, up over the incisal edges of the mandibular incisors, and then down to the floor of the mouth. The tongue-retracting coil should be loosened, or partially uncoiled, so that it extends posteriorly enough to hold the tongue away from the operating field. The Hygoformic saliva ejector is also used with absorbent cotton for maximum effectiveness.

Absorbent Paper and Cotton Products

Absorbent materials are important in dentistry. Vacuum apparatuses remove fluids from the operating field by suctioning them; cotton and paper products help control fluids by absorbing them. Several types of absorbent cotton rolls are available in various diameters and lengths. These are placed into areas of the mouth, where salivary gland ducts exit, to absorb saliva and prevent salivary contamination of the operating field.

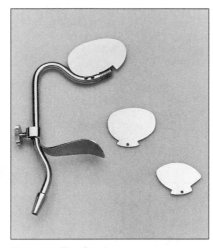

Fig 7-52a The Svedopter tongue-retracting evacuation device is supplied with three sizes of vertical blades.

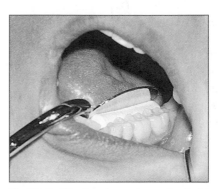

Fig 7-52b The Svedopter is used to hold the tongue away from the operating field.

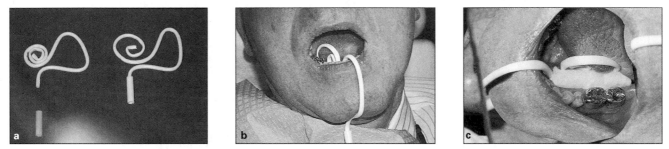

Figs 7-53a to 7-53c The Hygoformic saliva ejector should be routinely rebent to pass under the chin, over the incisal edges of the mandibular incisors, and then down to the floor of the mouth. The apparatus should usually be uncoiled slightly to extend further posteriorly. *(a, left)* Hygoformic saliva ejector as received; *(a, right)* Hygoformic saliva ejector that has been reshaped. Figs 7-53b and 7-53c show isolation achieved with the Hygoformic saliva ejector.

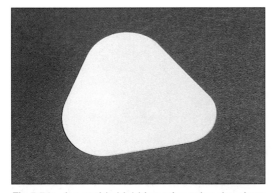

Fig 7-54a A parotid shield is a triangular absorbent paper.

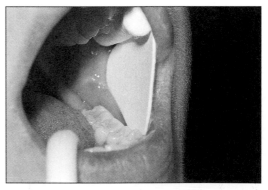

Fig 7-54b A parotid shield may supplement a cotton roll in the buccal vestibule or may be used alone.

Isolation using absorbent materials with suctioning devices is less effective than using the rubber dam with suction, but in many procedures, the more complete isolation provided by the dam is unnecessary. In these situations, absorbent products are useful.

Small gauze sponges may be folded or rolled to substitute for cotton rolls. In addition, absorbent paper triangles, or parotid shields, such as Dri-Aid (Lorvic), are useful on the facial aspect of posterior teeth to absorb saliva secreted by the parotid gland (Figs 7-54a and 7-54b).

References

1. Barghi N, Knight GT, Berry TG. Comparing two methods of moisture control in bonding to enamel: a clinical study. Oper Dent 1991;16:130–135.
2. Benavides R, Herrera H. Rubber dam with washed field evacuation: a new approach. Oper Dent 1992;17:26–28.
3. Brownbill JW. Double rubber dam. Quintessence Int 1987;18:699–670.
4. Childers JM, Marshall TD. Coolant evacuation; a solution for students working without dental assistance. Oper Dent 1995;20:130–132.
5. Christen AG, Sanford C. Barnum, discoverer of the rubber dam. Bull Hist Dent 1977;25:3–9.
6. Christensen GJ. Using rubber dams to boost quality, quantity of restorative services. J Am Dent Assoc 1994;125:81–82.
7. Drucker H, Wolcott RB. Gingival tissue management with Class V restorations. J Am Acad Gold Foil Oper 1970;13(1):34–38.
8. Fay MF, Beck WC, Checchi L, Winkler D. Gloves: new selection criteria. Quintessence Int 1995;26:27–29.
9. Gergely EJ. Rubber dam acceptance. Br Dent J 1989;167:249–252.
10. Knight GT, Barghi N, Berry T. Microleakage of enamel bonding as affected by moisture control methods [abstract]. J Dent Res 1991;70:561.
11. Knight GT, Barghi N. Effect of saliva contamination on dentin bonding agents in vivo [abstract 434]. J Dent Res 1992;71:160.
12. Lambert RL. Moisture evacuation with the rubber dam in place. J Prosthet Dent 1985;53:749–750.
13. March PJ. An allergic reaction to latex rubber gloves. J Am Dent Assoc 1988;117:590–591.
14. Rankin KV, Jones DL, Rees TD. Latex reactions in an adult dental population. Am J Dent 1993;6:274–276.
15. Reid JS, Callis PD, Patterson CJW. Rubber Dam in Clinical Practice. Chicago: Quintessence, 1990.
16. Reuter JE. The isolation of teeth and the protection of the patient during endodontic treatment. Int Endod J 1983;16:173–181.
17. Xhonga FA. Gingival retraction techniques and their healing effect on the gingiva. J Prosthet Dent 1971;26:640–648.

Enamel and Dentin Adhesion

Bart Van Meerbeek/Satoshi Inoue/Jorge Perdigão/
Paul Lambrechts/Guido Vanherle

After observing the industrial use of phosphoric acid to improve adhesion of paints and resin coatings to metal surfaces, Buonocore,[44] in 1955, applied acid to teeth to "render the tooth surface more receptive to adhesion." Buonocore's pioneering work led to major changes in the practice of dentistry. Today, we are in the age of adhesive dentistry. Traditional mechanical methods of retaining restorative materials have been replaced, to a large extent, by tooth-conserving adhesive methods. The concepts of large preparations and extension for prevention, proposed by Black[26] in 1917, have gradually been replaced by concepts of smaller preparations and more conservative techniques.

Advantages of Adhesive Techniques

Bonded restorations have a number of advantages over traditional, nonadhesive methods. Traditionally, retention and stabilization of restorations often required the removal of sound tooth structure. This is not necessary, in many cases, when adhesive techniques are used. Adhesion also reduces microleakage at the restoration-tooth interface. Prevention of microleakage, or the ingress of oral fluids and bacteria along the cavity wall, reduces clinical problems such as postoperative sensitivity, marginal staining, and recurrent caries, all of which may jeopardize the clinical longevity of restorative efforts.[72,249]

Adhesive restorations better transmit and distribute functional stresses across the bonding interface to the tooth and have the potential to reinforce weakened tooth structure.[74,131,200] In contrast, a traditional metal intracoronal restoration may act as a wedge between the buccal and lingual cusps and increase the risk of cuspal fracture. Adhesive techniques allow deteriorating restorations to be repaired and debonded restorations to be replaced with minimal or no additional loss of tooth material.

Adhesive techniques have expanded the range of possibilities for esthetic restorative dentistry.[142,291] Today's patient pays more attention to esthetics than ever before, and teeth are a key consideration in personal appearance. Tooth-colored restorative materials are used to esthetically restore and/or recontour teeth with little or no tooth preparation. Advances in dental adhesive technology have enabled the dentist to improve facial esthetics in a relatively simple and economic way.

Expanding Indications for Adhesive Dentistry

Adhesive techniques with resin composites were initially used for the replacement of carious and fractured tooth structure or for the filling of erosion or abrasion defects in cervical areas. Modern adhesive techniques also enable restorative material to be added to the tooth for the correction of unesthetic shapes, positions, dimensions, or shades. Resin composite can be placed mesiodistally to close diastemas, incisally to add length, or buccally to mask discoloration.[243-245] Because of the alleged mercury toxicity associated with silver amalgam,[172,179] substantial research is currently focused on the development of alternatives to amalgam.[343] Posterior resin composites can be directly or indirectly bonded into Class 1 and Class 2 preparations.

Adhesive techniques are also used to bond anterior and posterior ceramic restorations, such as veneers, inlays, and onlays, with adhesive luting composites. Adhesives can be used to bond silver amalgam restorations; to retain metal frameworks; to adhesively cement crowns and fixed partial dentures; to bond orthodontic brackets; for periodontal or orthodontic splints; to treat dentinal hypersensitivity; and to repair fractured porcelain, amalgam, and resin restorations. Pit and fissure sealants utilize adhesion as part of a preventive treatment program. Adhesive materials are often used with core buildup foundations.

Principles of Adhesion

The word *adhesion* is derived from the Latin word *adhaerere*, which is a compound of *ad*, or *to*, and *haerere*, or *to stick*.[216] Cicero used the expression *haerere in equo*, *to stick to a horse*, to refer to keeping a firm seat.

In adhesive terminology, *adhesion* or *bonding* is the attachment of one substance to another. The surface or substrate that is adhered to is termed the *adherend*. The *adhesive* or *adherent*, or in dental terminology the *bonding agent* or *adhesive system*, may then be defined as the material that, when applied to surfaces of substances, can join them together, resist separation, and transmit loads across the bond.[166,216] The *adhesive strength* or *bond strength* is the measure of the load-bearing capability of the adhesive. The time period during which the bond remains effective is referred to as *durability*.[4]

Adhesion refers to the forces or energies between atoms or molecules at an interface that hold two phases together.[216] In debonding tests, adhesion is often subjected to tensile or shear forces, and the mode of failure is quantified. If the bond fails at the interface between the two substrates, the mode of failure is referred to as *adhesive*. It is *cohesive* if failure occurs in one of the substrates, but not at the interface. The mode of failure is often mixed.

Table 8-1	Bond energy and bond distance (equilibrium length)[4]	
Bond type	**Bond energy (kJmol⁻¹)**	**Equilibrium length (Å)**
Primary		
Ionic	600–1200	2–4
Covalent	60–800	0.7–3
Secondary		
Hydrogen	~50	3
Dipole interactions*	~20	4
London dispersion*	~40	<10

*Dipole interactions and dispersion forces are often collectively referred to as *van der Waals* forces.

Four theories have been advanced to account for the observed phenomena of adhesion[4]:

1. *Mechanical* theories state that the solidified adhesive interlocks micromechanically with the roughness and irregularities of the surface of the adherend.

2. *Adsorption* theories encompass all kinds of chemical bonds between the adhesive and the adherend, including primary (ionic and covalent) and secondary (hydrogen, dipole interaction, and London dispersion) valence forces (Table 8-1). London dispersion forces are almost universally present, because they arise from and solely depend on the presence of nuclei and electrons. The other bond types require appropriate chemical groups to interact.

3. *Diffusion* theories propose that adhesion is the result of bonding between mobile molecules. Polymers from each side of an interface can cross over and react with molecules on the other side. Eventually, the interface will disappear and the two parts will become one.

4. *Electrostatic* theories state that an electrical double layer forms at the interface between a metal and a polymer, making a certain, yet obscure, contribution to the bond strength.

An important requirement for any of these interfacial phenomena to occur is that the two materials being joined must be in sufficiently close and intimate relation. Besides an intimate contact, sufficient wetting of the adhesive will occur only if its surface tension is less than the surface-free energy of the adherend.[89,92,265] Wetting of a surface by a liquid is characterized by the contact angle of a droplet placed on the surface.[217] If the liquid spreads completely on the solid

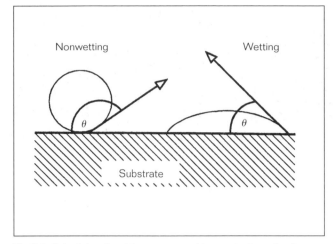

Fig 8-1 Principle of wetting measured by contact angle, θ.

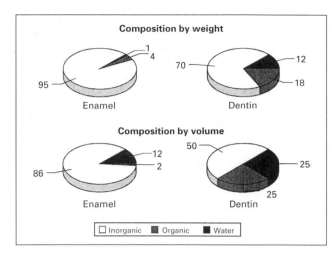

Fig 8-2 Composition of enamel and dentin by weight and volume.

surface, this indicates complete wetting, or a contact angle of 0 degrees (Fig 8-1).

According to this theory of wetting and surface-free energies, adhesion to enamel is much easier to achieve than is adhesion to dentin. Enamel contains primarily hydroxyapatite, which has a high surface-free energy, whereas dentin is composed of two distinct substrates, hydroxyapatite and collagen, and dentin has a low surface-free energy. In the oral environment, the tooth surface is contaminated by an organic saliva pellicle with a low critical surface tension (28 dynes/cm),[150] which impairs adequate wetting by the adhesive.[16] Likewise, instrumentation of the tooth substrate during cavity preparation produces a smear layer with a low surface-free energy. Therefore, the natural tooth surface should be thoroughly cleaned and pretreated before bonding procedures to increase its surface-free energy and hence to render it more receptive to bonding.

Several, if not all, of the mechanisms of adhesion described contribute to some extent to bond strength. Glass-ionomer cement is the only restorative material that has been reported to possess an intrinsic self-adhesive capacity to bond to tooth tissue without any pretreatment.[2,202] Other restorative materials with adhesive potential, such as resin composites, require the application of an intermediate resin to unite the tooth substrate with the restorative material. In the case of adhesion to enamel, a resin bonding agent is bonded primarily by micromechanical interlocking with the surface irregularities of the etched substrate. A micromechanical type of bonding is also largely involved in bonding to dentin.[31,81,204,229,326] Although there is some controversy about the contribution of primary chemical bonds to the resin-tooth attachment, secondary, weak London–van der Waals forces may play a contributing role because of the intimate contact between the resin and tooth substrate.[87,281,285,305,350]

Factors Affecting Adhesion to Tooth Tissue

The strength and durability of adhesive bonds depend on several factors. Important factors may include the physicochemical properties of the adherend and the adhesive; the structural properties of the adherend, which is heterogeneous; the formation of surface contaminants during cavity preparation; the development of external stresses that counteract the process of bonding and their compensation mechanisms; and the mechanism of transmission and distribution of applied loads through the bonded joint. Furthermore, the oral environment, which is subject to moisture, physical stresses, changes in temperature and pH, dietary components, and chewing habits, considerably influences adhesive interactions between materials and tooth tissues.[121]

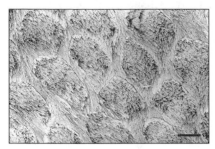

Fig 8-3 Field-emission scanning electron photomicrograph of an acid-etched (Non-Rinse Conditioner, Dentsply) enamel surface disclosing the typical keyhole-shaped enamel prisms or rods. Bar = 2.5 μm.

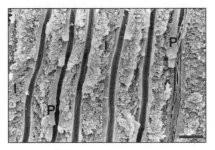

Fig 8-4 Field-emission scanning electron photomicrograph of longitudinally fractured dentinal tubules. I = intertubular dentin; P = peritubular dentin; bar = 5 μm.

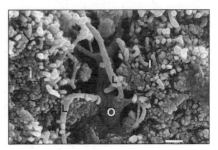

Fig 8-5 Scanning electron photomicrograph demonstrating an odontoblastic process (O) in a dentinal tubule with several lateral branches (L). I = intertubular dentin; bar = 1 μm.

Compositional and Structural Aspects of Enamel and Dentin

Because the composition and structure of enamel and dentin are substantially different, adhesion to the two tooth tissues is also different. The inorganic content of mature enamel is 95% to 98% by weight (wt%) and 86% by volume (vol%); the primary component is hydroxyapatite. The remainder consists of water (4 wt% and 12 vol%) and organic material (1 to 2 wt% and 2 vol%)[211] (Fig 8-2). The major inorganic fraction exists in the form of submicron crystallites, preferentially oriented in three dimensions, in which the spread and contiguous relationship of the crystallites contribute to the microscopic unit, called the *rod* or *prism*.[121,178] The natural surface of enamel is smooth, and the ends of the rods are exposed in what has been described as a keyhole pattern (Fig 8-3).[187] Operatively prepared surfaces expose rods in tangential, oblique, and longitudinal planes. Enamel is almost homogeneous in structure and composition, irrespective of its depth and location, except for some aprismatic (prismless) enamel at the outer surface,[121] in which the crystallites run parallel to each other and perpendicular to the surface.

Unlike enamel, dentin contains a higher percentage of water (12 wt%) and organic material (18 wt%), mainly type I collagen,[174] and only about 70 wt% hydroxyapatite (Fig 8-2).[196] Structurally more important to adhesion are the volumes occupied by the dentinal components. There is, combined, as much organic material (25 vol%) and water (25 vol%) as there is inorganic material (50 vol%).[196] In addition, these constituents are unevenly distributed in intertubular and peritubular dentin (Fig 8-4), so the dentinal tissue is heterogeneous.

Numerous dentinal tubules radiate from the pulp throughout the entire thickness of dentin, making dentin a highly permeable tissue.[109,220] These dentinal tubules contain the odontoblastic processes (Fig 8-5) and form a direct connection to the vital pulp. In contrast to enamel, dentin is a vital and dynamic tissue[223,351] that is able to develop specific defense mechanisms against external injuries. The diameter of the tubules decreases from 2.5 μm at the pulp side to 0.8 μm at the dentinoenamel junction. Likewise, the number of tubules decreases from about 45,000/mm² near the pulp to about 20,000/mm² near the dentinoenamel junction.[109] With an average of 30,000 tubules/mm² in the middle part of cut human dentin, a considerable volume of dentin consists of their lumina. Each tubule is surrounded by a collar of hypermineralized peritubular dentin (Fig 8-6). Intertubular dentin is less mineralized and contains more organic collagen fibrils. Besides an odontoblastic process in the deepest one third of the total tubule length, the tubules are filled with tissue fluid or so-called *dentinal fluid*, an organic membrane structure called *lamina limitans*, and intratubular collagen fibrils of yet unknown origin and function (Fig 8-7).

Because of the fan-shaped radiation of dentinal tubules (Fig 8-8), 96% of a superficial dentinal surface is composed of intertubular dentin; only 1% is occupied by fluid in the dentinal tubules, and 3% by peritubular dentin.[109,224] Near the pulp, peritubular dentin represents 66% and intertubular dentin only 12% of the area of a cut surface, while 22% of the surface area is occupied by water. Similar data demonstrate that 3% of the area of a cut surface consists of dentinal tubules in superficial dentin and 25% in deep dentin. A mean diameter of dentinal tubules ranging from 0.63 to 2.37 μm, depending on depth,

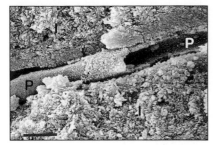

Fig 8-6 Field-emission scanning electron photomicrograph of a fractured dentinal substrate illustrating a tube of highly mineralized peritubular dentin. I = intertubular dentin; P = peritubular dentin; bar = 2 μm.

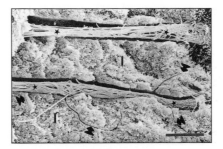

Fig 8-7 Field-emission scanning electron photomicrograph of a fractured dentinal substrate illustrating cross-banded collagen *(stars)* inside the lumen of two dentinal tubules. Note the microtubules branching off the main tubule *(black arrows)*. I = intertubular dentin; bar = 5 μm.

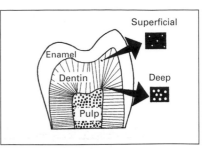

Fig 8-8 Dimension and concentration of dentinal tubules near the dentinoenamel junction (superficial dentin) and near the pulp (deep dentin). (Adapted from Heymann and Bayne.[136] Copyright © 1993 American Dental Association. Reprinted by permission of ADA Publishing, a Division of ADA Business Enterprises, Inc.)

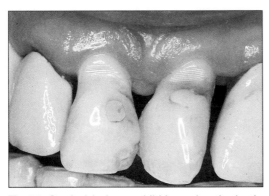

Fig 8-9 Cervical lesions exhibiting sclerotic dentin in combined abrasive (toothbrush) and stress-induced (tooth flexure) lesions.

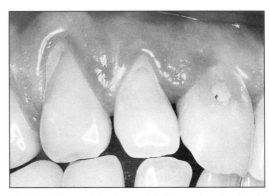

Fig 8-10 Cervical lesions exhibiting sclerotic dentin in chemically induced erosive lesions.

has been determined by image analysis of transmission electron microscopic and scanning electron microscopic (SEM) micrographs.[180] Hence, dentin is an intrinsically wet tissue. Dentinal fluid in the tubules is under a slight, but constant, outward pressure from the pulp. The intrapulpal fluid pressure is estimated to be 25 to 30 mm Hg[324] or 34 to 40 cm water.[215]

Changes in Dentinal Structure

Dentin is a dynamic substrate subject to continuous physiologic and pathologic changes in composition and microstructure.[223,288] Dentin that has been violated by caries or has undergone abrasion (Fig 8-9) or erosion (Fig 8-10) may be quite different from unaffected sound dentin. Dentin undergoes *physiologic dentinal sclerosis* as part of the aging process and *reactive sclerosis* in response to slowly progressive or mild irritations, such as mechanical abrasion or chem-

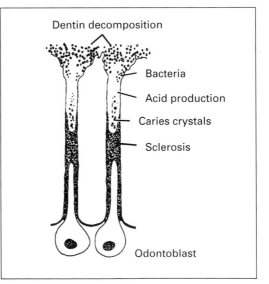

Fig 8-11 Obstruction of the dentinal tubules by "whitlockite" or caries crystals. (Adapted from Fusayama,[103] by permission of *Operative Dentistry*, and Ogawa et al.[212])

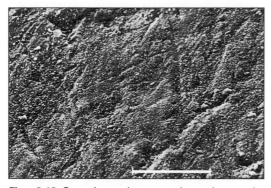

Fig 8-12 Scanning electron photomicrographs demonstrating heavily sclerotic dentin without exposed tubules, despite treatment with 10% citric acid. Bar = 20 µm. (From Van Meerbeek et al.[331] Reprinted with permission from Elsevier Science.)

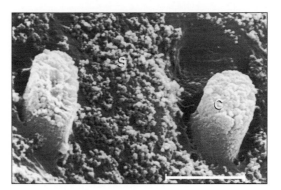

Fig 8-13 Two mineral sclerotic casts (C) extend from the tubules above the acid-etched dentinal surface, which is covered by silica particles (S) remaining from the etchant gel. Bar = 2 µm.

ical erosion.[288] *Tertiary*, or *reparative*, dentin is produced in the pulp chamber at the lesion site in response to insults such as caries, dental procedures, or attrition.[288] Hypermineralization, obstruction of tubules by whitlockite crystalline deposits (Fig 8-11), and apposition of reparative dentin adjacent to the pulp are well-documented responses to caries.[103,212] Less is known about the compositional and morphologic modifications of dentin that accompany the development of cervical abrasions and erosions.[69,70,331]

Dentinal sclerosis, or the formation of transparent, glasslike dentin, which occurs in the cervical areas of teeth, has several common characteristics. Sclerosis is reported to result from the obstruction of dentinal tubules by apposition of peritubular dentin and precipitation of rhombohedral mineral crystals. The refractive index of the obstructed tubules is similar to that of intertubular dentin, resulting in a glasslike appearance.[70,197,353,354]

Sclerotic dentin usually contains few, if any, patent tubules and, therefore, has low permeability[304,354] and tends to be insensitive to external stimuli.[70,331,353,354] The odontoblastic processes associated with sclerotic dentin often exhibit partial atrophy and mineralization.[100,288,351] Heavily sclerotic dentin has areas of complete hypermineralization[197,311] without tubule exposure, even when etched with an acid (Fig 8-12). Some areas show abundant mineral sclerotic casts, which extend from the tubule orifices above the dentinal surface and probably represent mineralized odontoblastic processes (Fig 8-13).

All of these morphologic and structural transformations of dentin, induced by physiologic and patho-

logic processes, result in a dentinal substrate that is less receptive to adhesive treatments than is normal dentin.[48,69,70,197]

The Smear Layer

When the tooth surface is altered by rotary and manual instrumentation during cavity preparation, cutting debris is smeared over the enamel and dentinal surfaces, forming what is termed the *smear layer*[78,227] (Figs 8-14a and 8-14b). The smear layer has been defined as "any debris, calcific in nature, produced by reduction or instrumentation of dentin, enamel or cementum,"[146] or as a "contaminant"[125] that precludes interaction with the underlying pure tooth tissue. This iatrogenically produced layer of debris has a great influence on any adhesive bond formed between the cut tooth and the restorative material.[79,227]

It has been suggested that the burnishing action of the cutting instrument generates considerable amounts of frictional heat locally and shear forces, so that the smear layer becomes attached to the underlying surface in a manner that prevents it from being rinsed off or scrubbed away.[24,220,222] In an in vivo study,[189] ethylenediaminetetraacetic acid (EDTA) was found to be the most potent conditioner for removing the smear layer and opening the orifices of the dentinal tubules. Acidic conditioners include, in order of increasing potential to remove the smear layer, citric, polyacrylic, lactic, and phosphoric acids. Cavity cleansers, such as Tubulicid (Dental Therapeutics) and hydrogen peroxide, were found to have only a slight effect.

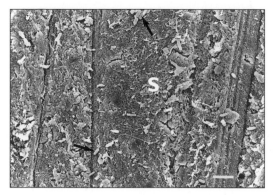

Fig 8-14a Note the bur tracks and the presence of bacteria *(arrows)*. S = smear debris; bar = 3 μm.

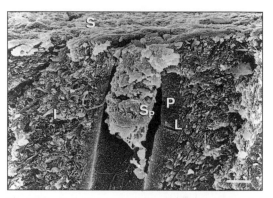

Fig 8-14b Note the smear plug (S$_p$). I = intertubular dentin; L = lateral tubule branch; P = peritubular dentin; S = smear debris; bar = 1 μm.

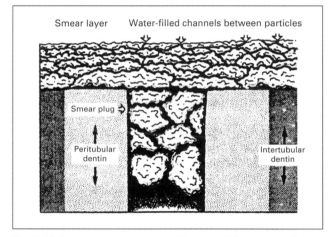

Fig 8-15 Porous smear layer with water-filled channels between the smear particles. (From Pashley et al.[228] Used by permission of *Operative Dentistry*.)

The morphologic features, composition, and thickness of the smear layer are determined to a large extent by the type of instrument used, by the method of irrigation employed, and by the site of dentin at which it is formed.[78,120,220,296] Its composition reflects the structure of the underlying dentin, mainly pulverized hydroxyapatite and altered collagen, mixed with saliva, bacteria (Fig 8-14a), and other grinding surface debris.[224] The thickness of the smear layer has been reported to vary from 0.5 to 5.0 μm.[78,227] Although smear debris occludes the dentinal tubules with the formation of smear plugs, the smear layer is porous and penetrated by submicron channels, which allow small amounts of dentinal fluid to pass through[228] (Figs 8-14b and 8-15). The smear layer is reported to reduce dentinal permeability by about 86%.[218]

Internal and External Dentinal Wetness

The dentinal permeability and, consequently, the internal dentinal wetness depend on several factors, including the diameter and length of the tubule, the viscosity of dentinal fluid and the molecular size of substances dissolved in it, the pressure gradient, the surface area available for diffusion, the patency of the tubules, and the rate of removal of substances by pulpal circulation[219,258] (Fig 8-16). Occlusal dentin is more permeable over the pulp horns than at the center of the occlusal surface, proximal dentin is more permeable than occlusal dentin, and coronal dentin is more permeable than root dentin.[221,226] High dentinal permeability allows bacteria and their toxins to easily penetrate the dentinal tubules to the pulp, if the tubules are not hermetically sealed.[279]

The variability in dentinal permeability makes dentin a more difficult substrate for bonding than enamel.[223,279] Removal of the smear layer creates a wet bonding surface on which dentinal fluid exudes from the dentinal tubules. This aqueous environment affects adhesion, because water competes effectively, by hydrolysis, for all adhesion sites on the hard tissue.[68,92] Early dentin bonding agents failed primarily because their hydrophobic resins were not capable of sufficiently wetting the hydrophilic substrate.[314] In addition, bond strengths of several adhesive systems were shown to decrease as the depth of the preparation increased, because dentinal wetness was greater.[193,240,264,284,296,303] No significant difference in bond strengths is observed between deep and superficial dentin when the smear layer is left intact.[306] Bond strengths of more recent adhesive systems that remove the smear layer appear to be less affected by differ-

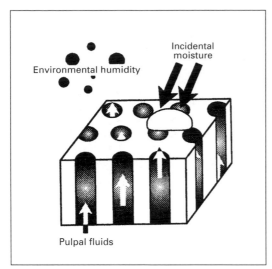

Fig 8-16 Sources of moisture. (From 3M. Reprinted with permission.)

Abbreviations for Chemicals Used in Dental Adhesive Technology*

AA	Acetic acid
4-AETA	4-Acryloxyethyl trimeric acid
bis-GMA	Bisphenol glycidyl methacrylate
BPDM	Biphenyl dimethacrylate
DMA	Dimethacrylate
DMAEMA	Dimethylaminoethyl methacrylate
GPDM	Glycerophosphoric acid dimethacrylate
HAMA	Hydroxyalkyl methacrylate
HDMA	Hexanediol dimethacrylate
HEMA	2-Hydroxyethyl methacrylate
HPMA	Hydroxypropyl methacrylate
MA	Methacrylate
MAC-10	11-Methacryloxy-1 1-undecadicarboxylic acid
10-MDP	10-Methacryloyloxy decyl dihydrogenphosphate
4-MET	4-Methacryloxyethyl trimellitic acid
4-META	4-Methacryloxyethyl trimellitate anhydride
MMA	Methyl methacrylate
MMEM	Mono-methacryloyloxyethylmaleate
MMEP	Mono-2-methacryloxy ethyl phthalate
MPDM	Methacryl propane diol monophosphate
NMENMF	N-Methacryloyloxyethyl-N-methyl formamide
5-NMSA	N-Methacryloyl-5-aminosalicylic acid
NPG	N-Phenylglycine
NPG-GMA	N-Phenylglycine glycidyl methacrylate
NTG-GMA	N-Tolylglycine glycidyl methacrylate
PEG-DMA	Polyethylene glycol dimethacrylate
PENTA	Dipentaerythritol penta acrylate monophosphate
Phenyl-P	2-Methacryloxy ethyl phenyl hydrogen phosphate
PMDM	Pyromellitic acid diethylmethacrylate
PMGDM	Pyromellitic acid glycerol dimethacrylate
PMO-MA	Polymethacryloligomaleic acid
TBB	Tri-n-butyl borane
TEG-DMA	Triethylene glycol dimethacrylate
TEG-GMA	Triethylene glycol-glycidyl methacrylate
UDMA	Urethane dimethacrylate

*Adapted from Van Meerbeek et al[326] and Perdigão.[234]

ences in dentinal depth,[48,267,307] probably because their increased hydrophilicity provides better bonding to the wet dentinal surface.

In addition to internal dentinal wetness, external dentinal wetness, or environmental humidity, has been demonstrated to negatively affect bond strengths to dentin[102,251] (Fig 8-16). This is discussed in more detail later in this chapter.

Wetting of the Adhesive

An ideal interface between dental restorative material and tooth tissue would be one that simulates the natural attachment of enamel to dentin at the dentino-enamel junction.[224] Intimate molecular contact between the two parts is a prerequisite for the development of strong adhesive joints.[166] This means that the adhesive system must sufficiently wet the solid surface, have a viscosity that is low enough to penetrate the micro-porosities, and be able to displace air and moisture during the bonding process.[312] In one study, the wetting characteristics of six adhesives were compared and judged to be sufficient with contact angles of less than 15 degrees[85] (see Fig 8-1). Primers in currently available systems usually contain hydrophilic monomers, such as 2-hydroxyethyl methacrylate (HEMA) (see list of abbreviations), as surface-active agents to enhance the wettability of the hydrophobic adhesive resins. In addition, solvents in modern primers, such as ethanol or acetone, ensure adequate removal of air and liquid by rapid evaporation.

From polymer chemistry, it is known that polarity and solubility characterize molecular interactions that determine many physical properties, such as wetting behavior.[13,14,191] If an adhesive monomer has a polarity and a solubility similar to those of a polymer substrate, the monomer may act as a solvent for the polymer and infiltrate it. If both parameters are sufficiently different, the monomer and polymer are immiscible.[14]

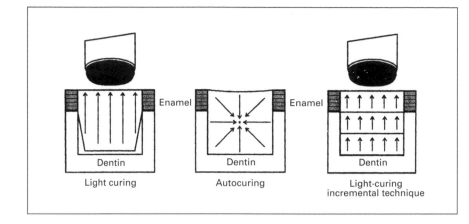

Fig 8-17 Effect of polymerization contraction *(arrows)* on the resin-enamel and resin-dentin bonds when a light-curing resin composite is applied *(left)*, an autocuring resin composite is applied *(middle)*, and a light-curing resin composite is applied with an incremental layering technique *(right)*. (Adapted from Davidson and de Gee,[64] Lutz et al,[175] and Imai et al.[143])

In dental adhesive technology, the collagen phase of dentin is a polymer, and both the primer and adhesive resin contain monomers that penetrate the exposed collagen layer to form a micromechanical bond. If a given conditioner conveys to the dentinal surface a specific polarity and solubility, the primer must match these to achieve penetration. The same is true for the adhesive resin applied to the primed dentinal surface.[13,191]

Polymerization Contraction of Restorative Resins

The dimensional rearrangement of monomers into polymer chains during polymerization inevitably leads to volume shrinkage.[37,94,95] Although high filler loading of the restorative resin matrix reduces polymerization contraction, current resin composites shrink 2.9 to 7.1 vol% during free polymerization.[94,151] Contraction stresses within resin of up to 7 MPa have been reported.[32,135]

In clinical situations, the curing contraction is restrained by the developing bond of the restorative material to the cavity walls.[162] This restriction induces polymerization contraction stress, which counteracts the developing resin-tooth bond by pulling the setting resin composite material away from the cavity walls[64,143,175] (Fig 8-17). If the weakest link is the bonding interface with the tooth, the resin-enamel bond may survive the shrinkage, but the weaker resin-dentin interface may not.[64] No dental resin composite material currently available is free of shrinkage during polymerization,[80] however, research is underway to develop nonshrinking materials.[79,80,97,289] A double ring-opening polymerization process, based on high-strength expandable resin composites used in industry, is being evaluated.[80,82,97,289]

Compensation for Polymerization Contraction

Flow

Throughout the entire polymerization process, plastic deformation, or flow, of the resin composite occurs and may partially compensate for the induced shrinkage stress.[64] This irreversible plastic deformation takes place during the early stages of the setting process, when the contraction stress exceeds the elastic limit of the restorative resin. As the setting proceeds, contraction and flow gradually decrease because stiffness increases. Fast-setting light-curing resin composites exhibit less flow-related stress relief, while self- or autocuring resin composites give the developing adhesive bond to dentin more time to survive. Only a fraction of the final stiffness is reached by most self-curing resin composites 10 minutes after mixing.[38] Consequently, the combination of a slow curing rate and rapid formation of an adhesive bond is considered favorable for the preservation of marginal integrity.[162]

The apparently superior marginal adaptation of autocuring resin composites can also be explained by the presence of air bubbles, which contribute to the amount of free surface and eventually increase the flow capacity of the resin composite.[5,96]

Restriction of flow is affected by the configuration of the restoration, known as the C-factor. The C-factor is the ratio of bonded (flow-inactive) to unbonded or free (flow-active) surfaces. An increase in the number of bonded surfaces results in a higher C-factor and greater contraction stress on the adhesive bond.[93] Only the free surface of a resin restoration, which is not restricted by bonding to the cavity walls, can act as a reservoir for plastic deformation in the initial stage of polymerization.[64] The higher the ratio of bonded to free resin surfaces, the less flow may compensate for contraction stress (Fig 8-18). For example, to improve marginal integrity of resin composite in a Class 5 restoration, a flatter and more wedge-shaped cavity design would be preferred to the typical butt-joint, five-walled preparation.[9,65,129] Carrying this a step farther, the use of a base material, such as glass-ionomer cement, within the cavity preparation (providing a so-called "sandwich" restoration) decreases the volume of the resin composite portion of the restoration, thus generating more free restorative surface relative to the smaller amount of resin.[175]

Other methods have been used to compensate for polymerization contraction. Bowen[34] has reported that the placement of glass or ceramic blocks into soft resin composite before light curing, displacing as much of the resin composite as possible, results in reduced microleakage. The improvement exhibited by megafilled resin composite restorations was attributed to a decrease in the overall curing contraction of the limited amount of resin composite and a decrease in the coefficient of thermal expansion of the restoration containing the inserts.[35,67]

Prepolymerized resin composite inserts may also be used to help offset polymerization contraction. One example is the addition of prepolymerized resin pieces in the manufacture of microfilled resin composites. At the other extreme are resin composite inlays, which are cemented in the cavity with a luting resin. The use of inlays avoids the direct adverse effect of polymerization contraction on the developing resin-tooth bond. However, the flow-active free surface of the luting resin composite is relatively small at the narrow inlay-tooth marginal gap, yielding a high C-factor. Consequently, the luting resin composite is not likely to provide enough compensation for the shrinkage stress induced by polymerization of the luting resin.[93] Nevertheless, the incorporation of pores by mixing of the two components and the slow autocuring rate of the dual-cured luting resin may still allow sufficient stress relaxation by flow.[5]

Another strategy to slow curing and thus allow more flow to compensate for shrinkage stress is the so-called *soft-start* or *ramped* light-curing technique.[188,266,323] Curing lights designed for this technique produce low-intensity light (400 mW/cm² or less) during a period of about 10 seconds, after which the light intensity is immediately or exponentially increased to about 800 mW/cm² or more.

The introduction of laser and xenon arc high-powered light-curing technology, a contrasting approach, has elicited much controversy. The theory behind this high-intensity light-curing technology is that curing

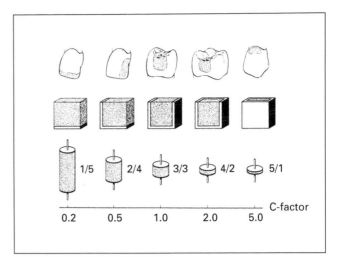

Fig 8-18 Diverse cavity configurations with different C-factors, or ratios of bonded to unbonded (free) surface, and their corresponding clinical cases. (From Feilzer et al.[93] Reprinted with permission.)

times can be reduced to 1 to 3 seconds without a decrease of physicomechanical material properties. Advocates of this new light-curing technique recommend placement of small resin composite increments to ensure sufficient polymerization. Evolution of curing technology is expected to continue. The recent development of long-lasting, high-intensity light-emitting diodes (LEDs) may become a useful adjunct to existing curing methods.[192]

Hygroscopic Expansion

The effect of polymerization shrinkage is somewhat tempered by fluid absorption, which causes resin composite to swell and may offset the residual elastic stress. Again, the configuration of the cavity determines the effectiveness of this compensation mechanism.[95,163] Overcompensation may even transform contraction stress into expansion stress. Microfilled resin composites have been shown to absorb nearly two and a half times more water than macrofilled materials because of the greater volume of resin in the microfills.[8]

However, hygroscopic expansion occurs during the days and weeks immediately following placement of the resin composite restoration, after the dentin bonding may already have failed. When this has occurred, hygroscopic expansion may force a Class 5 resin composite restoration to expand beyond the margin of the preparation.[163]

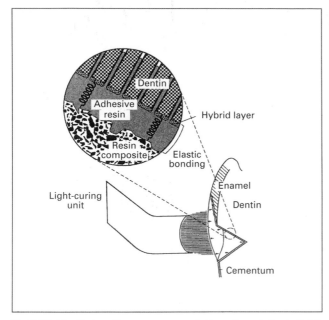

Fig 8-19 Elastic bonding area concept. Use of a relatively thick elastic adhesive may compensate for polymerization shrinkage that occurs in resin composite. Shown is an incrementally filled Class 5 resin composite restoration.

Elasticity

If the resin-tooth bond remains intact, the final stiffness or rigidity of a resin composite may play a compensating role in coping with remaining polymerization contraction stress. Stiffness is quantified by Young's modulus of elasticity, which represents the resistance of a material to elastic deformation.[37] The lower the Young's modulus of a restorative resin, the greater its flexibility and the more capacity it has to reduce remaining contraction stress. Resin composites with a high filler content have a higher Young's modulus of elasticity, which will reduce volumetric contraction (because of the higher filler content relative to the lower resin content), but have higher remaining contraction stress, which may affect the resin-dentin interface.

Viscous adhesive resins produce a rather thick resin bonding layer between the stiff dentinal cavity wall and the shrinking restorative resin composite. Stretching of this intermediate layer (with a low Young's modulus) may provide sufficient elasticity to relieve polymerization contraction stresses of the restorative resin composite[164,165,330] (Fig 8-19). Based on this theory, an "elastic bonding concept" has been advanced. It has been determined that a bonding layer thickness of 125 μm reduces shrinkage stresses below dentin bond strengths, preserving the bond.[199] A flexible in-termediate resin layer may also better transmit and distribute stresses induced by thermal changes, water absorption, and occlusal forces across the interface.[330] Also, a thick adhesive resin layer permits limited inhibition of polymerization by oxygen without impairing the resin-dentin bond.[263]

Support for the elastic bonding concept is provided by in vitro experiments conducted with Gluma (Bayer) resin. When Gluma was prepolymerized in a relatively thick layer,[63,132] less microleakage occurred than when it was left uncured prior to application of the resin composite. Lack of such a built-in polymerization contraction relaxation mechanism might have largely accounted for the high clinical failure rates recorded for Gluma, two experimental total-etch systems, and Gluma 2000.[332]

Cervical Sealing

Sealing of the cervical marginal gaps with an unfilled low-viscosity resin, after the restorative resin has been cured, is another technique that has been described to overcome the negative effects of polymerization shrinkage and obtain sealed cervical restorations.[34,161] Use of a restorative resin with high elasticity and low curing contraction in combination with such a low-viscosity resin layer may provide sufficient strain relief to compensate for the small curing contraction of the unfilled resin layer.[161] However, this technique is laborious and prone to failure in the event of contamination with blood or saliva.

Initial Polymerization

Initiation of polymerization at the resin-tooth interface, directing the shrinking resin material toward the cavity wall rather than away from it, is advantageous.[143] Contraction has always been claimed to occur toward the light source in light-curing resin composites, whereas initial setting has been said to occur in the center of the bulk of material in self-curing resin composites[175] (see Fig 8-17). For both light-curing and self-curing systems, tensile stresses operate across the resin composite–dentin interface, pulling the material away from the cavity walls. Countering the theory that contraction occurs toward the curing light in light-curing systems, a recent study[340] using finite element analysis showed that the direction of polymerization shrinkage was not significantly affected by the orientation of the incoming curing light. Instead, the cavity shape and the bond quality determined the direction of the polymerization vectors.

That study concluded that the contraction patterns between auto- and photocuring composites were similar.

For many years, Fusayama[108] has argued that the initial setting of autocuring resins starts at the dentinal wall because body heat accelerates the chemical reaction. In other words, the shrinking restoration is pulled toward, rather than away from, the cavity base.[64] Evaluation of premolar restorations in vivo showed that the use of chemically cured resin composite did not result in reduced gap formation relative to gaps produced when light-cured composites were used. This study could not confirm the supposed stress-relieving effect of self-curing resin composites.[236]

For light-initiated resin composite polymerization, there is general agreement that the unbonded resin material at the free surface of the restoration sets first when it is exposed to the light source; thus, its flow relaxation capacity is considerably diminished. Incremental layering techniques have been used to minimize the negative effects of light polymerization to increase the actual resin-free area relative to the resin-bonded area[130,176,316] (see Fig 8-17). This disciplined application technique promotes sufficient polymerization of the deepest material, in contrast to that achieved with the limited light penetration that occurs with bulk placement. The incremental technique has also been hypothesized to result in less stress caused by polymerization contraction, because the flow relaxation capacity is higher and can be used to direct polymerization shrinkage of each increment toward the cavity walls. But the theory that an incremental placement technique reduces stress effects of resin composite shrinkage is debated.[339] Completeness of cure, adequate adaptation to the cavity walls, and adequate bond formation may still be reasons to use a composite layering technique.[339] Furthermore, improved marginal adaptation of the critical gingivoproximal border of Class 2 resin composite restorations has been described with the use of a three-sited light-curing technique with laterally light-reflecting wedges.[175,177] Once again, however, the benefit of this directed curing technique is no longer generally accepted.[339]

Some adhesive systems are also designed so that chemical polymerization is initiated at the surface of dentin.[10,12] For example, the simplified Gluma 2000 System attempts to impregnate the dentinal surface with an amine part of the catalytic system in the form of glycine, which is claimed to establish a chemical bond to collagen.[11] Because camphoroquinone is incorporated as the other part of the catalytic system, and selected methacrylic monomers, such as HEMA and bisphenol glycidyl methacrylate (bis-GMA), are included in the adhesive resin, the polymerization was expected to be initiated at the adhesive interface. This simplified pretreatment technique has proved to be highly effective in reducing the marginal gap in cavities in both enamel and dentin.[11] However, several in vivo and in vitro reports on the use of amino acids have yielded contradictory results.[152,232,332]

A water-triggered polymerization has been described for the 4-methacryloxyethyl trimellitate anhydride/methyl methacrylate–tri-n-butyl borane (4-META/MMA-TBB) systems, such as Super-Bond D-Liner (Sun Medical) or AmalgamBond (Parkell).[206] Although water and oxygen, which are omnipresent in dentin, are normally expected to affect the polymerization process of bonding resins, they may apparently also act as coinitiators of the polymerization reaction.[144] Effective water-triggered polymerization in deep, tubule-rich dentin has been suggested to direct resin shrinkage toward the dentinal surface itself. Imai et al[143] hypothesized that the application of ferric chloride with these adhesive systems to acid etch dentin might promote and initiate resin polymerization at the interface. More research is needed to explore these mechanisms to initiate polymerization at the interface.

Thermal Expansion Coefficient and Thermal Conductivity

Because the coefficient of thermal expansion of resin is about four times that of tooth structure, any bonded resin restoration is likely to suffer from marginal gap formation.[8,260] The microfilled resin composites have a higher coefficient of thermal expansion than do hybrid-type resin composites.[37] However, Harper et al[133] suggested that the dimensional change that occurs in the clinical restoration as a result of temperature fluctuations may not be as great in magnitude as its relatively high coefficient of thermal expansion would suggest. The temperature transfer through resin composite restorations is slower, and the rate of temperature change is lower than in amalgam restorations.[133] Nevertheless, marginal adaptation and microleakage studies have shown that prolonged thermocycling induces percolation under resin composite restorations.[252,260]

Transmission of Stress Across the Restoration-Tooth Interface

The adhesive bond between a restorative material and tooth has a biomechanical role in the distribution of functional stress throughout the whole tooth.[68] A true

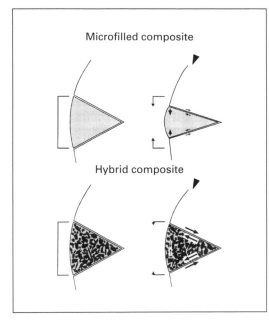

Fig 8-20 Tooth flexure concept. Microfilled resin composite flexes and absorbs some of the force, but the more rigid hybrid resin composite is more likely to be dislodged.

bond will transmit stress applied to the restoration to the remaining tooth structure, and bonded restorations may strengthen weakened teeth.[74,110] Displacement and bending of the cusps may compensate for the contraction stress in Class 2 resin composite restorations,[182] but polymerization contraction may also induce cuspal fracture.[68,151,169] In general, high masticatory stresses are known to reduce the longevity of adhesively bonded restorations.[203,279]

For wedge-shaped cervical lesions, transmission of occlusal loads may affect retention of Class 5 cervical restorations. Noncarious cervical lesions have a multifactorial etiology,[39,116,169,171] possibly including incisal or occlusal loads that induce compressive and tensile stresses at the dentinoenamel junction in the cervical region. Adhesively placed cervical restorations are subject to the same stresses,[137,138,330] which may progressively debond the resin restoration and eventually dislodge it. When resin composites with relatively low Young's moduli of elasticity, such as microfilled resin composites, are used, elastic deformation may partially compensate for the induced stress (Fig 8-20). The forces created by compression of the restoration are localized mainly in the bulk of the resin composite as compressive stress and to a lesser degree as shear

stress at the adhesive interface. When more rigid, denser resin composites are placed, the shear stress at the interface might exceed the compression stress, affecting the bond of resin to dentin. Naturally, this hypothesis can be valid only when the adhesive bond is sufficiently strong. In a clinical study involving Class 5 restorations placed with diverse dentin adhesive systems, the retention rate was found to improve as the Young's moduli of the resin composites declined.[332]

A similar concept of "tooth flexure" has been reported by Heymann et al.[138] It has been suggested that microfilled resin composites compress rather than dislodge during tooth flexure.[21] A high correlation between the modulus of elasticity and marginal leakage was found by Kemp-Scholte and Davidson.[165] They reported that the higher the modulus of elasticity of the resin composite used, the greater the number of cervical gaps.[162] Therefore, microfilled resin composites have commonly been preferred for restorations in wedge-shaped cervical lesions.[161] However, in recent clinical trials, performance of microfilled resin composites was comparable to that of hybrid resin composite materials in Class 5 noncarious cervical lesions at 2 years.[43,248] These findings cast some doubt on the advantages of flexible resin composites in stress-induced cervical lesions, though benefits may yet appear after a longer term.

Biocompatibility

To the physicochemical aspects of dentin and resin composite restorative materials must be added the biologic concern of pulpal compatibility. The dissemination of residual monomer molecules to the pulp chamber via the dentinal tubules has been reported to involve a significant degree of cytotoxicity, even in low concentrations.[6] However, in vivo biocompatibility studies have demonstrated that resin composites, whether fully or partially cured, cause little pulpal irritation if the cavities are sealed to prevent ingress of bacteria from the oral environment.[60,215,287,315] Fusayama[105] has argued that the fundamental factor involved in pulpal irritation is separation of the resin from dentin (see Fig 8-17). When debonding occurs, thermal and mechanical stresses on the restoration exert a pumping action on the fluid in the gap, pressing irritants or bacterial toxins into the tubules.[105,107]

Some general health concerns have been expressed related to the use of resin composite systems. One concern is that leakage of bisphenol-A from bis-GMA–based resin composites and sealants may have estrogenic effects.[181,210,214,241,271,280] Söderholm and Mariotti[280] concluded that, considering the dosages and routes of administration and the modest response of estrogenic-sensitive target organs, the short-term risk of estrogenic effects from treatment using bisphenol A–based resins is insignificant and therefore should not be of concern to the general public. Long-term effects need to be investigated further. A "three-finger" syndrome, or a contact allergy, at the fingertips of clinicians or dental assistants has been described, although there is currently little experimental data available.[158,159,271] A "noncontact" handling of diverse monomer-based materials, especially primers and adhesive resins, is therefore strongly advised.

Although the biologic evaluation of dentin adhesive systems has received a considerable amount of attention, the results and conclusions of these biocompatibility tests vary widely and do not cover all systems. Therefore, conclusions about the influence of chemical irritants on postoperative sensitivity must be considered premature.[279]

The use of acids on vital dentin has traditionally been avoided because of the fear of pulpal irritation, confusion over the protective function of the smear layer, and the lack in efficacy of the bonding agents.[90,106,190,257,283] Stanley et al[286] reported that acid etching of dentin causes pulpal reactions when the remaining dentin is less than 1.0 mm thick, but other histopathologic studies have shown that acid etching dentin has no adverse effects.[138,315] Fusayama has stated that, in the case of carious dentin, diffusion of penetrating acid is largely limited to 10 µm, because of the blocking action of odontoblast processes in the tubules of vital teeth and intertubular crystals.[107]

Adhesion to Enamel and Dentin

Concepts in restorative dentistry have been continually changing during the last four decades, and adhesive technology has become steadily more important. Today, clinicians are confronted with a continuous and rapid turnover in adhesive materials. The trend toward adhesive dentistry started in the mid-1960s with the advent of the first commercial restorative resin composites, followed in the early 1970s with the introduction of the acid-etch technique in clinical practice. Since then, there has been continuous progress in developing more refined and diversified restorative composites along with steady improve-

ment in bonding agents. Effective adhesion to enamel was achieved with relative ease and has repeatedly proven to be a durable and reliable clinical procedure. Although adhesion to dentin is not yet as reliable as that to enamel, today's adhesives produce superior results in laboratories,[99,301] along with an improved clinical effectiveness,[332,336] and the performance of dentin bonding has approached that of enamel bonding. Early one-step dentin bonding agents became multistep systems with more complicated, time-consuming, and technique-sensitive application procedures. Today, so-called universal, all-purpose, or multipurpose adhesive systems are available that purportedly bond to enamel, dentin, amalgam, metal, and porcelain. In the early 1990s, the selective enamel-etching technique was replaced by a total-etch concept. Since then, universal enamel-dentin conditioners are simultaneously applied to enamel and dentin. Now that total-etch adhesives have reached an acceptable bonding effectiveness, most recent efforts have been to simplify the multistep bonding process and to reduce its sensitivity to errors in clinical handling.

Bonding to tooth tissue can also be achieved directly with glass-ionomer cements. Glass-ionomer–based materials have an auto-adhesive capacity due to their specific chemical formula and structural nature. Parallel with the progress made in resin-based adhesives, glass-ionomer technology has undergone many improvements and modifications to the original chemistry, developed in the early 1970s by Wilson and Kent.[344] A recent trend in adhesive material development has been to combine glass-ionomer and resin composite technology in new adhesive systems and restorative materials with mixed characteristics.

Enamel Acid-Etching Technique

Adhesion to enamel is achieved through acid etching of this highly mineralized substrate, which substantially enlarges its surface area for bonding. This enamel-bonding technique, known as the acid-etching technique, was the invention of Buonocore[44] in 1955. He demonstrated a 100-fold increase in retention of small buttons of polymethylmethacrylate to incisors in vivo when enamel was etched with 85% phosphoric acid for 2 minutes. Further research into the underlying mechanism of the bond suggested that taglike resin extensions were formed and micromechanically interlocked with the enamel microporosities created by etching.[46,117,118]

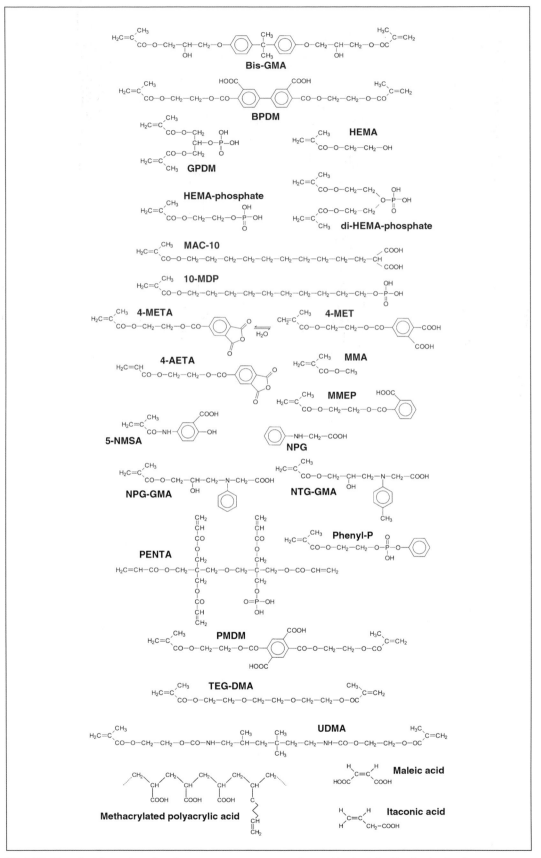

Fig 8-21 Chemical formulas of various monomers commonly used in dental adhesive technology.

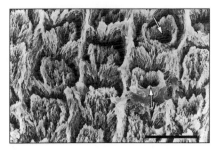

Fig 8-22a Type I enamel-etching pattern *(arrows)*. Etching of prism cores is predominant. Bar = 6 µm.

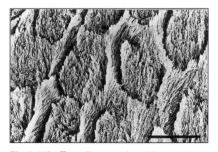

Fig 8-22b Type II enamel-etching pattern. Etching of prism peripheries is predominant. Bar = 6 µm.

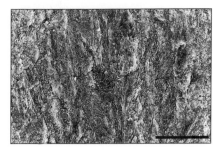

Fig 8-22c Type III enamel-etching pattern. No prism structures are evident. Bar = 6 µm.

Enamel etching transforms the smooth enamel surface into an irregular surface with a high surface-free energy (about 72 dynes/cm), more than twice that of unetched enamel.[150] An unfilled liquid acrylic resin with low viscosity, the enamel bonding agent, wets the high-energy surface and is drawn into the microporosities by capillary attraction. Enamel bonding agents are commonly based on bis-GMA, developed by Bowen[29] in 1962, or urethane dimethacrylate (UDMA) (Fig 8-21). Both monomers are viscous and hydrophobic and are often diluted with other monomers of higher hydrophilicity and lower viscosity, such as triethylene glycol dimethacrylate (TEG-DMA) and HEMA (Fig 8-21). The bond between enamel and the restorative material is established by polymerization of monomers inside the microporosities and by copolymerization of remaining carbon-carbon double bonds with the matrix phase of the resin composite, producing strong chemical bonds.[11] In addition, the potential for chemical interaction between specific monomers and the etched enamel surface cannot be excluded.[206]

Acid etching removes about 10 µm of the enamel surface and creates a microporous layer from 5 to 50 µm deep. Three enamel-etching patterns have been described.[119,277] These include type I, in which there is predominant dissolution of the prism cores; type II, in which there is predominant dissolution of the prism peripheries; and type III, in which no prism structures are evident (Figs 8-22a to 8-22c). Two types of resin tags have been described.[20,246] Macrotags are formed circularly between enamel prism peripheries; microtags are formed at the cores of enamel prisms, where the monomer cures into a multitude of individual crypts formed where hydroxyapatite crystals have dissolved (Fig 8-23). Microtags probably contribute most to the bond strength because of their greater quantity and large surface area.

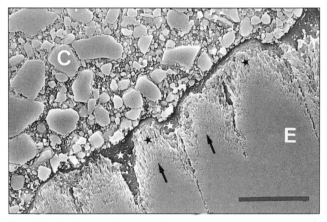

Fig 8-23 Field-emission scanning electron photomicrograph showing a resin-enamel interface subjected to an argon-ion–bombardment procedure when a "three-step total-etch" adhesive (Scotchbond Multi-Purpose Plus, 3M) was bonded to 35% phosphoric acid–etched enamel (E). Macrotags *(white stars)* are formed circularly between the longitudinally sectioned enamel prism *(black arrows)* peripheries. Microtags *(black stars)* are formed at the cores of the enamel prisms. C = luting composite; bar = 5 µm. (From Peumans et al.[246] Reprinted with permission from Elsevier Science.)

The effect of acid etching on enamel depends on several parameters[123,302]:

- The kind of acid used
- The acid concentration
- The etching time
- The form of the etchant (gel, semigel, or aqueous solution)
- The rinse time
- The way in which etching is activated (rubbing, agitation, and/or repeated application of fresh acid)
- Whether enamel is instrumented before etching
- The chemical composition and condition of enamel

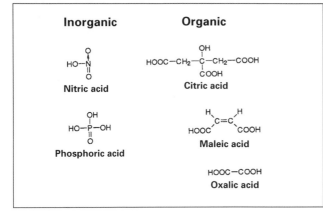

Fig 8-24 Chemical formulas of inorganic and organic acids supplied with total-etch adhesive systems.

- Whether enamel is on primary or permanent teeth
- Whether enamel is prism-structured or prismless
- Whether enamel is fluoridated, demineralized, or stained

An acid gel is generally preferred over a liquid because its application is easier to control.[12]

In vitro bond strengths of resin composite to phosphoric acid–etched enamel typically average 20 MPa.[81,113,124] This bond strength is thought to be sufficient to resist the shrinkage stress that accompanies the polymerization of resin composites.[65] Consequently, if the preparation is completely bordered by enamel, acid etching significantly reduces microleakage at the cavosurface interface.[62,273] This enamel-etching technique has proven to be a durable and reliable clinical procedure for routine applications in modern restorative dentistry.

Complete removal of the etchant and dissolved calcium phosphates, and preservation of the clean etched field without moisture and saliva contamination, are crucial to the longevity of the resin-enamel bond.[302] For this reason, isolation with a rubber dam is preferred over isolation with cotton rolls.[17]

Phosphoric Acid Etchants

Generally, use of a phosphoric acid concentration between 30% and 40%[276] (Fig 8-24), an etching time of not less than 15 seconds, and washing times of 5 to 10 seconds are recommended to achieve the most receptive enamel surface for bonding.[12,121,294,295]

Historically, some controversy existed about the concentration of phosphoric acid that would provide optimal etching efficacy, because some acids have been reported to form precipitates on the surface that might interfere with resin bonding.[117,160,249] One study showed that 50% phosphoric acid applied for 60 seconds on enamel produces a precipitate of monocalcium phosphate monohydrate that can be rinsed off. A precipitate of dicalcium phosphate dihydrate produced by etching with a less than 27% phosphoric acid was found not to be easily removable.[55] Calcium dissolution and etching depth increase as the concentration of phosphoric acid increases until the concentration reaches 40%; at higher concentrations, a reverse effect is obtained. Although most commercial enamel etchants have concentrations between 30% and 40%, lower concentrations are often used without compromising enamel bond strengths.[19,124,145,356]

The etching time has also been reduced from the traditional 60-second application with 30% to 40% phosphoric acid to etching times as brief as 15 seconds. Several laboratory and clinical studies have demonstrated bonding effectiveness to be equivalent with etching times from 15 to 60 seconds.[18,211,300]

Adequate rinsing is an essential step. Rinsing times of 1 to 3 seconds on flat surfaces have been shown to provide for adequate bond and seal.[294,295] For preparations with more geometric form, a rinse time of 5 to 10 seconds is recommended. The use of ethanol to remove residual water from the etched pattern has been reported to enhance the ability of resin monomers to penetrate the etched enamel surface irregularities.[121,256] Modern primers frequently contain drying agents, such as ethanol or acetone, with a similar effect.

In addition to phosphoric acid, other inorganic and organic acids (Fig 8-24) have been advocated for acid etching enamel (and dentin), as they were supplied with specific commercial adhesives.

Adhesion to Dentin

Successful bonding to enamel was achieved with relative ease, but the development of predictable bonding to dentin has been more problematic. Only recently have dentin adhesive systems produced laboratory results that approach those of enamel bonding[1,48,98,99,170] and achieve a predictable level of clinical success.[73,248,332,336]

The chronologic method of classifying dentin bonding systems, the "generational" classification system, is described below. A classification system based on bonding mechanism is described later in the chapter.

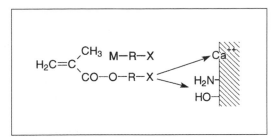

Fig 8-25 Claimed chemical bonding to inorganic and organic dentinal components. (From Asmussen and Munksgaard.[11] Reprinted with permission.)

Table 8-2	Chemical design of dentin adhesives with potential chemical bonding*
Potential Ca^{2+}–bonding dentin adhesives	
M-R$_1$-POYZ	Phosphate group
M-R$_2$-NZ-R$_3$-COOH	Amino acid
M-R$_3$-OH	Amino alcohol
M-R$_4$-COOH | COOH	Dicarboxylic acid
Potential collagen-bonding dentin adhesives	
M-R$_1$-NCO	Isocyanate group
M-R$_2$-COCl	Acid chloride
M-R$_3$-CHO	Aldehyde group
M-R$_4$-CO | COOH	Carboxylic acid anhydride

*M = methacrylate; R$_{1-4}$ = variable spacers; Y, Z = variable substituents. From Asmussen and Hansen.[14] Reprinted with permission.

Development of Resin Dentin Adhesives

First-Generation Adhesives

Imitating his enamel acid-etching technique, Buonocore et al[45] in 1956 reported that glycerophosphoric acid dimethacrylate (GPDM) (see Fig 8-21) could bond to hydrochloric acid–etched dentinal surfaces. The bond strengths attained with this primitive adhesive technique were only 2 to 3 MPa, however, in contrast to the 15 to 20 MPa bond strengths obtained to acid-etched enamel, and the bond was unstable in water.[9] Predating the experiments of Buonocore, other investigators used the same monomer, GPDM, in the early 1950s with the introduction of Sevriton Cavity Seal (Amalgamated Dental Company), an acrylic resin material that could be catalytically polymerized by the action of sulfinic acid.[183,186]

After the failures of this early dentin–acid-etching technique, numerous dentin adhesives with complex chemical formulas were designed and developed with the objective of promoting chemical adhesion. Dentin bonding agents were no longer unfilled resins intended purely to enhance wetting of the dentinal surface prior to the application of a stiff resin composite. They became bifunctional organic monomers with specific reactive groups that were claimed to react chemically with the inorganic calcium-hydroxyapatite and/or organic collagen component of dentin (Fig 8-25).[327] The traditional concept of molecules with chemical adhesive potential is based on a bifunctional molecule with a methacrylate group, M, linked to a reactive group, X, by an intermediary group, R, or spacer[9,14] (Fig 8-25). While X is designed for reaction with and/or bonding to dentin, M allows the molecule

to polymerize and copolymerize with resin composites. The spacer, R, must be of suitable length and polarity to keep the reactive groups separated.

The development of N-phenylglycine glycidyl methacrylate (NPG-GMA) (see Fig 8-21) was the basis of the first commercially available dentin bonding agent, Cervident (SS White).[30] This first-generation dentin bonding agent theoretically bonded to enamel and dentin by chelation with calcium on the tooth surface and had improved water resistance.[3,36]

Second-Generation Adhesives

Clearfil Bond System F (Kuraray), introduced in 1978, was the first product of a large second generation of dentin adhesives, such as Bondlite (Kerr/Sybron), J&J VLC Dentin Bonding Agent (Johnson & Johnson Dental), and Scotchbond (3M), among others. These products were based on phosphorous esters of methacrylate derivatives. Their adhesive mechanism involved enhanced surface wetting as well as ionic interaction between negatively charged phosphate groups and positively charged calcium.[51,85] Although diverse chemical interactions were postulated with either the inorganic or the organic part of dentin (Fig 8-25 and Table 8-2), and are theoretically possible, primary chemical adhesion is not thought to play a major role in the bonding process.[77,80,87,89,281,282,305,329,349] The second-generation systems had modest bond strengths, seldom exceeding 5 to 6 MPa.[14] In those instances in which higher bond strengths were measured,[31,204] other bonding mechanisms that were unknown at that time were probably involved. Clinical trials of these dentin bonding agents commonly met with poor results.[138,149,321,322,325] It was speculated that clinical failure was due to inadequate hydrolytic stability in the oral environment[86,139] and because their primary bonding was to the smear layer rather than to the underlying dentin.[355] The presence of an intermediate smear layer prevents intimate resin-dentin contact, which is a prerequisite for a chemical reaction.[166]

Third-Generation Adhesives

The basis for the third generation of dentin adhesives was laid when the Japanese philosophy of etching dentin to remove the smear layer gained acceptance.[104] This dentin–acid-etching technique was discouraged in America and Europe until the end of the 1980s because of concerns that acid etchants would induce pulpal inflammation.[25,61,259,286] The postulated bonding mechanism of the dentin-etching technique was that etched dentin would provide micromechanical retention for the restorative resin composite by allowing penetration of the resin bonding agent into the opened dentinal tubules. However, the counterpressure of dentinal fluid and its abundant presence on the bonding site hindered the micromechanical attachment of the early hydrophobic resins.[224,314] Based on this total-etch concept, Clearfil New Bond was introduced in 1984. It contained HEMA and 10-methacryloyloxy decyl dihydrogenphosphate (10-MDP) (see Fig 8-21), which had long hydrophobic and short hydrophilic components as active components.

Removal of the smear layer by the use of acids or chelating agents reduces the availability of calcium ions for interaction with chelating surface-active comonomers, such as NPG-GMA (see Fig 8-21). Bowen et al,[31] in 1982, tried to supplement the calcium ions by applying an acidic solution of 6.8% ferric oxalate to dentin as an acidic conditioner or cleanser. An insoluble precipitate of calcium oxalates and ferric phosphates was formed on the surface; the precipitate was also expected to seal the dentinal tubules and protect the pulp. The subsequent application of an acetone solution of pyromellitic acid diethylmethacrylate (PMDM) mixed with NPG-GMA or its alternative, N-tolylglycine glycidyl methacrylate (NTG-GMA) (see Fig 8-21), improved bonding to levels of clinical significance.[36] Ferric oxalate sometimes caused black interfacial staining, however, and was later replaced by aluminum oxalate.[33] The microretention created by etching dentin probably contributes more to bonding than does the oxalate precipitation,[279] however, and the precipitate may, in fact, interfere with the interaction of adhesive and dentin.[229]

Extensive research in Japan has demonstrated a favorable effect of 4-META (see Fig 8-21) on bonding to dentin.[204,206,207] 4-META contains both hydrophobic and hydrophilic chemical groups. In 1982, Nakabayashi et al[204] used this system to describe the micromechanical bonding mechanism that is used by current adhesive systems. With this system, dentin is etched with an aqueous solution of 10% citric acid and 3% ferric chloride, followed by the application of an aqueous solution of 35% HEMA and a self-curing adhesive resin containing 4-META, methyl methacrylate (MMA), and TBB, the last as a polymerization initiator (see Fig 8-21). Based on this technology, adhesive systems such as C&B Metabond (Sun Medical), Super-Bond D-Liner, and Amalgambond Plus (Parkell) are commercially available and have been reported to yield consistent results in in vitro experiments,[233,318] regardless of dentinal depth[307] (Table 8-3).

Removal of the smear layer with chelating agents such as EDTA was introduced with Gluma. However, irrespective of the use of EDTA, the effectiveness of this system, as mentioned, may have been impaired by the manufacturer's instructions to place the restorative resin composite over an uncured adhesive resin.[63,132,332] Denthesive (Heraeus-Kulzer) also used EDTA to pretreat dentin prior to bonding.

Another approach to smear layer treatment was the use of Scotchprep (3M), an aqueous solution of 2.5% maleic acid and 55% HEMA, followed by the application of an unfilled bis-GMA/HEMA adhesive resin (see Figs 8-21 and 8-24 and Table 8-3). The simultaneous etching and impregnation of the dentinal surface with this acidic hydrophilic monomer solution enabled more consistent and durable results.[332] In this way, Scotchbond 2 (3M) was in fact the precursor of current self-etching adhesives, though the self-etching primer Scotchprep at that time was advocated to be used solely on dentin. Supported by excellent clinical results in diverse clinical trials,[71,153,253] Scotchbond 2 was the first product to receive Provisional Acceptance from the American Dental Association, which was followed by Full Acceptance.[59] Other systems, such as Coltène ART Bond (Coltène), Superlux Universalbond 2 (DMG), and Syntac (Vivadent) are based on this smear layer–dissolving approach (Table 8-3).

Fourth-Generation Adhesives

Significant advances in adhesive dentistry were made with the development of the multistep dentin adhesive systems in the early-to-mid 1990s. Essential to the enhanced adhesive capacity and responsible for the

Table 8-3	Classification of modern adhesive systems according to their clinical application mode and the mechanism of adhesion to dentin		
Product	**Manufacturer**	**Product**	**Manufacturer**

One-step smear layer–modifying adhesives

Product	Manufacturer	Product	Manufacturer
Ariston Liner (Ariston)	Vivadent		
Compoglass SCA (Compoglass)	Vivadent		
Futurabond (Glasiosite)	Voco		
Hytac OSB (Hytac)	ESPE		
Prime&Bond 2.1 (Dyract)	Dentsply		
Prime&Bond NT* (Dyract)	Dentsply		
Solist (Luxat)	DMG		

One-step smear layer–dissolving adhesives/
One-step self-etch adhesives

Product	Manufacturer
Etch&Prime 3.0	Degussa
One-up Bond F	Tokuyama
Prompt L-Pop 1 (Hytac)	ESPE
Prompt L-Pop 2 (Composites)	ESPE
Syntac (self-etch)	Vivadent

Two-step glass-ionomer adhesives

Product	Manufacturer
FujiBond LC*	GC
FujiBond LC Liquid-Liquid	GC

Two-step smear layer–modifying adhesive

Product	Manufacturer
ProBOND	Dentsply

Two-step smear layer–dissolving adhesives/
Two-step self-etch adhesives

Product	Manufacturer
Clearfil Liner Bond 2*	Kuraray
Clearfil Liner Bond 2V*	Kuraray
Clearfil SE*	Kuraray
Imperva FL-Bond* (Fluorobond)	Shofu
Mac Bond 2	Tokuyama
NRC & Prime&Bond NT*	Dentsply
OptiBond (no-etch)*	Kerr
OptiBond FL (no-etch)*	Kerr
F2000 (Sustel)	3M
Unifil BOND	GC
Coltène ART Bond†	Coltène/Whaledent
Denthesive II†	Heraeus-Kulzer
Ecusit Primer-Mono†	DMG
Imperva Bond (no etch)†	Shofu
Scotchbond 2†	3M
Solid Bond†	Hereaus-Kulzer
Superlux Universalbond 2†	DMG
Syntac†	Vivadent
XR-Bond†	Kerr

Two-step smear layer–removing adhesives/
"One-bottle" total-etch adhesives

Product	Manufacturer
Bond 1	Jeneric/Pentron
Dentastic UNO	Pulpdent
EG Bond	Sun Medical
Everbond*	ESPE
Excite*	Vivadent
Gluma 2000	Bayer
Gluma One Bond	Heraeus-Kulzer
One Coat Bond*	Coltène/Whaledent
One-Step	Bisco
Optibond Solo*	Kerr
Optibond Solo Plus*	Kerr
Prime&Bond 2.1	Dentsply
Prime&Bond 2.1 Dual Cure	Dentsply
Prime&Bond NT*	Dentsply
Prime&Bond NT Dual Cure*	Dentsply
PQ1*	Ultradent
Scotchbond 1 (Single Bond)	3M
Snapbond	Cooley & Cooley
Solist	DMG
Solobond M	Voco
Stae	Southern Dental Industries
Syntac Single-Component	Vivadent
Syntac Sprint	Vivadent
Syntac 3 (total-etch)	Vivadent
Tenure Quik	Den-Mat
Tenure Quik with Fluoride	Den-Mat

Three-step smear layer–removing adhesives/Three-step total-etch adhesives

Product	Manufacturer	Product	Manufacturer
ABC Enhanced	Chameleon	OptiBond (total-etch)*	Kerr
Ælitebond	Bisco	OptiBond FL (total-etch)*	Kerr
All-Bond 2	Bisco	PAAMA2	Southern Dental Industries
Amalgambond Plus	Parkell		
Clearfil Liner Bond*‡	Kuraray	Permagen	Ultradent
Dentastic	Pulpdent	Permaquik*	Ultradent
Denthesive	Heraeus-Kulzer	Quadrant UniBond	Cavex Holland
EBS	ESPE	Restobond 3	Lee Pharmaceuticals
EBS Multi	ESPE	Scotchbond Multi-Purpose	3M
Gluma Bonding System	Bayer	Scotchbond Multi-Purpose Plus	3M
Gluma CPS	Bayer	Solid Bond	Heraeus-Kulzer
Imperva Bond (total-etch)	Shofu	Super-Bond D-Liner	Sun Medical
Mirage Bond	Chameleon	Tenure S	Den-Mat

*Systems providing filled adhesive resins.
†Early self-etch adhesives developed to be applied on dentin only; enamel is etched separately with a phosphoric acid (> 30%) conditioner.
‡Because of the application of a silica-filled low-viscosity resin (Protect Liner) in addition to the adhesive resin, Clearfil Liner Bond is applied in four steps.

improved clinical effectiveness of fourth-generation adhesive systems, still in wide use today, is the pretreatment of dentin with conditioners and/or primers that make the heterogeneous and hydrophilic dentin substrate more receptive to bonding. A final step in this relatively complex bonding technique involves the application of a low-viscosity adhesive resin, unfilled or semifilled, that copolymerizes with the primed dentinal surface layer and simultaneously offers bonding receptors for copolymerization with the restorative resin composite. With the multistep application procedure for the fourth-generation adhesives, the term *bonding agent* was replaced by the term *adhesive system*.

Fifth-Generation Adhesives

Because of the complexity and number of steps or compounds involved with the fourth-generation systems, researchers and manufacturers have worked to develop simpler adhesive systems. The objective has been to achieve similar or improved bonding and sealing to that provided by the fourth-generation materials, but to do it with fewer "bottles" and/or in less time. Although most of the fifth-generation systems have fallen somewhat short of this objective, the bond strengths achieved by some systems have been comparable to those of fourth-generation systems. Clinical testing and improvement of these systems continue. See the "Adhesive Strategies" section (page 207) for discussion and reclassification of the adhesive systems in use today, commonly called fourth- and fifth-generation systems.

Conditioning of Dentin

Conditioning of dentin can be defined as any chemical alteration of the dentinal surface by acids (or, previously, by the calcium chelator EDTA) with the objective of removing the smear layer and simultaneously demineralizing the dentinal surface. The use of the term *conditioner* found its origin in the early 1990s when the application of acid etchants to dentin, in particular in the United States and Europe, was taboo because of its alleged harmful effects on the underlying pulp. Conditioners are most commonly used as the initial step in the clinical application of total-etch systems and are therefore applied simultaneously to enamel and dentin following the so-called *total-etch* technique. Various acids, in varying concentrations, such as citric, maleic, nitric, and phosphoric acids, are supplied with various adhesive systems (see Fig 8-24).

After clinical application, these conditioners are generally rinsed off to remove any acid remnants and dissolved calcium phosphates. The only exception was the nitric acid included in ABC Enhanced (Chameleon); the excess etchant was blown off without rinsing. However, this procedure was found to be unfavorable for subsequent resin infiltration.[80,234]

In addition to removing the smear layer, this superficial demineralization process exposes a microporous scaffold of collagen fibrils (Figs 8-26 to 8-29), thus increasing the microporosity of intertubular dentin.[234] Because this collagen matrix is normally supported by the inorganic dentinal fraction, demineralization causes it to collapse[292,328] (Fig 8-30). On intertubular dentin, the exposed collagen fibrils are randomly oriented and are often covered by an amorphous phase with relatively few microporosities and of variable thickness (Figs 8-30 and 8-31). The formation of a relatively impermeable amorphous gel on top of the exposed collagen scaffold has been ascribed to the combined effect of denaturation and collapse of residual smear layer collagen.[80,229,328] Etchants thickened with silica leave residual silica particles deposited on the surface, but the silica does not appear to plug the intertubular microporosities[234] (Fig 8-27). Sometimes fibrous structures, probably remnants of odontoblastic processes, are pulled out of the tubules and smeared over the surface (Fig 8-32).

The depth of demineralization of the dentinal surface depends on several factors, such as the kind of acid and its application time, the acid concentration and pH, and the other components of the etchant such as surfactants, thickeners (silica vs polymer), and modifiers (Table 8-4). Parameters such as osmolality and viscosity may also be involved in the aggressiveness of demineralization.[228,234] The depth of demineralization also appears to be dependent on the distance between tubules. The closer the tubules, the deeper the demineralization. Because acid etching unplugs the dentinal tubules, acid is able to penetrate the tubule to a certain depth (Figs 8-28 to 8-30).

With increasing aggressiveness of the conditioning agent, a circumferential groove may be formed at the tubule orifice, separating a cuff of mineralized peritubular dentin from the surrounding intertubular dentin (Fig 8-33). Alternatively, the mineralized peritubular dentin may be completely dissolved to form a funnel shape (Fig 8-34). In this case, the underlying collagen network, made up primarily of circular collagen fibrils, is exposed (Figs 8-28 and 8-29). The characteristic collagen banding is most visible in the tubule wall.

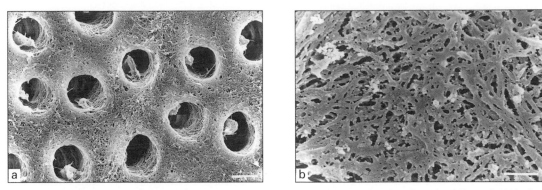

Figs 8-26a and 8-26b Field-emission scanning electron photomicrographs showing the effect of 10% phosphoric acid products All-Etch (Bisco) and Ultra-Etch (Ultradent), on dentin (top view). Note the exposed collagen fibril network almost completely denuded from hydroxyapatite. The pores represent the interfibrillar spaces that were occupied by hydroxyapatite and are now available for resin interdiffusion. The dentinal tubules were unplugged, and peritubular dentin was completely dissolved at the tubule orifices with exposure of circularly oriented collagen. Some remnants of odontoblastic processes remained inside the tubule orifices. Bar = 3 μm (a) and 500 nm (b).

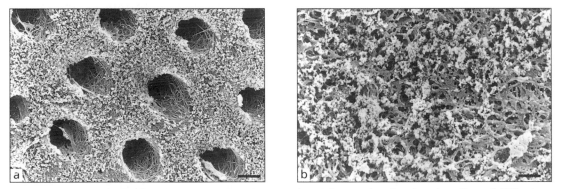

Figs 8-27a and 8-27b Field-emission scanning electron photomicrographs showing the effect of 36% phosphoric acid (DeTrey Etch) on dentin (top view). Note the deposition of silica particles that remained from the acid-etchant (thickener) despite it having been thoroughly rinsed off. Nevertheless, higher magnification disclosed that the interfibrillar spaces remained penetrable for resin. Bar = 2 μm (a) and 0.5 μm (b).

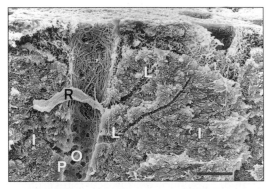

Fig 8-28 Field-emission scanning electron photomicrograph showing the effect of 37% phosphoric acid on dentin (lateral view). Intertubular dentin (I) was etched to a depth of about 2 to 3 μm. The acid penetrated the opened dentinal tubules, exposing primarily circularly oriented collagen fibrils at the dentinal tubule walls. L = lateral tubule branch; O = lateral tubule branch orifice; P = peritubular dentin; R = remnant of odontoblastic process; bar = 3 μm.

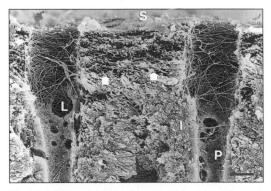

Fig 8-29 Field-emission scanning electron photomicrograph demonstrating the effect of 37.5% phosphoric acid (Kerr) on dentin (lateral view). Dentin was demineralized up to a depth of 4 to 5 μm *(arrows)*. The tubule orifice was funneled, with peritubular dentin (P) completely dissolved to a depth of about 6 to 7 μm. I = intertubular dentin; L = orifices of lateral tubule branches; S = silica remaining from the acid etchant; bar = 2 μm.

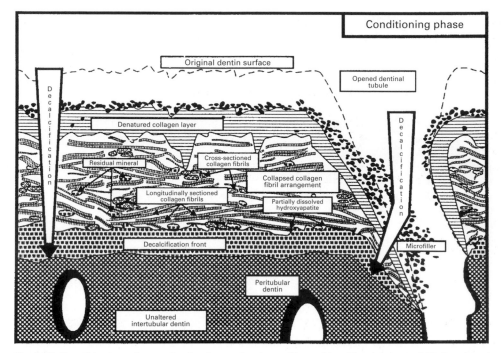

Fig 8-30 Conditioning phase of adhesive technology. (From Van Meerbeek et al.[328] Reprinted with permission.)

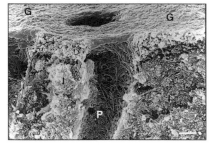

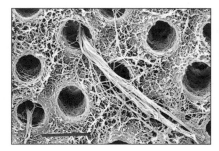

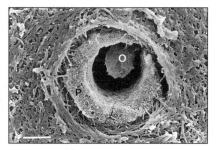

Fig 8-31 Field-emission scanning electron photomicrograph demonstrating the effect of 10% phosphoric acid (All-Etch, Bisco; 15 sec) on dentin (lateral view). Note the formation of a residual smear gel (G) with few microporosities on top of the exposed collagen fibril scaffold. I = intertubular dentin; P = peritubular dentin; bar = 1 μm.

Fig 8-32 Field-emission scanning electron photomicrograph demonstrating the effect of Non-Rinse Conditioner (Dentsply) on dentin (top view). Because of smear layer preparation, a bundle of intratubular collagen was pulled from the dentinal tubule and smeared over the exposed intertubular collagen fibril network. Bar = 5 μm.

Fig 8-33 Field-emission scanning electron photomicrograph demonstrating the effect of 10% citric acid and 3% ferric chloride (Amalgambond Universal Dentin Activator, Parkell). The etchant was not potent enough to dissolve peritubular dentin (P). O = odontoblast process; bar = 1 μm.

This demineralization process also changes the surface-free energy of dentin.[92] The high protein content exposed after conditioning with acidic agents is responsible for the low surface-free energy of etched dentin (44.8 dynes/cm), which differentiates it from etched enamel.[68] Wetting of such a low-energy surface is difficult, and adhesion is hard to achieve if the dentinal surface energy is not increased by the use of surface-active promoting agents, or primers.[23]

The dentinal surface may be alternatively modified by the use of hard tissue lasers or microabrasion.[25] With laser technology, the dentinal surface is modified by microscopic explosions caused by thermal transients, increasing the bondable fraction of inorganic dentin and micromechanical retention (Fig 8-35). Microabrasion is based on the removal of demineralized and discolored tooth tissue and results in the formation of a smear layer. It has been suggested that microabrasion may enhance the bonding capability of

Table 8-4	Etchants ranked by demineralization potency				
Etchant	**Composition**	**Etch time (sec)**	**pH**	**DID (μm)**	
				<2.0	
Clearfil CA Agent (Kuraray)	10% citric acid, 20% calcium chloride	15	–0.10	0.5	
Gluma 2000 Solution 1 (Bayer)	1.6% oxalic acid, 2.6% aluminum nitrate, 2.7% glycine	15	1.38	0.7	
Mirage ABC Conditioner (Den-Mat)	2.5% nitric acid	15	0.42	0.7	
Clearfil CA Agent (Kuraray)	10% citric acid, 20% calcium chloride	40	–0.10	0.9	
Amalgambond Universal Dentin Activator (Parkell)	10% citric acid, 3% ferric chloride	10	0.59	1.3	
Ultra-etch (Ultradent)	10% phosphoric acid	15	1.31	1.7	
Ultra-etch	35% phosphoric acid	15	0.02	1.9	
				2.0–3.0	
Scotchbond Multi-Purpose Etchant	10% maleic acid	15	0.87	2.1	
Mirage ABC Conditioner	2.5% nitric acid	60	0.42	2.2	
Mirage ABC Conditioner	10% phosphoric acid	15	*	2.2	
Ultra-etch	10% phosphoric acid	30	1.31	2.2	
All-etch (Bisco)	10% phosphoric acid	15	0.48	3.0	
All-etch without surfactantia (Bisco)	10% phosphoric acid	15	0.78	3.0	
All-etch	10% phosphoric acid with surfactans	15	*	3.0	
Scotchbond Etching Gel	35% phosphoric acid	15	–0.28	3.0	
				>3.0	
Aqueous phosphoric acid solution	10% phosphoric acid	15	0.48	3.2	
ESPE Etching Gel	32% phosphoric acid	15	*	3.9	
Uni-Etch (Bisco)	32% phosphoric acid with surfactans	15	*	4.0	
De Trey Etch	36% phosphoric acid	15	–0.26	4.3	
Mirage ABC Conditioner	10% phosphoric acid	30	*	4.5	
Etch-Rite (Pulpdent)	38% phosphoric acid	15	–0.29	4.6	
Uni-Etch	32% phosphoric acid	15	–0.17	4.8	
Aqueous phosphoric acid solution	37% phosphoric acid	15	–0.43	5.0	
Kerr Gel Etchant	37.5% phosphoric acid	15	*	5.6	

pH = acidity; DID = depth of intertubular demineralization. From Perdigão.[234]
*pH values not available.

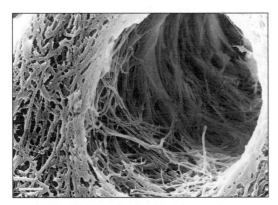

Fig 8-34 Field-emission scanning electron photomicrograph demonstrating the effect of 32% phosphoric acid (Uni-Etch, Bisco) on dentin (top view). The etchant was so aggressive that peritubular dentin was completely dissolved, exposing a circularly oriented network of collagen at the tubule orifice wall. Bar = 500 nm.

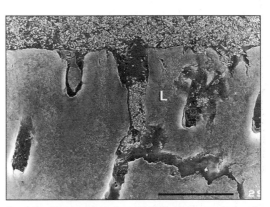

Fig 8-35 Field-emission scanning electron photomicrograph showing the surface of resin and laser-treated dentin (L). Clearfil Liner Bond System was used after preparation with a carbon dioxide laser. Bar = 3 μm.

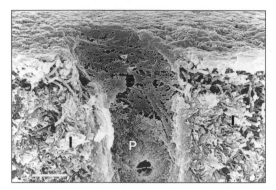

Fig 8-36 Field-emission scanning electron photomicrograph showing a dentinal surface etched with 10% phosphoric acid followed by the application of Permagen (Ultradent) primer. The primer did not plug the tubules; the individual collagen fibrils were coated by resin. I = intertubular dentin; P = peritubular dentin; bar = 1 μm.

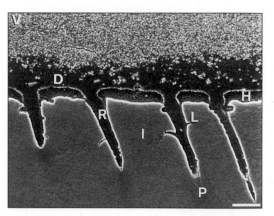

Fig 8-37 Scanning electron photomicrograph demonstrating the resin-dentin interface presented with Clearfil Liner Bond System after an argon-ion–beam etching technique.[326] D = dual-cured adhesive resin; H = hybrid layer; I = intertubular dentin; L = lateral tubule branch; P = peritubular dentin; R = resin tag; V = low-viscosity resin; bar = 5 μm. (From Van Meerbeek et al.[328] Reprinted with permission.)

smear layer–mediated dentin adhesive systems. More research is needed to investigate the potential of these alternative dentinal surface treatments to enhance bonding. They are not presently considered to be proven tooth surface pretreatments.

Primers

Primers serve as the actual adhesion-promoting agents and contain hydrophilic monomers dissolved in organic solvents, such as acetone or ethanol. Because of their volatile characteristics, these solvents can displace water from the dentinal surface and the moist collagen network, promoting the infiltration of monomers through the nanospaces of the exposed collagen network[147] (Figs 8-26 to 8-29 and 8-36). Effective primers contain monomers with hydrophilic properties that have an affinity for the exposed collagen fibril arrangement and hydrophobic properties for copolymerization with the adhesive resin.[92] The objective of this priming step is to transform the hydrophilic dentin surface into a hydrophobic and spongy state that allows the adhesive resin to wet and penetrate the exposed collagen network efficiently.[14,89,208,209]

HEMA, described as essential to the promotion of adhesion because of its excellent wetting characteristics,[208] is found in the primers of many modern adhesive systems. In addition to HEMA, primers con-

tain other monomers, such as NTG-GMA, PMDM, biphenyl dimethacrylate (BPDM), and dipentaerythritol penta acrylate monophosphate (PENTA) (see Fig 8-21). More recent primers, in All-Bond 2 (Bisco), OptiBond (Kerr), and Clearfil Liner Bond System (Kuraray), also include a chemical or photopolymerization initiator, so that these monomers can be polymerized in situ. More viscous primers, as provided by the so-called one-bottle adhesives, were developed to combine the priming and bonding function to simplify the bonding technique (see Table 8-3).

Primers have also been used to treat and prevent dentinal hypersensitivity.[299] Dentinal hypersensitivity is believed to be caused by pressure gradients of dentinal fluid within patent tubules that communicate with the oral environment.[41,354] Primers may induce denaturation and precipitation of proteins from the dentinal fluid and, consequently, decrease dentinal permeability and outward flow of pulpal fluid, reducing the clinical symptoms of hypersensitivity.[299]

Adhesive Resin

The adhesive resin, also called *bonding agent*, is equivalent to the enamel bonding agent and consists primarily of hydrophobic monomers, such as bis-GMA and UDMA, and more hydrophilic monomers, such as TEG-DMA as a viscosity regulator and

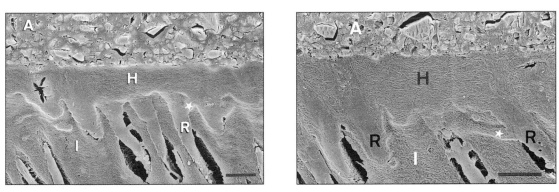

Figs 8-38a and 8-38b Field-emission scanning electron photomicrographs demonstrating the resin-dentin interface produced by Optibond Dual Cure (Kerr) when a 37.5% phosphoric acid was used. Dentin was removed during laboratory processing. A hybrid layer (H) of 4 to 5 μm was formed along with resin tags (R; often particle-filled) into the opened dentinal tubules. A = adhesive resin (particle-filled); I = intertubular dentin (unaffected); white star = micro–resin tag in lateral tubule branch; bar = 5 μm.

HEMA as a wetting agent (see Fig 8-21). The major role of the adhesive resin is to stabilize the hybrid layer and to form resin extensions into the dentinal tubules, called resin tags (Figs 8-37 and 8-38).

Adhesive resins can be light curing and/or autocuring. Autocuring adhesive resins have the theoretical advantage of initial polymerization at the interface due to the higher temperature produced by body heat,[108] but the disadvantage of slow polymerization. For light-curing bonding agents, it is recommended that the adhesive resin be polymerized before the application of the restorative resin. In this way, the adhesive resin is not displaced, and adequate light intensity is available to sufficiently cure and stabilize the resin-tooth bond to resist the stresses produced by polymerization shrinkage of the resin composite.[63,92,132] Because oxygen inhibits resin polymerization,[263] an oxygen-inhibited layer of about 15 μm will always be formed on top of the adhesive resin, even after light curing. This oxygen-inhibited layer offers sufficient double MMA bonds (see Fig 8-21) for copolymerization of the adhesive resin with the restorative resin.

Hybridization

Hybridization, or the formation of a hybrid layer, occurs following an initial demineralization of the dentinal surface with an acidic conditioner, exposing a collagen fibril network with interfibrillar microporosities that subsequently becomes interdiffused with low-viscosity monomers (Figs 8-39 and 8-40). This zone, in which resin of the adhesive system micromechanically interlocks with dentinal collagen, is termed the *hybrid layer* or *hybrid zone*.

Within the hybrid layer, three different layers or zones have been described.[328] In the Clearfil Liner Bond system, the top of the hybrid layer consists of an amorphous electron-dense phase, which has been ascribed to denatured collagen (Figs 8-39 and 8-40).[328] A more loosely arranged collagen fibril arrangement is seen at the top of the hybrid layer with OptiBond and Super-Bond D-Liner; in this layer, individual collagen fibrils are directed toward the adhesive resin, and the interfibrillar spaces are filled with resin (Figs 8-41 and 8-42). With Scotchbond Multi-Purpose and Single Bond (Scotchbond 1 in Europe, 3M), the hybrid layer was observed to be covered by an amorphous phase, which may have originated in a chemical reaction of a polyalkenoic acid copolymer of the primer with residual calcium (Fig 8-43). The middle part of the hybrid layer contains cross-sectioned and longitudinally sectioned collagen fibrils separated by electronlucent spaces (Fig 8-41b). These interfibrillar channels, which have typical dimensions of 10 to 20 nm, represent the areas wherein hydroxyapatite crystals had been deposited and have now been replaced by resin as a result of the hybridization process. Residual mineral crystals are sometimes scattered between the collagen fibrils (Figs 8-39 and 8-40). The base of the hybrid layer is characterized by a gradual transition to the underlying unaltered dentin, with a partially demineralized zone of dentin containing hydroxyapatite crystals enveloped by resin (Fig 8-39b), or by a more abrupt transition (Figs 8-41 and 8-42).

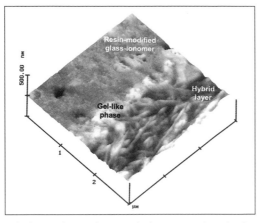

Fig 8-59 Atomic force photomicrograph demonstrating the interface formed at dentin by a glass-ionomer adhesive (Fuji Bond LC). The shallow hybrid layer of about 0.5 μm results from the short (10-second) application of a 20% polyalkenoic acid, by which collagen fibrils are exposed, but not completely denuded of hydroxyapatite. The hydroxyapatite crystals remaining around the collagen fibrils served as receptors for chemical bonding with the carboxyl groups of the polyalkenoic acid. On top of the hybrid layer, a 0.5-μm zone is demarcated from the glass-ionomer matrix. This phase represents the morphologic manifestation of a gelation reaction of the polyalkenoic acid with calcium that was extracted from the underlying dentin surface.

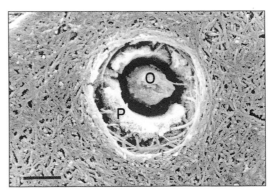

Fig 8-60 Field-emission scanning electron photomicrograph illustrating the effect of a 10-second application of 20% polyalkenoic acid (Cavity Conditioner, GC) to dentin. Note that although intertubular collagen was exposed, the fibrils were not completely denuded of hydroxyapatite. O = odontoblast process; P = peritubular dentin; bar = 1 μm.

Critical Steps in Adhesion

Isolation

Before any bonding procedure is begun, adequate isolation and moisture control of the substrate to be bonded to must be achieved. Bonding to acid-etched enamel theoretically requires an air-dried surface to allow the photopolymerizable hydrophobic bonding resin to be drawn by capillary attraction into the pits created by acid etching.

With bonding to dentin, a distinction should be made between an internal and external dentinal wetness. Internal dentinal wetness is caused by pulpal fluids that flow from the pulp through the dentinal tubules, if unplugged by acid etching, to exude onto the dentin cavity surface. This internal dentinal wetness and its effects on adhesion to dentin have been thoroughly documented in literature dealing with the aspects of dentin permeability, as published by Pashley and colleagues.[229,230] In this respect, first-generation adhesive systems were too hydrophobic to sufficiently wet the hydrophilic dentinal substrate that was etched with concentrated phosphoric acid in sim-

ulation of the successful enamel acid-etch technique.[314] As knowledge of the heterogeneous and hydrophilic nature of dentin has become more complete, newer adhesive formulations have been developed for enhanced hydrophilicity and improved wettability.

The external dentinal wetness is related to ambient or environmental humidity (see Fig 8-16) and has been demonstrated to negatively affect bond strengths to dentin.[49,102,250,251] The degree of environmental humidity is high and comparable to that of the oral cavity when no rubber dam is used, whereas with rubber dam use the environmental humidity will be similar to that of the ambient air in the operatory. Bond strengths obtained with most adhesive systems decrease as the level of humidity in air rises, but some systems appear to be more sensitive than others. In this respect, incorporation of polyalkenoic acid copolymers in the Scotchbond products, Scotchbond Multi-Purpose and its two-step successor Single Bond (Scotchbond 1 in Europe) (see Fig 8-43) have been reported to result in lower moisture sensitivity and better bonding stability over time.[88,102,333] The moisture-stabilizing effect of the polyalkenoic acid copolymer was explained by Eliades[88] following a concept introduced by Peters et al,[242] in which a reversible breaking and reforming of calcium–polyalkenoic acid complexes in the presence of water were suggested to develop a stress-relaxation capacity without rupture of adhesion at any time. Further study is needed to elucidate the effects of incorporating polyalkenoic acid copolymers in adhesive formulations. Other adhesives that contain methacrylated polyalkenoic acid copolymers are ART Bond (Coltène/Whaledent), Syntac Single-Component (Vivadent), and Syntac Sprint (Vivadent).

An accidental form of external dentinal wetness is contamination of the substrate with external fluids, impeding effective contact between the adhesive and the bonding substrate. Salivary contamination is detrimental because saliva contains proteins that may block adequate infiltration of resin in the microretentive porosities created on acid-etched enamel and dentin. Because maxillary teeth are more easily isolated, dentin adhesion appears more effective in maxillary than in mandibular teeth.[357] Consistent use of a rubber dam remains the most effective method of moisture control.

Dentin and Pulp Protection

Once the teeth in need of adhesive restoration have been adequately isolated, a decision must be made about the need for any kind of dentin protection.[334] The use of "nonadhesive" liners and bases beneath adhesive restorations is not recommended. Adhesive materials such as glass-ionomer cements can be used ("sandwich" restoration), but in most cases the simple application of an appropriate adhesive is effective. As mentioned, studies using microscopic examination have demonstrated that adhesives can hermetically seal tubules through tubule wall hybridization (see Figs 8-41a, 8-44, 8-50, 8-52, and 8-58b).

In a deep cavity with a remaining dentin thickness of less than 0.5 mm and very permeable dentin such as in young teeth, calcium hydroxide remains the material of choice due to its proven pulp-healing properties. Its major disadvantage is that it rapidly dissolves if the cavity is not adequately sealed. Therefore, when calcium hydroxide is used, it must be covered by a less-soluble traditional cement like a glass-ionomer cement. A resin-modified glass-ionomer cement is preferred. Unlike conventional glass-ionomer liners, resin-modified versions allow chemical copolymerization with the adhesive resin, uniting the restoration via the adhesive and liner to the remaining tooth structure. In addition, resin-modified glass-ionomer cements are more resistant to acid etching than are conventional

glass ionomers. Because of its high solubility, a calcium hydroxide liner should not be acid etched. It should be used sparingly and limited to the deepest areas of the cavity to preserve as much dentinal tissue as possible for bonding. (See Chapter 5 for an in-depth discussion of pulpal protection.)

Universal Enamel-Dentin Conditioning

Phosphoric Acid Alternatives

After the tooth in need of an adhesive restoration has been adequately isolated and cleaned, a proper etching or conditioning agent must be selected. As mentioned, in most modern adhesive systems, the selective enamel-etching technique used by older-generation bonding agents is replaced in smear layer–removing systems by a total-etch concept, in which the conditioner or acid etchant is applied simultaneously to enamel and dentin. As a result, two different microretentive surfaces are exposed in which the adhesive resin will become micromechanically interlocked. Although most research dealing with adhesive techniques has focused on producing good and stable bonds to dentin, the importance of enamel bonding cannot be neglected with the development of new adhesive systems.

Traditionally, enamel was selectively etched with phosphoric acid in a concentration between 30% and 40%. With the introduction of the total-etch technique, less concentrated phosphoric acids or weaker acids in varying concentrations, such as citric, maleic, nitric, and oxalic acid, have been supplied with various adhesive systems (see Fig 8-24). The objective of such universal enamel-dentin conditioning agents is to find the best compromise between etching enamel sufficiently to create a microretentive etch pattern and etching dentin mildly, avoiding exposure of collagen to a depth that is inaccessible for complete infiltration by resin.[326] However, a few years after the introduction of alternative total etchants into clinical practice, a steadily growing number of clinical trials,[332,336] as well as laboratory studies,[298,319] demonstrated a less consistent and inferior enamel bond with the use of these less aggressive alternative etchants. Two different etchants specifically adapted for enamel and dentin could be used, but this is clinically impractical. Using only a weak acid is acceptable if the enamel surface is mechanically roughened before etching or if the acid gel is rubbed vigorously on the enamel surface. Today, most adhesive systems again use conventional phosphoric acid etchants in concentrations

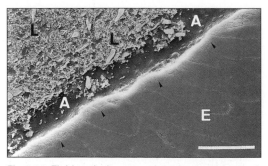

Fig 8-61 Field-emission scanning electron photomicrograph of an argon-ion–bombarded resin-enamel interface as produced by a "strong" self-etching adhesive (experimental Vivadent). Note that the self-etching approach resulted in a clearly detectable effect *(arrowheads)* at the enamel surface (E). No separation was observed between the adhesive resin (A) and enamel. The bonding mechanism is primarily based on the formation of micro–resin tags. L = low-viscosity resin cured on top of the adhesive resin; bar = 10 μm.

above 30% to etch both enamel and dentin in one application. It is recommended that these etchants be applied first to enamel, so that enamel is etched for at least 15 seconds. Only sclerotic dentin surfaces can be etched longer without the risk of etching too deeply. In fact, this hypermineralized tissue should be etched longer to make it more receptive to bonding.[331]

In all smear layer–removing systems, the conditioner and its by-products should be thoroughly rinsed away before application of the primer and the adhesive resin. For example, failure to rinse off the nitric acid conditioner, as recommended by the manufacturer of ABC Enhanced (Chameleon), resulted in an incomplete resin penetration of the demineralized dentin surface layer and minimal hybrid layer formation.[83,234,335] Properly rinsed, the conditioner was sufficient to achieve adequate hybridization.

Self-Etch Approach on Enamel

Another recent innovation in bonding to enamel is the use of self-etching primers on both enamel and dentin as part of one- and two-step smear layer–dissolving systems (Fig 8-61 and Table 8-3). Self-etching primers containing acidic monomers, like phenyl-P,[342] are air dispersed and not rinsed off, simplifying the application procedure. However, major controversy exists about the etching efficiency of these self-etching primers and the resultant enamel bond strength and stability. Perdigão et al[237] recently concluded, from a

combined enamel shear bond strength and SEM study, that although the phenyl-P self-etching primer did not etch enamel as deeply as conventional etchants, Clearfil Liner Bond 2 demonstrated good bond strengths to enamel.

In the measurement of the microtensile bond strength (μTBS) to enamel,[145a] two self-etching adhesives, the relatively severe self-etching NRC/Prime&Bond NT and even the moderate self-etching Clearfil SE Bond provided bond strengths comparable to those of the conventional three-step total-etch adhesive Optibond FL. It is noteworthy that in this study all adhesives were bonded to enamel, which had been prepared with 600-grit sandpaper leaving a smear layer. Similar results were reported in another study by Kanemura et al,[157] which revealed that two other self-etching adhesives (Clearfil Liner Bond 2; Mac Bond 2, Tokuyama) produced μTBSs to ground enamel that were comparable to those measured for two one-bottle adhesives (One-Step and Single Bond) that involved a separate phosphoric acid treatment. When the self-etching adhesives were directly bonded to unground, intact enamel, the resultant μTBS values were, however, significantly lower.

Long-term clinical trials are needed to confirm this promising enamel bonding effectiveness recorded in vitro. Until then, it remains clinically advisable to use this simplified application technique only on enamel that has been coarsened by bur. Additionally, the self-etching primer should be applied for at least 30 seconds and actively applied by rubbing the dentin surface with repeated application of fresh material. Alternatively, a separate conventional etchant can be applied before application of the self-etching primer.

Compomers

Modification of the monomer backbone of conventional resin composites by adding acidic carboxylic groups has recently led to a new group of adhesive restorative materials. On the basis of their composition, they should be regarded as polyacid-modified resin composites,[185] but products such as Dyract (Dentsply), Dyract AP (Dentsply), Hytac (ESPE), Luxat (DMG), and F2000 (3M) are commercially advertised as so-called compomers. This term does not encompass the true characteristics of these materials, however, since it suggests that they originate from combined resin composite and glass-ionomer technology. These materials, in fact, behave more like resin composites. The popularity of the compomers among clinicians must be attributed to their superb clinical handling and simple application method, with only a

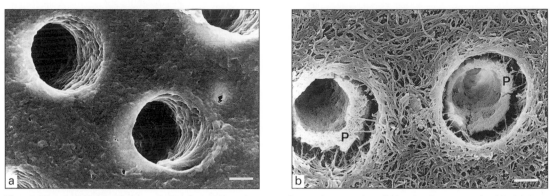

Figs 8-62a and 8-62b Field-emission scanning electron photomicrographs of dentin that was air dried (a) or kept moist (b) after conditioning (top view). P = peritubular dentin; bar = 1 µm.

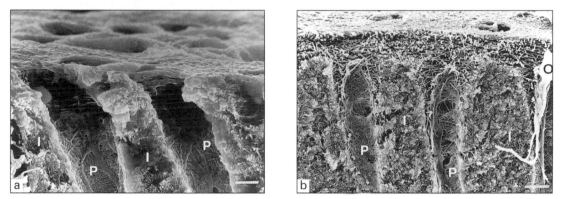

Figs 8-63a and 8-63b Field-emission scanning electron photomicrographs of dentin that was air dried (a) or kept moist (b) after conditioning (lateral view). I = intertubular dentin; O = remnants of odontoblast process or lamina limitans; P = peritubular dentin; bar = 1 µm.

self-etching primer required to pretreat the enamel and dentin surface. The primers, which usually contain acidic monomers dissolved in acetone, like most one-bottle primer/adhesive combinations, are only mildly acidic. They interact superficially, to a depth of about 200 nm, with dentin (comparable effect as that seen in Fig 8-48) and are not aggressive enough to expose a highly retentive etch pattern on enamel surfaces. Moreover, recent clinical trials reported the occurrence of minimal to severe enamel margin chipping after only 6 months of clinical service, which, if left untreated, could rapidly lead to marginal discoloration and even caries.[114,115] These early enamel margin defects are due to ineffective etching of enamel using only the mild, self-etching primers. These clinical results were confirmed in vitro, where the primer provided with Dyract produced relatively low bond strengths to enamel.[58,101] Most likely, the clinical effectiveness of these polyacid-modified composites could be substantially improved by supplementary acid etching of the enamel before primer application.

Wet Vs Dry Bonding

After conditioning, the enamel and dentin surfaces should be properly treated to allow full penetration of adhesive monomers. On the enamel surface, a dry condition is theoretically preferred. On the dentin site, a certain amount of moisture is needed to avoid collapse of the exposed collagen scaffold, which impedes effective penetration of adhesive monomers (Figs 8-62 and 8-63). Consequently, in the treatment of enamel and dentin, it is difficult to achieve the optimal environment for both substrates. One way to achieve this goal is to keep the substrate field dry and to use adhesive systems with water-based primers to rehydrate, and thus re-expand, the collapsed collagen network, enabling the resin monomer to interdiffuse efficiently.[337] The alternative is to keep the acid-etched dentin surface moist and to rely on the water-chasing capacity of acetone-based primers. This clinical technique, commonly referred to as "wet bonding," was introduced by Kanca[154–156] and Gwinnett[122] in the early 1990s.

217

It is fundamentally important to effective hybridization that the collagen fibril web, deprived of its mineral support following acid treatment, keeps its spongelike quality, allowing interdiffusion of resin monomers in the subsequent priming and bonding steps. Dehydration of the acid-conditioned dentin surface through air drying is thought to induce surface tension stress, causing the exposed collagen network to collapse, shrink, and form a compact coagulate that is impenetrable to resin.[229,230,313] If some water remains inside the interfibrillar spaces, the loose quality of the collagen matrix is maintained and the interfibrillar spaces are left open.[155,231,234–236] An appropriate amount of moisture on the dentin surface has also been reported to promote the polymerization reaction of specific monomers.[144] The wet-bonding technique has repeatedly been reported to increase in vitro bond strengths.[122,154,155,231,297]

Clinically, a shiny, hydrated surface is seen with moist dentin. Pooled moisture should be removed by blotting or be wiped off with a slightly damp cotton pellet. Excess water might dilute the primer and render it less effective.[300] It should, however, be emphasized that this wet-bonding technique can guarantee efficient resin interdiffusion only if all of the remaining water on the dentin surface is eliminated as completely as possible and replaced by monomers during the subsequent priming step. In some of the currently available adhesive systems, hydrophilic primer monomers are therefore dissolved in volatile solvents, such as acetone and ethanol. These solvents may aid in displacement of the remaining water as well as carrying the polymerizable monomers into the opened dentinal tubules and through the nanospaces of the collagen web.[309] The primer solvents are then evaporated by gently air drying, leaving the active primer monomers behind. These monomers have hydrophilic ends with an affinity for the exposed collagen fibrils and hydrophobic ends that form receptors for copolymerization with the adhesive resin. When the water inside the collagen network is not completely displaced, the polymerization of resin inside the hybrid layer may be affected or, at least, the remaining water will compete for space with resin inside the demineralized dentin.[148] The risk that all of the moisture on an overwet dentin surface may not be completely replaced by hydrophilic primer monomers has been well documented for adhesive systems that provide water-free acetone-based primers.[309] In such overwet conditions, excessive water that was incompletely removed during priming appeared to cause phase separation of the hydrophobic and hydrophilic monomer components, resulting in blister and globule formation at the resin-dentin interface. Such interface deficiencies undoubtedly weaken the resin-dentin bond and result in incompletely sealed tubules.[309] On the other hand, even gentle drying of the dentin surface, for times as short as 3 seconds prior to the application of a water-free, acetone-based primer, has been shown to result in incomplete intertubular resin infiltration. Ineffective resin penetration due to collagen collapse has been observed ultramorphologically as the formation of a so-called hybridoid zone (Figs 8-64 and 8-65).[308,309] These hybridoid zones inside the hybrid layer do not appear electron dense on demineralized TEM sections. Consequently, this wet-bonding technique appears technique-sensitive, especially in terms of the precise amount of moisture that should be kept on the dentin surface after conditioning. In other words, acid-etched dentin should not be kept too wet but also should not be dried too long. A short air blast or blotting of the excess water with a dry sponge or small piece of tissue paper have been recommended as most effective in wet-bonding procedures.

This wet-bonding technique has two other disadvantages of clinical importance. First, acetone quickly evaporates from the primer bottle so that, after the primer solution is dispensed in a dappen dish, the primer bottle should be immediately closed and the primer solution immediately applied to the etched surface. Despite careful handling, the composition of the primer solution may change after several uses due to rapid evaporation of solvent. This will increase the ratio of monomers to the acetone content and will eventually affect the penetrability of monomers into the exposed collagen network. To reduce the problem of rapid primer solvent volatilization, special delivery systems have been developed. Examples are the "bubble mixer" syringe system of Permagen (Ultradent), a syringe system with a disposable application brush for Permaquik and PQ1 (Ultradent), or a delivery system with predose, single-use capsules introduced with Optibond Solo, Optibond Solo Plus, and Excite (Vivadent). Another disadvantage of keeping the cavity walls wet after conditioning is that one cannot observe the white, frosted appearance of the enamel that indicates that it has been properly etched.

Adhesive systems that provide water-dissolved primers have been demonstrated to bond equally effectively to dry or wet dentin. In one study,[337] the hybridization effectiveness of two three-step smear layer–removing adhesive systems, Optibond Dual Cure and Scotchbond Multi-Purpose, were examined by TEM. No substantial difference in the ultrastructure

Fig 8-64 Transmission electron photomicrograph of the resin-dentin interface produced by Clearfil Liner Bond System when applied to 35% phosphoric acid–etched dentin. Due to insufficient resin infiltration, a typical hybridoid zone (H') was formed underneath the top area of the hybrid layer (H), which stained more electron dense indicating adequate resin infiltration. Compare to Fig 8-39, which shows the resin-dentin interface when Clearfil Liner Bond System was applied, per manufacturer's instructions, following a 20% citric acid solution and resulted in complete resin infiltration. A = adhesive resin; I = lab-demineralized intertubular dentin; L = micro–resin tag in hybridized lateral tubule branch; R = resin tag; W = hybridized tubule wall; bar = 1 μm.

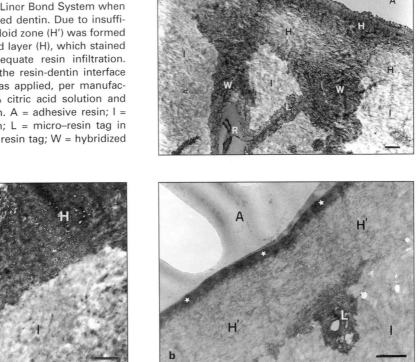

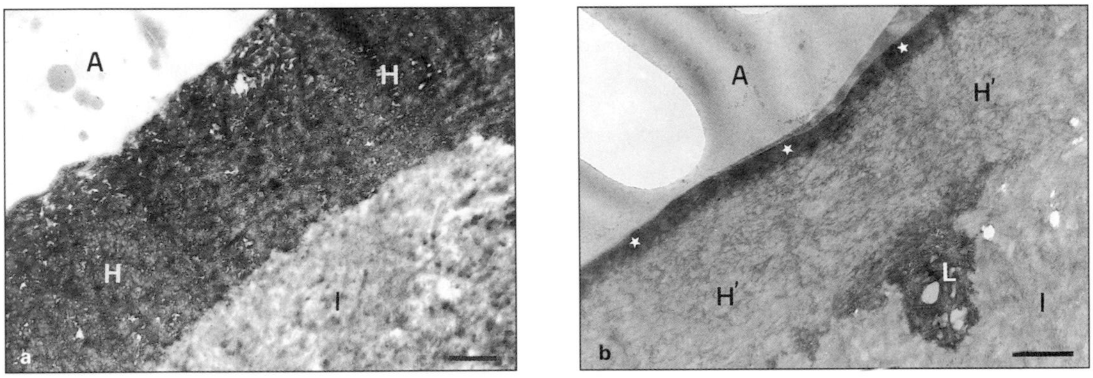

Figs 8-65a and 8-65b Transmission electron photomicrographs of resin-dentin interfaces produced by Prime&Bond applied to moist or blot-dried dentin (a) or air-dried dentin (b). Whereas a homogeneously stained hybrid layer (H) is formed with a wet-bonding technique (a), air drying dentin prior to application of the primer/adhesive resin combination resulted in the formation of a collapsed, non-resin-infiltrated collagen or hybridoid zone (H') (b). In the latter case, resin penetrated only the top part of the exposed collagen fibrils *(white stars)* and at the bottom through a lateral tubule branch (L). A = adhesive resin; I = lab-demineralized intertubular dentin; bar = 1 μm.

of the hybrid layer, nor signs of incomplete resin penetration or collagen collapse, were detected when these water-based adhesives were applied following a wet- or dry-bonding technique. Even excessive postconditioning air drying of the dentin surface for 15 seconds did not result in the formation of a hybridoid zone.[310] When both adhesives were bonded to wet dentin, no morphologic evidence of the overwetting phenomenon was observed.[310] This indicates that the two water-based primers were capable of displacing the water that remained as part of the wet-bonding technique as well as the additional amount of water that was introduced with the primers themselves. A self-rewetting effect of the primer, which evidently provides sufficient water to re-expand the air-dried and collapsed collagen scaffold, has been advanced as a reasonable explanation as to why these systems perform equally well in wet or dry conditions. Air drying of demineralized dentin reduces its volume by 65%, but the original dimensions can be regained after rewetting.[50]

Alternatively, conditioned dentin may be air dried and remoistened with water or an antibacterial solution such as chlorhexidine.[122,154] A recent study by Perdigão et al[239] has shown that an aqueous HEMA (35%) solution (Aquaprep, Bisco) is effective for rewetting etched dentin. The postconditioning application of the rewetting agent significantly improved the bonding of some simplified adhesives.

In contrast to adhesive systems that provide acetone-based primers, adhesive systems that provide water-based primers appear less technique-sensitive and bond equally well to varying degrees of surface dryness and wetness. Bonding to dry dentin has the advantage of being clinically accepted and familiar to most clinicians. In addition, dry bonding permits the clinician to verify the frosted appearance of enamel following conditioning. In addition, dry bonding does not involve any risk for overwetting. Clinically, a standard dry-bonding procedure is recommended that involves gentle air drying of the dentin surface after

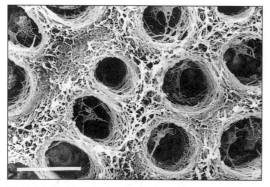

Fig 8-66 Field-emission scanning electron photomicrograph of dentin that was treated with Non-Rinse Conditioner. By actively rubbing the dentin surface, a typical "shag-carpet" appeared with well-opened pores available for interdiffusion. Bar = 5 μm.

conditioning for about 5 seconds, or until the glossy wet surface turns dull and the acid-etched enamel surface appears white and frosted. Future research should clarify and further define this self-rewetting effect in other adhesive systems that include water-based primers.

Primer Application

Primers should clinically be applied with care to ensure that resin effectively infiltrates the network of interfibrillar collagen channels. A primer application time of at least 15 seconds, as recommended by most manufacturers, should be respected to allow monomers to interdiffuse to the complete depth of surface demineralization. When a dry-bonding technique is followed with self-rewetting water-based primers, this 15-second primer application time should allow the gently air-dried and thus collapsed collagen scaffold to re-expand. With a wet-bonding technique, the primer should be applied for at least 15 seconds to displace all remaining surface moisture through concurrent evaporation of the primer solvent carrier. Moreover, water-free, acetone-based primers, provided with three- and two-step (single-bottle) smear layer–removing adhesive systems, should be applied copiously in multiple layers. After brief, gentle air drying, the primed surface should appear glossy. The primer should be actively rubbed into the dentin surface with disposable brushes or sponge applicators. This may improve and accelerate the monomer interdiffusion process. The typical "shag carpet" appear-

ance of collagen fibrils, which are directed up toward the adhesive resin and appear to be frayed into their microfibrils (Figs 8-41b, 8-50, 8-55, and 8-66), has been attributed to this active rubbing application method.[310,335,337] A similar pattern of deeply tufted collagen fibrils has been observed to result from citric-acid burnishing of a root surface as part of a tissue regenerative periodontal treatment.[290] The physical rubbing action, combined with the chemical action of citric acid, was found to enhance the removal of chemically dissolved inorganic dentin material and surface debris, exposing a deeply tufted collagen fibril surface topography. Likewise, the combined mechanical/chemical action of rubbing the dentin surface with a slightly acidic primer probably dissolves additional inorganic dentin material, while fluffing and separating the entangled dentin collagen at the surface.

Acid-etched enamel does not need a separate primer application to achieve effective bonding when an unfilled or low-filled hydrophobic enamel bonding agent is applied on air-dried enamel. On the other hand, primers can be applied on acid-etched enamel without harming the enamel bonding process. In the wet-bonding technique, primers should always be applied on acid-etched enamel to displace any residual surface moisture through concurrent evaporation of the primer's solvent carrier. The primer application should be completed by short and gentle air drying to volatilize any remaining solvent excess before application of the adhesive resin.

Adhesive Resin Application

In the final step of the bonding process, the adhesive layer is placed. Spreading of the adhesive resin over the surface to be bonded should be done by brush thinning rather than by air thinning. The adhesive should be placed and then evenly spread with a brush tip that can be blotted repeatedly with a paper tissue. In this way, the adhesive resin layer will reach an optimal thickness of about 100 μm.[199] When placed in a sufficiently thick layer, the adhesive resin may act as a stress-relaxation buffer (see Fig 8-19) and absorb some of the tensile stresses imposed by polymerization contraction of the resin composite placed over the adhesive resin.[22,28,164,330] Thinning the adhesive resin layer with an air syringe may reduce its thickness too much, decreasing its elastic buffer potential. In support of this elastic bonding concept, dentin adhesive systems that provide a low-viscosity resin have been reported to produce higher bond strengths and less microleakage.[66,98,99] Microleakage was also found to be reduced when a filled low-viscosity resin was used as an intermediate liner.[301] This elastic bonding concept can be regarded as an efficient means not only to counteract the polymerization contraction stress of the resin composite, but to aid in absorbing masticatory forces, tooth flexure effects, and thermal cycling shocks, all of which may jeopardize the integrity of the resin-tooth bond.

This innovative concept for relaxation of polymerization shrinkage by elastic compensation was adopted by several modern adhesive systems. Clearfil Liner Bond systems 1 and 2 provide a low-viscosity resin, filled with silanated microfiller and prepolymerized filler at 42 wt%. Optibond DC, Optibond FL, Optibond Solo, and Optibond Solo Plus provide a light-polymerizable adhesive resin that contains radiopaque, fluoride-releasing glass filler particles at 48 wt% (see Figs 8-38, 8-41, 8-49, 8-50, and 8-52).[330] A filled adhesive resin is also supplied with other modern adhesives (see Table 8-3). In addition to alleviating stress, these semifilled adhesive resins undergo less polymerization contraction. They have superior physical properties, with a compressive strength approximating that of microfilled resin composites, and a Young's modulus of elasticity closer to that of resin composites. They form particle-reinforced resin tags as anchors in the dentinal tubules (see Figs 8-38, 8-41, 8-50, and 8-52). Some may release fluoride to the surrounding demineralized dentin and may provide improved esthetics by preventing the formation of a prism effect or a translucent line around the restoration's margins.[234]

Apart from adhesives that provide low-viscosity particle-filled resins (see Table 8-3), thick adhesive layers are also placed with polyalkenoic acid–based adhesive systems, such as Scotchbond Multi-Purpose and Single Bond, and with the more recently developed glass-ionomer–based adhesive system, Fuji Bond LC. Excellent clinical results have been reported for Clearfil Liner Bond, Scotchbond Multi-Purpose, and Optibond Dual Cure in clinical trials.[22,28,317,336]

Other materials also have stress-relaxing properties. In theory, chemical- and dual-cured adhesive systems that allow small porosities to be mixed in the resin layer and that polymerize more slowly than light-cured materials may also contribute to this stress-relaxation mechanism.[5,236] Adhesive lining cements used under resin composite restorations also act as stress absorbers. The use of an intermediate glass-ionomer liner will reduce the total stiffness and increase the stress-absorption capacity of the restoration. In this respect, resin-modified glass-ionomer cements are preferred over conventional glass-ionomer cements because they can chemically copolymerize with the restorative resin composite placed over the intermediate cement layer. This so-called sandwich technique has been demonstrated to significantly reduce the loss rate of restorations placed with an earlier-generation adhesive, Scotchbond 2, when a resin-modified glass-ionomer liner, Vitrebond (3M), was used as an intermediate liner.[254]

For light-cured bonding agents, the adhesive resin should always be cured before the application of the restorative resin composite. In this way, the adhesive resin is not displaced when the restorative resin composite is applied, and adequate light intensity is provided to sufficiently cure the adhesive resin layer.[92] Curing the adhesive resin prior to inserting resin composite will stabilize the resin-tooth bond and consequently activate the elastic stress-relaxation mechanism.

Because of oxygen inhibition, the top 15 μm of the adhesive resin will not polymerize,[263] but will provide sufficient double methacrylate bonds for copolymerization with the restorative resin. Again, brush thinning rather than air thinning may prevent the film thickness from being reduced to an extent that the air-inhibited layer permeates the whole resin layer, reducing the stress-relaxation capacity and bond effectiveness.[92,320]

Restorative Procedure

As long as resin composites shrink during polymerization, additional clinical measures will be needed to compensate for the polymerization shrinkage.[79,80,97,289] In addition to building in a flexible stress-absorbing bonding interface, the restorative material should be placed in such a manner that the polymerization contraction stress is clinically reduced as much as possible. An in vivo study by Perdigão showed that, in bulk-filled Class 1 cavities, the dentin-adhesive was not able to withstand polymerization shrinkage stress.[236] Almost consistent detachment of the adhesive resin from the underlying hybrid layer was observed. In that study, porosities incorporated in relatively thick adhesive resin layers were found to result in less frequent resin-dentin interface separation, providing support for the elastic bonding concept. These observations also confirm the influence of the cavity geometry or configuration on the eventual bond integrity, with Class 1 cavities having the most unfavorable geometry, as previously described[93] (see Fig 8-18).

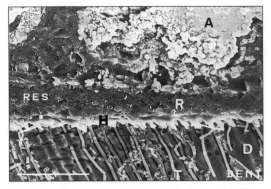

Fig 8-67a Scanning electron photomicrograph illustrating the interface of amalgam (A) and dentin (D). Note the formation of a hybrid layer (H) with resin tags when All-Bond 2 and Dispersalloy are used. Bar = 30 μm.

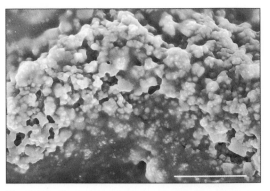

Fig 8-67b Scanning electron photomicrograph revealing the mixture of amalgam particles with resin when All-Bond 2 and Tytin are used. Bar = 7.5 μm.

Amalgam Bonding

The use of adhesive technology to bond amalgam to tooth tissue is an application of universal or multipurpose adhesive systems. Adhesive systems such as All-Bond 2 (Bisco), Amalgambond Plus (Parkell), Panavia (Kuraray), and Scotchbond Multi-Purpose Plus have been advocated for bonding amalgam to enamel and dentin. The nature of the bond between resin and amalgam is yet unclear, but appears to involve at least micromechanical mixing of amalgam with resin during condensation (Fig 8-67).[300] Because amalgam does not allow light transmission, these amalgam-bonding systems must have autopolymerizing capability. In vitro bond strengths of amalgam to dentin are generally less than 10 MPa, which is less than bond strengths of resin composite to dentin.[15,57,134,225] A possible problem with the incorporation of resin into amalgam is potential weakening of the mechanical properties of the bonded amalgam.[53]

The use of amalgam-bonding techniques has several potential benefits.[300] Retention gained by bonding lessens the need for removal of tooth structure to gain retention or for retentive devices such as dovetails,[26] grooves, and parapulpal pins.[54,141] Bonded amalgam may increase the fracture resistance of restored teeth,[75] and adhesive resin liners may seal the margins better than traditional cavity varnishes, with decreased risks for postoperative sensitivity and caries recurrence.[54,76,128,225] Although these amalgam-bonding techniques have been advocated for repair of existing amalgam restorations with either resin or fresh amalgam,[293] several studies have reported poor results in the strengthening of old amalgam restorations.[127,168,261]

Ceramic Bonding

Bonding resin to a ceramic surface, whether porcelain or glass ceramic, is based on the combined effects of micromechanical interlocking and chemical bonding.[246,247] Porcelain and glass-ceramic surfaces are generally etched with hydrofluoric acid and ammonium bifluoride, respectively, to increase the surface area and create microporosities. The adhesive resin flows into the porosities and interlocks, forming strong micromechanical bonds (Figs 8-68 and 8-69).

Thorough rinsing followed by ultrasonic cleaning is recommended to remove any remaining acid gel, precipitates, or loose particles, which may weaken the final bond (Fig 8-70). Complete drying of the etched ceramic surface can be obtained by brief immersion in a highly concentrated solution of ethanol.[262]

Chemical bonding to ceramic surfaces is achieved by silanization with a bifunctional coupling agent. A silane group at one end chemically bonds to the hydrolyzed silicon dioxide at the ceramic surface, and a methacrylate group at the other end copolymerizes with the adhesive resin (Fig 8-71). Single-component systems contain silane in alcohol or acetone and require prior acidification of the ceramic surface with hydrofluoric acid to activate the chemical reaction. With two-component silane solutions, the silane is mixed with an aqueous acid solution to hydrolyze the silane so that it can react with the ceramic surface. If not used within several hours, the silane will polymerize to an unreactive polysiloxane.[293]

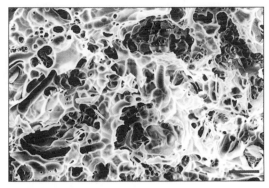

Fig 8-68 Field-emission scanning electron photomicrograph of porcelain etched with 9.6% hydrofluoric acid (Porcelain Etch, Ultradent). Bar = 5 μm.

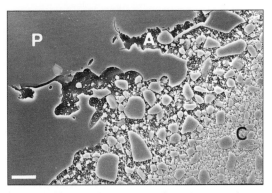

Fig 8-69 Field-emission scanning electron photomicrograph of the porcelain-lute interface. A = adhesive resin (Scotchbond Multi-Purpose Plus); C = luting composite (Opal Luting Composite); P = porcelain (Cosmotech, GC); bar = 5 μm. (From Peumans et al.[246] Reprinted with permission from Elsevier Science.)

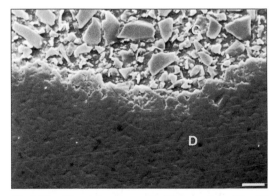

Fig 8-70a Dicor glass ceramic (D) was etched for 60 seconds with 10% ammonium bifluoride, ultrasonically cleaned, and luted with Dicor MGC (C). Post-etching ultrasonic cleaning is necessary to remove loose and weakened crystals at the surface to prevent cohesive subsurface failure (see Fig 8-70b).

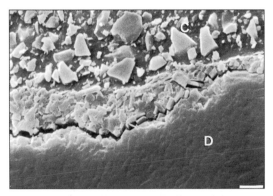

Fig 8-70b Dicor glass ceramic (D) was etched for 60 seconds with 10% ammonium bifluoride and luted with Dicor MGC (C) without ultrasonic cleaning.

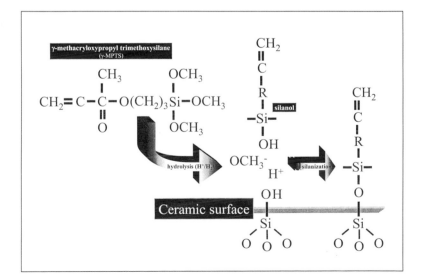

Fig 8-71 Silanization of a ceramic surface.

Glass-Ionomer Cements

Conventional Glass-Ionomer Cements

Glass-ionomer cements were developed in the early 1970s by Wilson and Kent,[344,345] who combined the technology of silicate and zinc carboxylate cements (Fig 8-72). Since that time, glass-ionomer cements have undergone many improvements and modifications of their original chemistry. Conventional glass-ionomer cements contain the ion-leachable fluoroaluminosilicate glass of the silicate cements but avoid their susceptibility to dissolution by substitution of the carboxylic acids from zinc carboxylate cements for phosphoric acid.[195] As stated by McLean et al,[185] a more accurate term for this type of material is *glass-polyalkenoate cement*, because these cements are not true ionomers chemically, but the term *glass-polyalkenoate cement* has never been as widely used as *glass-ionomer cement*.

The glass is high in aluminum and fluoride, with significant amounts of calcium, sodium, and silica.[275,278,347] The liquid is typically polyacrylic acid, but may contain polymers and copolymers of polyacrylic, itaconic, maleic, or vinyl phosphonic acid.[185,278]

The setting reaction of glass-ionomer cements has been characterized as an acid-base reaction between the glass powder and the polyacid liquid (Fig 8-73). When the powder and liquid are mixed, the fluoroaluminosilicate glass is attacked by hydrogen ions (H^+) from the polyalkenoic acid, liberating Al^{3+}, Ca^{2+}, Na^+, and F^- ions. A layer of silica gel is slowly formed on the surface of unreacted powder, with the progressive loss of metallic ions (Fig 8-74) (Ellison S, Warrens C. Solid-State NMR Study of Aluminosilicate Glasses and Derived Dental Cements. Report of the Laboratory of the Government Chemist. 1987).[47] When the free calcium and aluminum ions reach saturation in the silica gel, they diffuse into the liquid and cross-link with two or three ionized carboxyl groups (COO^-) of the polyacid to form a gel. As the crosslinking increases through aluminum ions and the gel is sufficiently hydrated, the crosslinked polyacrylate salt begins to precipitate until the cement is hard (Fig 8-75).

Conventional glass-ionomer cements offer several advantages over other restorative materials. They provide long-term release of fluoride ions, with cariostatic potential, and inherent adhesion to tooth tissue.[47,202,275] Because they possess a coefficient of thermal expansion closely approximating that of tooth structure and a low setting shrinkage, they are

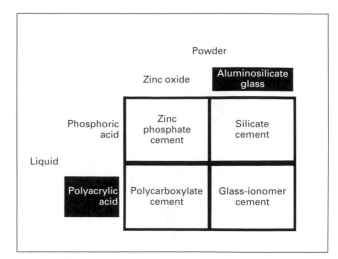

Fig 8-72 Development of glass-ionomer cements from combined technology of silicate and zinc polycarboxylate cements.

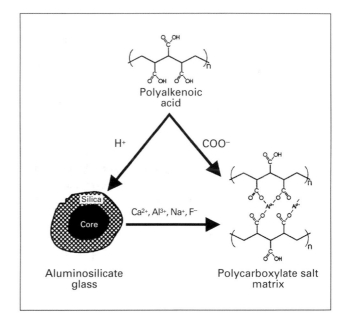

Fig 8-73 Acid-base setting reaction of conventional glass-ionomer cements.

reported to provide good marginal sealing, little microleakage at the restoration-tooth interface, and a high retention rate.[47,195] They are biocompatible and have esthetic potential.[47,195]

Despite these important biotherapeutic and clinical advantages, practical difficulties have limited their clinical use.[47,140,195] The material is technically demanding and highly sensitive to changes in its water content. Early moisture contamination disrupts its surface and removes metallic ions, while desiccation causes shrinkage and crazing. Glass-ionomer cements have a short working time but a long setting time,

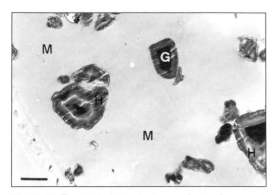

Fig 8-74 Transmission electron photomicrograph showing the ultrastructure of the resin-modified glass-ionomer adhesive Fuji Bond LC. G = core of fluoroaluminosilicate glass filler; H = hydrogel representing the link formed between the matrix and the filler core during the acid-base reaction; M = polycarboxylate salt matrix; bar = 1 μm.

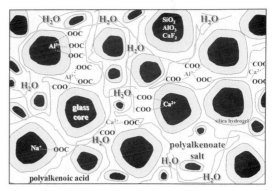

Fig 8-75 The structure of a set glass-ionomer cement.

which requires delayed finishing of the restoration. In addition, their physical properties and esthetic potential are inferior to those of resin composites.

Resin-Modified Glass-Ionomer Cements

To overcome the practical limitations of conventional glass-ionomer cements, yet preserve their clinical advantages, conventional glass-ionomer chemistry was combined with methacrylate resin technology; this led to the creation of resin-modified glass-ionomer systems.[7,275] They are often incorrectly referred to as light-cured glass-ionomer cements.[185,195,202] The term *dual-cured* is more appropriate, because the original acid-base reaction is supplemented by light-activated polymerization.[194,275]

Generally, these materials still have ion-leachable fluoroaluminosilicate glass in the powder, but they also contain monomers, primarily HEMA, and a photoinitiator, camphorquinone, which are added to the aqueous polyacid liquid.[195,202] In the simplest form of resin-modified glass-ionomer cement, some of the water content of the conventional glass-ionomer cement is replaced by a water-HEMA mixture, while more complex formulations comprise modified polyacids with methacrylate side chains, which can be light polymerized.[275] The first setting reaction is a slow acid-base reaction, typical of conventional glass-ionomer cements (see Fig 8-73). The photoinitiated setting reaction occurs much faster through homopolymerization and copolymerization of methacrylate groups grafted onto the polyacrylic acid

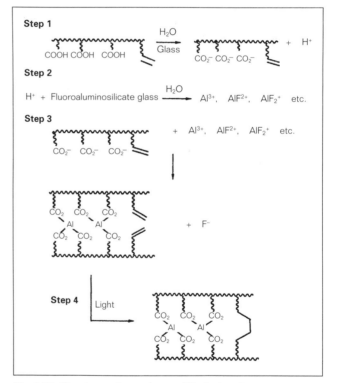

Fig 8-76 Structure of a resin-modified glass-ionomer cement and its probable setting reaction. (From Mitra.[194] Reprinted with permission.)

chain and methacrylate groups of HEMA (Figs 8-21 and 8-76). With certain materials, such as Fuji II LC and Vitremer, a third polymerization initiation is claimed to occur through chemically initiated, free-radical methacrylate curing of the polymer system and HEMA (Table 8-5).[47,195,300]

Table 8-5	Hybrid restorative materials according to their setting mechanism				
		Setting mechanism			
Material	**Manufacturer**	**Acid-base reaction**	**Visible light–initiated polymerization**	**Chemically initiated polymerization**	
Resin-modified glass-ionomer cements					
Fuji II LC	GC	✓	✓	✓	
Ionosit	DMG	✓	✓		
Photac-Fil Quick	ESPE	✓	✓		
Vitremer	3M	✓	✓	✓	
Polyacid-modified resin composites (compomers)					
Compoglass	Vivadent	*	✓		
Dyract	Dentsply	*	✓		
Dyract AP	Dentsply	*	✓		
Elan	Kerr	*	✓		
Hytac Aplitip	ESPE	*	✓		
Freedom	SDI	*	✓		
F2000	3M	*	✓		
Geristore	Den-Mat	*	✓		
Glasiosite	Voco	*	✓		
Luxat	DMG	*	✓		

* Claimed but unproven.

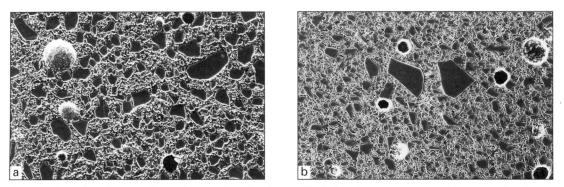

Fig 8-77 Scanning electron photomicrographs of resin-modified glass-ionomer cements after argon-ion–beam etching. (a) Photac Bond. (b) Vitremer. (From Van Meerbeek et al.[326] Reprinted with permission.)

A diverse group of materials is marketed as resin-modified glass-ionomer cements (Table 8-5). The products vary from those that closely resemble conventional glass-ionomer cements to those that approximate light-curing resin composites and cure almost exclusively by light-initiated polymerization of free radicals.[47,114,185,300] For the latter, no or little water is present in the system to allow the acid-base reaction, typical of glass-ionomer cements.[275] A true resin-modified glass-ionomer cement, then, is defined as a two-part system, characterized by an acid-base reaction critical to its cure, diffusion-based adhesion between the tooth surface and the cement, and continuing fluoride release.[185,275]

The underlying mechanism of adhesion of glass-ionomer cements to tooth structure has always been thought to be an ion-exchange process, in which the polyalkenoic acid softens and infiltrates the tooth surface, displacing calcium and phosphate ions (Figs 8-78 and 8-79).[2,173,202,348] It has been postulated that an intermediate adsorption layer of calcium and aluminum phosphates and polyacrylates is formed at the glass-ionomer cement–hydroxyapatite interface.[201,275,346] A reversible breaking and reforming of calcium-carboxyl

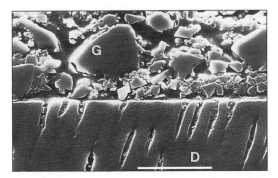

Fig 8-78 Scanning electron photomicrograph of the resin-modified glass-ionomer cement–dentin interface with Fuji II LC. The dentinal tubules appear to be occluded by smear debris. D = dentin; G = resin-modified glass-ionomer cement; bar = 20 μm.

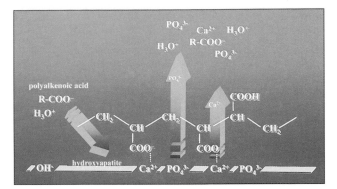

Fig 8-79 The ion-exchange process induced by the application of a polyalkenoic acid on hydroxyapatite, which results in the formation of an ionic bond of the carboxyl groups of the polyalkenoic acid with calcium of hydroxyapatite.

complexes in the presence of water is suggested to form a dynamic bond.[42] It was only recently that direct evidence of primary chemical bonding of the carboxyl groups of the polyalkenoic acid to calcium of hydroxyapatite could be provided.[352] The interfacial ultrastructure as formed by a resin-modified glass-ionomer adhesive has been documented as well (Fig 8-80).[338]

Clinically, glass-ionomer cement can be used as a luting agent, as a cavity liner or base, as a core buildup material, as a direct restorative material in permanent and primary teeth, as a pit and fissure sealant, as a provisional restorative material, and as a retrograde root filling material.[184,275,300]

Resin-modified glass ionomers are easier to use than conventional glass-ionomer cements. The supplementary light polymerization allows a longer working time, a rapid hardening on command, and a more rapid early development of strength and resistance against aqueous attack than are found with conventional glass-ionomer cements.[114,275,300] Mechanical properties such as compressive, tensile, and flexural strengths; fracture toughness; wear resistance; fatigue resistance; bond strengths to enamel, dentin, and other resin-based restorative materials; marginal adaptation; and microleakage are reported to be better than those of conventional glass-ionomer cements.[40,47,114,275,300] They appear to be less sensitive to water, are radiopaque, and offer better esthetic possibilities than do conventional glass-ionomer cements. The fluoride release of resin-modified glass-ionomer cements is reported to be equal to or higher than that of conventional glass-ionomer cements, and fluoride potential may even be rechargeable.[198,275] However, their physical properties remain inferior to those of resin composites. At this time, although the long-term clinical

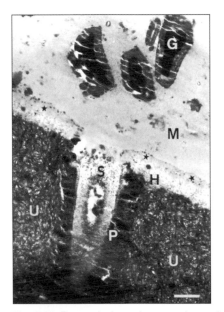

Fig 8-80 Transmission electron photomicrograph of an unstained, nondemineralized section demonstrating the interface formed at dentin by a glass-ionomer adhesive (Fuji Bond LC). The shallow hybrid layer (H) of about 0.5 μm results from the short (10-second) application of a 20% polyalkenoic acid, by which collagen fibrils are exposed but not completely denuded from hydroxyapatite (collagen is not visible on this image as the section was not positively stained). The hydroxyapatite crystals remaining around the collagen fibrils served as receptors for chemical bonding with the carboxyl groups of the polyalkenoic acid. On top of the hybrid layer, a 0.5-μm gray zone *(black stars)* typically contains small black globules of yet unknown origin and is clearly demarcated from the glass-ionomer matrix (M). This phase represents the morphologic manifestation of a gelation reaction of the polyalkenoic acid with calcium that was extracted from the underlying dentin surface. G = fluoroaluminosilicate glass filler surrounded by a silica hydrogel; P = peritubular dentin; S = smear occluding the tubule orifice; U = unaffected intertubular dentin; bar = 1 μm.

performance of resin-modified glass-ionomer cements is still not very well known, the currently available materials appear promising. They are best used in clinical practice for specific indications such as in patients at high risk for caries, in areas where esthetics is not a primary concern, in technically difficult areas requiring a capsule application technique, or in the so-called ART concept (atraumatic restorative treatment).

References

1. Abdalla AI, Davidson CL. Shear bond strength and microleakage of new dentin bonding systems. Am J Dent 1993; 6:295.

2. Akinmade AO, Nicholson JW. Glass-ionomer cements as adhesives. Part I. Fundamental aspects and their clinical relevance. J Mater Science Mater Med 1993;4:95.

3. Alexieva C. Character of the hard tooth tissue-polymer bond. II. Study of the interaction of human tooth enamel and dentin with N-phenylglycine-glycidyl methacrylate adduct. J Dent Res 1979;58:1884.

4. Allen KW. Adsorption theory of adhesion. Theories of adhesion. In: Packham DE (ed). Handbook of Adhesion, ed 1. Essex, England: Longman, 1992:39, 473.

5. Alster D, Feilzer AJ, de Gee AJ, et al. The dependence of shrinkage stress reduction on porosity concentration in thin resin layers. J Dent Res 1992;71:1619.

6. Anderson DAF, Ferracane JL, Zimmerman E, Kaga M. Cytotoxicity of variably cured light-activated dental composites [abstract 905]. J Dent Res 1988;67:226.

7. Antonucci JM, McKinney JE, Stansbury JW [inventors]. Resin-modified glass-ionomer cement. US patent 160856, 1988.

8. Asmussen E. Clinical relevance of physical, chemical, and bonding properties of composite resins. Oper Dent 1985;10:61.

9. Asmussen E, Munksgaard EC. Adhesion of restorative resins to dentinal tissues. In: Vanherle G, Smith DC (eds). Posterior Composite Resin Dental Restorative Materials, ed 1. Utrecht, The Netherlands: Peter Szulc, 1985:217.

10. Asmussen E, Antonucci JM, Bowen RL. Adhesion to dentin by means of Gluma resin. Scand J Dent Res 1988;96:584.

11. Asmussen E, Munksgaard EC. Bonding of restorative resins to dentine: status of dentine adhesives and impact on cavity design and filling techniques. Int Dent J 1988;38:97.

12. Asmussen E, de Araujo PA, Peutzfeldt A. In-vitro bonding of resins to enamel and dentin: an update. Trans Acad Dent Mater 1989;2:36.

13. Asmussen E, Uno S. Solubility parameters, fractional polarities, and bond strengths of some intermediary resins used in dentin bonding. J Dent Res 1993;72:558.

14. Asmussen E, Hansen EK. Dentine bonding agents. In: Vanherle G, Degrange M, Willems G (eds). State of the Art on Direct Posterior Filling Materials and Dentine Bonding. Proceedings of the International Symposium Euro Disney, ed 2. Leuven, Belgium: Van der Poorten, 1994:33.

15. Bagley A, Wakefield CW, Robbins JW. In vitro comparison of filled and unfilled universal bonding agents of amalgam to dentin. Oper Dent 1994;19:97.

16. Baier RE. Principles of adhesion. Oper Dent 1992;suppl 5:1.

17. Barghi N, Knight GT, Berry TG. Comparing two methods of moisture control in bonding to enamel: a clinical study. Oper Dent 1991;16:130.

18. Barkmeier WW, Shaffer SE, Gwinnett AJ. Effects of 15 vs 60 second enamel acid conditioning on adhesion and morphology. Oper Dent 1986;11:111.

19. Barkmeier WW, Erickson RL. Shear bond strength of composite to enamel and dentin using Scotchbond Multi-Purpose. Am J Dent 1994;7:175.

20. Bayne SC, Flemming JE, Faison S. SEM-EDS analysis of macro and micro resin tags of laminates [abstract 1128]. J Dent Res 1982;61:304.

21. Bayne SC, Heymann HO, Sturdevant JR, et al. Contributing co-variables on clinical trials. Am J Dent 1991;4:247.

22. Bayne SC, Wilder AD, Heymann HO, et al. 1-year clinical evaluation of stress-breaking class V DBA design. Trans Acad Dent Mater 1994;7:91.

23. Benediktsson S, Retief DH, Russel CM, Mandras RS. Critical surface tension of wetting of dentin [abstract 777]. J Dent Res 1991;70:362.

24. Berry EA III, von der Lehr WN, Herrin HK. Dentin surface treatments for the removal of the smear layer: an SEM study. J Am Dent Assoc 1987;115:65.

25. Bertolotti RL. Conditioning of the dentin substrate. Oper Dent 1992;suppl 5:131.

26. Black GV. A Work on Operative Dentistry in Two Volumes, ed 3. Chicago: Medico-Dental Publishing, 1917.

27. Blunck U, Roulet J-F. Effect of one-bottle-adhesives on the marginal adaptation of composite resins and compomers in Class V cavities in vitro [abstract 2231]. J Dent Res 1998;77:910.

28. Boghosian A. Clinical evaluation of a filled adhesive system in Class 5 restorations. Compend Contin Educ Dent 1996;17:750.

29. Bowen RL [inventor]. Dental filling material comprising vinyl silane, treated fused silica and a binder consisting of the reaction product of bisphenol and glycidyl acrylate. US patent 3066.112, 1962.

30. Bowen RL. Adhesive bonding of various materials to hard tooth tissues. II. Bonding to dentin promoted by a surface-active comonomer. J Dent Res 1965;44:895.

31. Bowen RL, Cobb EN, Rapson JE. Adhesive bonding of various materials to hard tooth tissues: improvement in bond strength to dentin. J Dent Res 1982;61:1070.

32. Bowen RL, Nemoto K, Rapson JE. Adhesive bonding of various materials to hard tooth tissue: forces developing in composite materials during hardening. J Am Dent Assoc 1983;106:475.

33. Bowen RL, Tung MS, Blosser RL, Asmussen E. Dentine and enamel bonding agents. Int Dent J 1987;37:158.

34. Bowen RL. Bonding agents and adhesives: reactor response. Adv Dent Res 1988;2:155.

35. Bowen RL, Eichmiller FC, Marjenhoff WA. Glass-ceramic inserts anticipated for "megafilled" composite restorations. J Am Dent Assoc 1991;122:71.

36. Bowen RL, Marjenhoff WA. Development of an adhesive bonding system. Oper Dent 1992;suppl 5:75.

37. Braem M. An In-Vitro Investigation into the Physical Durability of Dental Composites [thesis]. Leuven, Belgium: Catholic University of Leuven, 1985.

38. Braem M, Lambrechts P, Vanherle G, Davidson CL. Stiffness increase during the setting of dental composite resins. J Dent Res 1987;66:1713.

39. Braem M, Lambrechts P, Vanherle G. Stress-induced cervical lesions. J Prosthet Dent 1992;67:718.

40. Braem MJA, Gladys S, Lambrechts P, et al. Flexural fatigue limit of several restorative materials [abstract 47]. J Dent Res 1995;74:17.

41. Brännström M, Linden LA, Astrom A. The hydrodynamics of the dentinal tubule and of pulp fluid. A discussion of its significance in relation to dentinal sensitivity. Caries Res 1967;1:310.

42. Brook IM, Craig GT, Lamb DJ. Initial in-vitro evaluation of glass-ionomer cements for use as alveolar bone substitutes. Clin Mater 1991;7:295.

43. Browning WD, Brackett WW, Gilpatrick RO. Two-year clinical comparison of a microfilled and a hybrid resin-based composite in noncarious Class V lesions. Oper Dent 2000;25:50.

44. Buonocore MG. A simple method of increasing the adhesion of acrylic filling materials to enamel surfaces. J Dent Res 1955;34:849.

45. Buonocore M, Wileman W, Brudevold F. A report on a resin composition capable of bonding to human dentin surfaces. J Dent Res 1956;35:846.

46. Buonocore MG, Matsui A, Gwinnett AJ. Penetration of resin dental materials into enamel surfaces with reference to bonding. Arch Oral Biol 1968;13:61.

47. Burgess J, Norling B, Summitt J. Resin ionomer restorative materials: the new generation. J Esthet Dent 1994;6:207.

48. Burrow MF, Takakura H, Nakajima M, et al. The influence of age and depth of dentin on bonding. Dent Mater 1994;10:241.

49. Burrow MF, Taniguchi Y, Nikaido T, et al. Influence of temperature and relative humidity on early bond strengths to dentine. J Dent 1995;23:41.

50. Carvalho RM, Pashley EL, Yoshiyama M, et al. Dimensional changes in demineralized dentin [abstract 171]. J Dent Res 1995;74:33.

51. Causton BE. Improved bonding of composite restorative to dentine. Br Dent J 1984;156:93.

52. Chappell RP, Cobb CM, Spencer P, Eick JD. Dentinal tubule anastomosis: a potential factor in adhesive bonding? J Prosthet Dent 1994;72:183.

53. Charlton DG, Murchison DF, Moore BK. Incorporation of adhesive liners in amalgam: effect on compressive strength and creep. Am J Dent 1991;4:184.

54. Charlton DG, Moore BK, Swartz ML. In vitro evaluation of the use of resin liners to reduce microleakage and improve retention of amalgam restorations. Oper Dent 1992;17:112.

55. Chow LC, Brown WE. Phosphoric acid conditioning of teeth for pit and fissure sealants. J Dent Res 1973;52:1158.

56. Ciucchi B, Sano H, Pashley DH. Bonding to sodium hypochlorite treated dentin [abstract 1556]. J Dent Res 1994;73:296.

57. Cooley RL, Tseng EY, Barkmeier WW. Dentinal bond strengths and microleakage of a 4-META adhesive to amalgam and composite resin. Quintessence Int 1991;22:979.

58. Cortes O, Garcia-Godoy F, Boj JR. Bond strength of resin-reinforced glass ionomer cements after enamel etching. Am J Dent 1993;6:299.

59. Council on Dental Materials, Instruments, and Equipment. ADA Clinical Protocol Guidelines for Dentin and Enamel Adhesive Restorative Materials. Chicago: American Dental Association, 1987.

60. Cox CF, Keall CL, Keall HJ, et al. Biocompatibility of surface-sealed dental materials against exposed pulp. J Prosthet Dent 1987;57:1.

61. Cox CF. Effects of adhesive resins and various dental cements on the pulp. Oper Dent 1992;suppl 5:165.

62. Crim GA, Shay JS. Effect of etchant time on microleakage. J Dent Child 1987;54:339.

63. Crim GA. Prepolymerization of Gluma 4 sealer: effect on bonding. Am J Dent 1990;3:25.

64. Davidson CL, de Gee AJ. Relaxation of polymerization contraction stress by flow in dental composites. J Dent Res 1984;63:146.

65. Davidson CL, de Gee AJ, Feilzer A. The competition between the composite-dentin bond strength and the polymerization contraction stress. J Dent Res 1984;63:1396.

66. Davidson CL, Abdalla AI. Effect of occlusal load cycling on the marginal integrity of adhesive class V restorations. Am J Dent 1994;7:111.

67. Donly KJ, Wild TW, Bowen RL, Jensen ME. An in vitro investigation of the effects of glass inserts on the effective composite resin polymerization shrinkage. J Dent Res 1989;68:1234.

68. Douglas WH. Clinical status of dentine bonding agents. J Dent 1989;17:209.

69. Duke ES, Lindemuth JS. Polymeric adhesion to dentin: contrasting substrates. Am J Dent 1990;3:264.

70. Duke ES, Lindemuth JS. Variability of clinical dentin substrates. Am J Dent 1991;4:241.

71. Duke ES, Robbins JW, Snyder DE. Clinical evaluation of a dentinal adhesive system: three-year results. Quintessence Int 1991;22:889.

72. Duke ES. Adhesion and its application with restorative materials. Dent Clin North Am 1993;37:329.

73. Duke ES, Robbins JW, Trevino D. The clinical performance of a new adhesive resin system in class V and IV restorations. Compend Contin Educ Dent 1994;15:825.

74. Eakle WS. Fracture resistance of teeth restored with Class II bonded composite resin. J Dent Res 1986;65:149.

75. Eakle WS, Staninec M, Lacy AM. Effect of bonded amalgam on the fracture resistance of teeth. J Prosthet Dent 1992;68:257.

76. Edgren BN, Denehy GE. Microleakage of amalgam restorations using Amalgambond and Copalite. Am J Dent 1992;5:296.

77. Edler TL, Krikorian E, Thompson VP. FTIR surface analysis of dentin and dentin bonding agents [abstract 1534]. J Dent Res 1991;70:458.

78. Eick JD, Wilko RA, Anderson CH, Sorenson SE. Scanning electron microscopy of cut tooth surfaces and identification of debris by use of the electron microprobe. J Dent Res 1970;49:1359.

79. Eick JD. Smear layer–materials surface. Proc Finn Dent Soc 1992;88(suppl 1):8.

80. Eick JD, Robinson SJ, Byerley TJ, Chappelow CC. Adhesives and nonshrinking dental resins of the future. Quintessence Int 1993;24:632.

81. Eick JD, Robinson SJ, Chappell RP, et al. The dentinal surface: its influence on dentinal adhesion. Part III. Quintessence Int 1993;24:571.

82. Eick JD, Byerley TJ, Chappell RP, et al. Properties of expanding SOC/epoxy copolymers for dental use in dental composites. Dent Mater 1993;9:123.

83. Eick JD, Robinson SJ, Byerley TJ, et al. Scanning transmission electron microscopy/energy-dispersive spectroscopy analysis of the dentin adhesive interface using a labeled 2-hydroxyethylmethacrylate analogue. J Dent Res 1995;74:1246.

84. El Feninat F, Ellis TH, Sacher E, Stangel I. Moisture-dependent renaturation of collagen in phosphoric acid etched human dentin. J Biomed Mater Res 1998;42:549.

85. Eliades GC, Caputo AA, Vougiouklakis GJ. Composition, wetting properties and bond strength with dentin of 6 new dentin adhesives. Dent Mater 1985;1:170.

86. Eliades GC, Vougiouklakis GJ. ^{31}P-NMR study of P-based dental adhesives and electron probe microanalysis of simulated interfaces with dentin. Dent Mater 1989;5:101.

87. Eliades G, Palaghias G, Vougiouklakis G. Surface reactions of adhesives on dentin. Dent Mater 1990;6:208.

88. Eliades GC. Reaction paper: dentine bonding systems. In: Vanherle G, Degrange M, Willems G (eds). Proceedings of the International Symposium on State of the Art on Direct Posterior Filling Materials and Dentine Bonding. Leuven, Belgium: Van der Poorten, 1993:49–74.

89. Eliades G. Clinical relevance of the formulation and testing of dentine bonding systems. J Dent 1994;22:73.

90. Ericksen HM. Protection against harmful effects of a restorative procedure using an acid cavity cleanser. J Dent Res 1976; 55:281.

91. Erickson RL. Mechanism and clinical implications of bond formation for two dentin bonding agents. Am J Dent 1989;2:117.

92. Erickson RL. Surface interactions of dentin adhesive materials. Oper Dent 1992;suppl 5:81.

93. Feilzer AJ, de Gee AJ, Davidson CL. Setting stress in composite resin in relation to configuration of the restoratives. J Dent Res 1987;66:1636.

94. Feilzer AJ, de Gee AJ, Davidson CL. Curing contraction of composites and glass ionomer cements. J Prosthet Dent 1988; 59:297.

95. Feilzer AJ. Polymerization Shrinkage Stress in Dental Composite Resin Restorations—An In-Vitro Investigation [thesis]. Amsterdam, The Netherlands: University of Amsterdam (ACTA), 1989.

96. Feilzer AJ, de Gee AJ, Davidson CL. Increased wall-to-wall curing contraction in thin bonded resin layers. J Dent Res 1989;68:48.

97. Ferracane JL. Current trends in dental composites. Crit Rev Oral Biol Med 1995;6:302.

98. Fortin D, Perdigão J, Swift EJ Jr. Microleakage of three new dentin adhesives. Am J Dent 1994;7:315.

99. Fortin D, Swift EJ, Denehy GE, Reinhardt JW. Bond strength and microleakage of current dentin adhesives. Dent Mater 1994;10:253.

100. Frank RM, Voegel JC. Ultrastructure of the human odontoblast process and its mineralization during dental caries. Caries Res 1980;14:367.

101. Fritz U, Finger W, Uno S. Resin-modified glass ionomer cements: bonding to enamel and dentin. Dent Mater 1996; 12:161.

102. Fundingsland JW, Aasen SM, Bodger PD, Cernhous JJ. The effect of high humidity on adhesion to dentine [abstract 1199]. J Dent Res 1992;72:665.

103. Fusayama T. Two layers of carious dentin: diagnosis and treatment. Oper Dent 1979;4:63.

104. Fusayama T, Nakamura M, Kurosaki N, Iwaku M. Non-pressure adhesion of a new adhesive restorative system. J Dent Res 1979;58:1364.

105. Fusayama T. Factors and prevention of pulp irritation by adhesive composite resin restorations. Quintessence Int 1987; 18:633.

106. Fusayama T. The problems preventing progress in adhesive restorative dentistry. Adv Dent Res 1988;2:158.

107. Fusayama T. A new dental caries treatment system developed in Japan. Proc Jpn Acad 1990;66:121.

108. Fusayama T. Biological problems of the light-cured composite resin. Quintessence Int 1993;24:225.

109. Garberoglio R, Brännström M. Scanning electron microscopic investigation of human dentinal tubules. Arch Oral Biol 1976; 21:355.

110. Gelb MN, Barouch E, Simonsen RJ. Resistance to cusp fracture in class II prepared and restored premolars. J Prosthet Dent 1986;55:184.

111. Gerzina TM, Hume WR. Effect of dentine on release of TEGDMA from resin composite in vitro. J Oral Rehabil 1994;21:463.

112. Gerzina TM, Hume WR. Effect of hydrostatic pressure on the diffusion of monomers through dentin in vitro. J Dent Res 1995;74:369.

113. Gilpatrick RO, Ross JA, Simonsen RJ. Resin-to-enamel bond strengths with various etching times. Quintessence Int 1991; 22:47.

114. Gladys S, Van Meerbeek B, Braem M, et al. Comparative physico-mechanical characterization of new hybrid restorative materials with conventional glass-ionomer and resin composite restorative materials. J Dent Res 1997;76:883.

115. Gladys S, Van Meerbeek B, Lambrechts P, Vanherle G. Marginal adaptation and retention of a glass-ionomer, resin-modified glass-ionomers and a polyacid-modified resin composite in cervical Class-V lesions. Dent Mater 1998;14:294.

116. Goel VK, Khera SC, Ralston JL, Chang KH. Stresses at the dentinoenamel junction of human teeth—a finite element investigation. J Prosthet Dent 1991;66:451.

117. Gwinnett AJ, Buonocore MG. Adhesion and caries prevention. A preliminary report. Br Dent J 1965;119:77.

118. Gwinnett AJ, Matsui A. A study of enamel adhesives. The physical relationship between enamel and adhesive. Arch Oral Biol 1967;12:1615.

119. Gwinnett AJ. Histologic changes in human enamel following treatment with acidic adhesive conditioning agents. Arch Oral Biol 1971;16:731.

120. Gwinnett AJ. Smear layer: morphological considerations. Oper Dent 1984;suppl 3:3.

121. Gwinnett AJ. Interactions of dental materials with enamel. Trans Acad Dent Mater 1990;3:30.

122. Gwinnett AJ. Moist versus dry dentin: its effect on shear bond strength. Am J Dent 1992;5:127.

123. Gwinnett AJ. Structure and composition of enamel. Oper Dent 1992;suppl 5:10.

124. Gwinnett AJ, Kanca J. Micromorphology of the bonded dentin interface and its relationship to bond strength. Am J Dent 1992;5:73.

125. Gwinnett AJ. Quantitative contribution of resin infiltration/ hybridization to dentin bonding. Am J Dent 1993;6:7.

126. Gwinnett AJ. Altered tissue contribution to interfacial bond strength with acid conditioned dentin. Am J Dent 1994;7:243.

127. Hadavi F, Hey JH, Ambrose ER, Elbadrawy HE. The influence of an adhesive system on shear bond strength of repaired high copper amalgams. Oper Dent 1991;16:175.

128. Hadavi F, Hey JH, Ambrose ER, Elbadrawy HE. Effect of different adhesive systems on microleakage at the amalgam/composite resin interface. Oper Dent 1993;18:2.

129. Hansen EK, Asmussen E. Cavity preparation for restorative resins used with dentin adhesives. Scand J Dent Res 1985; 93:474.

130. Hansen EK. Effect of cavity depth and application technique on marginal adaptation of resins in dentin cavities. J Dent Res 1986;65:1319.

131. Hansen EK. In vivo cusp fracture of endodontically treated premolars restored with MOD amalgam or MOD resin fillings. Dent Mater 1988;4:169.

132. Hansen SE, Swift EJ. Microleakage with Gluma: effects of unfilled resin polymerization and storage time. Am J Dent 1989; 2:266.

133. Harper RH, Schnell RJ, Swartz ML, Phillips RW. In vivo measurements of thermal diffusion through restorations of various materials. J Prosthet Dent 1980;43:180.

134. Hasegawa T, Retief DH, Russell CM, Denys FR. A laboratory study of the Amalgambond Adhesive System. Am J Dent 1992;5:181.

135. Hegdahl T, Gjerdet NR. Contraction stresses of composite filling materials. Acta Odontol Scand 1987;35:191.

136. Heymann HO, Bayne SC. Current concepts in dentin bonding: focusing on dentinal adhesion factors. J Am Dent Assoc 1993;124:27.

137. Heymann HO, Sturdevant JR, Brunson WD, et al. Twelve-month clinical study of dentinal adhesives in Class V cervical lesions. J Am Dent Assoc 1988;116:179.

138. Heymann HO, Sturdevant JR, Bayne S, et al. Examining tooth flexure effects on cervical restorations: a two-year clinical study. J Am Dent Assoc 1991;122:41.

139. Huang GT, Söderholm K-JM. In vitro investigation of shear bond strength of a phosphate based dentinal bonding agent. Scand J Dent Res 1989;97:84.

140. Hunt PR, ed. Glass Ionomers: The Next Generation. Proceedings of the 2nd International Symposium on Glass Ionomers. Philadelphia: International Symposia in Dentistry, 1994.

141. Ianzano JA, Mastrodomenico J, Gwinnett AJ. Strength of amalgam restorations bonded with Amalgambond. Am J Dent 1993;6:10.

142. Ibsen R, Ouellet D, Strassler H. Clinically successful dentin and enamel bonding. Am J Dent 1991;2:125.

143. Imai Y, Kadoma Y, Kojima K, et al. Importance of polymerization initiator systems and interfacial initiation of polymerization in adhesive bonding of resin to dentin. J Dent Res 1991;70:1088.

144. Imai Y, Suzuki A. Effects of water and carboxylic acid monomer on polymerization of HEMA in the presence of N-phenylglycine. Dent Mater 1994;10:275.

145. Inoue M, Finger WJ, Mueller M. Effect of filler content of restorative resins on retentive strength to acid-conditioned enamel. Am J Dent 1994;7:161.

145a. Inoue S, Van Meerbeek B, Vargas M, et al. Adhesion mechanism of self-etching adhesives. In: Tagami J, Toledano M, Prati C (eds). Third International Kuraray Symposium of Advanced Dentistry, 3–4 December 1999, Granada, Spain. Como, Italy: Graphice Erredue, 2000 (in press).

146. Ishioka S, Caputo AA. Interaction between the dentinal smear layer and composite bond strengths. J Prosthet Dent 1989;61:180.

147. Jacobsen T, Ma R, Söderholm K-J. Dentin bonding through interpenetrating network formation. Trans Acad Dent Mater 1994;7:45.

148. Jacobsen T, Söderholm K-J. Some effects of water on dentin bonding. Dent Mater 1995;11:132.

149. Jendresen MD. Clinical performance of a new composite resin for class V erosion [abstract 1057]. J Dent Res 1978;57:339.

150. Jendresen MD, Glantz P-O. Microtopography and clinical adhesiveness of an acid etched tooth surface. Acta Odontol Scand 1981;39:47.

151. Jensen ME, Chan DCN. Polymerization shrinkage and microleakage. In: Vanherle G, Smith DC (eds). Posterior Composite Resin Dental Restorative Materials, ed 1. Utrecht, The Netherlands: Szulc, 1985:243.

152. Jordan RE, Suzuki M, MacLean DF. Early clinical evaluation of Tenure and Scotchbond 2 for conservative restoration of cervical erosion lesions. J Esthet Dent 1989;1:10.

153. Jordan RE, Suzuki M, Davidson DF. Clinical evaluation of a universal dentin bonding resin: preserving dentition through new materials. J Am Dent Assoc 1993;124:71.

154. Kanca J III. Effect of resin primer solvent and surface wetness on resin composite bond strength to dentin. Am J Dent 1992;5:213.

155. Kanca J III. Resin bonding to wet substrate. I. Bonding to dentin. Quintessence Int 1992;23:39.

156. Kanca J. Improving bond strength through acid etching of dentin and bonding to wet dentin surfaces. J Am Dent Assoc 1992;123:35.

157. Kanemura N, Sano H, Tagami J. Tensile bond strength to and SEM evaluation of ground and intact enamel surfaces. J Dent 1999;27:523.

158. Katsuno K, Manabe A, Itoh K, et al. A delayed hypersensitivity reaction to dentine primer in the guinea-pig. J Dent 1995;23:295.

159. Katsuno K, Manabe A, Kurihara A, et al. The adverse effect of commercial dentine-bonding systems on the skin of guinea pigs. J Oral Rehabil 1998;25:180.

160. Kellar M, Duke ES. Neutralizing phosphoric acid in the acid etch resin technique. J Oral Rehabil 1988;15:625.

161. Kemp-Scholte CM, Davidson CL. Marginal sealing of curing contraction gaps in class V composite resin restorations. J Dent Res 1988;67:841.

162. Kemp-Scholte CM. The Marginal Integrity of Cervical Composite Resin Restorations [thesis]. Amsterdam, The Netherlands: University of Amsterdam (ACTA), 1989.

163. Kemp-Scholte CM, Davidson CL. Overhang of Class V composite resin restorations from hygroscopic expansion. Quintessence Int 1989;20:551.

164. Kemp-Scholte CM, Davidson CL. Complete marginal seal of class V resin composite restorations effected by increased flexibility. J Dent Res 1990;69:1240.

165. Kemp-Scholte CM, Davidson CL. Marginal integrity related to bond strength and strain capacity of composite resin restorative systems. J Prosthet Dent 1990;64:658.

166. Kinloch AJ. Adhesion and Adhesives. Science and Technology, ed 1. London: Chapman and Hall, 1987.

167. Labella R, Van Meerbeek B, Yoshida Y, et al. Marginal gap distribution of two-step versus three-step adhesive systems [abstract P35]. Trans Acad Dent Mat 1998;12:237.

168. Lacy AM, Rupprecht R, Watanabe L. Use of self-curing composite resins to facilitate amalgam repair. Quintessence Int 1992;23:53.

169. Lambrechts P, Braem M, Vanherle G. Evaluation of clinical performance for posterior composite resins and dentin adhesives. Oper Dent 1987;12:53.

170. Lee S-Y, Greener EH, Mueller HJ, Chiu C-H. Effect of food and oral simulating fluids on dentine bond and composite strength. J Dent 1994;22:352.

171. Lee WC, Eakle WS. Possible role of tensile stress in the etiology of cervical erosive lesions of teeth. J Prosthet Dent 1984;52:374.

172. Leinfelder KF. After amalgam, what? Other materials fall short. J Am Dent Assoc 1994;125:586.

173. Lin A, McIntyre NS, Davidson RD. Studies on the adhesion of glass ionomer cements to dentin. J Dent Res 1992;71:1836.

174. Linde A. The extracellular matrix of the dental pulp and dentin. J Dent Res 1985;64:523.

175. Lutz F, Krejci I, Oldenburg TR. Elimination of polymerization stresses at the margins of posterior composite resin restorations: a new restorative technique. Quintessence Int 1986;17:659.

176. Lutz F, Krejci I, Barbakow F. Quality and durability of marginal adaptation in bonded composite restorations. Dent Mater 1991;7:107.

177. Lutz, Krejci I, Luescher B, Oldenburg TR. Improved proximal margin adaptation of Class II composite resin restorations by use of light-reflecting wedges. Quintessence Int 1986;17:777.

178. Lyon D, Darling AI. Orientation of the crystallites in human dental enamel. Br Dent J 1957;102:483.

179. Mackert JR. Dental amalgam and mercury. J Am Dent Assoc 1991;122:54.

180. Marchetti C, Piacentini C, Menghini P. Morphometric computerized analysis on the dentinal tubules and the collagen fibers in the dentine of human permanent teeth. Bull Group Int Rech Sci Stomatol Odontol 1992;35:125.

181. Mariotti A, Söderholm KJ, Johnson S. The in vivo effects of bisGMA on murine uterine weight, nucleic acids and collagen. Eur J Oral Sci 1998;106:1022.

182. McCullock AJ, Smith BGN. In vitro studies of cuspal movement produced by adhesive restorative materials. Br Dent J 1986;161:405.

183. McLean JW, Kramer IRH. A clinical and pathological evaluation of a sulphinic acid activated resin for use in restorative dentistry. Br Dent J 1952;93:255.

184. McLean JW. Clinical applications of glass-ionomer cements. Oper Dent 1992;suppl 5:184.

185. McLean JW, Nicholson JW, Wilson AD. Proposed nomenclature for glass-ionomer dental cements and related materials [guest editorial]. Quintessence Int 1994;25:587.

186. McLean JW. Bonding to enamel and dentin [letter]. Quintessence Int 1995;26:234.

187. Meckel AH, Grebstein WJ, Neal RJ. Structure of mature human enamel as observed by electron microscopy. Arch Oral Biol 1965;10:775.

188. Mehl A, Manhart J, Kremers L. Physical properties and marginal quality of class-II composite fillings after softstart-polymerization [abstract 2121]. J Dent Res 1997;76:279.

189. Meryon SD, Tobias RS, Jakeman KJ. Smear removal agents: a quantitative study in vivo and in vitro. J Prosthet Dent 1987; 57:174.

190. Michelich V, Schuster GS, Pashley DH. Bacterial penetration of human dentin, in vitro. J Dent Res 1980;59:1398.

191. Miller RG, Bowles CQ, Chappelow CC, Eick JD. Application of solubility parameter theory to dentin-bonding systems and adhesive strength correlations. J Biomed Mater Res 1998;41: 237.

192. Mills RW, Jandt KD, Ashworth SH. Dental composite depth of cure with halogen and blue light emitting diode technology. Br Dent J 1999;186:388.

193. Mitchem JC, Gronas DG. Effects of time after extraction and depth of dentin on resin dentin adhesives. J Am Dent Assoc 1986;113:285.

194. Mitra SB. Adhesion to dentin and physical properties of a light-cured glass-ionomer liner/base. J Dent Res 1991;70:72.

195. Mitra S. Curing reactions of glass ionomer materials. In: Hunt PR, ed. Glass Ionomers: The Next Generation. Proceedings of the 2nd International Symposium on Glass Ionomers. Philadelphia: International Symposia in Dentistry, 1994:13.

196. Mjör IA, Fejerskov O, eds. Human Oral Embryology and Histology, ed 1. Copenhagen: Munksgaard, 1986.

197. Mjör I. Reaction patterns of dentin. In: Thylstrup A, Leach SA, Qvist V (eds). Dentine and Dentine Reactions in the Oral Cavity. Oxford, England: IRL Press, 1987:27.

198. Momoi Y, McCabe JF. Fluoride release from light-activated glass ionomer restorative cements. Dent Mater 1993;9:151.

199. Moon PC, Chang YH. Effect of DBA layer thickness on composite resin shrinkage stress [abstract 1357]. J Dent Res 1992; 71:275.

200. Morin D, DeLong R, Douglas WH. Cusp reinforcement by the acid-etch technique. J Dent Res 1984;63:1075.

201. Mount GJ. An Atlas of Glass-Ionomer Cements. London: Martin Dunitz, 1990.

202. Mount GJ. Glass-ionomer cements: past, present and future. Oper Dent 1994;19:82.

203. Munksgaard EC, Itoh K, Jorgensen KD. Dentin-polymer bond in resin fillings tested in vitro by thermo- and load-cycling. J Dent Res 1985;64:144.

204. Nakabayashi N, Kojima K, Masuhara E. The promotion of adhesion by the infiltration of monomers into tooth substrates. J Biomed Mater Res 1982;16:265.

205. Nakabayashi N. Bonding of restorative materials to dentine: the present status in Japan. Int Dent J 1985;35:145.

206. Nakabayashi N, Nakamura M, Yasuda N. Hybrid layer as a dentin-bonding mechanism. J Esthet Dent 1991;3:133.

207. Nakabayashi N. Adhesive bonding with 4-META. Oper Dent 1992;suppl 5:125.

208. Nakabayashi N, Takarada K. Effect of HEMA on bonding to dentin. Dent Mater 1992;8:125.

209. Nikaido T, Burrow MF, Tagami J, Takatsu T. Effect of pulpal pressure on adhesion of resin composite to dentin: bovine serum versus saline. Quintessence Int 1995;26:221.

210. Noda M, Komatsu H, Sano H. HPLC analysis of dental resin composites components. J Biomed Mat Res 1999;47:374.

211. Nordenvall K-J, Brännström M, Malmgren O. Etching of deciduous teeth and young and old permanent teeth. A comparison between 15 and 60 seconds of etching. Am J Orthod 1980;78:99.

212. Ogawa K, Yamashita Y, Ichijo T, Fusayama T. The ultrastructure and hardness of the transparent layer of human carious dentin. J Dent Res 1983;62:7.

213. Okamoto Y, Heeley JD, Dogon IL, Shintani H. Effects of phosphoric acid and tannic acid on dentine collagen. J Oral Rehabil 1991;18:507.

214. Olea N, Pulgar R, Perez P, et al. Estrogenicity of resin-based composites and sealants used in dentistry. Environ Health Perspect 1996;104:298.

215. Otsuki M. Histological study on pulpal response to restorative composite resins and their ingredients. J Stomatol Soc Jpn 1988;55:203.

216. Packham DE. Adhesion. In: Packham DE (ed). Handbook of Adhesion, ed 1. Essex, England: Longman, 1992:18.

217. Padday JF. Contact angle measurement. In: Packham DE, ed. Handbook of Adhesion, ed 1. Essex, England: Longman, 1992:88.

218. Pashley DH, Livingstone MJ, Greenhill JD. Regional resistances to fluid flow in human dentin in vitro. Arch Oral Biol 1978;23:807.

219. Pashley DH. The influence of dentin permeability and pulpal blood flow on pulpal solute concentrations. J Endod 1979; 5:355.

220. Pashley DH. Smear layer: physiological considerations. Oper Dent 1984;suppl 3:13.

221. Pashley DH, Andringa HJ, Derkson GD, et al. Regional variability in the permeability of human dentine. Arch Oral Biol 1987;32:519.

222. Pashley DH, Tao L, Boyd L, et al. Scanning electron microscopy of the substructure of smear layers in human dentine. Arch Oral Biol 1988;33:265.

223. Pashley DH. Dentin: a dynamic substrate—a review. Scan Microsc 1989;3:161.

224. Pashley DH. Interactions of dental materials with dentin. Trans Acad Dent Mater 1990;3:55.

225. Pashley EL, Comer RW, Parry EE, Pashley DH. Amalgam buildups: shear bond strength and dentin sealing properties. Oper Dent 1991;16:82.

226. Pashley DH, Pashley EL. Dentin permeability and restorative dentistry: a status report for the American Journal of Dentistry. Am J Dent 1991;4:5.

227. Pashley DH. Smear layer: an overview of structure and function. Proc Finn Dent Soc 1992;88:215.

228. Pashley DH, Horner JA, Brewer PD. Interactions of conditioners on the dentin surface. Oper Dent 1992;suppl 5:137.

229. Pashley DH, Ciucchi B, Sano H, Horner JA. Permeability of dentin to adhesive agents. Quintessence Int 1993;24:618.

230. Pashley DH, Carvalho RM. Dentine permeability and dentine adhesion. Review. J Dent 1997;25:355.

231. Perdigão J, Swift EJ, Cloe BC. Effects of etchants, surface moisture, and composite resin on dentin bond strengths. Am J Dent 1993;6:61.

232. Perdigão J, Swift EJ. Analysis of dentin bonding systems using the scanning electron microscope. Int Dent J 1994;44:349.

233. Perdigão J, Swift EJ, Denehy GE, et al. In vitro bond strengths and SEM evaluation of dentin bonding systems to different dentin substrates. J Dent Res 1994;73:44.

234. Perdigão J. An Ultra-Morphological Study of Human Dentine Exposed to Adhesive Systems [thesis]. Leuven, Belgium: Catholic University of Leuven, 1995.

235. Perdigão J, Lambrechts P, Van Meerbeek B, et al. A field emission SEM comparison of four post-fixation drying techniques for human dentin. J Biomed Mater Res 1995;29:1111.

236. Perdigão J, Lambrechts P, Van Meerbeek B, et al. The interaction of adhesive systems with human dentin. Am J Dent 1996;9:167.

237. Perdigão J, Lopes L, Lambrechts P, et al. Effects of self-etching primer on enamel shear bond strengths and SEM morphology. Am J Dent 1997;10:141.

238. Perdigão J, Ramos CJ, Lambrechts P. In vitro interfacial relationship between human dentin and one-bottle dental adhesives. Dent Mater 1997;13:218.

239. Perdigão J, Van Meerbeek B, Lopes MM, Ambrose WW. The effect of a re-wetting agent on dentin bonding. Dent Mater 1999;15:282.

240. Pereira PNR, Okuda M, Sano H, et al. Effect of intrinsic wetness and regional difference on dentin bond strength. Dent Mater 1999;15:46.

241. Perez P, Pulgar R, Olea-Serrano F, et al. The estrogenicity of bisphenol A–related diphenylalkanes with various substituents at the central and carbon and the hydroxy groups. Environ Health Perspect 1998;106:167.

242. Peters WJ, Jackson RW, Smith DC. Studies of the stability and toxicity of zinc polyacrylate (polycarboxylate) cements (PAZ). J Biomed Mater Res 1974;8:53.

243. Peumans M, Van Meerbeek B, Lambrechts P, Vanherle G. The five-year clinical performance of direct composite additions to correct tooth form and position. Part I: esthetic qualities. Clin Oral Invest 1997;1:12.

244. Peumans M, Van Meerbeek B, Lambrechts P, Vanherle G. The five-year clinical performance of direct composite additions to correct tooth form and position. Part II: marginal qualities. Clin Oral Invest 1997;1:19.

245. Peumans M, Van Meerbeek B, Lambrechts P, et al. The influence of direct composite additions for the correction of tooth form and/or position on periodontal health. A retrospective study. J Periodont 1998;69:422.

246. Peumans M, Van Meerbeek B, Yoshida Y, et al. Porcelain veneers bonded to tooth structure: an ultra-morphological FE-SEM examination of the adhesive interface. Dent Mater 1999;15:105.

247. Peumans M, Van Meerbeek B, Lambrechts P, Vanherle G. Factors affecting the efficacy of porcelain veneers: a literature review. J Dent 2000;28:163.

248. Peumans M, Van Meerbeek B, Lemaire V, et al. One-year clinical effectiveness of two total-etch dentin adhesive systems in cervical lesions [abstract 17 (IADR-CED)]. J Dent Res. In press.

249. Phillips RW. Skinner's Science of Dental Materials, ed 8. Philadelphia: Saunders, 1982:25.

250. Plasmans PJ, Creugers NH, Hermsen RJ, Vrijhoef MM. Intraoral humidity during operative procedures. J Dent 1994;22:89.

251. Plasmans PJJM, Reukers EAJ, Vollenbrock-Kuipers L, Vollenbrock HR. Air humidity: a detrimental factor in dentine adhesion. J Dent 1993;21:228.

252. Porte A, Lutz F, Lund MR, et al. Cavity designs for composite resins. Oper Dent 1984;9:50.

253. Powell LV, Gordon GE, Johnson GH. Clinical comparison of class 5 resin composite and glass ionomer restorations. Am J Dent 1992;5:249.

254. Powell LV, Johnson GH, Gordon GE. Factors associated with clinical success of cervical abrasion/erosion restorations. Oper Dent 1995;20:7.

255. Prati C. Reaction paper: mechanisms of dentine bonding. In: Vanherle G, Degrange M, Willems G (eds). Proceedings of the International Symposium on State of the Art on Direct Posterior Filling Materials and Dentine Bonding, ed 2. Leuven, Belgium: Van der Poorten, 1994:171.

256. Qvist V, Qvist J. Effect of ethanol and NPG-GMA on replica patterns on composite restorations performed in vivo in acid-etched cavities. Scand J Dent Res 1985;93:371.

257. Qvist V, Thylstrup A. Pulpal reactions to resin restorations. In: Anusavice KJ (ed). Quality Evaluation of Dental Restorations: Criteria for Placement and Replacement. Chicago: Quintessence, 1989:291.

258. Reeder OW, Walton RE, Livingston MJ, Pashley DH. Dentin permeability: determinants of hydraulic conductance. J Dent Res 1978;57:187.

259. Retief DH, Austin JC, Fatti LP. Pulpal response to phosphoric acid. J Oral Pathol 1974;3:114.

260. Retief DH. Dentin bonding agents: a deterrent to microleakage? In: Anusavice KJ (ed). Quality Evaluation of Dental Restorations: Criteria for Placement and Replacement. Chicago: Quintessence, 1989:185.

261. Roeder LB, Deschepper EJ, Powers JM. In vitro bond strength of repaired amalgam with adhesive bonding systems. J Esthet Dent 1991;3:126.

262. Roulet J-F, Herder S. Bonded Ceramic Inlays. Chicago: Quintessence, 1991.

263. Rueggeberg FA, Margeson DH. The effect of oxygen inhibition on an unfilled/filled composite system. J Dent Res 1990;69:1652.

264. Rueggeberg FA. Substrate for adhesion testing to tooth structure—review of literature: a report of the ASC MD156 Task Group on test methods for the adhesion of restorative materials. Dent Mater 1991;7:2.

265. Ruyter IE. The chemistry of adhesive agents. Oper Dent 1992;suppl 5:32.

266. Sakaguchi RL, Berge HX. Effect of light intensity on polymerization contraction of posterior composite [abstract 481]. J Dent Res 1997;76:74.

267. Sano H, Shono T, Sonoda H, et al. Relationship between surface area for adhesion and tensile bond strength—evaluation of a micro-tensile bond test. Dent Mater 1994;10:236.

268. Sano H, Shono T, Takatsu T, Hosoda H. Microporous dentin zone beneath resin-impregnated layer. Oper Dent 1994;19:59.

233

269. Sano H, Takatsu T, Ciucchi B, et al. Nanoleakage: leakage within the hybrid layer. Oper Dent 1995;20:18.

270. Sano H, Yoshikawa T, Pereira PN, et al. Long-term durability of dentin bonds made with a self-etching primer. J Dent Res 1999;78:906.

271. Schuurs AHB, van Amerongen JP. Algemene gezondheidsschade door composietrestauraties. Ned Tijdschr Tandheelk 1996;103:444.

272. Scott PG, Leaver AG. The degradation of human collagen by trypsin. Connect Tissue Res 1974;2:299.

273. Shaffer SE, Barkmeier WW, Kelsey WP. Effects of reduced acid conditioning time on enamel microleakage. Gen Dent 1987;35:278.

274. Shimokobe H, Honda T, Kobayashi Y, et al. Denaturation of dentin collagen by phosphoric acid treatment [abstract 908]. J Dent Res 1988;67:226.

275. Sidhu SK, Watson TF. Resin-modified glass ionomer materials. A status report for the American Journal of Dentistry. Am J Dent 1995;8:59.

276. Silverstone LM. Fissure sealants: laboratory studies. Caries Res 1974;8:2.

277. Silverstone LM, Saxton CA, Dogon IL, Fejerskov O. Variation in pattern of etching of human dental enamel examined by scanning electron microscopy. Caries Res 1975;9:373.

278. Smith DC. Polyacrylic acid–based cements: adhesion to enamel and dentin. Oper Dent 1992;suppl 5:177.

279. Söderholm K-JM. Correlation of in vivo and in vitro performance of adhesive restorative materials: a report of the ASC MD156 Task Group on test methods for the adhesion of restorative materials. Dent Mater 1991;7:74.

280. Söderholm KJ, Mariotti A. Bis-GMA-based resins in dentistry: are they safe? J Am Dent Assoc 1999;130:201.

281. Spencer P, Byerley TJ, Eick JD, Witt JD. Chemical characterization of the dentin/adhesive interface by Fourier transform infrared photoacoustic spectroscopy. Dent Mater 1992;8:10.

282. Spencer P, Wieliczka DM, Meeske J, et al. The resin-dentin interface—morphological and chemical characterization [abstract 44]. J Dent Res 1994;73:107.

283. Stanford JW. Bonding of restorative materials to dentine. Int Dent J 1985;35:133.

284. Stanford JW, Sabri Z, Jose S. A comparison of the effectiveness of dentine bonding agents. Int Dent J 1985;35:139.

285. Stangel I, Ostro E, Domingue A, et al. Photoacoustic Fourier transform IR spectroscopy study of polymer-dentin interaction. In: Pireaux JJ, Bertrand P, Bredas JL (eds). Polymer-Solid Interfaces. Philadelphia: Institute of Physics Publishing, 1991:157.

286. Stanley HR, Going RE, Chauncey HH. Human pulp response to acid pretreatment of dentin and to composite restoration. J Am Dent Assoc 1975;91:817.

287. Stanley HR, Bowen RL, Folio J. Compatibility of various materials with oral tissues. II. Pulp responses to composite ingredients. J Dent Res 1979;58:1507.

288. Stanley HR, Pereira JC, Spiegel E, et al. The detection and prevalence of reactive and physiologic sclerotic dentin, reparative dentin and dead tracts beneath various types of dental lesions according to tooth surface and age. J Oral Pathol 1983;12:257.

289. Stansbury JW. Synthesis and evaluation of new oxaspiro monomers for double ring-opening polymerization. J Dent Res 1992;71:1408.

290. Sterrett JD, Murphy HJ. Citric acid burnishing of dentinal root surfaces. A scanning electron microscopy report. J Clin Periodontol 1989;16:98.

291. Strassler HE. Insights and innovations. J Esthet Dent 1991;3:114.

292. Sugizaki J. The effect of the various primers on the dentin adhesion of resin composites—SEM and TEM observations of the resin-impregnated layer and adhesion promoting effect of the primers. Jpn J Conserv Dent 1991;34:228.

293. Suh BI. All-Bond—fourth generation dentin bonding system. J Esthet Dent 1991;3:139.

294. Summitt JB, Chan DCN, Burgess JO, Dutton FB. Effect of air/water rinse versus water only and of five rinse times on resin-to-etched enamel shear bond strength. Oper Dent 1992;17:142.

295. Summitt JB, Chan DCN, Dutton FB, Burgess JO. Effect of rinse time on microleakage between composite and etched enamel. Oper Dent 1993;18:37.

296. Suzuki T, Finger WJ. Dentin adhesives: site of dentin vs bonding of composite resins. Dent Mater 1988;4:379.

297. Swift EJ, Triolo PT. Bond strengths of Scotchbond Multi-Purpose to moist dentin and enamel. Am J Dent 1992;5:318.

298. Swift EJ, Cloe BC. Shear bond strengths of new enamel etchants. Am J Dent 1993;6:162.

299. Swift EJ, Hammel SA, Perdigão J, Wefel JS. Prevention of root surface caries using a dental adhesive. J Am Dent Assoc 1994;125:571.

300. Swift EJ, Perdigão J, Heymann HO. Bonding to enamel and dentin: a brief history and state of the art, 1995. Quintessence Int 1995;26:95.

301. Swift EJ Jr, Triolo PT Jr, Barkmeier WW, et al. Effect of low-viscosity resins on the performance of dental adhesives. Am J Dent 1996;9:100.

302. Tagami J, Hosoda H, Fusayama T. Optimal technique of etching enamel. Oper Dent 1988;13:181.

303. Tagami J, Tao L, Pashley DH. Correlation among dentin depth, permeability, and bond strength of adhesive resin. Dent Mater 1990;6:45.

304. Tagami J, Hosoda H, Burrow MF, Nakajima M. Effect of aging and caries on dentin permeability. Proc Finn Dent Soc 1992;88(suppl 1):149.

305. Tam LE, Pilliar RM. Fracture surface characterization of dentin-bonded interfacial fracture toughness specimens. J Dent Res 1994;73:607.

306. Tao L, Pashley DH. Shear bond strengths to dentin: effects of surface treatments, depth and position. Dent Mater 1988;4:371.

307. Tao L, Tagami J, Pashley DH. Pulpal pressures and bond strengths of Superbond and Gluma. Am J Dent 1991;4:73.

308. Tay FR, Gwinnett AJ, Pang KM, Wei SHY. Structural evidence of a sealed tissue interface with a total-etch wet-bonding technique in vivo. J Dent Res 1994;73:629.

309. Tay FR, Gwinnett AJ, Pang KM, Wei SH. Resin permeation into acid-conditioned, moist, and dry dentin: a paradigm using water-free adhesive primers. J Dent Res 1996;75:1034.

310. Tay FR, Gwinnett AJ, Wei SHY. Micromorphological spectrum from overdrying to overwetting acid-conditioned dentin in water-free acetone-based, single-bottle primer/adhesives. Dent Mater 1996;12:236.

311. Ten Cate JM, Jongebloed WL, Simons YM. Adaptation of dentin to the oral environment. In: Thylstrup A, Leach SA, Qvist V (eds). Dentine and Dentine Reactions in the Oral Cavity. Oxford, England: IRL Press; 1987:67.

312. Terkla LG, Brown AC, Hainisch AP, Mitchem JC. Testing sealing properties of restorative materials against moist dentin. J Dent Res 1987;66:1758.

313. Titley K, Chernecky R, Maric B, Smith D. Penetration of a dentin bonding agent into dentin. Am J Dent 1994;7:190.

314. Torney D. The retentive ability of acid-etched dentin. J Prosthet Dent 1978;39:169.

315. Torstenson BC, Nordenvall KJ, Brännström M. Pulpal reaction and microorganisms under Clearfil composite resin in deep cavities with acid etched dentin. Swed Dent J 1982; 6:167.

316. Torstenson BC, Odén A. Effects of bonding agent types and incremental techniques on minimizing contraction gaps around resin composites. Dent Mater 1989;5:218.

317. Trevino DF, Duke ES, Robbins JW, Summitt JB. Clinical evaluation of Scotchbond Multi-Purpose Adhesive System [abstract 3037]. J Dent Res 1996;75:397.

318. Triolo PT, Swift EJ. Shear bond strengths of ten dentin adhesive systems. Dent Mater 1992;8:370.

319. Triolo PT, Swift EJ, Mudgil A, Levine A. Effect of etching time on enamel bond strengths. Am J Dent 1993;6:302.

320. Tsai YH, Swartz ML, Phillips RW, Moore BK. A comparative study: bond strength and microleakage of dentin bond systems. Oper Dent 1990;15:53.

321. Tyas MJ, Burns GA, Byrne PF, et al. Clinical evaluation of Scotchbond: three-year results. Aust Dent J 1989;34:277.

322. Tyas MJ. Three-year clinical evaluation of dentine bonding agents. Aust Dent J 1991;36:298.

323. Uno S, Asmussen E. Marginal adaptation of a restorative resin polymerised at reduced rate. Scand J Dent Res 1991;99:440.

324. Van Hassel HJ. Physiology of the human dental pulp. Oral Surg Oral Med Oral Pathol 1971;32:126.

325. Vanherle G, Lambrechts P, Braem M. An evaluation of different adhesive restorations in cervical lesions. J Prosthet Dent 1991;65:341.

326. Van Meerbeek B, Inokoshi S, Braem M, et al. Morphological aspects of the resin-dentin interdiffusion zone with different dentin adhesive systems. J Dent Res 1992;71:1530.

327. Van Meerbeek B, Vanherle G, Lambrechts P, Braem M. Dentin- and enamel-bonding agents. Curr Opin Dent 1992; 2:117.

328. Van Meerbeek B, Dhem A, Goret-Nicaise M, et al. Comparative SEM and TEM examination of the ultrastructure of the resin-dentin interdiffusion zone. J Dent Res 1993;72:495.

329. Van Meerbeek B, Mohrbacher H, Celis JP, et al. Chemical characterization of the resin-dentin interface by micro-Raman spectroscopy. J Dent Res 1993;72:1423.

330. Van Meerbeek B, Willems G, Celis JP, et al. Assessment by nano-indentation of the hardness and elasticity of the resin-dentin bonding area. J Dent Res 1993;72:1434.

331. Van Meerbeek B, Braem M, Lambrechts P, Vanherle G. Morphological characterization of the interface between resin and sclerotic dentine. J Dent Res 1994;73:141.

332. Van Meerbeek B, Peumans M, Verschueren M, et al. Clinical status of ten dentin adhesive systems. J Dent Res 1994;73: 1690.

333. Van Meerbeek B, Conn LJ Jr, Duke ES, et al. Correlative transmission electron microscopy examination of nondemineralized and demineralized resin-dentin interfaces formed by two dentin adhesive systems. J Dent Res 1996;75:879.

334. Van Meerbeek B, Perdigão J, Inokoshi S, et al. Pulpareacties en pulpabescherming: traditionele onderlagen versus dentine hechtlakken. Ned Tijdschr Tandh 1996;103:439.

335. Van Meerbeek B, Perdigão J, Lambrechts P, Vanherle G. The clinical performance of adhesives. J Dent 1998;26:1.

336. Van Meerbeek B, Peumans M, Gladys S, et al. Three-year clinical effectiveness of four total-etch dentinal adhesive systems in cervical lesions. Quintessence Int 1996;27:775.

337. Van Meerbeek B, Yoshida Y, Lambrechts P, et al. A TEM study of two water-based adhesive systems bonded to dry and wet dentin. J Dent Res 1998;77:50.

338. Van Meerbeek B, Yoshida Y, Lambrechts P, Vanherle G. Mechanisms of bonding of a resin-modified glass-ionomer adhesive with dentin [abstract 2236]. J Dent Res 1998;77:911.

339. Versluis A, Douglas WH, Cross M, Sakaguchi RL. Does an incremental filling technique reduce polymerization shrinkage stresses? J Dent Res 1996;75:871.

340. Versluis A, Tantbirojn D, Douglas WH. Do dental composites always shrink toward the light? J Dent Res 1998;77:1435.

341. Wakabayashi Y, Kondou Y, Suzuki K, et al. Effect of dissolution of collagen on adhesion to dentin. Int J Prosthod 1994; 7:302.

342. Watanabe I, Nakabayashi N, Pashley DH. Bonding to ground dentin by a phenyl-P self-etching primer. J Dent Res 1994;73: 1212.

343. Willems G. Multistandard Criteria for the Selection of Potential Posterior Composites [thesis]. Leuven, Belgium: Catholic University of Leuven, 1985.

344. Wilson AD, Kent BE. The glass-ionomer cement, a new translucent cement for dentistry. J Appl Chem Biotechnol 1971;21:313.

345. Wilson AD, Kent BE. A new translucent cement for dentistry. The glass ionomer cement. Br Dent J 1972;132:133.

346. Wilson AD, Prosser HJ, Powis DM. Mechanism of adhesion of polyelectrolyte cement to hydroxyapatite. J Dent Res 1983; 62:590.

347. Wilson AD, McLean JW. Glass Ionomer Cement. Chicago: Quintessence, 1988.

348. Wilson AD, Nicholson JW. Acid-Base Cements. Their Biomedical and Industrial Applications. Cambridge, England: Cambridge University Press, 1993.

349. Wolinsky LE, Armstrong RW, Seghi RR. The determination of ionic bonding interactions of N-phenyl glycine and N-(2-hydroxy-3-methacryloxypropyl)-N-phenyl glycine as measured by carbon-13 NMR analysis. J Dent Res 1993;72:72.

350. Xu J, Butler IS, Gilson DFR, Stangel I. The HEMA interface with dentin and collagen by FT-Raman spectroscopy [abstract 615]. J Dent Res 1995;74:88.

351. Yamada T, Nakamura K, Iwaku M, Fusayama T. The extent of the odontoblast process in normal and carious human dentin. J Dent Res 1983;62:798.

352. Yoshida Y, Van Meerbeek B, Nakayama Y, et al. Evidence of chemical bonding at biomaterial-hard tissue interfaces. J Dent Res 2000;79:709.

353. Yoshiyama M, Masada J, Uchida A. Scanning electron microscope characterization of sensitive vs. insensitive human radicular dentin. J Dent Res 1989;68:1398.

354. Yoshiyama M, Noiri Y, Ozaki K, et al. Transmission electron microscopic characterization of hypersensitive human radicular dentin. J Dent Res 1990;69:1293.

355. Yu XY, Joynt RB, Wieczkowski G, Davis EL. Scanning electron microscopic and energy dispersive x-ray evaluation of two smear layer–mediated dentinal bonding agents. Quintessence Int 1991;22:305.

356. Zidan O, Hill G. Phosphoric acid concentration: enamel surface loss and bonding strength. J Prosthet Dent 1986;55:388.

357. Ziemiecki TL, Dennison JB, Charbeneau GT. Clinical evaluation of cervical composite resin restorations placed without retention. Oper Dent 1987;2:27.

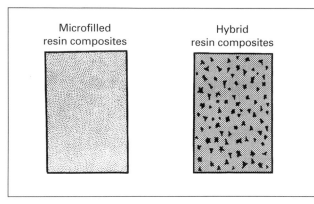

Fig 9-1 Most commonly used classes of resin composite. The microfilled resins contain only submicron particles, while the hybrids contain a combination of submicron particles and particles up to 4 µm in diameter.

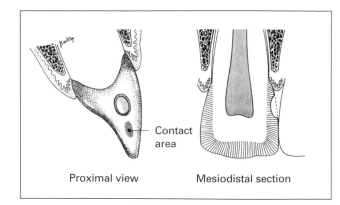

Fig 9-2 Saucer-shaped preparation in enamel. The carious lesion is usually located slightly gingival to the contact area. Every attempt should be made to maintain natural tooth contact between the adjacent teeth during restoration. If no cavitation is present, remineralization is preferable to restoration.

Glass-Ionomer Restorative Materials

Glass-ionomer restorative materials are not commonly used when esthetics is a major consideration in anterior restorations. They are often recommended for patients with high rates of caries.[47] The traditional chemically cured glass-ionomer material is not esthetic, but this quality has been greatly improved in the resin-modified glass-ionomer materials. Recent clinical trials of 5 years' duration have reported high retention rates in Class 5 restorations.[9,10,76] Though not as color stable as resin composites, these materials are suitable for use in visible anterior areas when dentin margins are prevalent or the patient has been identified as being at high risk for new caries lesions. Glass-ionomer restorative materials are discussed in more depth in Chapter 13.

Class 3 Restorations

Class 3 caries is smooth-surface caries found on the proximal surfaces of anterior teeth, usually slightly gingival to the proximal contact, but does not involve the incisal angle of the tooth. It can usually be detected with an explorer, radiographically, or with transillumination. Clinical changes in translucency may be evident and may be enhanced if a light source is placed against the proximal area (transillumination). Carious areas appear more opaque than does sound enamel.

The penetration through the enamel and the pattern of spread is typical of smooth-surface lesions. Incipient lesions tend to be V-shaped and confined to enamel; deeper lesions tend to spread along the dentinoenamel junction and penetrate dentin.

Incipient Enamel Caries

The proximal lesion that is located within enamel and is not cavitated may not need a restoration. Although there is no doubt that the lesion is pathologic, research and clinical experience have shown that this lesion is often dormant. Charting it as a lesion that could potentially reactivate and necessitate restorative treatment is a valid and acceptable procedure.[30,63] With proper home care, there is evidence that enamel caries lesions can be remineralized.[81] Chapter 4 contains a more complete discussion of caries and remineralization processes.

Cavitated Enamel Caries

When the enamel surface is cavitated, it is past the point of remineralization. If the cavitation is very shallow and deeper enamel has been remineralized, a restoration may not be necessary unless the lesion is esthetically displeasing. If the lesion is confined to enamel, a cavity preparation may be made with a round tungsten carbide bur or diamond used in a

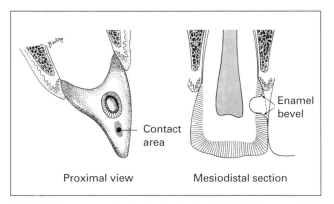

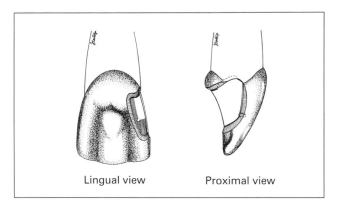

Fig 9-3 This preparation is similar to that in Fig 9-2, except that the axial wall is extended into dentin and the external enamel margins are beveled.

Fig 9-4 Mechanical retention is not necessary, but can be added if desired. A retentive groove may be placed with a No. ¼ round bur on the gingival floor, and a retentive point may also be placed at the same depth at the facioincisoaxial point angle. Reinforcement of remaining dental structure, eg, thinned incisal edge, may be obtained from internal etching and bonding to the resin composite.

high-speed handpiece. The finished preparation resembles a saucer and has no retentive undercuts (Fig 9-2). Adhesion to acid-etched enamel provides the necessary retention. Both laboratory and 3-year clinical data have demonstrated the durability of these saucer-shaped restorations.[54,77]

Dentinal Caries with Peripheral Enamel Margins

The preparation necessitated by dentinal caries lesions is similar to that for enamel caries except that the axial wall extends into dentin, and carious dentin, and in many areas, overlying fragile enamel, is removed (Fig 9-3). Bevels have been advocated by some authors,[38,71] but enamel bonds have been demonstrated clinically to be adequate without bevels.[74,94] An in vitro study using a silver nitrate tracer revealed no significant difference in marginal microleakage between beveled and nonbeveled Class 3 restorations.[49] Margins should receive short bevels or chamfers when the gradual blending of enamel and restorative shades would benefit esthetics or when maximum retention is desired (Fig 9-4). If the cervical enamel will be eliminated or compromised by a bevel with a resultant margin in or near dentin, the beveling procedure

should be avoided in the cervical area. If the peripheral margin is entirely composed of enamel, no undercuts, retentive points, or grooves are necessary, as the restoration will be retained by adhesion.[85]

Dentinal Caries with Margin Extending Onto the Root Surface

In areas where there is little or no enamel for bonding, the marginal adaptation of the restoration may be optimized in two distinct ways. An open sandwich technique, using a resin-modified glass-ionomer restorative material, may be used to seal the cervical portion of the restoration. The remaining cavity is then filled with resin composite for improved esthetics.[87] If a dentin bonding agent is the sole form of adhesion at the cervical margin, placement of a retentive groove may help to minimize gap formation in this area. The groove may be placed to the depth of a No. ⅛ or ¼ round bur (0.4 and 0.5 mm, respectively), 0.5 to 1.0 mm inside the cementoenamel junction (Fig 9-5).[17] A more complete discussion of gap formation is found in Chapters 8 and 10. As dentin bonding agents continue to improve, mechanical undercut retention may become unnecessary.

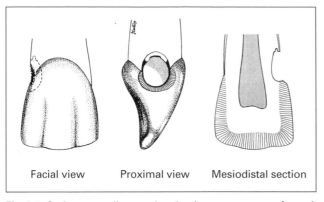

Facial view   Proximal view   Mesiodistal section

Fig 9-5 Caries extending to the dentin-cementum surface. A retentive groove is placed 0.5 to 0.7 mm from the external surface of the root.

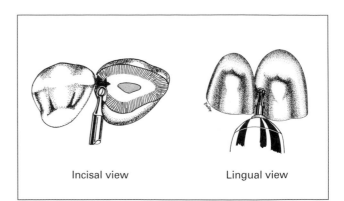

Incisal view   Lingual view

Fig 9-6 Initial penetration should be made through the marginal ridge, away from the adjacent tooth surface. Note the angulation of the long axis of the bur in relation to the location of the lesion.

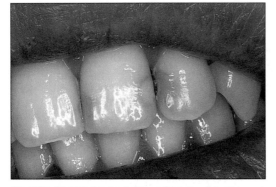

Fig 9-7a Moderate-sized Class 3 carious lesions on the mesial and distal surfaces of the maxillary left central incisor and mesial surface of the lateral incisor.

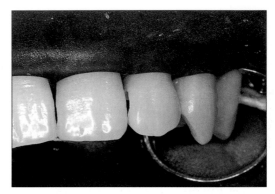

Fig 9-7b After cavity preparation, the labial margins are only slightly visible, and the labial enamel is unsupported by dentin.

Preparation Approach and Instrumentation

Resin Composite Restorations

Outline form for resin composite restorations is determined solely by access and by the extent of the caries lesion(s). There is no need for extension for prevention, and the removal of sound tooth structure to gain mechanical undercut retention is contraindicated. The lingual approach is preferred for Class 3 restorations, but it is not always possible, depending on the location of the caries lesion. The number of burs used for cavity preparation should be kept to a minimum. A No. 2 round bur or a No. 329 pear-shaped carbide bur in a high-speed handpiece can be used for initial access to the lesion. Initial penetration should be made through the marginal ridge, away from the adjacent tooth surface (Fig 9-6). The outline form of the preparation is then extended to provide access to the dentinal caries lesion. A larger round bur may be used in

the low-speed handpiece to excavate demineralized dentin.

The need for enamel bevels has not been clearly demonstrated, but narrow bevels (0.5 to 1.0 mm) may be placed on accessible enamel margins to remove fragile enamel, to make margins smooth, and to enhance esthetics if the margin is in a visible location. For placing bevels, a flame-shaped finishing bur, a gingival margin trimmer, or another hand instrument may be used.

Enamel is more natural and esthetic than the best restorative materials. To preserve facial esthetics, the preparation should not be extended onto the facial surface unless necessitated by the lesion (Figs 9-7a and 9-7b). Unsupported facial enamel may be left for internal etching and bonding to resin composite[33] (Figs 9-8a to 9-8f). The facial approach is indicated only when the caries lesion already involves the facial surface or when the adjacent tooth overlaps the tooth

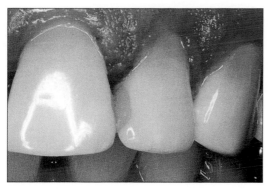

Fig 9-8a A discolored anterior resin composite restoration to be replaced to improve esthetics.

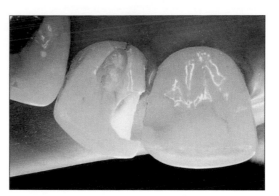

Fig 9-8b Lingual view after existing resin composite was removed, revealing unsupported facial enamel.

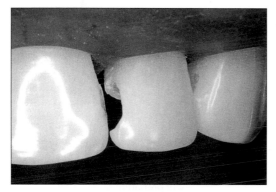

Fig 9-8c Completed preparation with no attempt to remove labial unsupported enamel.

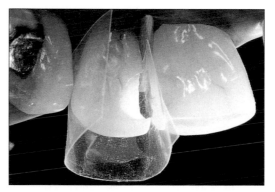

Fig 9-8d Clear matrix and interproximal wedge in place.

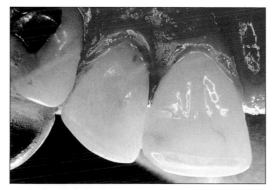

Fig 9-8e Lingual view of the finished and polished resin composite restoration.

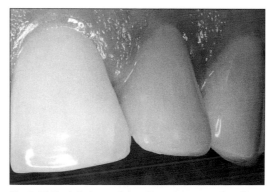

Fig 9-8f Facial view of the Class 3 restoration illustrates the improved esthetic outcome.

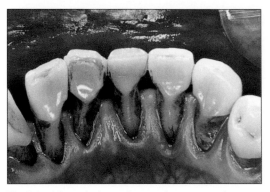

Fig 9-9a Lingual view of extensive root surface exposure and root caries; teeth to be restored with resin-modified glass-ionomer material.

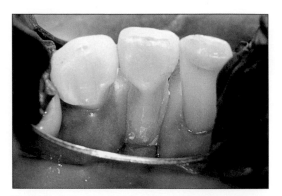

Fig 9-9b Completed caries excavation; the adhesive nature of the restorative material does not demand preparation of mechanical resistance and retention features. (Figs 9-9a and 9-9b courtesy of Dr Robert H. Poindexter.)

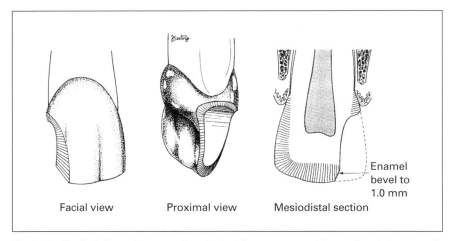

Facial view   Proximal view   Mesiodistal section

Enamel bevel to 1.0 mm

Fig 9-10a Typical Class 4 preparation. Incisal fracture caused by undermining associated with a Class 3 lesion may necessitate a Class 4 cavity preparation, which is similar to a Class 3 preparation but includes a portion of the incisal edge.

being restored, preventing a lingual approach. The outline should be as conservative as possible, preserving the facial enamel.

Glass-Ionomer Cement Restorations

Because of their anticaries potential, glass-ionomer restorative materials may be used in Class 3 restorations for patients with a high risk of caries.[47] Preparations for these materials should resemble those for resin composite; no bevels are necessary. Only the tooth structure required to allow access for excavation of the carious dentin should be removed (Figs 9-9a and 9-9b). Because these materials bond to enamel and dentin, the placement of retention grooves or points is not necessary.[88]

Class 4 Restorations

Class 4 restorations are usually necessitated by the fracture of an incisal angle, a situation plainly visible on clinical examination. If caries is present, radiographs may be helpful to determine the extent of the carious lesion and its proximity to the pulp chamber.

Etiology and Treatment Rationale

A caries-induced Class 4 restoration is usually the result of a large Class 3 carious lesion that has undermined the incisal edge. The need for Class 4 restorations due to traumatic fracture occurs most often among children or young adults. The frequency of fractures of perma-

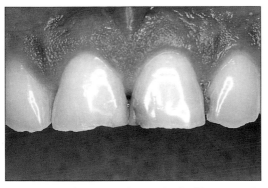

Fig 9-10b Defective and unesthetic Class 4 resin composite restoration.

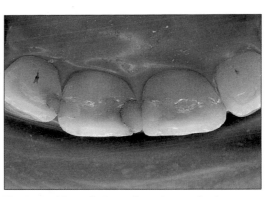

Fig 9-10c Lingual view of moderate-sized restoration requiring replacement due to caries and unacceptable esthetics.

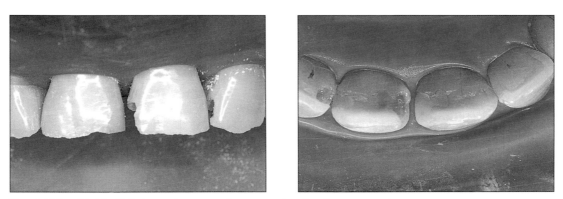

Figs 9-10d and 9-10e Existing resin composite removed and caries excavated.

nent incisors in children is reported to range from 5%[32] to 20%.[46] Traumatic fractures are likely to be more horizontal than vertical.

For Class 4 carious lesions, the cavity design follows the conventional form of the Class 3 preparation and includes a portion of the incisal edge. Carious tooth structure and weak incisal enamel are removed, and all enamel margins are beveled, with wider bevels placed in the incisal portion of the tooth where the enamel is thicker and the stresses on the restoration are likely to be greater (Figs 9-10a to 9-10f). A modified Class 4 preparation with extensive loss of incisal enamel is shown in Fig 9-11.

For fractures, if there is no carious or pulpal involvement, a bevel is often the only preparation necessary[6] (Fig 9-12). An enamel bevel of at least 1.0 mm should be placed around the periphery of the cavity where enamel thickness allows. Increasing the width of the bevel beyond 1.0 mm has been shown to provide no additional strength,[4] but a wider bevel can achieve a more harmonious esthetic blend between

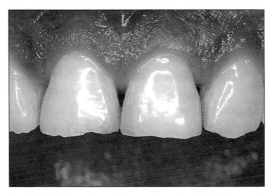

Fig 9-10f Completed Class 4 restoration after adjustments for occlusion and finishing/polishing.

Figs 9-15a and 9-15b Direct composite veneering technique with the body shade deposited in bulk and distributed by plastic instrument. A brush slightly wetted with liquid resin adhesive may also be used for contouring.

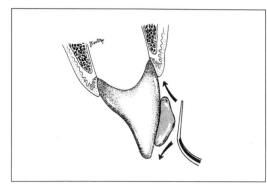

Fig 9-15a Lateral view.

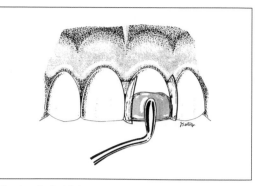

Fig 9-15b Labial view showing the use of clear plastic matrix strips in both interproximal areas.

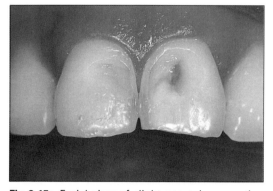

Fig 9-15c Facial view of slight enamel preparation and extent of margins for direct resin composite veneers on maxillary central incisors.

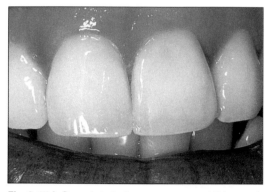

Fig 9-15d Completed direct veneers exhibit excellent esthetics and mask intrinsic stains. (Figs 9-15c and 9-15d courtesy of Dr Nasser Barghi.)

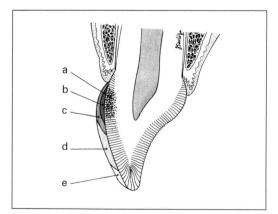

Fig 9-16 Facial veneering and masking of heavy stain/fluorosis using a combination of opaque, cervical, body, and translucent shades. a = stain/fluorosis; b = opaque shade; c = cervical shade; d = body shade; e = translucent shade.

characterization of the incisal edge may be added in the incisal third of the veneer. The resin composite is built to slightly oversized proportions and is finished and polished to the proper contours (Fig 9-16).

Diastema Closure

The technique for diastemata closure is similar to that for placement of direct veneers, and the two techniques may be used in combination. In most cases, no tooth structure has to be removed, and the resin composite is retained solely by a resin adhesive (Figs 9-17a to 9-17c). For a small- to moderate-sized diastema, resin composite added to the proximal surfaces of the two adjacent teeth will usually suffice (Figs 9-18a to 9-18c). If the diastema exceeds 2.5 mm,

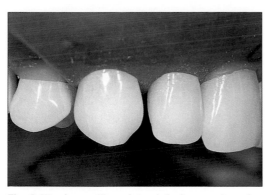

Fig 9-17a A maxillary lateral incisor and canine with an existing diastema to be closed with resin composite.

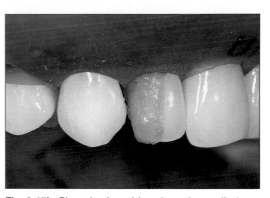

Fig 9-17b Phosphoric acid etchant is applied; no preparation of natural tooth structure is required for adhesion.

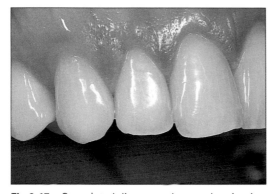

Fig 9-17c Completed diastema closure showing improved esthetics and imperceptible blend of resin composite and natural enamel. Note the translucency of the incisal edge.

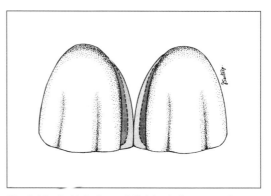

Fig 9-18a Labial view of finished diastema closure showing the use of body and translucent shades to simulate natural tooth color and translucency.

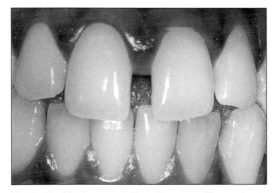

Fig 9-18b Moderate midline diastema. The patient's desire for esthetic improvement may be met with resin composite.

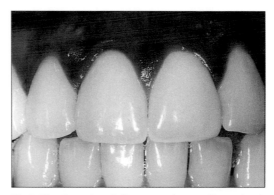

Fig 9-18c Completed diastema closure. Note physiologic contouring of the cervical aspect of the restorations and the homogenous luster of the composite material and natural tooth surface. (Figs 9-18b and 9-18c courtesy of Dr Robert H. Poindexter.)

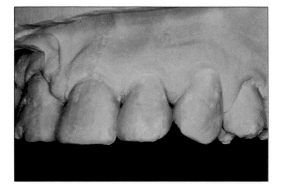

Fig 9-19 Diagnostic waxup of proposed recontouring and closure of diastemata. This treatment planning procedure may assist in identifying tooth-size discrepancies, areas requiring esthetic recontouring, and gingival height and contour considerations. The cast may also be used for patient education and communication of treatment goals, as well as for a chairside guide for direct restorations.

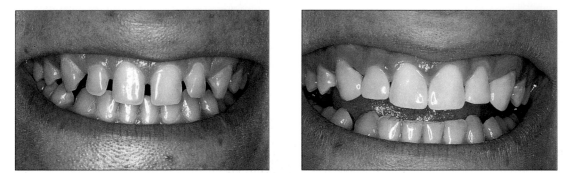

Figs 9-20a and 9-20b Diastema closures frequently require bonding of resin composite to two to six teeth to achieve proper esthetic relationships. Multiple veneers were needed in this case.

Clinical Steps for a Direct Resin Composite Veneer

1. Select resin shades prior to initiation of dehydration.
2. Place a rubber dam and No. 212 (retractor) clamp if desired. If a rubber dam is not used, place gingival retraction cord to control sulcular fluid and retract the gingival tissue.
3. In most cases, the composite material is bonded directly to the tooth surface. If it is necessary to remove tooth structure to establish proper tooth alignment or to create space to mask dark tooth structure, a blunt-ended diamond is recommended. Remove as little tooth structure as necessary to achieve the desired objective.
4. Etch the tooth surface with an appropriate etchant, such as 37% phosphoric acid. Protect the adjacent teeth with clear plastic strips.
5. Rinse the tooth thoroughly and dry the etched tooth surface with a stream of air.
6. Place a clear-plastic strip or other matrix and wedge interproximally.
7. Apply opaque resin, if indicated, and light cure.
8. Add the selected composite and adapt and contour the material. Light cure for at least 40 seconds.
9. Add additional composite as necessary to achieve the proper shape, color, and translucency. Light cure each increment for at least 40 seconds.
10. Contour the gingival margins and remove flash with a No. 12 or 12b scalpel blade.
11. Contour and finish the composite material with a carbide or diamond finishing bur.
12. Repeat the above process on adjacent teeth if indicated.
13. Remove the rubber dam, if used.
14. Check the occlusion and adjust as necessary with finishing burs.
15. Finish and polish with disks, polishing points, etc.
16. Apply low-viscosity rebonding resin (surface sealer) to restoration surface and margins.

it may be necessary to use a combination of direct veneering and orthodontic movement to position the teeth into a more easily managed and esthetically pleasing location.

When diastema closure is performed, occlusal relationships and esthetic proportion, as well as the overall facial esthetics, must be considered. When anterior teeth are widened, it may also be necessary to lengthen them to preserve natural anatomic proportions. If occlusal relationships and facial appearance will allow it, the proper tooth length can be established by adding to the incisal edge. It is also possible to improve the length-to-width ratio by surgical crown lengthening in some patients. The desired lengths and widths of teeth should be determined using a diagnostic waxup before the treatment is begun (Fig 9-19). A trial application, assessing esthetic alteration of the shape and color of the proposed veneer, may be accomplished with resin composite applied to unetched teeth.[60,93]

Maintenance of the proper length and width relationships in anterior teeth is very important to achieving an esthetic result for resin composite veneers, porcelain veneers, and diastema closures. A study evaluating the length and width of anterior teeth revealed that, on average, central incisors and canines are approximately equal in length and are 20% longer than lateral incisors.[42] The proper dimensions, length-to-width ratios, and width-to-width ratios are shown in Tables 9-1 and 9-2.

A periodontal probe or caliper may be used as a measuring device to evenly divide the space to be closed. Diastema closures frequently require augmenting two to six teeth with resin composite to achieve optimal esthetic relationships (Figs 9-20a and 9-20b).

Matching the appearance of the natural tooth structure when adding resin composite to proximal surfaces can be difficult because of the disparity in the optical properties of the resin composite material and the tooth structure. Even when diastema closure is combined with direct facial veneering, the proximal additions tend to be more translucent. To avoid this "shine-through" effect, a relatively opaque dentin shade or a heavily filled hybrid resin composite may be used to build the lingual portion of the resin composite that is added to the proximal surface. The facial and incisal contours can then be established with an enamel shade or microfilled resin composite to reproduce the surface gloss and translucence of natural tooth structure.

Table 9-1	Dimensional averages (in mm) for maxillary incisors and canines*			
	Males		Females	
Tooth	Length	Width	Length	Width
Central incisor	10.7	9.4	9.6	9.1
Lateral incisor	9.1	7.5	8.2	7.1
Canine	10.7	8.5	9.2	8.0

*From Gillen et al.[42]

Table 9-2	Length/width and width/width ratios for maxillary incisors and canines*			
Males				
	Length/Width	Width/Width Central	Width/Width Lateral	Width/Width Canine
Central incisor	1.15:1	—	1.25:1	1.1:1
Lateral incisor	1.2:1		—	
Canine	1.25:1	—	1.15:1	—
Females				
	Length/Width	Width/Width Central	Width/Width Lateral	Width/Width Canine
Central incisor	1.05:1	—	1.3:1	1.15:1
Lateral incisor	1.15:1		—	
Canine	1.15:1		1.15:1	—

The length-to-width ratios are for the teeth in the first column.

The width-to-width ratios are between different teeth. Only the larger-to-smaller ratios are listed. For example, the central incisor–to–lateral incisor width ratio is listed, but not the lateral incisor–to–central incisor ratio.

*From Gillen et al.[42]

Diastema closure can usually be accomplished without the use of a matrix to separate the two restorations, thus avoiding the need for a wedge and allowing better control of contours in the gingival aspects. The resin composite on one proximal surface should be built slightly over the desired contours, then finished back to desired contours and polished. Then, without a separating matrix, resin composite is added to the adjacent proximal tooth surface to establish desired contours and contact area, then polished. There should be definite contact between the two restorations, but floss should slide through with appropriate resistance.

Shade or Color Selection

Selection of the shade or color of resin composite restorative material is an important and sometimes demanding step in completing an anterior restoration.

Factors Influencing Shade Selection

Proper Lighting

One of the first requirements for a good color match is proper lighting. Commonly used fluorescent tubes emit light with a green tint that can distort color perception. Color-corrected fluorescent tubes that approximate natural daylight are available and are recommended for dental treatment rooms. The objective is to obtain shadow-free, color-balanced illumination without distracting glare or false colors (see box).[21,98]

Color-Corrected Lighting[90]

Overhead lights (fluorescent tubes)

Color Rendering Index (CRI): 90 or higher
Spectral energy distribution (SED): natural daylight
Color temperature: 5,500°K
Illumination intensity: approximately 150 to 200 foot-candles at 30 inches above floor

Dental operating light

Illumination intensity: 1,000 to 2,000 foot-candles
Color temperature: optimum 5,000°K, should be adjustable from 4,500°K to 5,500°K to assist in color matching

---

If such lighting is not available, color selection can be made near a window. However, even daylight varies considerably from day to day and throughout the day. It is wise to use multiple light sources to choose the best shade and to avoid problems with metamerism when shade selection is critical. Metamerism is a complication observed when the perceived color of objects (in this case teeth and resin composite restorations) is different in different light sources.

Color Acuity and Eye Fatigue

When selecting color or shade, the operator should avoid staring at the tooth and shade guide for long periods of time. Staring at these objects during shade selection will cause the colors to blend, resulting in a loss of color acuity. The shade guide should be placed adjacent to the tooth to be restored and then viewed briefly to determine which shade or shades match the color of the tooth; then the eyes should be moved away. Ideally, the eyes should be "rested" by viewing the horizon through a window or by looking at an object with muted blue, violet, or gray color.

The dental assistant and patient can also assist in shade selection. By viewing the shade guide and tooth from several positions and accepting input from the assistant and patient, the dentist can achieve an acceptable color match.

Achieving Optimal Color Match

The color or shade selection should be accomplished before the restorative procedure is initiated. Therefore, selection is made while the tooth is moist, prior to rubber dam placement or cavity preparation. Desiccation of the tooth causes significant lightening of the shade, and the presence of a rubber dam can distort color perception.

Most manufacturers of resin composites provide or recommend a shade guide for their products to offer an approximation of the colors available. The selected shade can be confirmed with a small amount of resin composite (test shade) placed directly on or adjacent to the tooth and cured. This procedure should be performed on an unetched tooth surface to make removal easy after shade verification. For Class 4 restorations and others in which no tooth structure will remain lingual or facial to the planned restoration, the test shade should be placed in the approximate thickness of the tooth structure to be replaced to ensure adequate opacity or color density.

Tinting and Opaquing

Many manufacturers of resin composites provide accessory shades that contain a number of intense colors and opaques, premixed in syringes, ampules, or bottles. These materials are normally not necessary in conservative Class 3 restorations but can play an important role in large Class 4 restorations, diastema closures, and direct veneers. Opaque shades, or hybrid resin materials, can be used to block the reflection of darkness from the mouth that may cause a Class 4 restoration to appear too dark or low in value, or too translucent (Fig 9-21). Opaque resins may also be needed to mask discolored tooth structure.

Use of the proper accessory shades can create the appearance of dentin overlaid with enamel. Accessory shades can also be used to recreate the yellow color seen in cervical areas or the translucency that appears in incisal areas. Tints may be used to imitate white or

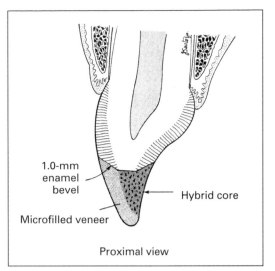

Fig 9-21 Opaque resin or a hybrid core may be used to block the shine-through effect.

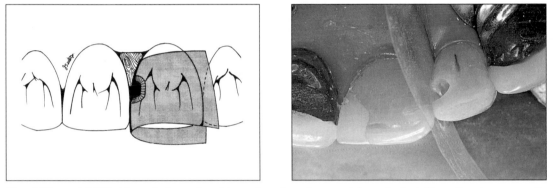

Figs 9-22a and 9-22b Lingual view of matrix and wedge placement for a typical Class 3 resin composite restoration.

brown spots that appear on adjacent teeth, although with the current ability to bleach teeth, the spots can usually be bleached out or their appearance neutralized with bleaching (see Chapter 15).

Matrices

For Class 3 Restorations

With Class 3 restorations, the most commonly used matrix is the clear plastic strip (Figs 9-22a and 9-22b). The clear plastic matrix, when properly wedged, will reduce flash (excess material) at the gingival margin. It is placed between the teeth and adjacent to the cavity preparation. The resin composite may be shaped with a plastic instrument, or the matrix strip may be pulled snugly around the tooth and held in place

manually to provide shape to the restoration and intimately adapt the resin composite. An excellent contouring instrument for resin composite is the interproximal carver (IPC) described in Chapter 6.

For Class 4 Restorations

The majority of Class 4 restorations must be built up incrementally, to avoid resin thicknesses of greater than 2.0 mm that would prevent an adequate degree of polymerization of the resin composite. This method usually requires placement of several increments. A clear plastic matrix strip and wedge may be used to achieve proximal contact and contours.

Another option, on the lingual and proximal aspects, is the use of a portion of a thin, clear plastic crown form, positioned to provide support until the lingual and proximal resin has been polymerized. The

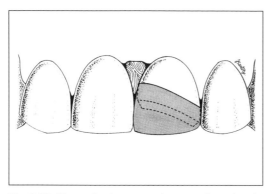

Fig 9-23 Clear plastic crown form and wedge in place for a Class 4 restoration.

Placement and Curing of Resin Composite Restorations

Light-cured resin composites are packaged in bulk form in syringes or in unit-dose ampules. The main advantage of purchasing material in bulk is that each unit costs less. However, for direct placement into the preparation, bulk material requires more handling because it must be dispensed and then loaded into a resin composite syringe. Unit-dose ampules allow ejection of the material directly into the preparation, minimizing entrapped air bubbles.[64] The ampules also make infection control procedures easier because they are discarded after use and require no disinfection.

Incremental Placement and Curing

Incremental placement and curing of the resin composite may be necessary for large light-cured restorations.[70] Most resin composite should be placed in thicknesses not greater than 2.0 mm. In restorations greater than 2.0 mm in thickness, incremental placement will produce a higher degree of polymerization for the material. Incremental placement has been shown in some studies to offset some of the effects of polymerization stresses,[12,23] but other studies show no difference in bulk placement vs incremental filling techniques.[91,95]

Incremental placement without loss of restoration strength is possible because of a phenomenon referred to as the *air- (or oxygen-) inhibited layer*. Polymerization of resin composite is initiated and progresses because of free radicals that are formed in the resin monomers. These free radicals are highly reactive to oxygen, and when they come in contact with air at the surface of the resin composite, an unpolymerized, air-inhibited layer is formed.[78] The air-inhibited layer is reactive to new resin composite, however, and forms a cohesive bond to additional increments. Even when the air-inhibited layer is removed, if the restoration is freshly placed, some free radicals remain that can induce a degree of chemical attachment of a succeeding increment. However, if new resin composite must be added to a resin composite surface that is very smooth, such as one that was in contact with a clear plastic strip, the surface should first be roughened with a bur and a layer of adhesive resin should be placed and polymerized to enhance attachment of the new increment.

crown form should be trimmed to fit 1.0 mm past the prepared margins. If the crown form is thicker than a clear plastic matrix strip, the contact areas should be thinned with an abrasive disk to allow contact of the restoration with the adjacent tooth.

For Class 4 restorations in which the restoration will not be more than 2 mm thick, some clinicians prefer to use a crown form to completely enclose a bulk of resin and carry it to the prepared tooth, and thereby to shape facial as well as lingual and proximal contours (Fig 9-23).

Wedging

Wooden wedges are inserted between the teeth and against the matrix to seal the gingival margin, separate the teeth, protect interproximal gingiva, ensure proximal contact, and push the rubber dam and proximal tissue gingivally to open the gingival embrasure.

Prewedging, or placement of the wedge prior to tooth preparation, may be helpful in some situations. This is generally not needed with Class 3 restorations but may be with Class 4 restorations. Prewedging allows greater separation of the teeth and more space to build a contact. Resin composite cannot be condensed against the adjacent tooth, as can amalgam, and depends on the space created by the wedge for achieving contact with the adjacent tooth.

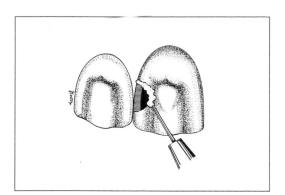

Fig 9-24 Application of gel etchant using a syringe tip. A matrix strip should be placed first to protect the adjacent tooth from the acid.

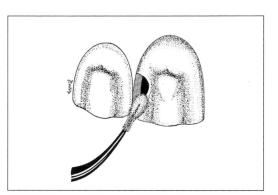

Fig 9-25 The primer and adhesive are placed with disposable brushes or applicators, and the adhesive is light cured in accordance with the manufacturer's protocol.

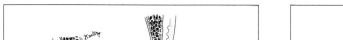

Figs 9-26a and 9-26b Incremental insertion of composite in a Class 3 restoration.

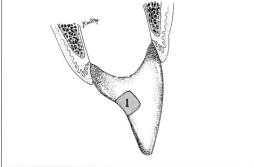

Fig 9-26a Small restorations may be filled in a single increment.

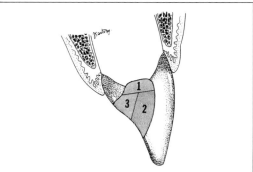

Fig 9-26b Large cavities require multiple increments to minimize the effects of polymerization shrinkage and ensure adequate polymerization.

Placement Technique

Class 3 Restorations

The enamel margins are etched, usually with phosphoric acid with a concentration of 30% to 40%.[80] Phosphoric acid is most easily dispensed in a gel form with a small syringe (Fig 9-24). The dentin may also be etched, depending on the adhesive system used. (See Chapter 8 for a discussion of dentin adhesives.) The dentin adhesive system may be applied and polymerized either before or after the matrix and wedge have been placed (Fig 9-25).

The resin composite–dispensing tip should be inserted into the preparation and the resin composite slowly injected until there is a slight overfill. Small Class 3 preparations can be filled in a single step without incremental placement. For larger Class 3 restorations, placement of multiple increments is recommended to optimize the degree of conversion of the resin composite in deep areas and to minimize the effects of polymerization shrinkage (Figs 9-26a and 9-26b).

After placement, the resin composite is shaped with a plastic instrument or interproximal carver or by pulling the matrix strip tightly around the tooth. The material is light cured for a minimum of 40 seconds. Sixty seconds of light exposure is recommended for deeper preparations or those receiving a darker shade of resin composite. When the material has been light cured, the wedge and matrix strip are removed, and the restoration is inspected for voids. If voids are present, they may be filled with additional resin composite material, which is then light cured.

Clinical Steps for a Class 3 or Class 4 Resin Composite Restoration

1. Select a shade before initiation of dehydration.
2. Place a rubber dam.
3. Prewedge if difficulty in achieving proximal contact is anticipated.
4. Initiate the cavity preparation by accessing the caries lesion through the marginal ridge with a No. 329 or 330 bur in a high-speed handpiece. Remove the proximal plate of enamel. Be careful to avoid damaging the adjacent tooth.
5. Remove the carious dentin with a round bur in a low-speed handpiece.
6. Remove unsupported enamel if appropriate, and place bevels with a finishing bur and/or gingival margin trimmer.
7. Etch the enamel. Be careful not to etch the adjacent tooth; protect it with a matrix strip.
8. Place the primer and adhesive, following the manufacturer's instructions.
9. Light cure as indicated.
10. If the preparation is large, place resin composite into the deep areas.
11. Light cure for at least 40 seconds
12. Place a clear plastic strip or other matrix and wedge.
13. Add composite and contour the clear plastic matrix strip to contain the material in the proper shape.
14. Light cure for at least 40 seconds.
15. Remove the wedge and matrix strip, and inspect the restoration for voids. Add composite if necessary.
16. Remove gingival flash with a No. 12 or 12b scalpel blade.
17. Remove flash from the other margins, and contour the restoration with a finishing bur, finishing diamond, or abrasive disk.
18. Remove the rubber dam.
19. Check the occlusion and adjust as necessary.
20. Finish and polish with disks, rubber points, etc.
21. Apply etchant to surface and margins. Rinse, then apply and cure rebonding resin.

Class 4 Restorations

Etching procedures are performed and the adhesive system applied. In most cases, resin composite is built up incrementally and polymerized. Each increment should be exposed to the curing light for a minimum of 40 seconds from the facial aspect and 40 seconds from the lingual aspect. Short curing times will result in resin composite restorations with inferior physical properties and an increased chance that unreacted monomer will leach out of the restoration with time. The incremental placement technique allows the clinician to closely shape the restoration to the desired form and contours. The cavity should be slightly overfilled to allow contouring and finishing.

If a section of a clear plastic crown form is to be used, it may be filled with resin composite, placed over the preparation, and wedged in place. After the crown form and wedge are in position, excess material is removed with an explorer or interproximal carver. The restoration is then exposed to a curing light for a minimum of 60 seconds on the facial aspect and 60 seconds on the lingual aspect.

As described previously, another option is to use only the proximal and lingual aspects of the crown form, leaving the facial aspect open for incremental insertion of the resin composite. This allows layering of more opaque and translucent materials to closely mimic the natural appearance of dentin and enamel.

An overlay technique may be used for Class 4 restorations to obtain both strength and a very smooth surface.[99] The bulk of the restoration is built with a hybrid resin composite to provide strength. The final layer is a veneer of microfilled resin composite to provide a smooth, glossy surface. The final layer should be contoured and shaped before polymerization until it closely resembles the desired shape. It is then light polymerized. After any voids are eliminated, the restoration is contoured, finished, and polished.

Visible Light–Curing Units

Any light-curing unit with the prescribed wavelength may be used with any resin composite. However, the various commercially available units do not have the same curing capacity. Some units have been shown to cure greater thicknesses of material than others.[67] A light's effectiveness depends on several factors: (1) the wavelength of the emitted light (it should be 450 to 500 nm),[18] (2) the intensity of the bulb, (3) light exposure time, (4) distance from light tip to composite surface, and (5) shade of resin composite. Studies of light-curing units have found that some do not have the correct wavelength, which reduces the effectiveness of the unit.[68]

As curing units age, the bulb and its reflector degrade, reducing light output and curing effectiveness. Friedman[37] examined 67 curing lights in use by dentists around the United States and found bulb blackening in 21 lamps, frosted glass envelopes in 33 lamps, and reflector degradation in 3 lamps.

Light-curing units can rapidly lose their effectiveness. Every office should have a light analyzer (curing radiometer) to evaluate curing lights at least weekly. The bulb and reflector should be examined regularly for signs of degradation, and the light tip should be checked for clarity. The tip should also be cleaned of any resin composite or bonding resin that may have touched and adhered to the tip in the course of restoration placement. Some authorities recommend that bulbs be replaced periodically or when any discoloration is noted.

High-intensity curing lights such as lasers and plasma arc lights have been evaluated for curing resin composite. *Laser* is an acronym for *light amplification by stimulated emission of radiation*. Both lasers and plasma arc curing (PAC) light units are able to cure much faster and to a greater degree than the regular halogen light–curing units.[7] However, at present, lasers are expensive to own and maintain, and many practitioners consider them impractical to purchase for light-curing alone. The potential advantages and disadvantages of PAC lights are still being investigated. A more complete discussion on the new curing lights can be found in Chapter 10.

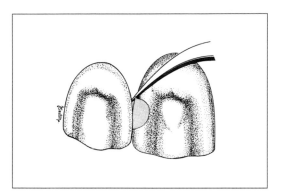

Fig 9-27 Gingival flash is removed with a No. 12 or 12b scalpel blade.

face staining, plaque accumulation, and wear characteristics of the resin composite.[50] Either traumatic finishing technique or overheating can damage the surface of resin composite[58,97] and result in accelerated wear.[58,75] The finishing technique may be one reason that wear of resin composite is often reported to be greatest in the first 6 to 12 months after placement. A low-viscosity surface sealer or rebonding resin, applied after finishing the resin composite, may help stop crack propagation, improve wear resistance, add color stability, and enhance marginal integrity over time.[28]

Finishing and Polishing

Finishing includes the shaping, contouring, and smoothing of the restoration, while polishing imparts a shine or luster to the surface. Sharp amalgam carvers and scalpel blades, such as the No. 12 or 12b, or specific resin carving instruments made of carbide, anodized aluminum, or nickel titanium, are useful for shaping polymerized resins (Fig 9-27). There are many products available for finishing and polishing, including diamond and carbide burs, various types of flexible disks, abrasive-impregnated rubber points and cups, metal and plastic finishing strips, and polishing pastes. The smoothest possible surface is obtained, however, when the resin composite polymerizes against a clear plastic strip without subsequent finishing or polishing.[72,84]

The finishing and polishing process can affect many aspects of the final restoration, including sur-

Instruments

Diamond vs Carbide Burs

The 12-fluted carbide burs have traditionally been used to perform gross finishing of resin composite (Fig 9-28). These finishing burs may be used to develop the proper anatomy for the restoration. The transition from resin to enamel should be slowly smoothed until it is undetectable. These burs can be used dry to better visualize the margins and anatomy being developed but should be used with light pressure to avoid overheating and possibly damaging the resin composite surface.

Fine finishing diamonds are also available for finishing resin composite restorations and have been found to impart less surface damage to microfilled resin composites than carbide finishing burs.[8,50] They are used in a series of progressively finer abrasive particle sizes.

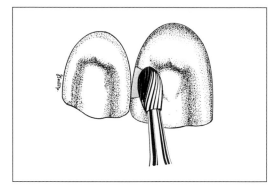

Fig 9-28 A finishing bur or fine diamond is used for gross finishing.

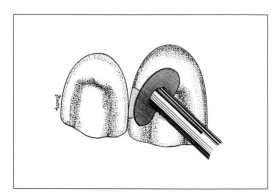

Fig 9-29 Polishing of the final restoration may be accomplished with flexible disks or impregnated rubber points.

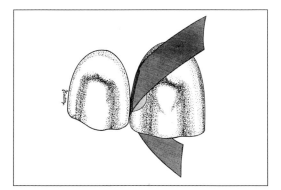

Fig 9-30 Polishing strips are used to contour and polish the proximal surface and margin.

Disks

One brand of flexible disks (Sof-Lex, 3M) has practically become the standard in finishing and polishing. The disks in one Sof-Lex series have a soft, flexible backing and a series of grits that can provide a smooth, even finish. Another Sof-Lex series, and similar disks made by other manufacturers, have thin plastic or polymeric backings that allow access of the abrasive side into embrasures and interproximal areas. When all four grits are used in sequence, these flexible finishing disks are reported to provide the best surface of any finishing system.[5,14] Sequential use of disks to a fine grit produces a smooth, durable finish (Fig 9-29).

Dry finishing with disks used in sequence is reported to be superior or equal to wet finishing for smoothness, hardness, and color stability.[29] However, dry finishing tends to clog the abrasive particles and makes the disks work less efficiently. If the restoration is finished dry, the resin composite surface should be rinsed, before a finer disk is used, to remove the larger particles and abrasive debris left by the previous disk.

Impregnated Rubber Points and Cups

A wide variety of rubber points and cups are available that are impregnated with abrasive materials. Like disks, rubber cups and points are used sequentially from coarse to fine grit. The coarse grits are effective for gross reduction and finishing, while the fine grits create a smooth, shiny surface. The primary advantage of rubber points and cups over disks is for providing access to grooves, desirable surface irregularities, and the concave lingual surfaces of anterior teeth.

Finishing Strips

Finishing strips are used to contour and polish the proximal surfaces and margins gingival to the interproximal contact (Fig 9-30). They are available with metal or plastic backings. Most metal strips are used for gross reduction, but care must be taken not to overreduce the restoration; these metal strips will also remove enamel, cementum, and dentin. Plastic strips come in various widths and grits and can be used for both finishing and polishing. Like the flexible disks, finishing strips come in a series of grits, which should be used in series from coarsest to finest.

Procedures

A No. 12 or 12b scalpel blade is effective for removing interproximal flash, carving the proximal margins, and otherwise shaping the polymerized resin. Gross reduction and shaping are then performed with diamonds, carbide burs, and/or coarse abrasive disks and strips. Finishing should be done carefully to avoid damaging the surface or margin of the resin composite restoration, and water or air should be applied as a coolant. Finishing strips can be used on the proximal surfaces and margins so that floss snaps through the contact smoothly without shredding. After the resin composite is polished with fine abrasive-impregnated disks, strips, or rubber cups or points, a high shine can be added with aluminum oxide or diamond polishing pastes.

Many operators have observed the development of a "white line" at the margins of resin composite restorations during finishing. The exact cause of this phenomenon is not known, but several investigators and clinicians have put forward possible explanations. One explanation[1,15,52,93] implicates traumatic finishing leading to microfractures at the margins of the resin composite or tooth structure. Other proposed causes include improperly rotating abrasive disks,[34,44] inadequate polymerization of the resin composite material,[1] and polymerization shrinkage causing microfracture of unsupported or fragile enamel at the margins.[48] When the white line presents an esthetic problem, if more conservative procedures such as rebonding do not resolve it, the white area must be removed with a bur and additional composite must be bonded and finished.

Rebonding

Rebonding (also called glazing) is performed after the restoration is finished and polished. The enamel margins are re-etched, and a coat of unfilled or lightly filled low-viscosity resin is placed over the restoration surface and polymerized. Rebonding has been reported to improve marginal integrity,[39] aid color stability, improve early wear resistance, and help reduce staining of the restoration.[28,40,41,53] A number of low-viscosity resins, called surface sealers, are now available for use in the rebonding procedure.

References

1. Albers HF. Tooth-Colored Restoratives, ed 8. Santa Rosa: Alto, 1996.
2. Alster D, Feilzer AJ, De Gee AJ, et al. The dependence of shrinkage stress reduction on porosity concentration in thin resin layers. J Dent Res 1992;71:1619–1622.
3. Andreasen FM, Noren JG, Andreasen JO, et al. Long term survival of fragment bonding in the treatment of fractured crowns. Quintessence Int 1995;26:669–681.
4. Bagheri J, Denehy GE. Effect of enamel bevel and restoration length on Class 4 acid-etch retained composite resin restorations. J Am Dent Assoc 1983;107:951–953.
5. Berastegui E, Canalda C, Brau E, Miquel C. Surface roughness of finished composite resins. J Prosthet Dent 1992, 68:742–790.
6. Black JB, Retief DH, Lemmons JE. Effect of cavity design on the retention of Class 4 composite resin restorations. J Am Dent Assoc 1981;103:42–46.
7. Blankenau RJ, Kelsey WP, Powell GL, et al. Degree of composite resin polymerization with visible light and argon laser. Am J Dent 1991;4:40–42.
8. Boghosian AA, Randolph RG, Jekkals VJ. Rotary instrument finishing of microfilled and small-particle hybrid composite resins. J Am Dent Assoc 1987;115;299–301.
9. Boghosian AA, Ricker J, McCoy R. Clinical evaluation of a resin-modified glass-ionomer restorative: 5-year results [abstract 1436]. J Dent Res 1999;78 (special issue):285.
10. Brackett WW, Gilpatrick RO, Browning WD, Gregory PN. Two-year clinical performance of a resin-modified glass-ionomer restorative material. Oper Dent 1999;24:9–13.
11. Buda M. Form and color reproduction for composite resin reconstruction of anterior teeth. Int J Periodont Rest Dent 1994;14:34–47.
12. Burke FJT. Reattachment of a fractured central incisor tooth fragment. Br Dent J 1991;170:223–225.
13. Cavalleri G, Zerman N. Traumatic crown fractures in permanent incisors with immature roots: a follow-up study. Endod Dent Traumatol 1995;11:294–296.
14. Chen RCS, Chan DCN, Chan KC. A quantitative study of finishing and polishing techniques for a composite. J Prosthet Dent 1988;59:292–298.
15. Christensen GJ. Overcoming challenges with resin in Class II situations. J Am Dent Assoc 1997;128:1579–1580.
16. Cipalla AJ. Laser Curing of Photoactivated Restorative Materials. Salt Lake City: ILT Systems, 1994.
17. Coli P, Blixt M, Brännström M. The effect of cervical grooves on the contraction gap in Class 2 composites. Oper Dent 1993;18:33–36.
18. Cook WD. Spectral distributions of dental photopolymerization sources. J Dent Res 1982;61:1436–1438.
19. Craig RG. Restorative Dental Materials, ed 10. St. Louis: Mosby, 1997:253–254.
20. Craig RG. Restorative Dental Materials, ed 10. St. Louis: Mosby, 1997:261, 275.
21. Crigger LP, Foster CD, Young JM, Stockman TD. Visible-Light Curing Units. Aeromedical Review. San Antonio, TX: USAF School of Aerospace Medicine, 1984.
22. Crim G, Chapman K. Effect of placement techniques on microleakage of a dentin-bonded composite resin. Quintessence Int 1986;17:21–24.

257

23. Crim GA. Microleakage of three resin placement techniques. Am J Dent 1991;4:69–72.

24. Croll TP. Emergency repair followed by complete-coronal restoration of a fractured mandibular incisor. Quintessence Int 1992;23:817–822.

25. Darveniza M. Cavity design for Class 4 composite resin restorations—a systematic approach. Aust Dent J 1987;32:270–275.

26. Davidson CL, DeGee AJ. Relaxation of polymerization contraction stresses by flow in dental composites. J Dent Res 1984;63:16–48.

27. Davidson CL, Feilzer AJ. Polymerization shrinkage and polymerization shrinkage stress in polymer-based restoratives. J Dent 1997;25:435–440.

28. Dickinson GL, Leinfelder KF. Assessing the long term effects of a surface penetrating sealant. J Am Dent Assoc 1993;124:68–72.

29. Dodge WW, Dale RA, Cooley RL, Duke ES. Comparison of wet and dry finishing of resin composites with aluminum oxide discs. Dent Mater 1991;7:18–20.

30. Eames WB. When not to restore. J Am Dent Assoc 1988;117:429–432.

31. Eick JD, Welch F. Polymerization shrinkage of posterior composite resins and its possible influence on postoperative sensitivity. Quintessence Int 1986;17:103–111.

32. Eick JD, Robinson SJ, Byerley TJ, Chappelow CC. Adhesives and nonshrinking dental resins of the future. Quintessence Int 1993;24:632–640.

33. Espinosa HD. In vitro study of resin-supported internally etched enamel. J Prosthet Dent 1979;40:526–529.

34. Farah J, Powers J. Composite finishing and polishing. The Dental Advisor 1998;15:3.

35. Feilzer AJ, De Gee AJ, Davidson CL. Curing contraction of composites and glass-ionomer cements. J Prosthet Dent 1988;59:297–300.

36. Feilzer AJ, De Gee AJ, Davidson CL. Influence of light intensity on polymerization shrinkage and integrity of restoration-cavity interface. Eur J Oral Sci 1995;103:322–326.

37. Friedman J. Variability of lamp characteristics in dental curing lights. J Esthet Dent 1990;1:189–190.

38. Fusayama T. Ideal cavity preparation for adhesive composites. Asian J Aesthet Dent 1993;1:55–62.

39. Galan JR, Mondelli J, Coradazzi JL. Marginal leakage of two composite restorative systems. J Dent Res 1976;55:74–76.

40. Garman TA, Fairhurst CW, Hewer GA, et al. A comparison of glazing materials for composite restorations. J Am Dent Assoc 1977;95:950–956.

41. Gibson GB, Richardson AS, Patton RE, Waldman R. A clinical evaluation of occlusal composite and amalgam restorations: one-year and two-year results. J Am Dent Assoc 1992;104:335–337.

42. Gillen RJ, Schwartz RS, Hilton TJ, Evans DB. Analysis of selected normative tooth proportions. Int J Prosthodont 1994;7:410–417.

43. Goldman M. Fracture properties of composite and glass ionomer dental restorative materials. J Biomed Mater Res 1985;19:771–783.

44. Goldstein RE. Finishing of composites and laminates. Dent Clin North Am 1989;33:305–318.

45. Gordon M, Plasschaert A, Saiku J, Plezner R. Microleakage of posterior composite resin materials and an experimental urethane restorative material, tested in vitro above and below the cementoenamel junction. Quintessence Int 1986;17:11–15.

46. Gutz DP. Fractured permanent incisors in a clinical population. J Dent Child 1971;38:94–95.

47. Haveman C, Burgess J, Summitt J. Clinical comparison of restorative materials for caries in xerostomic patients [abstract 1441]. J Dent Res 1999;78 (special issue):286.

48. Heath JR, Jordan JH, Watts DC. The effect of time of trimming on the surface finish of anterior composite resins. J Oral Rehabil 1993;20:45–52.

49. Ireland E, Xu X, Burgess JO. Microleakage of beveled and nonbeveled Class 3 resin restorations [abstract 207]. J Dent Res 1998;77 (special issue):131.

50. Jeffries SR. The art and science of abrasive finishing and polishing in restorative dentistry. Dent Clin North Am 1998;42:613–627.

51. Jokstad A, Mjör IA, Qvist V. The age of restorations in situ. Acta Odontol Scand 1994;52:234–242.

52. Jordan RE. Esthetic Composite Bonding, ed 2. St. Louis: Mosby, 1993:48.

53. Kawai K, Leinfelder KF. Effect of surface-penetrating sealant on composite wear. Dent Mater 1993;9:108–113.

54. Kidd EAM, Roberts GT. The saucer preparation. Part 2. Laboratory evaluation. Br Dent J 1982;153:138–140.

55. Krejci I, Sparr D, Lutz F. A three sited light curing technique for conventional Class II composite resin restorations. Quintessence Int 1987;18:125–131.

56. Lambrechts PP, Willems G, Vanherle G, Braem M. Aesthetic limits of light-cured composite in anterior teeth. Int Dent J 1990;40:149–158.

57. Lambrechts PP, Ameye C, Vanherle G. Conventional and microfilled composite resins. Part II: chip fractures. J Prosthet Dent 1982;48:527–538.

58. Leinfelder KF, Wilder AD, Teixeira AC. Wear rates of posterior composite resins. J Am Dent Assoc 1986;112:829–833.

59. Leinfelder KF, Suzuki S. In vitro wear device for determining posterior composite wear. J Am Dent Assoc 1999;130:1347–1353.

60. Levin JB. Esthetic diagnosis. Curr Opin Cosmet Dent 1995;1:9–17.

61. Lutz F, Krejci I, Oldenburg TR. Elimination of polymerization stresses at the margins of posterior composite resin restorations: a new restorative technique. Quintessence Int 1986;17:777–784.

62. Lutz F, Krejci I, Barbakow F. Quality and durability of marginal adaptation in bonded composite restorations. Dent Mater 1991;7:107–113.

63. McDonald SP, Sheiham A. A clinical comparison of non-traumatic methods of treating dental caries. Int Dent J 1994;44:465–470.

64. Medlock JW, Zinck JH, Norling BK, Sisca RF. Composite resin porosity with hand and syringe insertion. J Prosthet Dent 1985;54:47–51.

65. Mehl A, Hickel R, Kunzelmann KH. Physical properties and gap formation of light-cured composite with and without "soft-start" polymerization. J Dent 1997;25:321–330.

66. Mjör IA. Placement and replacement of restorations. Oper Dent 1981;6:49–54.

67. Mjör IA, Toffenetti F. Placement and replacement of resin-based restorations in Italy. Oper Dent 1992;17:82–85.

68. Nuemeyer S, Wolfgang G, Kappert HF, et al. PCR pin-anchored anterior fracture restorations. Gen Dent 1992;40:200–202.

69. Newman SM, Murray GA, Yates JL. Visible lights and visible light–activated composite resins. J Prosthet Dent 1983;50:31–35.

70. Podshadley AG, Gullett G, Crim G. Interface seal of incremental placement of visible light-cured composite resins. J Prosthet Dent 1985;53:625–626.

71. Porte A, Lutz F, Lund MR, et al. Cavity designs for composite resins. Oper Dent 1984;9:50–55.

72. Pratten DH, Johnson GH. An evaluation of finishing instruments for an anterior and posterior composite. J Prosthet Dent 1988;60:154–158.

73. Qvist V, Thystrup A, Mjör IA. Restorative treatment pattern and longevity of resin restorations in Denmark. Acta Odontol Scand 1986;44:351–356.

74. Qvist V, Strom C. 11-year assessment of Class III resin restorations completed with two restorative procedures. Acta Odontol Scand 1993;51:253–262.

75. Ratanapridakul K, Leinfelder KF, Thomas J. Effect of finishing on the in vivo wear rate of a posterior composite resin. J Am Dent Assoc 1989;118:524–526.

76. Robbins JW, Duke ES, Schwartz RS, Trevino D. Clinical evaluation of a glass ionomer restorative in cervical abrasions [abstract 171]. J Dent Res 1996;75 (special issue):39.

77. Roberts GT. The saucer preparation. Part 1: Clinical evaluation over 3 years. Br Dent J 1982;153:96–98.

78. Ruyter IE. Unpolymerized surface layers on sealants. Acta Odontol Scand 1981;39:27–32.

79. Sakaguchi RL, Berge H-X. Reduced light energy density decreases post-gel contraction while maintaining degree of conversion in composites. J Dent 1998;26:695–700.

80. Silverstone LM, Saxton CA, Dogon JL, Fejerskov O. Variation in the pattern of acid etching of human dental enamel examined by scanning electron microscopy. Caries Res 1975;9:373–387.

81. Silverstone LM. Fluorides and Remineralization: Clinical Uses of Fluorides. Philadelphia: Lea & Febiger, 1985:153–175.

82. Simonsen RJ. Restoration of a fractured central incisor using the original tooth fragment. J Am Dent Assoc 1982;105:646–648.

83. Smales RJ. Effects of enamel bonding, type of restoration, patient age and operator on the longevity of an anterior composite resin. Am J Dent 1991;4:130–133.

84. Stoddard JW, Johnson GH. An evaluation of polishing agents for composite resins. J Prosthet Dent 1991;65:491–495.

85. Summitt JB, Chan DCN, Dutton FB. Retention of Class 3 composite restorations: retention grooves versus enamel bonding. Oper Dent 1993;18:88–93.

86. Tyas MJ. Correlation between fracture properties and clinical performance of composite resins in Class IV cavities. Aust Dent J 1990;35:46–49.

87. van Dijken JW, Kieri C, Carlen M. Longevity of extensive Class II open-sandwich restorations with a resin-modified glass-ionomer cement. J Dent Res 1999;78:1319–1325.

88. van Dijken JW. 3-year clinical evaluation of a compomer, a resin-modified glass-ionomer and a composite in Class III cavities. Am J Dent 1996;9:195–198.

89. van Dijken JW, Olofsson AL, Holm C. 5-year evaluation of Class III composite resin restorations in cavities pre-treated with an oxalic- or a phosphoric acid conditioner. J Oral Rehabil 1999;26:364–371.

90. van Noort R, Davis LG. A prospective study of the survival of chemically activated anterior resin composite restorations in general practice: 5-year results. J Dent 1993;21:209–215.

91. Versluis A, Douglas WH, Cross M, Sakaguchi RL. Does an incremental filling technique reduce polymerization shrinkage stresses? J Dent Res 1996;75:871–878.

92. Watts DC, Al Hindi A. Intrinsic "soft-start" polymerisation shrinkage-kinetics in an acrylate-based resin composite. Dent Mater 1999;15:39–45.

93. Weinstein AR. Esthetic applications of restorative materials and techniques in the anterior dentition. Dent Clin North Am 1993;37:391–409.

94. Wilson NH, Wastell MA, Wastell DG, Smith GA. Performance of Occlusin in butt-joint and bevel-edged preparations: five year results. Dent Mater 1991;7:92–98.

95. Winkler MM, Katona TR, Paydar NH. Finite element stress analysis of three filling techniques for Class V light-cured restorations. J Dent Res 1996;75:1477–1483.

96. Worthington RB, Murchison DF, Vandewalle KS. Incisal edge reattachment: the effect of preparation utilization and design. Quintessence Int 1999;30:637–643.

97. Wu W, Toth EE, Ellison JA. Subsurface damage layer of in vivo worn dental composite restorations. J Dent Res 1984;63:675–680.

98. Young JM, Satrom KD, Berrong JM. Intraoral dental lights: test and evaluation. J Prosthet Dent 1987;57:99–107.

99. Zalkind M, Heling I. Composite resin layering: an esthetic technique for restoring fractured anterior teeth. J Prosthet Dent 1992;68:204–205.

10 Direct Posterior Esthetic Restorations

Thomas J. Hilton

The use of resin composite as a material for restoring posterior teeth has increased greatly in recent years. Patients are attracted to a restoration that matches the color of natural teeth.[136,162] Resin composite meets this demand and has become the most frequently used esthetic restorative material in dentistry.[163] In addition, resin composites contain no mercury, are thermally nonconductive,[136] and bond to tooth structure with the use of adhesives.[66,141,192] There are problems associated with using resin composite in posterior restorations, however, including shrinkage that occurs on setting,[83] occasional postoperative sensitivity,[247] and less-than-ideal resistance to wear.[111,147,166,176,180] Minimizing these negative aspects requires meticulous operative technique. Technique is the most important variable governing the success of posterior resin composite restorations.[82,165]

Although some questions about longevity remain,[29] there is increasing evidence that properly accomplished posterior resin composite restorations can be quite durable. Tables 10-1 to 10-3 are compilations of clinical studies on posterior amalgam, cast gold, and resin composite restorations, respectively. Because studies use different methods to assess restoration survival, an annual failure rate for each study has been computed to allow a means of comparison. As can be seen, study duration and the range of annual failure rates are comparable among the three materials. Considering that the materials used in the resin composite studies, particularly the studies

of longer duration, are of earlier formulations, and that materials have improved considerably in recent years, it is reasonable to conclude that resin composites can provide very successful posterior restorations. Key to the long-term success of resin composite posterior restorations is cavity size, restoration type, and tooth type.[15,22,179,227,298] Properly used, resin composite has demonstrated the ability to perform as well as amalgam in posterior restorations for up to 10 years.[91,179,227]

It is interesting to note the contrast in annual failure rates for amalgam, cast gold, and resin composite in a private practice setting (Fig 10-1) vs controlled clinical studies (Fig 10-2). As can be seen, there is a marked difference among material longevity in private practices, whereas the controlled clinical trials show similar results among the materials. No doubt there are a variety of explanations for these differences, including patient selection, technique sensitivity, and differences in approach related to practice setting. Although the clinical studies are often accomplished in relatively controlled environments, they clearly demonstrate the potential for the materials. With appropriate case selection and clinical technique, posterior resin composite restorations can serve very acceptably. It is the purpose of this chapter to present the factors that will lead to clinical success by examining the advantages, disadvantages, indications, and placement procedures for resin composite as a posterior restorative material.

Table 10-1	Longevity of amalgam restorations		
Investigators	Study time (y)	No. of restorations	Annual failure rate (%)
Smales et al, 1991[241a]	18	1,801	2.5
Smales et al, 1991[241b]	18	1,680	1.5–6.0
Osborne et al, 1991[202a]	14	320	0.9
Crabb, 1981[50a]	10	407	6.3
Collins et al, 1998[50]	8	52	0.7
Letzel et al, 1989[166a]	7	2,431	1.3–2.4
Fukushima et al, 1992[91]	5	73	0.8

Table 10-2	Longevity of cast-gold restorations		
Investigators	Study time (y)	No. of restorations	Annual failure rate (%)
Fritz et al, 1992[90a]	1–30	2,717	3.0–4.0
Bentley and Drake, 1986[22]	1–25	1,207	0.9
Crabb, 1981[50a]	10	86	5.9

Table 10-3	Longevity of posterior resin composite restorations		
Investigators	Study time (y)	No. of restorations	Annual failure rate (%)
Wilder et al, 1996[289]	17	60	1.3
Pallesen and Qvist, 1995[203]	10	93	1.6
Barnes et al, 1991[15]	8	28	2.9
Collins et al, 1998[50]	8	161	1.2–2.0
Wilson et al, 1991[298]	5	94	3.4
Fukushima et al, 1992[91]	5	432	1.0
Letzel et al, 1989[166]	4	696	1.5
Rowe, 1989[227]	4	266	1.5
Geurtsen et al, 1994[98]	4	1,214	3.0

Advantages of Resin Composite as a Posterior Restorative Material

Esthetics

Manufacturers have developed sophisticated resin composite systems with multiple shades, tints, and opaque resins that allow the practitioner to place highly esthetic restorations (Fig 10-3). Clinical studies often report excellent color match of resin composite with tooth structure. One study found that 98% of resin composite restorations still provided excellent color match at 2 years.[184] Visible light–cured (VLC) composites have less amine content than the auto-cured systems, resulting in less yellowing of the restoration and greater color stability over time.[296] Microfilled resin composites have the smoothest surface finish of all the systems and tend to stain less than other systems.[296] Because they are more heavily filled, hybrid composites tend to impart a more opaque appearance to restorations (Figs 10-4a and 10-4b).[293]

Conservation of Tooth Structure

In the past, it was recommended by some that preparation design for posterior resin composite restorations be patterned after the traditional amalgam preparation[165] as described by Dr G. V. Black. Researchers today recommend a more conservative approach.[37,252,283] To take advantage of resin composite's positive properties and to minimize its negative ones, the adhesive preparation has evolved. This design limits the removal of tooth structure to that needed to eliminate carious lesions and fragile enamel[122] (Figs 10-5a to 10-5f).

The adhesive preparation for posterior Class 2 resin composite restorations differs from the traditional amalgam design of G. V. Black in several ways[25]:

1. The preparation tends to be shallower. Because retention is provided through bonding to tooth structure rather than mechanical undercuts, there is no need to penetrate to dentin if the carious lesion does not. This conserves tooth structure and expands the area of enamel available for bonding (Fig 10-5a).

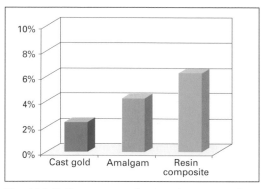

Fig 10-1 Failure rates of posterior restorations placed in private practices.[135]

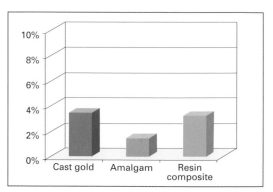

Fig 10-2 Median annual failure rate ranges for posterior restorations evaluated in 17 clinical studies.[16,22,50,50a,90,91,98,166,166a,202a,203,226,227,241a,241b,289,298]

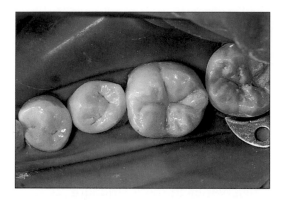

Fig 10-3 Modern resin composite materials can provide an esthetic restoration, such as the mesio-occlusal restoration in the mandibular first molar. (Courtesy of Dr Bill Dunn.)

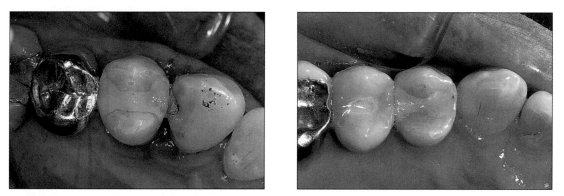

Figs 10-4a and 10-4b Heavily filled resin composite formulations tend to give the restoration a more opaque appearance.

2. The preparation tends to have a narrower outline form, which allows less occlusal contact on the restoration and reduces wear.[15,99,176,227,298] A less bulky restoration helps to decrease the adverse effects of resin composite polymerization shrinkage, resulting in improved marginal integrity[122] and less cuspal deflection[251] (Fig 10-5b).

3. The preparation has rounded internal line angles; this conserves tooth structure, decreases stress concentration associated with sharp line angles,[296] and enhances resin adaptation during placement[65,132] (Fig 10-5c).

4. There is no extension for prevention (Fig 10-5d). The occlusal fissures are included in the prepara-

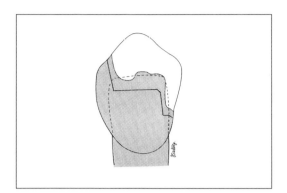

Fig 10-5a The adhesive preparation is extended only enough to provide access and to remove carious tooth structure. It may not penetrate the dentinoenamel junction *(upper solid line)*, unlike the traditional preparation *(lower solid line)*. *Dotted line* represents the dentinoenamel junction.

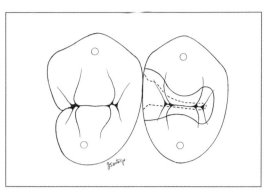

Fig 10-5b The more conservative outline form of the adhesive resin composite restoration *(dotted line)* compared to that of the traditional restoration *(solid line)*.

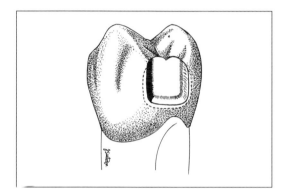

Fig 10-5c In the adhesive preparation, internal angles are rounded.

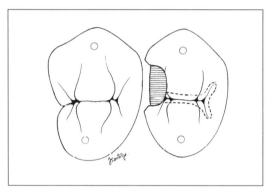

Fig 10-5d If there is no occlusal caries lesion, a Class 2 preparation for a resin composite restoration can be very conservative, similar to a Class 3 preparation. The occlusal fissures can be sealed *(dotted line)* after restoration placement.

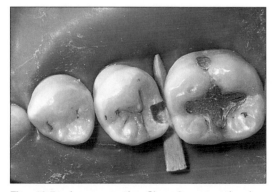

Figs 10-5e A conservative Class 2 preparation has been made. The occlusal fissures are stained but not carious.

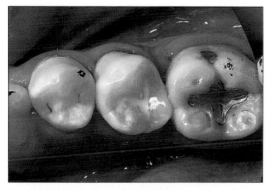

Fig 10-5f After the restoration is completed, a sealant is placed in the fissures.

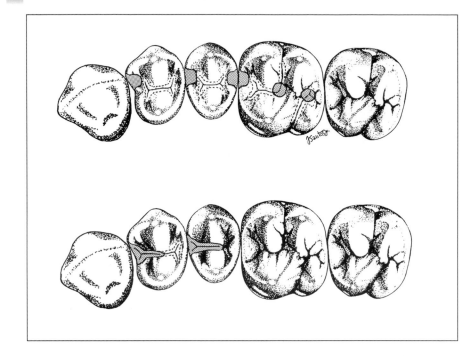

Fig 10-6 Outline of various Class 2 resin composite restorations. Access is limited to that required for removal of carious tooth structure and/or previous restoration(s), so outline form will vary based on extent of carious lesions. Occlusal pits and fissures that are not carious may be treated with sealants. Deeply stained or demineralized fissures may be opened with a small bur or air abrasion prior to sealing. (*Dashed outlines* indicate sealant; *dotted areas* indicate composite.)

tion only if the presence of caries lesions dictates this need. Extending the Class 2 preparation through occlusal grooves does not make the restoration more resistant to fracture than the more conservative proximal slot restoration.[41,252] In clinical studies, use of a proximal slot preparation for posterior resin composite restorations showed no failures after over 2 years in service[156] and 70% success after up to 10 years.[195] In this long-term study,[195] no restorations were lost due to loss of retention or to wear. Adjacent pits and fissures can be treated with sealants to enhance caries prevention[296] (Figs 10-5e and 10-5f). Figure 10-6 shows some examples of outline form of posterior resin composite restorations; each is designed to treat the pathosis presented, and none has a "standard" shape.

Adhesion to Tooth Structure

The clinical success of bonded resin composite restorations is well documented.[1,52,107,208] The bond between resin composite and tooth structure achieved with bonding systems offers the potential to seal the margins of the restoration[92] and reinforce remaining tooth structure against fracture.[66,141,192] Although not all studies have found teeth with bonded restorations to have an increased resistance to fracture,[138,246] and the longevity of the bond is shortened by increased occlusal forces,[88] it has been suggested that less cuspal flexure occurs with bonded resin composite restorations under subcatastrophic occlusal loads, providing protection against the propagation of cracks, which can ultimately lead to fatigue failure.[246]

Low Thermal Conductivity

Because resin composites do not readily transmit temperature changes, there is an insulating effect that helps to reduce postoperative temperature sensitivity.[83]

Elimination of Galvanic Currents

Resin composite does not contain metal and so will not initiate or conduct galvanic currents.[296]

Radiopacity

Radiopaque restorative materials are necessary to allow the practitioner to evaluate the contours and marginal adaptation of the restoration as well as to distinguish among the restoration, caries lesions, and sound tooth structure.[73,266] Most modern resin composites have a radiopacity in excess of that of enamel[266] and greater than that of an equal thickness of aluminum,[5] the criterion the American Dental Association uses to allow a manufacturer to claim its material is radiopaque.

Alternative to Amalgam

Amalgam, despite having a long track record of clinical success,[56,149,225] has declined in use as a restorative material due to its unesthetic appearance and its mercury content. Although concerns about mercury in amalgam are more psychological than scientific, there is an increasing desire to find mercury-free alternatives.[27] Patients are aware of indictments against amalgam, and some express concern over potential health hazards.[35] Amalgam is also less attractive to dental professionals as government agencies consider classifying it as hazardous waste[64] and requiring that dental offices install expensive systems to remove mercury from waste water.[27,75] For these reasons, resin composite use in posterior restorations continues to gain popularity in the profession.[27]

Disadvantages of Resin Composite as a Posterior Restorative Material

Polymerization Shrinkage

Despite improvements in resin composite formulations over the years, modern systems are still based on variations of the bis-GMA molecule, which has been used for more than 30 years.[29] One of the major drawbacks of this material is the polymerization shrinkage that occurs during the setting reaction. Modern resin composites undergo volumetric polymerization shrinkage of 2.6% to 7.1%.[78]

Most of the problems associated with posterior resin composite restorations can be related directly or indirectly to polymerization shrinkage. During polymerization, resin composite may pull away from the least retentive cavity margins (usually those with little or no enamel on them), resulting in gap formation.[69,159,175] Tensile forces developed in enamel margins can result in marginal degradation from mastication.[184] Contraction forces on cusps can result in cuspal deformation,[207] enamel cracks and crazes,[183] (Figs 10-7a and 10-7b), and ultimately decreased fracture resistance of the cusps.[288]

Polymerization shrinkage occurs regardless of the system used to initiate the setting reaction, but there is a difference in opinion regarding the direction of the force vectors developed. For many years, it was believed that autocured resin composite polymerizes toward the center of the mass of the resin composite, while visible light–cured resin composite polymerizes toward the light source (Figs 10-8a and 10-8b).[83,175] Recent research has questioned this assertion, and provides evidence that polymerization shrinkage occurs toward walls of cavity preparations to which it is bonded, regardless of the initiator mode.[278]

A number of techniques have been suggested to decrease the adverse effects of polymerization shrinkage. The most commonly used is incremental placement of VLC composite, which decreases the effect of setting contraction by reducing the bulk of resin composite cured at one time.[175] In addition, incremental insertion reduces the ratio of bonded to unbonded surface area, which helps to relieve the stress developed at the bond between tooth and resin composite.[77] The incremental placement technique is discussed later in this chapter.

Beta-quartz inserts, which can be incorporated into the resin composite during insertion, have been developed to reduce the bulk of composite and resultant polymerization shrinkage.[67] While little clinical evidence is available on the efficacy of the inserts, early indications were that wear was not adversely affected.[142] However, studies have shown that inserts have not reduced cuspal strain[63] or marginal leakage.[8,49]

Autocured resin composites are sometimes recommended for posterior restorations because an autocured composite tends to induce less polymerization stress than does a comparable bulk of VLC composite. This is due in part to greater porosity being incorporated into the autocured resin composite as a result of mixing. The incorporated oxygen inhibits the set of resin immediately adjacent to the voids and decreases the ratio of bonded to unbonded surface area.[7] The voids increase the free surface area for stress compensation by flow of the resin during the

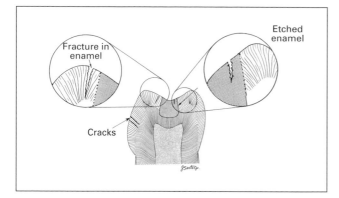

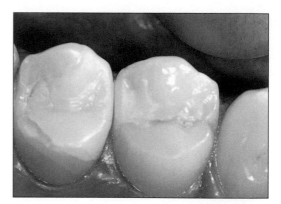

Fig 10-7a Polymerization shrinkage can cause crazing in the enamel or fractures within the resin composite.

Fig 10-7b Craze lines are evident in the lingual cusp of the maxillary right second premolar after placement of a very large Class 2 resin composite restoration.

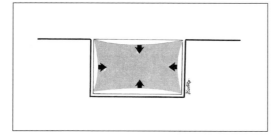

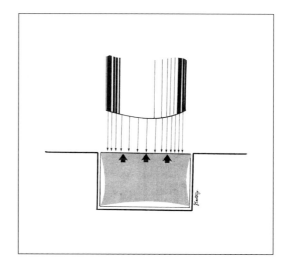

Figs 10-8a Polymerization shrinkage was thought to occur toward the center of the mass of resin in autocuring resin composites.

Fig 10-8b Polymerization shrinkage was thought to occur toward the light in light-curing resin composites.

setting reaction.[79] In addition, autocured resin composites develop shrinkage stresses more slowly than do VLC materials because of a slower polymerization rate. This allows for increased restorative material flow during polymerization.[78,144] However, a number of problems associated with the use of autocured resin composite in posterior restorations argue against its use. These problems are discussed in subsequent sections.

Decreasing the rate of polymerization of VLC resin composite can be accomplished by varying the curing light intensity. This has resulted in a form of curing for VLC resin composites variously referred to as "two-step" or "soft-start" polymerization. Research has shown that, by reducing the initial irradiance (to approximately 150 mW/cm²), followed by high level

irradiance (650 mW/cm² or greater), the curing reaction is slowed, marginal integrity is enhanced, and physical properties are not adversely affected.[80,103,153,185,272] The best hope for overcoming the problems of polymerization shrinkage lies in the future development of tooth-colored materials that do not contract during setting, an area of vigorous research.[68,100,292]

Secondary Caries

Several clinical studies have demonstrated that secondary caries is a significant cause of failure of posterior resin composite restorations.[16,50,135,166,218] It is believed that the marginal gap formed at the gingival margin as a result of polymerization shrinkage allows

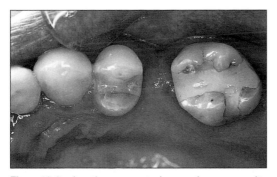

Figs 10-9a In these posterior resin composite restorations, the dark shadowing adjacent to the occlusal margins was caused by recurrent caries lesions.

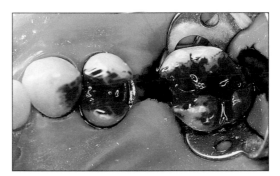

Fig 10-9b After placement of a rubber dam, the resin composite restorations are removed and caries-detecting solution is placed.

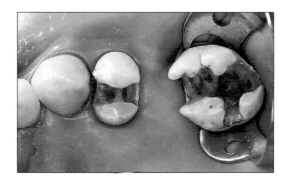

Fig 10-9c Stained areas confirm the presence of demineralized tooth structure.

the ingress of cariogenic bacteria[166] (Figs 10-9a to 10-9c). Because marginal degradation has been demonstrated to increase with time,[15,16,58,287] the risk of secondary caries also increases with time.

Studies have shown that levels of mutans streptococcus, the organism linked most closely to the incidence of dental caries,[302] are significantly higher in the plaque adjacent to proximal surfaces of posterior resin composite restorations than in plaque adjacent to either amalgam or glass-ionomer restorations. A retrospective study by Qvist et al[218] revealed that less secondary caries occurred in all classes of amalgam restorations than in resin composite restorations. In addition, the organic acids of plaque have been found to soften bis-GMA polymers, and this in turn could have an adverse effect on wear and surface staining.[11] These facts emphasize the need for regular recall and close follow-up of patients with posterior resin composite restorations.

Postoperative Sensitivity

Postoperative sensitivity has been associated with the placement of posterior resin composite restorations. One clinical study noted that 29% of teeth suffered from sensitivity following placement of the restorations.[247] Reports of postoperative sensitivity have diminished somewhat with improvements in dentin adhesives.[13,18] However, studies continue to report postoperative sensitivity following the placement of even conservative posterior resin composite restorations.[156]

A number of reasons have been postulated for the occurrence of postoperative sensitivity, but the most commonly accepted theories relate to polymerization shrinkage. As previously discussed, polymerization shrinkage results in gap formation, which allows bacterial penetration and fluid flow under the restoration. The bacteria or their noxious products may

At the present time, the best wear characteristics of resin composites for posterior use are generally exhibited by heavily filled materials (more than 60% by volume) with a mean filler particle size between 1 and 3 μm.[161,176,292] Clinical studies show that resin composite formulations have acceptable wear characteristics for up to 17 years.[18,179,289] In fact, some studies have indicated that posterior resin composite restorations wear as well as amalgam.[112,179,227] However, other studies report that composites have significantly higher wear rates than amalgam,[50,111,147,166,176,180] and no composite has been shown to exhibit less wear than amalgam.

Other Mechanical Properties

Generally, the more closely the mechanical properties of a restorative material simulate those of enamel and dentin, the better the restoration's longevity.[163,292,297] A number of the mechanical properties of resin composite are inferior to those of tooth structure and other restorative materials. These inferior properties can have an adverse effect on the durability of the restoration.

Resin composite materials have low fracture toughness relative to metallic restorative materials.[159,166] Indeed, bulk fracture of posterior resin composite restorations has been noted as a significant cause of failure in many clinical studies.[18,50,98,203,298] Increased filler loading of resin composite leads to improved fracture toughness.[84,85] Research in altering resin composite formulation to increase fracture toughness is ongoing.[117]

Resin composite has a relatively high degree of elastic deformation (ie, low modulus of elasticity) that exceeds that of amalgam by six to eight times.[37] Failures of resin composite restorations associated with its high elastic deformation have included bulk fracture,[159] microcrack formation,[85] and relatively low resistance to occlusal loading.[247] As with fracture resistance, more highly filled composites exhibit less elastic deformation than their less filled counterparts.[292]

The coefficient of thermal expansion of resin composite is another property that differs significantly from that of tooth structure.[51,277] Because the coefficient of thermal expansion of resin composite is higher than that of tooth structure, composite tends to expand and contract more than enamel and dentin when subjected to variations in temperature. This can increase marginal gap formation and exacerbate the effects of polymerization shrinkage on cuspal deformation, and it may result in the fracture of composite or enamel.[159,297] It has been demonstrated that as the mismatch in thermal expansion properties between restorative material and the tooth structure increases, so does marginal leakage.[38] As the filler content of resin composite increases, however, the mismatch decreases.[51]

Water Sorption

Water sorption is another factor in the clinical performance of resin composites. Water is absorbed preferentially into the resin component of composite, and water content is therefore increased when resin content is increased.[29,159] Because of the swelling of the resin matrix from water sorption, the filler particle bond to resin is weakened. If the resulting stress is greater than the bond strength, the resulting debond is referred to as hydrolytic breakdown.[159,243] Incompletely cured resin composite will exhibit more water sorption and greater resultant hydrolytic degradation.[189]

It has been suggested that the swelling of resin composite caused by water sorption can be beneficial due to closing of the marginal gap caused by polymerization shrinkage. However, studies have shown that the swelling from moisture absorption usually is not enough to overcome the polymerization shrinkage gap.[75,184] Even if water sorption did result in a closed marginal gap, it would only provide a close adaptation, without adhesion between the resin composite and tooth.[152]

It has been demonstrated that resin composites containing strontium and barium, added to increase radiopacity, tend to have an increased incidence of hydrolytic breakdown and crack formation.[243]

Variable Degree of Cure

Analysis of the polymerization, or cure, of resin composites reveals that certain characteristics of this material are at odds with one another. As the degree of cure of a resin composite material increases, the mechanical properties improve.[7,19,29] Clinical research has clearly demonstrated that a reduced degree of cure causes significantly increased wear.[86] However, polymerization shrinkage also increases with a more thorough cure.[276] Resins with decreased filler content exhibit decreased viscosity and improved diffusion of reactive groups during the polymerization reaction, and, thereby, improved cure.[81] However, a decreased filler content also results in inferior mechanical properties[51,84,85,292] and

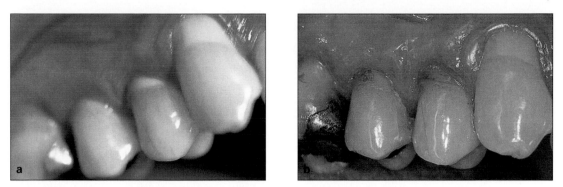

Figs 10-13a and 10-13b Marginal staining/discoloration indicating degradation of adhesion between resin composite and cavity preparation that occurs with aging. (a) Facial Class 5 resin composite restorations in teeth 4 and 5. (b) The same restorations 3 years later. Discoloration is evident, particularly at the gingival (dentin) margins of the restorations.

poorer clinical performance.[58,176,184,247,287] Achieving the best balance among these factors is a challenge for both the manufacturers of resin composites and clinicians.

Visible light–cured composites have been shown to achieve a somewhat higher degree of cure than autocured materials.[10,81] Several factors influence the extent of polymerization of VLC composites. Lighter shades cure more easily and in less time than darker shades.[83] Resin composites with larger filler particles tend to transmit light throughout the material more effectively than those with smaller filler particles.[229] The longer the composite is subjected to the curing light, the more effective the cure,[212] but the thickness of each increment should be limited to 2.0 mm.[83] The degree of cure is inversely related to the distance of the light tip from the resin composite,[212] and tip distances greater than 6 mm away from the surface of the increment can significantly decrease resin composite cure.[230] The condition of the curing unit can, of course, also impact the effectiveness of the cure.[90]

Inconsistent Dentin Bonding (Marginal Leakage)

Polymerization shrinkage causes the composite to pull away from cavity margins, resulting in gap formation.[69,159,175] Despite advances in dentin bonding systems, they still do not consistently and reliably achieve bond strengths to dentin and cementum that are high enough to prevent this occurrence (Figs 10-13a and 10-13b).[223,244,270] This sometimes results in open margins, sensitivity, interfacial staining, and bacterial invasion.[48] In addition, the bond between adhesive and tooth has been shown to degrade with aging, both in vitro[284] and in vivo.[106,233]

Technique Sensitivity

Because of the negative aspects of using resin composite as a posterior restorative material described previously, the most important variable in clinical success is the placement technique.[293] There is little room for error.[82] Technique may account for the great variability reported in clinical success rates for posterior resin composite restorations.[166] The meticulous operative procedures demanded for placing these restorations require increased chair time. Clinical research has shown that posterior resin composite restorations require significantly more time to place than do comparable amalgam restorations.[179]

Indications for Resin Composite as a Posterior Restorative Material

Results of clinical studies demonstrate that resin composite can serve adequately when used in posterior restorations. Restorations placed in occlusal surfaces of molars fare worse than those in premolars, Class 2 restorations fare worse than Class 1 restorations, and large restorations fare worse than small-to-moderate–sized restorations. Therefore, limiting the size of the outline form and ensuring that most of the occlusal forces are absorbed by tooth structure are im-

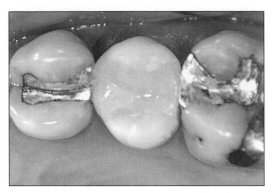

Fig 10-14 A resin composite restoration that exceeds one third the intercuspal distance. There is a greater likelihood of increased wear and fracture in a resin composite restoration this large.

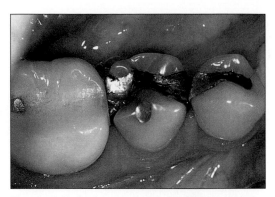

Fig 10-15 Defective mesio-occlusodistal amalgam restoration in the mandibular second premolar. Excessive width and need for cusp replacement precludes this amalgam restoration from being replaced with resin composite. A discolored fracture line running from the MOD amalgam to the amalgam in the facial cusp tip would necessitate making the replacement restoration to include the facial cusp.

portant to the clinical success of these restorations.[178,227,298] Based on these facts and the foregoing discussion, several factors should be considered before a posterior resin composite restoration can be recommended to a patient:

1. Esthetics should be a prime consideration.[283] There are few indications for resin composite in areas in which esthetics is not important.
2. The faciolingual width of the cavity preparation should be restricted to no more than one third of the intercuspal distance (Fig 10-14),[82,298] and, if possible, the gingival cavosurface margin in Class 2 restorations should be located on intact enamel.[87,117,119] Cuspal replacement with resin composite is not recommended (Fig 10-15).[4,119,283,295]
3. Centric occlusal stops should be located primarily on tooth structure.[283]
4. The patient should not exhibit excessive wear from clenching or grinding.[82]
5. The tooth should be amenable to rubber dam isolation.[2,82]

Autocured vs Light-Cured Resin Composites

Autocured resin composite restorative materials largely disappeared from clinical practice in the 1980s because of the popularity of the light-cured materials.

In recent years, some clinicians have recommended the use of autocured resin composites, either alone or in combination with VLC resin composites, for posterior applications.[24,93,94] The primary advantage of an autocured material is that it can be placed in bulk, saving time compared to the incremental insertion technique used with VLC materials.

Although more time-consuming, use of VLC resin composites has a number of advantages over use of autocured resin composites. Visible light–cured composites achieve more complete polymerization,[10] resulting in superior physical properties,[7,29,230] and they exhibit better color stability.[7,269] Autocured composites tend to incorporate voids as a result of mixing in two-paste systems,[79] and the increased porosity decreases tensile strength and surface smoothness,[57] accelerating wear.[161] Mixing interrupts the polymerization process and may compromise the size and configuration of the final polymer molecule, resulting in reduced strength and wear resistance.[290]

Visible light–cured composites should be used with an incremental placement technique to reduce the overall polymerization shrinkage of the final restoration.[262] This technique allows the practitioner to build up and sculpt the restoration. Research has shown VLC composite increments to have adequate interfacial strength.[213] Perhaps most important, VLC resin composites performed better in clinical trials than autocured materials over 1 year[176] and 3 years.[53]

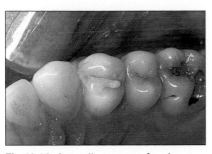

Fig 10-16 A small amount of resin composite is placed on the unprepared tooth to verify the shade prior to isolation with a rubber dam.

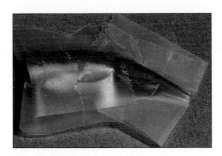

Fig 10-17 An appropriate resin is selected and placed into a light-protected syringe tip, the ends taped or the tip placed in a sealed plastic bag, and the protected syringe tip placed in a warm (60°C/140°F) water bath to reduce viscosity.

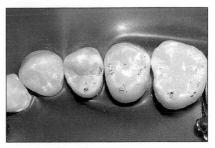

Fig 10-18 The occlusion is marked and rubber dam isolation achieved. The rubber dam has been inverted around the teeth to ensure moisture control.

Direct Posterior Resin Composite Restorations

Preoperative Evaluation

The factors noted previously as indications should be considered in the preoperative evaluation. The occlusion should be marked with articulating paper as a guide to preparation design. The best type of resin composite for the restoration should be chosen. At present, the heavily filled hybrid composites, with a mean particle size of 1 to 3 μm, are considered best suited for posterior use.[176,292]

For many posterior resin composite restorations, shade selection is not critical. In fact, some clinicians prefer a deliberate shade mismatch to aid in subsequent finishing and future evaluation procedures. But when shade is important, shade selection should be performed before isolation of the tooth, because isolated teeth become dehydrated, and dehydration changes the shade of the enamel. A shade is chosen from the shade guide that accompanies the composite, and then a small portion of the composite is placed on the unprepared and unetched tooth and polymerized (Fig 10-16). The resin "test shade" can be easily removed because the tooth surface has not been etched or primed prior to its placement.

If the resin composite material is in syringes rather than ampules, an appropriate amount of resin composite may be transferred to a syringe tip (Centrix) that is amber-colored or opaque to prevent premature polymerization. If a more fluid consistency of resin

composite is desired, the Centrix syringe tip, or single-use ampule, may be placed in a sealed plastic bag (eg, resealable sandwich bag) and placed in a warm water bath (60°C/140°F). This will reduce the resin composite's viscosity and aid in subsequent placement (Fig 10-17). The rationale for this technique is discussed in the section, "Class 2 Resin Composite Restorations" (page 278).

Isolation

Placement of a rubber dam is mandatory; failure to maintain a dry field will result in clinical failure.[165] In a clinical study, the margins of all Class 2 resin composite restorations placed without a rubber dam demonstrated marginal leakage 4 to 6 weeks after placement.[2] The rubber dam prevents moisture contamination and protects gingival tissues (Fig 10-18).[2]

Sealants and Preventive Resin Restorations

Sealants

While not normally considered to be posterior resin composite restorations, fissure sealants have been in use as a preventive restorative procedure for several decades. Sealants provide an effective means of reducing caries. Sealed teeth compared to unsealed teeth have demonstrated a reduction in caries by 35% over

5 years,[127] 43% over 4 years,[101] and 55% over 7 years.[187] However, there are a number of factors that must be considered regarding fissure sealant effectiveness. Numerous clinical studies have demonstrated that sealants tend to fail at a rate of 5% to 10% per year.[17,43,226,238,286] This is significant because the caries rate for teeth in which sealants are partially or totally lost increases significantly, in many cases equaling the caries rate of unsealed teeth.[43,101,127,187,238] The key to sealant success in preventing caries is total retention of the sealant.[127,187,238] Enhancing complete sealant retention will therefore enhance the caries reduction benefit. Some factors that affect sealant retention and effectiveness include:

1. Mandibular teeth show higher retention rates than maxillary teeth; premolars show higher retention rates than molars.[43,71,118]
2. Annual recall of patients and repair of partially or totally lost sealants improves effectiveness.[43,226,286]
3. Use of bonding agents prior to sealant placement helps to wet fissures,[55] improve sealant penetration into fissures,[258] increase bond strength,[123,267] improve sealant adhesion to saliva-contaminated enamel,[44,123,267] and improve clinical retention of sealants.[76,167]
4. Slight mechanical preparation of fissures with a No. 1/16 or 1/8 bur or air abrasion, to provide sound, unstained enamel prior to sealant placement, enhances sealant penetration and attachment, decreases bubble formation and improves marginal adaptation,[32,181,237] decreases marginal leakage,[109] improves microbial elimination,[154] and increases clinical retention compared to unprepared fissures.[237]
5. Clinical studies of resin-modified glass-ionomer sealants show good caries prevention but very poor retention compared to resin sealants. However, these studies are of very short duration, and the long-term effectiveness of resin-modified glass ionomers used as sealants remains unknown.[209,242]
6. Flowable resin composite materials may prove to perform well as fissure sealants. One clinical study has demonstrated improved performance of a flowable resin composite material when compared to a traditional resin sealant.[26]
7. The level of caries activity is critical to the cost-effectiveness of sealants; if a patient exhibits a low caries index, then the value of this procedure is low.[70] Clinical parameters including occlusal fissure morphology; number of decayed, missing, or filled surfaces (DMFS); and the clinician's subjective judgment are all significant predictors of future occlusal caries activity.[12,61] Therefore, sealant use should be based on a diagnosis of the patient's disease level and determination of the potential for future fissure caries; sealants should not be placed universally.

Preventive Resin Restorations

A restoration that maximizes the benefits of conservative, adhesive dentistry is the preventive resin restoration (PRR). Suggested by Ulvestad[271] in 1975 and popularized by Simonsen et al,[239–241] the PRR was developed to overcome problems associated with traditional "extension for prevention" in restorations necessitated by minimal occlusal caries lesions.

The PRR limits preparation to pits and fissures that are carious. Once the lesion is eliminated, no further preparation is performed. If the resultant preparation is restricted to narrow and shallow opening of the fissure, a resin sealant (or flowable resin composite material) is placed. If additional tooth structure is removed, a posterior resin composite is placed in that area, and the remaining fissures and the surface of the resin composite restoration(s) are sealed with resin sealant material or flowable composite. A number of advantages have been ascribed to this technique. They include:

1. Conservation of tooth structure: One 5-year clinical study determined that the average occlusal amalgam occupied 25% of the occlusal surface compared to just 5% for an average PRR.[285]
2. Enhanced esthetics: This is provided by the tooth-colored restorative material.[245]
3. Improved seal of restorative material to tooth structure: This is through the bond of resin composite to etched enamel with an adhesive resin.[148]
4. Minimal wear: This is due to restricted cavity preparations, so that occlusal contacts on the restoration are limited.[128]
5. No progression of sealed caries lesions: If a caries lesion is inadvertently allowed to remain in or at the base of a sealed fissure, it will not progress, because the seal prevents nutrients from supplying cariogenic bacteria.[186]
6. Good longevity: Clinical studies have demonstrated that PRRs are successful over periods up to 10 years[104,128,148,186,245] and can equal[285] or exceed the performance of amalgam restorations.[186]

The same provisos concerning sealants must be applied to PRRs; that is, the sealants placed in association with PRRs will tend to be lost at a rate of 5% to 10% per year.[104,128,245] Therefore, these restorations must be monitored over time, and the sealants and/or restorations must be repaired or replaced as needed.[245]

Indications and Contraindications

Preventive resin restorations are indicated when there are minimally or moderately carious fissures. The extent of the anticipated restoration should be minimal such that occlusal forces will be primarily limited to tooth structure. Such restorations are not indicated for restorations that will occupy a large area of the occlusal surface.

Technique

The preoperative evaluation, marking of occlusion, shade selection, and rubber dam isolation should be accomplished (Fig 10-19a). After the resin composite is selected, it may be used directly from a unit-dose ampule, or, if it is in a syringe, it should be placed into a light-protected syringe tip (see Fig 10-17). If desired, the viscosity of the resin composite may be further reduced by heating in a water bath to enhance adaptation to the cavity preparation as described in the section on Class 2 restorations.

The conservative adhesive preparation eliminates demineralized dentin, overlying unsupported enamel, and associated demineralized enamel. The preparation should be initiated with the smallest instrument that will accomplish this limited preparation, such as a No. 1/16 or 1/8 round bur (Fig 10-19b) or air abrasion. Larger instrumentation is used only as the size of the caries lesion dictates. Any fragile or unsupported enamel remaining on the occlusal surface after removal of the demineralized dentin should be removed. No bevels should be placed on the occlusal margins of the preparation.

Typically, these restorations are limited in size and depth, so no pulpal protection is needed (Fig 10-19c). Etching and application of a dentin bonding agent are the same as with other adhesive restorative procedures. Those areas of the preparation that have extended into dentin are filled with a posterior restorative resin composite that is cured in increments no greater than 2 mm in depth (Fig 10-19d). If the preparation is narrow and shallow, sealant material, flowable resin composite, or warmed resin composite may be used. Prior to curing the final increment, occlusal anatomy is developed with a hand instrument (Fig 10-19e). If, after curing the final increment, excess restorative material is present, the surface should be adjusted to provide desired contours and anatomy. If no adjustment is required, sealant is placed over the resin composite, through remaining prepared or unprepared etched fissures, and cured (Fig 10-19f). If adjustment is required, the entire fissure system, including the resin composite and its margins, should be re-etched and adhesive resin reapplied prior to sealant placement.[33,235] After completion of the restoration (Fig 10-19g), the rubber dam is removed and correct occlusion verified or obtained.

Figures 10-20a through 10-20o present an alternative technique for placing preventive resin restorations. In this technique, an occlusal stent is fabricated before tooth preparation and is used to form the occlusal anatomy.[275]

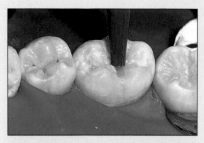

Fig 10-20j Warmed resin composite is syringed into deeper areas of the preparation.

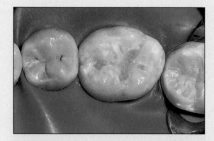

Fig 10-20k Maximum increment thickness is 2.0 mm; an initial increment is placed and cured in any area of the preparation deeper than 2.0 mm.

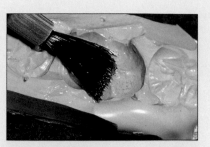

Fig 10-20l Impression is painted with a thin layer of adhesive resin.

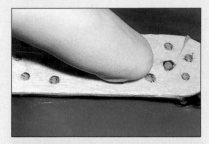

Fig 10-20m After syringing remaining warmed resin composite into the preparation, the impression is repositioned on the teeth.

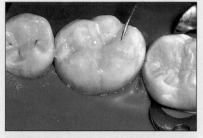

Fig 10-20n The impression is removed, and an explorer is used to remove excess resin composite material. With the flowability achieved by warming the resin composite and perfect adaptation of the impression to the teeth, all pits and fissures are filled with resin composite, making subsequent sealant placement unnecessary.

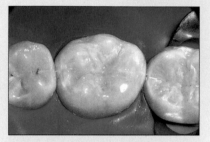

Fig 10-20o Completed restoration. A surface-penetrating sealant is placed and cured to ensure that all aspects of the occlusal surface are sealed. Close reproduction of the original occlusal surface with this technique often minimizes the need for occlusal adjustment.

Other Class 1 Resin Composite Restorations

When a Class 1 restoration is being placed due to initial carious lesion(s), the PRR is usually the technique of choice. If there was a previous restoration, the outline form and depth of the preparation will be determined by the previous restoration and any new pathosis. Margins of occlusal preparations for resin composite should not be beveled.[159a] Lining and bonding techniques should be used as described for Class 2 restorations.

Class 2 Resin Composite Restorations

As with preventive resin restorations, Class 2 restorations should be limited to obtaining access to the carious dentin, its removal, and the removal of any overlying fragile enamel and associated demineralized enamel.

Prewedging

Obtaining adequate interproximal contact in the final restoration starts at this stage of the restorative procedure, not at matrix placement or condensation, as is the norm for amalgam restorations. Uncured resin

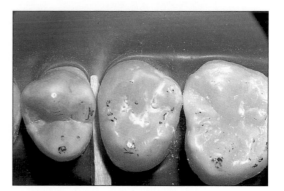

Fig 10-21 A wedge is placed before preparing the mesial surface of the maxillary second premolar; it provides tooth separation to help ensure adequate interproximal contact in the final restoration, and it helps prevent damage to the adjacent tooth, rubber dam, and gingival tissues.

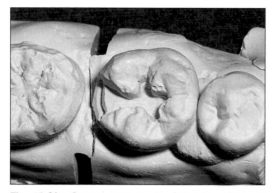

Fig 10-22a Stone cast made following Class 2 preparation involving the distal surface of a mandibular first molar.

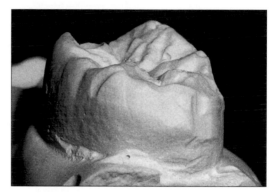

Fig 10-22b View of the mesial surface of the mandibular second molar shows the damage that resulted from inadequate protection during preparation of the distal surface of the first molar.

composites, even the so-called "packable" composites, do not have the ability to hold the matrix band in close adaptation to an adjacent tooth.[42,116] This makes obtaining an adequate interproximal contact one of the more difficult aspects of placing a Class 2 resin composite restoration. Placement of an interproximal wedge at the start of the procedure is recommended to open the contact with the adjacent tooth and to compensate for the thickness of the matrix band.[285] It has been demonstrated that multiple wedging, ie, inserting a wedge initially and then reapplying seating pressure several times during the course of the procedure, is more effective in opening the contact than is a single placement of a wedge.[281] In addition, the wedge can protect the rubber dam from damage and gingival tissues from laceration, and it can reduce leakage into the operative site.[283] Tooth separation obtained from prewedging promotes more conservative preparation and helps protect adjacent teeth from damage during preparation (Fig 10-21). Failure to take measures to protect adjacent teeth during proximal surface preparation with rotary instruments will usually result in damage to the adjacent teeth (Figs 10-22a and 10-22b).[170] Furthermore, this damage makes it significantly more likely that the damaged surface will require subsequent restoration.[217]

Preparation

As a general principle, preparation should be limited to eliminating carious tooth structure and providing access for restoration placement and finishing (Figs 10-23a to 10-23c). If there are one or more areas of fissure caries lesions in the tooth, in addition to the proximal surface lesion(s), they should be treated separately if possible, as described in the section on preventive resin restorations.

Bevel placement is a point of controversy with this preparation. When used in conjunction with adhesive agents and composite, bevels in enamel provide more area for acid etching and bonding. In addition, the

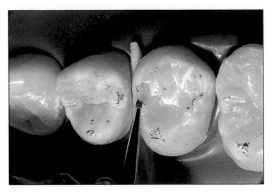

Fig 10-23a Preparation is initiated just inside the marginal ridge with a small round bur (No. ¼).

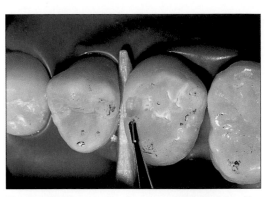

Fig 10-23b The preparation is extended with a No. 329 bur. Note that the proximal surface is left intact.

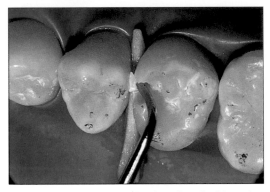

Fig 10-23c After the proximal surface is thinned, a spoon excavator is used to fracture and remove the thinned enamel.

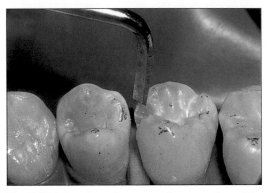

Fig 10-23d Bevels at the cavosurface margins of the proximal walls are placed with hand instruments.

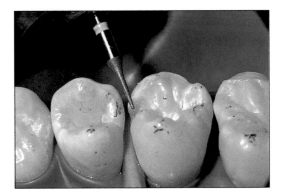

Fig 10-23e Alternatively, fine grit diamonds or carbide finishing burs can be used to place bevels.

bevel is designed to expose enamel rods transversely (cross cut, or "end-on") to achieve a more effective etching pattern. Research has shown that etching of transversely exposed enamel results in a bond that is significantly greater than that attained with a longitudinal etching (lengthwise) pattern.[193] Clinical research has demonstrated favorable results with the use of acid-etched beveled preparations in Class 3 resin composite restorations.[219]

Following are recommendations regarding bevel placement in Class 2 preparations for posterior resin composite restorations:

Facial and Lingual Proximal Margins

Conservative bevels (0.5 mm) should be placed, at approximately a 45-degree angle to the surface, on the facial and lingual cavosurface margins of the proximal box preparation (Figs 10-23d and 10-23e). This will achieve the benefits of beveling, as well as aid in placing the margins in a more accessible location for finishing and polishing. Research has demonstrated that bevels on these margins significantly reduce marginal leakage.[117,198,199]

Gingival Margins

The decision to place a gingival margin bevel requires clinical judgment. The gingival margin should be beveled only if the margin is well above the cementoenamel junction and an adequate band of enamel remains (Figs 10-5c and 10-24). When sufficient dentin-supported enamel remains for adequate bevel placement, resin composite adaptation is enhanced.[60] As the preparation nears the cementoenamel junction, the enamel layer is thinner than in other regions of the crown, and beveling the preparation increases the potential for removing the little enamel that remains. Because of the presence of prismless enamel in this region, acid etching is often less effective.[182] When a cavity preparation approaches within approximately 1 mm of the cementoenamel junction, adhesion is essentially no better than bonding to dentin (Figs 10-25a to 10-25c).[87,117,119]

Use of an inverse bevel, or so-called internal bevel, leaving enamel that is not supported by dentin at the gingival cavosurface margin (Fig 10-26), has been shown to significantly reduce microleakage compared to a butt margin[125] (Fig 10-26b) and would be preferable to placing the gingival margin on, or near, the cementoenamel junction. This type of marginal configuration should not be created with a bur, but if a lip of unsupported enamel remains after removal of demineralized dentin, it should be configured to an inverse bevel rather than planing the unsupported enamel off to form a butt margin in cementum or dentin. A groove in the gingival floor has been demonstrated to reduce microleakage if the gingival margin lies below the cementoenamel junction, and the so-called cervical groove should be considered when there is no enamel at the gingival cavosurface margin.[47]

Occlusal Margins

The use of occlusal cavosurface margin bevels is not indicated. Some have advocated the use of bevels on occlusal cavosurface margins to maximize the exposure of end-cut enamel rods.[182] However, it has been

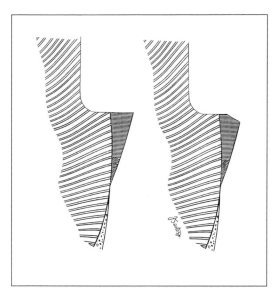

Fig 10-24 When enamel is adequate, a bevel is placed to enhance resin composite adaptation and seal.

noted that a normal preparation in the occlusal surface will result in end-cut enamel rods because of the orientation of the enamel rods in cuspal inclines[100] (Fig 10-27). Avoidance of bevels on the occlusal surface prevents the loss of sound tooth structure, decreases the surface area of the final restoration, lessens the chance of occlusal contact on the restoration, eliminates a thin area of composite that would be more susceptible to fracture, and presents a well-demarcated marginal periphery to which resin composite can be more precisely finished.[16,136,165,295]

Placement of occlusal bevels has demonstrated no benefit to clinical longevity of Class 2 resin composite restorations.[298] The most significant factor predicting the survivability of posterior resin composite restorations is the proportion of the occlusal surface restored; this factor is increased by occlusal beveling.[131,298] Therefore, occlusal cavosurface margin bevels should be avoided (Fig 10-28).

Use of Cavity Liners

If used, calcium hydroxide liner should be limited to those areas of the preparation that are believed to be very close to the pulp, where there is the possibility of

Figs 10-25a to 10-25c When adequate enamel remains at the gingival margin, a cavosurface margin bevel is placed to expose the ends of the enamel rods for etching.

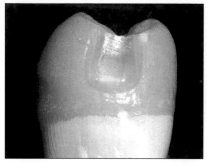
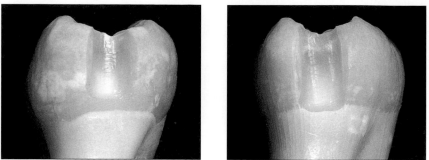

Fig 10-25a Appropriate proximal cavosurface margin bevels when the enamel is well above the cementoenamel junction. Gingival as well as facial and lingual vertical cavosurface margins are beveled.

Figs 10-25b and 10-25c As the gingival margin approaches 1 to 1.5 mm of the cementoenamel junction (CEJ) (b), or is apical to the CEJ (c), no gingival bevel is placed. Note that the facial and lingual vertical cavosurface margins are still beveled.

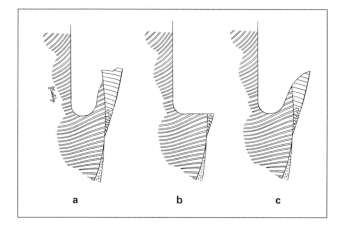

Fig 10-26 Excavation of a proximal caries lesion will sometimes result in a more gingival extent of the preparation in dentin than in enamel (a). If the preparation is extended straight out to the cavosurface, remaining enamel for bonding is compromised (b). Refining the preparation to eliminate very thin enamel and prepare an inverse bevel will expose enamel rods for etching on their internal ends and secure better adhesion to the gingival margin (c). Assuming removal of carious dentin created the situation shown in (a), the marginal configuration shown in (c) is preferable to that in (b).

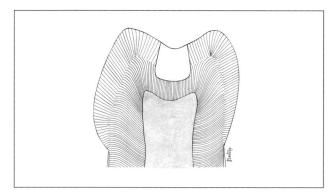

Fig 10-27 The enamel rods on the occlusal surface are oriented in such a way that the ends are exposed without beveling.

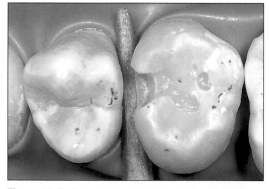

Fig 10-28 Finished preparation. The tooth has been prepared only in those areas where carious dentin was present. The preparation has not penetrated to dentin in other areas of the occlusal surface. Proximal facial, lingual, and gingival cavosurface margins have been beveled; occlusal cavosurface margins have not been beveled.

a minute pulpal exposure.[18] Placement of a calcium hydroxide liner over an extensive area of dentin provides no benefit to the pulp and decreases the surface area for adhesion. Dissolution of the liner during acid etching can interfere with a sound bond to enamel and dentin.[166] If the preparation is conservative in size, no liner is required in addition to adhesive agent. In deeper preparations and those in which the gingival margin approaches or extends beyond the cementoenamel junction, a glass-ionomer liner may be beneficial. Pulpal considerations are discussed in depth in Chapter 5.

Glass-ionomer liners are reported to offer a number of potential advantages when used under posterior resin composite restorations. Glass-ionomer materials bond to both tooth structure and overlying resin composite,[246] and they introduce less polymerization stress into tooth structure than does resin composite.[78] Glass-ionomer releases fluoride into adjacent tooth structure,[36] which may be advantageous because of the tendency for secondary caries lesions to occur adjacent to posterior resin composite restorations.[165] Use of a glass-ionomer liner has been demonstrated to improve marginal integrity[173] and decrease marginal leakage.[2,110,214] Less bulk of resin composite material is required to fill the preparation, reducing the amount of polymerization shrinkage[15,155] and improving marginal adaptation.[175] Glass-ionomer liners, particularly the autocuring versions, have excellent rigidity,[39] which helps to decrease deformation of resin composite under load. This results in reduced wear and improved marginal integrity. Glass-ionomer cement can reinforce the preparation walls by adhering to dentin and minimizing cuspal deformation under load.[155] Glass-ionomer liners also reduce the rise in pulpal temperature associated with application of the curing light during incremental insertion procedures.[102] However, with improvements in dentin adhesives, the use of glass ionomer under posterior resin composite restorations has been greatly reduced in recent years. If an adequate band of enamel surrounds the entire preparation, a glass-ionomer liner is usually not necessary.

If the gingival margin of a Class 2 preparation is in enamel but within 1 mm of the cementoenamel junction, or if it is in dentin, and an alternative restorative material cannot be used, a resin-modified glass-ionomer material should be placed as the initial increment in the proximal box. This technique, known as the "bonded base" or "open sandwich" technique, has been demonstrated to reduce in vitro marginal leakage[3,188] as well as in vivo demineralization adjacent to the gingival margin.[40a]

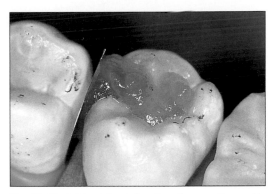

Fig 10-29 Acid etchant is placed over the entire preparation. A small piece of matrix has been placed to protect the adjacent proximal surface.

Acid Etching

The walls of the preparation should be etched with 37% phosphoric acid for 15 seconds and rinsed.[35] A small piece of metal matrix band material is placed to protect the adjacent proximal surface from being etched. This will prevent inadvertent bonding to this surface in subsequent resin composite placement procedures (Fig 10-29). The enamel is examined for a frosted matte appearance to confirm proper enamel conditioning (see Fig 10-20h).

Application of Bonding Resin

The manufacturer's instructions for the particular bonding system should be followed. In most fourth-generation (multicomponent) adhesive systems, a primer is placed after etching, followed by an adhesive. The primer is usually a hydrophilic resin contained in a volatile liquid carrier. After application of the primer, the carrier evaporates, leaving behind a very thin layer of resin. It is imperative that the solvent be thoroughly evaporated with compressed air before adhesive placement; failure to do so will significantly impair the quality of adhesion, particularly to dentin.[261] The adhesive is then applied in a thin layer (Fig 10-30a) and thinned further with a blotted brush (Fig 10-30b). Care should be taken not to overly thin the adhesive layer. Research has demonstrated that increased adhesive resin thickness results in reduced

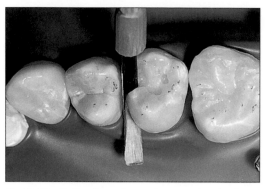

Fig 10-30a Following primer placement and solvent evaporation, adhesive resin is placed with a brush.

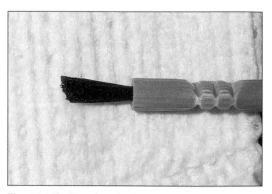

Fig 10-30b The brush is blotted with a gauze sponge and then used to absorb excess adhesive resin from the preparation. Air thinning of the adhesive component of fourth-generation (multiple component) dentin bonding systems should be avoided.

polymerization shrinkage stress,[191] decreased gap formation,[202] and decreased microleakage.[257] Compressed air should not be used to thin the adhesive resin because this has been shown to significantly reduce bond strength.[118] However, it is possible to leave adhesive layers that are too thick, which can also reduce bond strength.[160] In addition, layers of adhesive that are 42 μm thick or greater can be detected on bite-wing radiographs[202] and mistaken for a marginal defect or a caries lesion.

In fifth-generation, or "single-bottle," adhesive systems, in which the primer and adhesive components have been combined, a different placement technique is required. Air thinning is needed to ensure adequate evaporation of the solvent; however, the air stream also thins the adhesive. Additional applications of these adhesive systems (double the number noted by the manufacturer) are recommended to maximize the bond to dentin.[120]

If the preparation is etched and the bonding resin is placed before application of the matrix, visualization and access to all areas of the preparation are better, and it is easier to brush thin the adhesive and avoid pooling. A small piece of matrix band material, used to protect the adjacent proximal surface, may be kept in place. However, the wedge should either not be replaced at this time or it should be placed between the piece of matrix material and the preparation. This enables the resin adhesive access to all areas of the preparation and provides an escape for the adhesive resin at the margin, to prevent it from pooling. Placement of a matrix after applying the adhesive sometimes results in contamination of the preparation with blood or saliva, so the operator may prefer to place the matrix and

wedge prior to etching and application of the adhesive. If so, special care must be taken to ensure the absence of pooling of the resin adjacent to the matrix. Enamel and dentin adhesives are discussed at length in Chapter 8.

Matrix Application

Several useful matrices are available, including the clear plastic matrix, the ultrathin (0.001-inch) Tofflemire metal matrix (Figs 10-31a and 10-31b), the thin (0.0015-inch) sectional matrix, and the Tofflemire metal matrix with photoetch-thinned (0.0005-inch) contact areas.

The clear matrix can be used in conjunction with a light-reflecting wedge (Fig 10-31b) and offers the advantage of allowing penetration of the curing light from multiple directions. This allows the clinician to cure the increments of resin composite from the proximal and gingival directions, rather than from the occlusal aspect only, to ensure adequate polymerization of each increment. In addition, it has been reported that this technique allows more favorable direction of the polymerization shrinkage. One study showed enhanced gingival margin adaptation using this technique when the proximal box was prepared in enamel,[173] although another study failed to show a similar benefit when the gingival margin was in dentin.[119] However, the clear matrix is thicker than the thinnest metal matrices, and its lack of rigidity makes placement through tight interproximal contacts difficult.[16] In addition, the rigidity and smoothness of the plastic, light-reflecting wedge makes it less effective in gaining the slight tooth separation needed to ensure adequate interproximal

Figs 10-31a and 10-31b *Two common matrices for Class 2 resin composite restorations.*

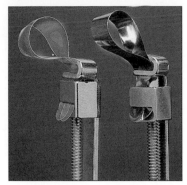

Fig 10-31a Clear and metal matrix bands are shown with Tofflemire retainers.

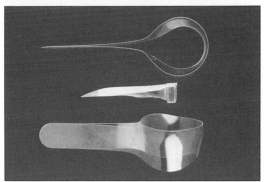

Fig 10-31b The clear matrix is usually used with a light-reflecting wedge.

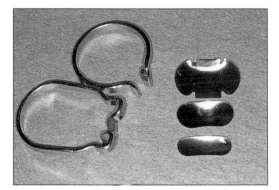

Fig 10-32a Palodent sectional matrix system (Darway).

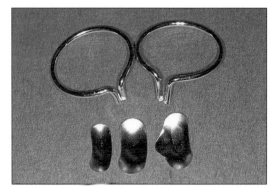

Fig 10-32b Composi-Tight sectional matrix system (Garrison Dental Solutions).

contact. Methods to compensate for this lack of separation are described later in this chapter.

Tight interproximal contacts are more easily developed with the ultrathin metal matrices than with the clear matrices, because they are easier to place, maintain their shape better, and can be burnished against the adjacent tooth.[16] One disadvantage of a metal matrix that wraps around the facial and lingual surfaces of the tooth is that increments must be initially cured only from the occlusal aspect. After removal of the matrix, the proximal resin composite may be further polymerized from the facial and lingual aspects. To avoid flat proximal surface contours, metal matrices should be shaped or contoured by burnishing before they are placed.

Other devices that are helpful in developing adequate interproximal contact are the sectional matrix systems, used with metal rings with springlike properties (Figs 10-32a and 10-32b). After the sectional matrix and wooden wedge are placed, the ring is placed using rubber dam clamp forceps, or similar forceps, so that the vertical points of the ring are positioned in the facial and lingual embrasures adjacent to the box preparation. The ring holds the ends of the sectional matrix tightly against the tooth and exerts a continuous separating force between the teeth. These systems have a number of advantages (Fig 10-33): they provide wedging to ensure good interproximal contact; they provide better proximal contour for posterior resin composite restorations than traditional matrices; and they simplify matrix placement for single proximal surface restorations, compared to a circumferential band.[114,115] It should be recognized that the ring provides progressive tooth separation, so, if it is left in place for a long period of time, excess separation can occur, resulting in a contact that is too tight.

Yet another type of sectional matrix involves a short piece of thin, stainless steel matrix material that is con-

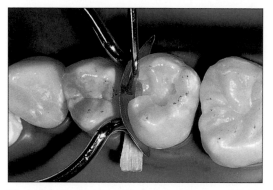

Fig 10-33 Sectional matrix and ring in place. Matrix is burnished in the contact area to enhance proximal contour and contact.

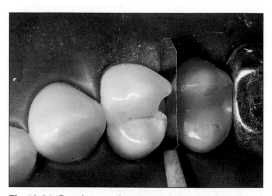

Fig 10-34 Passive sectional matrices are placed and wedged. Resin composite will be sculpted in facial and lingual embrasures with a thin instrument such as an interproximal carver.

toured only occlusogingivally and does not surround the tooth at all (Fig 10-34). This allows some light curing from facial and lingual aspects. The contoured matrix is secured with a wooden wedge and lies passively against the adjacent tooth surface or is held there with an instrument during curing of the first increment. That increment then holds the matrix against the adjacent tooth during placement of succeeding increments. When this technique is used, resin composite in facial and lingual embrasures must be contoured or sculpted with a thin-bladed instrument, such as an interproximal carver (IPC), prior to curing.

Resin Composite Placement: Incremental Technique

Visible light–cured resin composite should be placed in successive, laminated increments to ensure proper curing and prevent excessive polymerization shrinkage.[15,234] Incremental curing decreases the effects of polymerization shrinkage, enhances marginal adaptation, decreases gap formation, reduces marginal leakage, decreases cuspal deformation, makes the cusps more resistant to subsequent fracture, and decreases postoperative sensitivity.[52,63,69,137,173,175,196]

First Increment

Some general guidelines should be followed for the placement of the resin composite. Proper handling of the bonding system and resin composite at the gingival margin is critical because of the tendency for microleakage to occur in that area.[214] A clinical study that assessed gingival margin quality in Class 2 resin composite restorations showed that only 27% were

satisfactory.[197] Therefore, techniques must be used to enhance the bond and reduce the adverse effects of polymerization shrinkage. First, an increment no thicker than 1.0 mm is placed against the gingival floor.[36] A thin first layer will ensure proper light irradiation throughout the increment. A light, translucent shade should be used in the box to maximize polymerization.[296] Because this portion of the restoration is rarely critical from an esthetic standpoint, a shade mismatch with the tooth will not adversely affect the final appearance of the restoration.

If a clear matrix and light-reflecting wedge are being used, the initial curing should be directed through the flat end of the wedge. The amount of light that a reflecting wedge will transmit varies in the literature. One study indicated that 90% to 95% of the incident light is transmitted,[173] while another showed that it could be as low as 66%.[46] Because of the possible attenuation of light through the wedge, exposure time should be increased by 50% (to 60 seconds) to ensure adequate polymerization. It has been suggested that the light-reflecting wedge will direct the curing light to the gingival margin of the restoration and draw the polymerization shrinkage toward that margin. When the gingival margin is on enamel, this method has been shown to result in better marginal adaptation than curing from an occlusal direction.[172–175] However, when the gingival margin is on dentin, this technique failed to reduce gingival margin microleakage compared to other techniques.[119]

Because the plastic wedges are rigid and smooth, they may slip out of proper position easily and may not maintain the pressure necessary to ensure proper adaptation of the gingival aspect of the matrix band

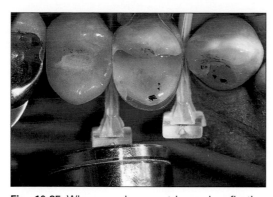

Fig 10-35 When a clear matrix and reflecting wedge are used, the initial cure for the gingival resin composite increment is through the wedge. The end of the light guide can be used to maintain pressure on the smooth plastic wedge during initial polymerization to help ensure interproximal contact. Due to loss of irradiance when curing through a wedge, cure times should be increased by one half.

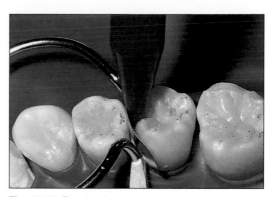

Fig 10-36 Previously warmed resin composite is syringed into the preparation via a Centrix placement tip to maximize adaptation to the cavity walls.

and separation from the adjacent tooth. Two suggestions may help to overcome this problem. After the plastic wedge is positioned, a wooden wedge is inserted beside it on the side away from the tooth being restored. Alternatively, the plastic wedge can be maintained in proper position with the light-curing tip during curing of the initial increment (Fig 10-35). After this is completed, the plastic wedge has accomplished its purpose and may be replaced with a wooden wedge for succeeding increments.

If a metal matrix that surrounds the tooth has been chosen, all increments must be cured from the occlusal direction. The tip of the light should be positioned as close as possible to the resin being cured.[19,83] After the metal matrix is removed, all proximal areas of the restoration should receive additional curing with the light.

Resin composites that are marketed for posterior use vary widely in their viscosity.[200] This can have an impact on adaptation of resin composite to the walls of a cavity preparation.[201] Thicker-consistency resin composites have significantly increased cavity wall voids compared to medium or thinner viscosity materials.[200] Resin composites that are supplied in preloaded resin composite tips, or ampules, tend to have a higher viscosity than do composites that are supplied in syringes.[200] Placement technique can also determine how well the resin composite adapts to the cavity preparation walls. Use of a placement tip (Centrix) (Fig 10-36) for resin composite decreases the viscosity of the material[200] and significantly decreases voids adjacent to the preparation walls compared to either smearing the material into place with a plastic instrument or "condensing" it.[201] A technique that will further enhance the flow of the resin composite into a cavity preparation is to use resin composite that is supplied in a syringe, transfer the required amount of material into a Centrix syringe tip, put the tip in a small sealed plastic bag (see Fig 10-17), and place it into a warm water bath (140°F/60°C) to reduce the viscosity. This material can then be more easily syringed into place, and the lowered viscosity enhances resin composite adaptation to the cavity walls (Fig 10-36). This prewarming of the resin composite does not adversely affect either the strength or degree of cure.[168]

Another method that has been suggested is the use of low-viscosity or "flowable" resin composites for the first increment.[21] The rationale is that these materials flow more readily than standard hybrid formulations and will therefore easily and thoroughly adapt to all areas of the cavity preparation. Also, because of their lower filler content and reduced elastic modulus, it is theorized that these materials could act as "stress breakers" to absorb forces of polymerization shrinkage or cyclic loading.[20] However, the efficacy of this method has not been demonstrated.[20]

There are a number of problems associated with these materials. Because of their higher resin content,[20] flowable resin composites demonstrate up to three times greater polymerization shrinkage than do standard hybrid resin composite formulations.[157,264] This would likely result in significantly greater polymeriza-

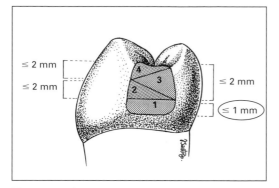

Fig 10-37a If a metal matrix is used with a light-curing resin composite, the minimal (1.0 mm) gingival increment is placed and cured. The material is then layered in alternating oblique increments. No increment exceeds 2.0 mm in thickness. To minimize cuspal deformation and polymerization stress, an oblique increment should not contact both facial and lingual cavity walls. This placement technique can also be used with a clear matrix and reflecting wedge.

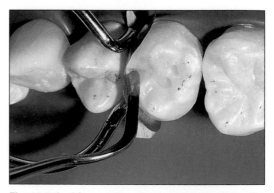

Fig 10-37b After curing the initial increment, the next increment is syringed into place and "ramped" obliquely with a plastic instrument or interproximal carver. Here the Composi-Tight matrix and ring are being used, and an oblique increment is being shaped with an interproximal carver.

tion shrinkage forces generated at the restoration–cavity preparation interface. The use of a flowable resin composite in conjunction with Class 2 resin composite restorations has failed to produce reduced marginal leakage in studies.[231,280] In addition, due to their lower filler loading, flowable resin composites have inferior physical properties compared to traditional resin composites.[20] This leads to concern that the occlusal forces may introduce increased deflection of the overlying hybrid resin composite, which has a higher modulus of elasticity, due to the inability of the flowable resin composite to provide adequate support.[20] In fact, the use of a flowable resin liner in conjunction with a high-viscosity (packable) resin composite has been shown to weaken the strength of the packable material.[220]

A final and significant concern with flowable resin composites pertains to their radiopacity. Most flowable resin composites have not met the standard of being at least as radiopaque as enamel, the guideline that enables adequate distinction of tooth demineralization due to caries from the restorative material.[194] Given this research data and the resultant concerns generated, it would be prudent to wait until this technique has been proven effective in controlled clinical trials before using it.

Additional Increments

Subsequent increments should be placed in thicknesses no greater than 2.0 mm. If a surrounding metal matrix is employed, an oblique layering technique should be used (Figs 10-37a and 10-37b), and the restoration should be cured from the facial and lingual aspects after removal of the matrix (Fig 10-38). If a clear matrix is employed, the oblique technique (Fig 10-37a) or a vertical technique (Fig 10-39) should be used. Use of these techniques allows initial curing to occur from the facial or lingual direction and for polymerization shrinkage to be directed toward the facial or lingual proximal preparation walls and margins. This has been shown to improve marginal integrity[105,262] and decrease cuspal deformation.[159,234]

When the proximal boxes have been filled and the resin polymerized, the occlusal channel, if present, is filled and cured incrementally. With the exception of the initial increment in the gingival aspect of the proximal box, subsequent resin composite increments should not contact both the facial and lingual preparation walls simultaneously; this is to minimize cuspal deformation.[63] Figures 10-40a to 10-40d present posterior resin composite restorations placed using a clear matrix and light-reflecting wedges.

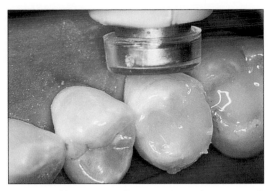

Fig 10-38 If a surrounding metal matrix was used, the restoration should be cured from the facial and lingual aspects after matrix removal.

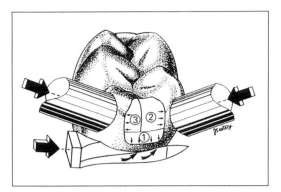

Fig 10-39 If a clear matrix is used with a light-reflecting wedge, after the initial increment, succeeding increments may be placed using a wide and a narrow vertical increment, as shown. Alternatively, succeeding increments may be placed obliquely as shown in Fig 10-37a.

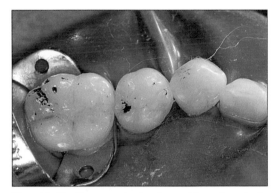

Figs 10-40a Preoperatively, the rubber dam is in place and the occlusion is marked.

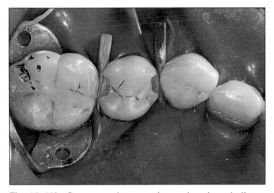

Fig 10-40b Conservative mesio-occlusal and disto-occlusal preparations have been made in the mandibular left second premolar. Wooden wedges are in place for prewedging.

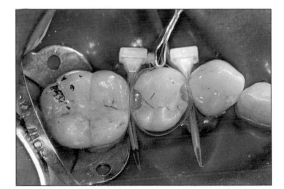

Fig 10-40c A clear matrix and reflecting wedges in place.

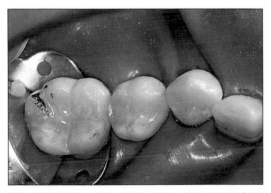

Fig 10-40d When the resin composite restorations are completed, a surface sealer is placed.

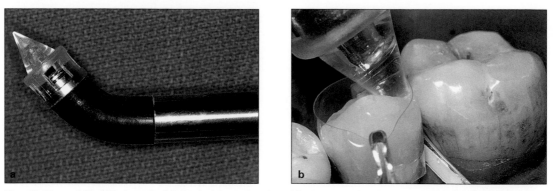

Figs 10-41a and 10-41b A conical light tip (a) can be placed into uncured resin composite increment (b) to provide curing while also pushing the matrix against the adjacent tooth to enhance proximal contact.

An alternative to the layering techniques is the use of a conical light-curing tip (Figs 10-41a and 10-41b). The proximal box is filled with composite to just gingival to the contact area, and the conical tip is wedged into the resin composite. The cone is used to apply pressure to the matrix band and push it against the adjacent tooth during curing. Subsequent increments restore the cone-shaped gap formed by the tip. This technique is designed to ensure adequate interproximal contact and to minimize the thickness of resin composite that the light must penetrate. While the technique is relatively untested, initial study results have shown formation of fewer marginal gaps than in the more traditional incremental techniques,[72] as well as improved hardness and decreased porosity.[279]

A similar technique to help establish interproximal contact is to place the first increment into the proximal box as with the conical light-curing tip technique, but instead of the matrix being pushed with the conical tip, it is held against the adjacent tooth during the polymerization with a plastic instrument, condenser, or similar instrument. That increment, after it is hardened, will then hold the matrix against the tooth as successive increments are placed.

The use of prepolymerized resin composite "balls" has also been suggested to aid in establishing interproximal contact. The normal incremental technique is used until the proximal box is filled to just before the proximal contact. A small, slightly flattened ball of composite is precured on the tip of an instrument (eg, a Hollenback No. ½ carver). An additional increment of uncured resin composite is placed into the proximal box. The precured ball is pushed into this increment to wedge the matrix tightly against the adjacent tooth, then the resin composite is cured (Fig 10-42).[282]

If both the mesial and distal surfaces of a tooth are being restored with resin composite, it is sometimes difficult to obtain adequate interproximal separation for both proximal surfaces simultaneously. When mesio-occlusal and disto-occlusal restorations (or a mesio-occlusodistal restoration) are being placed, one proposed remedy is to remove the wedge from one interproximal area, reapply pressure to the remaining wedge to maximize separation, and incrementally place resin composite to fill that box only. The wedge is then removed from the interproximal area adjacent to the restored surface and inserted adjacent to the unrestored surface, and that box is incrementally filled. Sectional matrix systems with rings may be used in a similar manner, or simultaneously, on the mesial and distal aspects (Fig 10-43).

Final Increment

Careful control of the final increment will minimize the amount of finishing. A rounded cone-shaped instrument (eg, PKT3), slightly moistened with some resin adhesive, may be used to shape and form the occlusal surface before curing (Fig 10-44). Some clinicians recommend use of a resin composite that has a slightly different shade from the tooth to aid in locating margins during finishing procedures.[93] After removal of the wedge and matrix, the resin composite is

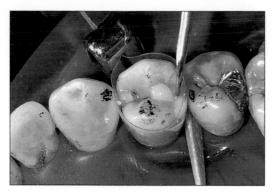

Fig 10-42 Use of a precured resin composite "ball" to establish proximal contact. A small amount of composite is placed on the tip of an instrument (such as the Hollenback No. ½ carver) and cured. It is then pushed into uncured resin composite material in the proximal box. While the precured ball is wedged tightly against the contact, the composite in the proximal box is cured.

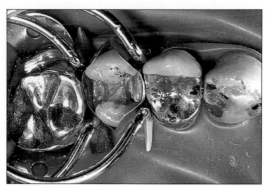

Fig 10-43 Simultaneous mesial and distal placement of sectional matrices and rings for an MOD restoration.

cured from the facial and lingual aspects to help ensure adequate polymerization throughout the entire restoration (see Fig 10-38).

Resin Composite Placement: Other Techniques

Materials other than visible light–cured resin composites have been suggested for placement in the proximal box preparation. Autocured (or self-curing) resin composites are available for this purpose in both low- and high-viscosity formulations. It has been suggested that the portion of the autocured resin composite adjacent to the cavity preparation walls cures first, especially if used in conjunction with an autocured (or dual-cured) adhesive. The shrinkage of the autocured composite is said to be directed toward the cavity walls due to initiation of the curing reaction by the ongoing polymerization of the adhesive resin, and the reaction is said to be accelerated in that area by the higher temperature of the preparation walls due to body heat. This supposedly results in less polymerization shrinkage stress at the cavity margins,[24,93] thus improving marginal adaptation. However, research has failed to demonstrate either enhanced marginal adaptation[274] or reduced marginal leakage when this technique has been compared to VLC incremental placement techniques.[119]

Another class of materials that is sometimes suggested for use in the proximal box is the dual-cured resin-modified glass ionomers. The self-curing glass ionomers are placed in a manner similar to that used

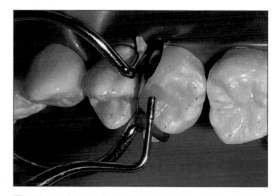

Fig 10-44 A small condenser or burnisher, lightly moistened with adhesive, is used to establish preliminary occlusal contours in the final resin composite increment before light curing.

for the autocured resin composites and allowed to polymerize. The VLC or dual-cured resin-modified glass ionomers should be placed using a technique similar to that used for VLC resin composites. A significant benefit to the use of a restorative glass ionomer in the gingival portion of the proximal box is the protection it provides against carious demineralization.[40a] All of the glass-ionomer materials should be veneered occlusally with a VLC resin composite.

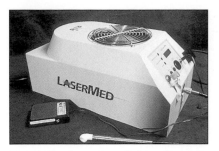

Fig 10-45a Argon laser light-curing unit.

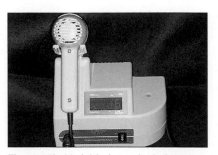

Fig 10-45b Variable-intensity halogen light–curing unit.

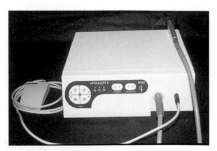

Fig 10-45c Plasma arc high-intensity light-curing unit.

Resin Composite Placement: Alternative Polymerization Techniques

A number of alternative techniques and devices have been introduced for curing visible light–cured resin composites in recent years, including lasers, plasma arc high-intensity units, and halogen units that allow variable curing intensity (Figs 10-45a to 10-45c).

Argon laser units have demonstrated the ability to produce an increased degree of cure of resin composite compared to standard halogen light–curing units.[260] In addition, the depth of cure with the laser is improved,[260] and bond strength is less affected as the light guide is moved further from the surface of the resin composite.[121] However, when the light guide is kept approximated to the composite increment, and increment depth is limited to 1.5 to 2 mm, no difference in bond strength is seen between laser and standard halogen lights.[121,236] Laser light is monochromatic,[121] with the band width of the laser being much narrower than that of the halogen light, and centered at approximately 470 nm, the maximal absorption wavelength for camphorquinone, the photoinitiator used in most resin composites.[28,260] However, some manufacturers are starting to use proprietary photoini- tiators with absorption spectra differing from that of camphorquinone, making it possible that the argon laser curing unit would be less likely to initiate the polymerization reaction than a halogen unit.

Plasma arc units generate notably higher irradiance levels than do standard halogen units. The purpose of this increased intensity is to increase the resin composite polymerization rate. Argon laser units also cure resin composite at a faster rate than do the halogen curing lights.[260] Considerable evidence has been accumulated to show that this increased rate of cure does not enhance adhesion of resin composite to cavity walls. Class 5 restorations cured with argon lasers or plasma arc units showed significantly increased microleakage[216] and poorer marginal adaptation[40] compared to similar restorations cured with a standard halogen curing light. This is likely due to the fact that the rate at which the modulus of elasticity, or stiffness, of the setting composite develops has a significant impact on marginal integrity. Decreasing the polymerization reaction rate allows additional time for molecular conformational changes and material flow that can relieve polymerization shrinkage stress.[78,144] This has led to research in which the polymerization reaction rate is slowed even further by reducing the irradiance of halogen curing units. Lowering irradiance to 250 mW/cm² has been shown to significantly improve marginal adaptation in cavity preparations vs irradiating the resin composite in those same preparations at either 450 mW/cm²,[273] or 650 mW/cm².[80] There has been some concern, however, that simply reducing the irradiance to these levels, while enhancing marginal adaptation, might adversely affect physical properties.[273] This has led to the "two-step," "soft-start," or "ramped" curing technique. Regardless of the name, the underlying principle is the same: initial cure at diminished irradiance to initiate the polymerization reaction at a slower rate to minimize polymerization stress, followed by a period of higher irradiance to maximize degree of cure and physical properties. This technique has proven to significantly enhance marginal adaptation without impairing physical properties.[40,153,185]

A recent evaluation of dental practices revealed that 46% of the halogen visible light–curing units provided inadequate output to cure resin composite.[211] It is important for the practitioner to ensure that the curing light unit is in proper working condition and provides adequate and accurate irradiance. This can be conveniently accomplished with a radiometer (Fig 10-46).

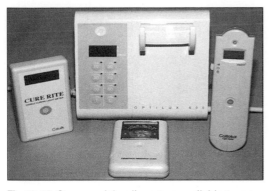

Fig 10-46 Commercial radiometers available to monitor adequacy of visible light–curing unit irradiance. (Courtesy of USAF Dental Investigation Service.)

Packable Resin Composites

A relatively recent introduction is the category known as "condensable" or "packable" resin composites, specifically designed for posterior use. In these materials, the manufacturers have altered the filler type, size, and/or particle distribution[44a,259] to increase viscosity and impart a consistency that more closely mimics that of dental amalgam. In addition, claims of enhanced clinical performance, reduced polymerization shrinkage, and enhanced wear characteristics have been made. The term *condensable* is not appropriate for these materials, since condensation, by definition, denotes an increase in density, as occurs when dental amalgam is condensed into a cavity preparation. Such a volume reduction does not occur with resin composites when they are pushed into a preparation.[44a]

Considerable in vitro research has been accomplished to test these materials. In general, properties such as wear,[14,44a,54,151,253] flexural modulus,[143,228] flexural strength,[143,177,228] fracture toughness,[143,145] and polymerization shrinkage[44a] of the packable resin composites are comparable, but not superior, to those of other hybrid or reinforced microfilled resin composites currently available. One clinical study of a packable composite showed extreme and unacceptable wear.[89] Of particular concern with the packable resin composites is the claim by some manufacturers that these materials can be bulk-cured in thicknesses of 5 mm or greater. Independent research has clearly demonstrated that this is not the case, and adequate polymerization of the resin composite can be accomplished only in thicknesses of 2 mm or less.[116,145]

In general, practitioners can anticipate that the handling characteristics of the packable resin composite formulations may vary somewhat from other hybrid or microfilled materials. In particular, they may have a heavier consistency with a "drier" feel. However, current research seems to indicate that, with proper technique, the clinical performance of these materials can be comparable to that of other resin composites. The decision to use these materials should be based on individual operator preference concerning handling characteristics and not on expectations of improved clinical performance.

Finishing

Placement procedures that minimize the need for finishing and polishing should be used. The smoothest surface that can be obtained is that of unfinished resin composite that has been cured against a smooth matrix.[45,124,126,215] Finishing and polishing procedures are inherently destructive to the restoration surface[4] and may result in the formation of microcracks below the surface.[164,299] Because cracks may also be produced or exacerbated during mastication, the fracture toughness of the resin composite may be significantly reduced by destructive finishing techniques.[84]

Early finishing of resin composite (3 minutes after placement) has been shown to significantly increase microleakage.[92] Therefore, finishing should be delayed as long as is practical to minimize adverse effects. Delaying finishing for 10 to 15 minutes will allow approximately 70% of maximal polymerization to occur during the "dark-curing" phase following application of the curing light.[6,7]

A variation of the previously described "soft-start" technique for posterior resin composite restorations is the so-called "pulse delay" technique. With this technique, the final composite increment is cured for a brief period (3 to 5 seconds) at very low irradiance (150 mW/cm^2) to initiate the curing reaction at a reduced rate. After 3 to 5 minutes, the composite is again cured with a high level of irradiance. During the interim between the two curing periods, the occlusal surface is shaped and finished.[139] It should be noted, however, that the effects of manipulating this incompletely cured resin composite on physical properties and clinical performance have not been determined by independent research.

The finishing and polishing process for posterior resin composite restorations is similar to that used with other composites. A No. 12 or 12b scalpel blade,

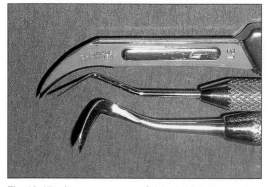

Fig 10-47a Instruments useful in initial contouring and removal of flash: *(top)* No. 12b scalpel blade; *(middle)* interproximal carver; *(bottom)* No. 14L carver.

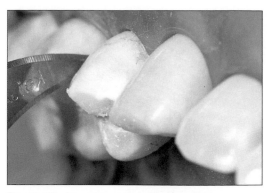

Fig 10-47b No. 12b scalpel blade used to remove flash from a resin composite restoration in the distal aspect of a maxillary first premolar.

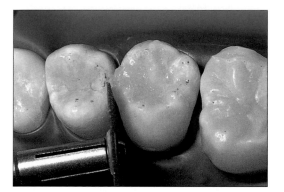

Fig 10-48 Aluminum oxide disk used to contour and polish the proximal surface of a resin composite restoration.

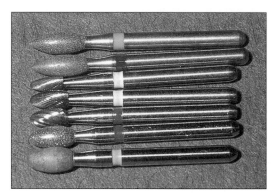

Fig 10-49 Fine diamonds and multifluted carbide burs for finishing resin composite restorations come in a variety of sizes, shapes, and grits.

sharp No. 14L carver, Wedelstaedt chisel, or other thin, sharp-edged hand instrument is useful for removing flash from the proximal and gingival margins and for shaping proximal surfaces of resin composite (Figs 10-47a and 10-47b). The composite material can then be finished and blended to the tooth with successively finer grits of polishing points, cups, or disks. Aluminum oxide disks, used in series from coarse to very fine, tend to impart among the smoothest finishes to resin composite.[23,124,126] These work well for restoration contours that are relatively flat or convex, such as those found in the facial and lingual proximal embrasure areas (Fig 10-48).

Abrasive disks are not practical for finishing occlusal surfaces. Shaping of these surfaces may be accomplished with multifluted carbide finishing burs or fine diamonds (Figs 10-49 and 10-50a). There is some controversy as to which of these instruments provides

the smoothest surface and/or minimizes trauma-induced microleakage. Studies indicate that carbide finishing burs perform better,[23] finishing diamonds perform better,[9,140] or both perform equally well.[30,126] It is clear that the use of burs with 18 or fewer flutes leaves a significantly roughened surface, so these burs should not be the final rotary instruments used in the finishing process.[126] Rubber or silicone disks, points, and cups, impregnated with aluminum oxide, have been found to provide very acceptable results[45,124,126] and can be used to smooth the resin composite surface after initial finishing (Fig 10-50b). Finishing strips coated with aluminum oxide can be used to finish proximal surfaces (Fig 10-50c). As with the disks, these strips should be used in series, from coarse to very fine grit. A final high polish may be accomplished using a rubber prophylaxis cup with aluminum oxide polishing pastes.

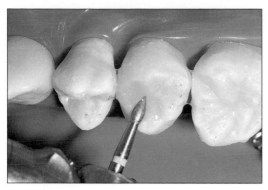

Fig 10-50a Finishing diamond used to refine occlusal anatomy in a resin composite restoration.

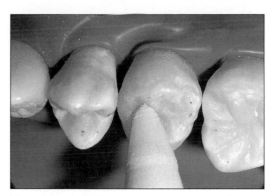

Fig 10-50b A flexible point impregnated with aluminum oxide is used for smoothing the resin composite of an occlusal surface.

Rebonding and Final Cure

As previously mentioned, finishing procedures are destructive to the resin composite restoration and have been shown to adversely affect wear.[128] In addition, the composite surface that was closest to the light tip during curing, and therefore has the best physical properties, is removed during finishing procedures. Finishing procedures can also exacerbate the marginal gaps formed during polymerization.[69,159,175]

For these reasons, the occlusal surface and all accessible restoration margins should be rebonded with an unfilled VLC resin. The lower the viscosity of the rebonding resin, the more effective it will be in penetrating interfacial gaps and microcracks.[222,261] Several low-viscosity resins, called surface sealers, are being marketed for use in rebonding. Rebonding, the application of a low-viscosity resin to the finished surface and margins of a restoration, has been shown to improve the marginal integrity of resin composite restorations in vitro[59] and in vivo,[142] significantly reduce microleakage in vitro,[95,222,263,265] and reduce marginal staining in vivo.[99] Rebonding has been demonstrated in clinical studies to significantly reduce wear and prolong marginal integrity; it may be performed yearly for maximal effectiveness.[59,99,142]

Although the need for etching before rebonding is somewhat controversial, phosphoric acid is usually applied to the marginal areas for 10 seconds (Fig 10-51a), rinsed off, and the area thoroughly dried. The rebonding resin is placed, thinned with a blotted brush (Fig 10-51b) or applicator, and light cured for 20 to 40 seconds. This will not only polymerize the rebonding resin, but may also provide additional

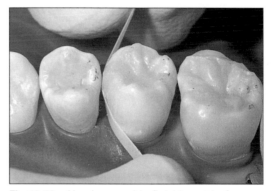

Fig 10-50c Aluminum oxide finishing strip for contouring/finishing/polishing the proximal surface gingival to the interproximal contact.

polymerization of the resin composite restoration.[19,229,230] To prevent the rebonding resin from joining the restored tooth to the adjacent tooth, a piece of matrix or other thin material may be placed interproximally prior to performing the rebonding procedure. Alternatively, floss is passed through the interproximal contact after the rebonding resin has been applied and before it is cured. After curing, any ledges of excess rebonding resin should be removed with a sharp-bladed instrument.

The proximal contact and contours are verified with dental floss (Fig 10-52). The rubber dam is removed, and the occlusion is checked. If further occlusal adjustment is required, rebonding resin should be reapplied in the areas that were adjusted.

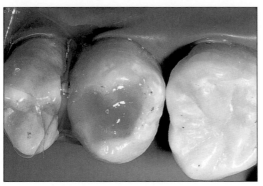

Fig 10-51a Etching the restoration margins prior to rebonding. Note the thin plastic shim placed interproximally to protect the adjacent tooth.

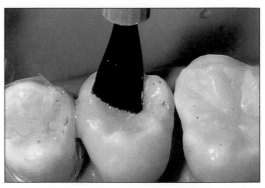

Fig 10-51b Rebonding resin is brushed onto the restoration surface and margins.

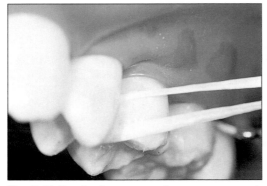

Fig 10-52 Proximal contact and contours are verified with dental floss. Floss is wrapped around the proximal contact to confirm appropriate contact area.

Advantages

Several advantages are claimed for this technique. The outer surface of the proximal enamel is removed only if cavitated by caries, so there is less potential for a restorative overhang. Overhangs have been shown to occur 25% to 76% of the time with traditional Class 2 restorations, resulting in gingivitis and bone loss.[34] With an occlusal approach, the marginal ridge is preserved, and destruction of tooth structure is minimized. A two-surface, Class 2 cavity preparation has been shown to reduce tooth stiffness by 46%; only a 20% reduction occurs with an occlusal preparation.[221] The perimeter of the restoration is reduced, decreasing the potential for microleakage.[206] Because minimal preparation is required interproximally, the potential for disturbance of the adjacent tooth is reduced. If the carious tooth structure is more extensive than originally thought and greater access is required, the preparation can easily be extended into a more traditional Class 2 design.[130]

■ The Tunnel Restoration

An alternative to the traditional approach for gaining access to proximal carious dentin has been termed the *tunnel preparation*. It was first suggested by Jinks[133] in 1963 as a method for placing a silver alloy mixed with sodium silicofluoride in the distal aspect of primary second molars to "inoculate" permanent first molars with fluoride as they erupted. Hunt[129] and Knight[150] later modified this procedure for use as a conservative technique for restoring teeth with small proximal carious lesions.

Disadvantages

Despite seemingly attractive benefits of the tunnel procedure, it remains largely unused in practice. It is a difficult procedure, demanding careful control of the preparation by the operator. The angulation of the bur for the preparation causes it to pass near the pulp. Studies have shown that the tunnel preparation often invades to within 1.0 mm of the pulp. A more traditional Class 2 preparation, in which penetration toward the pulp is determined by the depth of the carious lesion, tends to leave greater remaining dentinal thickness between the preparation and the pulp.[205,249] Because of the small entrance to the tunnel preparation, visibility is decreased, and removal of carious dentin is more uncertain.[129,130,301] In vitro studies on the effectiveness of carious lesion removal in the tunnel preparation have shown that there is a high rate of residual carious tooth structure after completion of the preparation.[204,249,250] For this reason, a caries-detecting solution should be used to disclose remaining carious tooth structure.

There is also concern that the marginal ridge is undermined and its strength reduced. As the diameter of the preparation increases, the marginal ridge strength decreases.[5,74,113] Although use of an adhesive restorative material has been shown to restore much of the strength of the marginal ridge,[5,74,113] this is not always the case,[205] and the degree to which marginal ridge strength is restored can depend on the size of the preparation.[7]

A number of clinical studies of tunnel restorations have been published (Table 10-4). Tunnel restorations tend to fail at a considerably higher rate than do other types of posterior restorations. Other problems noted in these studies include the fact that 34% to 41% of the restorations show either untreated carious dentin or progression of enamel caries.[210,248] The most common causes of restoration failure are marginal ridge fracture and secondary caries. In an evaluation of tunnel restorations compared to slot amalgam restorations, 21% of tunnel restorations failed over 7 years compared to zero failures for the slot restorations.[169]

Indications and Contraindications

Tunnel restorations are rarely indicated. Consideration of the tunnel preparation should be limited to those patients with high esthetic demands and a low caries index, who exhibit small, noncavitated proximal caries lesions that can be removed without penetrating the proximal surface.[108,248] This preparation should be avoided when large carious lesions are diagnosed, where access is particularly difficult, or when the overlying marginal ridge is subject to heavy occlusal loads or demonstrates a crack.

Preoperative Evaluation

The above factors must be assessed before the tunnel preparation is initiated. The occlusion should be marked with articulating paper.

Table 10-4	Longevity of tunnel restorations		
Investigators	Study time (y)	No. of restorations	Annual failure rate (%)
Pilebro et al, 1999[210]	3	262	6.7
Strand et al, 1996[248]	3	161	10.0
Lumley and Fisher, 1995[169]	7	33	3.0
Hasselrot, 1998[108]	7	282	7.1

Rubber Dam Isolation

For the reasons mentioned previously, use of a rubber dam is very important for this procedure.

Preparation

Access may be gained through the occlusal surface with a No. 2 round bur used in a high-speed handpiece and directed toward the carious lesion. The preparation should be started about 2.0 mm into the occlusal surface from the crest of the marginal ridge (Figs 10-53a and 10-53b). Removal of carious dentin can be accomplished with a No. 2 round bur in a low-speed handpiece. Because of the limited access, a caries-disclosing solution is needed to improve visualization of carious dentin.[130] Dentin stained with a caries-disclosing solution, unless very near the pulp, is removed.[232] Magnifying loupes help the clinician ascertain the completeness of removal of carious dentin.

After the carious dentin has been removed, the proximal enamel lesion is evaluated. If the proximal surface is intact, it is left alone.[130] The early enamel lesion is more resistant to carious attack than sound enamel[146] and should be left intact and allowed to remineralize. Tunnel restorations in which the proximal enamel is perforated, the so-called "open" tunnel restoration, tend to fail at a higher rate due to marginal ridge fracture.[108,248] If the clinician determines that the marginal ridge has been undermined, the tunnel preparation should be converted to a traditional Class 2 preparation.

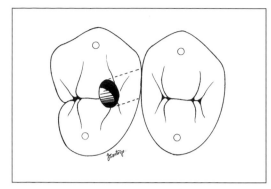

Figs 10-53a In the tunnel preparation, access is made in the occlusal fossa adjacent to the marginal ridge.

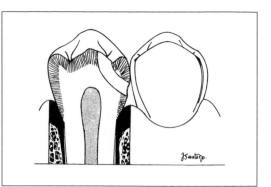

Fig 10-53b A "tunnel" is made under the marginal ridge to the carious dentin, usually just below the interproximal contact.

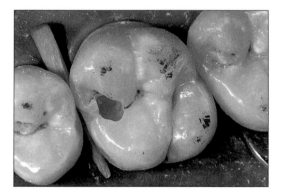

Fig 10-53c Tunnel preparation access opening in the maxillary first molar.

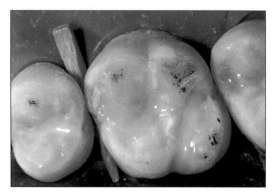

Fig 10-53d Tunnel restoration. Occlusal fissures have been sealed.

Restoration

Glass ionomer was the original restorative material of choice. Cermet glass ionomers were originally used because of their radiopacity and fluoride release. Compared to amalgam, they have been shown to reduce recurrent caries around the restoration as well as in the adjacent tooth surface.[254] In addition, mutans streptococci levels in plaque adjacent to proximal glass-ionomer restorations are lower than levels adjacent to either resin composite or amalgam restorations.[255,256] Although one study showed good sealing in tunnel restorations with a glass-ionomer cermet,[96] another did not.[224] A different study showed that the use of cermet glass ionomer did not prevent lesion progression in many cases.[210]

Resin-modified glass ionomers are the current materials of choice for this restoration. They are radiopaque and have been shown to prevent microleakage.[62] The glass ionomer should be placed in accordance with the manufacturer's recommendations, to approximately the level of the occlusal dentinoenamel junction.

Glass ionomer has shown a marked propensity to fail under occlusal stress.[291] Resin composites are more wear resistant than glass ionomer and may help to increase the fracture resistance of the restored tooth.[10] Therefore, the occlusal 1.5 to 2.0 mm of the preparation should be filled with a VLC resin composite, using the techniques previously described. Finishing and rebonding should be accomplished as described previously in this chapter. Figures 10-53c and 10-53d show a tunnel preparation and restoration.

References

1. Abdalla AI, Davidson CL. Comparison of the marginal and axial wall integrity of in vivo and in vitro made adhesive Class V restorations. J Oral Rehabil 1993;20:257–269.

2. Abdalla AI, Davidson CL. Comparison of the marginal integrity of in vivo and in vitro Class II composite restorations. J Dent 1993;21:158–162.

3. Aboushala A, Kugel G, Hurley E. Class II composite resin restorations using glass-ionomer liners: microleakage studies. J Clin Pediatr Dent 1996;21:67–71.

4. ADA Council on Scientific Affairs, ADA Council on Dental Benefit Programs. Statement on posterior resin-based composites. J Am Dent Assoc 1998;129:1627–1628.

5. Akerboom HBM, Dreulen CM, van Amerongen WE, Mol A. Radiopacity of posterior composite resins, composite resin luting cements, and glass ionomer lining cements. J Prosthet Dent 1993;70:351–355.

6. Albers HE. Direct composite restoratives. Adept Report 1991; 2:53–64.

7. Alster D, Feilzer AJ, de Gee AJ, et al. The dependence of shrinkage stress reduction on porosity concentration in thin resin layers. J Dent Res 1992;71:1619–1622.

8. Applequist EA, Meiers JC. Effect of bulk insertion, prepolymerized resin composite balls, and beta-quartz inserts on microleakage of Class V resin composite restorations. Quintessence Int 1996;27:253–258.

9. Ashe MJ, Tripp GA, Eichmiller FC, et al. Surface roughness of glass-ceramic insert-composite restorations: assessing several polishing techniques. J Am Dent Assoc 1996;127:1495–1500.

10. Asmussen E. Factors affecting the quantity of remaining double bonds in restorative resin polymers. Scand J Dent Res 1982;90:490–496.

11. Asmussen E. Softening of BISGMA-based polymers by ethanol and by organic acids of plaque. Scand J Dent Res 1984;92:257–261.

12. Bader JD, Graves RC, Disney JA, et al. Identifying children who will experience high caries increments. Community Dent Oral Epidemiol 1986;14:198–201.

13. Bailey SJ, Swift EJ Jr. Effects of home bleaching products on composite resins. Quintessence Int 1992;23:489–494.

14. Barkmeier WW, Wilwerding TM, Latta MA, Blake SM. In vitro wear assessment of high density composite resins [abstract 2737]. J Dent Res 1999;78:448.

15. Barnes DM, Blank LW, Thompson VP, et al. A 5- and 8-year clinical evaluation of a posterior composite resin. Quintessence Int 1991;22:143–151.

16. Barnes DM, Holston AM, Strassler HE, Shires PJ. Evaluation of clinical performance of twelve posterior composite resins with a standardized placement technique. J Esthet Dent 1990; 2:36–43.

17. Barrie AM, Stephen KW, Kay EJ. Fissure sealant retention: a comparison of three sealant types under field conditions. Community Dent Health 1990;7:273–277.

18. Bayne SC, Heymann HO, Swift EJ Jr. Update on dental composite restorations. J Am Dent Assoc 1994;125:687–701.

19. Bayne SC, Taylor DF, Heymann HO. Protection hypothesis for composite wear. Dent Mater 1992;8:305–309.

20. Bayne SC, Thompson JY, Swift EJ Jr, et al. A characterization of first-generation flowable composites. J Am Dent Assoc 1998;129:567–577.

21. Behle C. Flowable composites: properties and applications [news]. Pract Periodontics Aesthet Dent 1998;10:347, 350–347, 351.

22. Bentley C, Drake CW. Longevity of restorations in a dental school clinic. J Dent Educ 1986;50:594–600.

23. Berastegui E, Canalda C, Brau E, Miquel C. Surface roughness of finished composite resins. J Prosthet Dent 1992;68: 742–749.

24. Bertolotti RL. Posterior composite technique utilizing directed polymerization shrinkage and a novel matrix. Pract Periodontics Aesthet Dent 1991;3(4):53–58.

25. Black GV. A Work on Operative Dentistry. Chicago: Medico Dental Publishing, 1908.

26. Boksman L, Carson B. Two-year retention and caries rates of UltraSeal XT and FluoroShield light-cured pit and fissure sealants. Gen Dent 1998;46:184–187.

27. Bonner P. Advances in dental materials: an exclusive interview with Dr. Karl Leinfelder. Dent Today 1994;March:32–34.

28. Bouschlicher MR, Vargas MA, Boyer DB. Effect of composite type, light intensity, configuration factor and laser polymerization on polymerization contraction forces. Am J Dent 1997; 10:88–96.

29. Bowen RL, Marjenhoff WA. Dental composites/glass ionomers: the materials. Adv Dent Res 1992;6:44–49.

30. Brackett WW, Gilpatrick RO, Gunnin TD. Effect of finishing method on the microleakage of Class V resin composite restorations. Am J Dent 1997;10:189–191.

31. Brannstrom M. Infection beneath composite resin restorations: can it be avoided? Oper Dent 1987;12:158–163.

32. Brocklehurst PR, Joshi RI, Northeast SE. The effect of air-polishing occlusal surfaces on the penetration of fissures by a sealant. Int J Paediatr Dent 1992;2:157–162.

33. Brosh T, Pilo R, Bichacho N, Blustein R. Effect of combinations of surface treatments and bonding agents on the bond strength of repair composites. J Prosthet Dent 1997;77: 122–126.

34. Brunsvold MA, Lane JJ. The prevalence of overhanging dental restorations and their relationship to periodontal disease. J Clin Periodontol 1990;17:67–72.

35. Bryant RW. Direct posterior composite resin restorations: a review. 1. Factors influencing case selection. Aust Dent J 1992; 37(2):81–87.

36. Bryant RW. Direct posterior composite resin restorations: a review. 2. Clinical technique. Aust Dent J 1992;37(3):161–171.

37. Bryant RW, Mahler DB. Modulus of elasticity in bending of composites and amalgams. J Prosthet Dent 1986;56:243.

38. Bullard RH, Leinfelder KF, Russell CM. Effect of coefficient of thermal expansion on microleakage. J Am Dent Assoc 1988;116:871–874.

39. Burgess JO, Barghi N, Chan DCN, Hummert T. A comparative study of three glass ionomer base materials. Am J Dent 1993;6:137–141.

40. Burgess JO, DeGoes M, Walker R, Ripps AH. An evaluation of four light-curing units comparing soft and hard curing. Pract Periodontics Aesthet Dent 1999;11:125–132.

40a. Burgess JO, Summit JB, Robbins JW, et al. Clinical evaluation of base, sandwich and bonded Class 2 composite restorations [abstract 3405]. J Dent Res 1999;78:531.

41. Castillo MD. Class II composite marginal ridge failure: conventional vs. proximal box only preparation. J Clin Pediatr Dent 1999;23:131–136.

42. Charlton D. SureFil high density posterior restorative. USAF Dental Items of Significance 1999;58:11.

43. Chestnutt IG, Schafer F, Jacobson APM, Stephen KW. The prevalence and effectiveness of fissure sealants in Scottish adolescents. Br Dent J 1994;177:125–129.

44. Choi JW, Drummond JL, Dooley R, et al. The efficacy of primer on sealant shear bond strength. Pediatr Dent 1997;19:286–288.

44a. Choi KK, Ferracane JL, Hilton TJ, Charlton D. Properties of packable dental composites. J Esthet Dent 2000;12:224–234.

137. Joynt RB, Davis EL, Wieczkowski G Jr, Laura J. Bond strength durability between dentinal bonding agents and tooth structure [abstract 2134]. J Dent Res 1988;67:379.

138. Joynt RB, Wieczkowski G, Klockowski R, Davis EL. Effects of composite restorations on resistance to cuspal fracture in posterior teeth. J Prosthet Dent 1987;57:431.

139. Kanca IJ, Suh B, Vinson W. Pulse activation of resin composite: reducing stresses at cavosurface interfaces. J Dent Res 1998;77:190.

140. Kaplan BA, Goldstein GR, Vijayaraghavan TV, Nelson IK. The effect of three polishing systems on the surface roughness of four hybrid composites: a profilometric and scanning electron microscopy study. J Prosthet Dent 1996;76:34–38.

141. Kasloff Z, Galan D, Williams PT. Cuspal deflection studies using an electronic probe [abstract 2264]. J Dent Res 1993; 72:386

142. Kawai K, Leinfelder KF. Effect of surface-penetrating sealant on composite wear. Dent Mater 1993;9:108–113.

143. Kelsey WP, Latta MA, Barkmeier WW. Physical properties of high density composite restorative materials [abstract 810]. J Dent Res 1999;78:207.

144. Kemp-Scholte CM, Davidson CL. Marginal integrity related to bond strength and strain capacity of composite resin restorative systems. J Prosthet Dent 1990;64:658–664.

145. Kerby R, Lee J, Knobloch L, Seghi R. Hardness and degree of conversion of posterior condensable composite resins [abstract 414]. J Dent Res 1999;78:157.

146. Kidd EA, Joyston-Bechal S. Susceptibility of natural carious lesions in enamel to an artificial caries-like attack in vitro. Br Dent J 1986;160:345–348.

147. Kilpatrick NM. Durability of restorations in primary molars. J Dent 1993;21:67–73.

148. King NM, Yung LKM, Holmgren CJ. Clinical performance of preventive resin restorations placed in a hospital environment. Quintessence Int 1996;27:627–632.

149. Klausner LH, Green TG, Charbeneau GT. Placement and replacement of amalgam restorations. Oper Dent 1987;12:105–111.

150. Knight GM. The use of adhesive materials in the conservative restoration of selected posterior teeth. Aust Dent J 1984;29: 324–331.

151. Knoblach L, Kerby R, Seghi R. Wear resistance of posterior condensable composite resins [abstract 2735]. J Dent Res 1999;78:447.

152. Koike T, Hasegawa T, Manabe A, et al. Effect of water sorption and thermal stress on cavity adaptation of dental composites. Dent Mater 1990;6:178–180.

153. Koran P, Kurschner R. Effect of sequential versus continuous irradiation of a light-cured resin composite on shrinkage, viscosity, adhesion, and degree of polymerization. Am J Dent 1998;11:17–22.

154. Kramer PF, Zelante F, Simionato MR. The immediate and long-term effects of invasive and noninvasive pit and fissure sealing techniques on the microflora in occlusal fissures of human teeth. Pediatr Dent 1993;15:108–112.

155. Krejci I, Lutz F, Krejci D. The influence of different base materials on marginal adaptation and wear of conventional Class II composite resin restorations. Quintessence Int 1988;19:191–198.

156. Kreulen CM, van Amerongen WE, Akerboom HB, Borgmeijer PJ. Two-year results with box-only resin composite restorations. ASDC J Dent Child 1995;62:395–400.

157. Labella R, Lambrechts P, Van Meerbeek B, Vanherle G. Polymerization shrinkage and elasticity of flowable composites and filled adhesives. Dent Mater 1999;15:128–137.

158. Lambrechts P, Braem M, Vuylsteke-Wauters M, Vanherle G. Quantitative in vivo wear of human enamel. J Dent Res 1989; 68:1752–1754.

159. Lambrechts P, Braem M, Vanherle G. Evaluation of clinical performance for posterior composite resins and dentin adhesives. Oper Dent 1987;12:53–87.

159a. Lang LA, Burgess JO, Lang BR, Wang R-F. Wear of composite resin restorations in beveled and nonbeveled preparations [abstract 1226]. J Dent Res 1995;74(special issue):165.

160. Langdon RS, Moon PC, Barnes RF. Effect of dentin bonding adhesive thickness on bond strength [abstract 244]. J Dent Res 1994;73:132.

161. Leinfelder KF. Composite resins. Dent Clin North Am 1985; 29:359–371.

162. Leinfelder KF. Posterior composite resins. J Can Dent Assoc 1989;55:34–39.

163. Leinfelder KF. Composite resin systems for posterior restorations. Pract Periodontics Aesthet Dent 1993;suppl 1:23–27.

164. Leinfelder KF, Wilder AD, Teixeira ER. Wear rates of posterior composite resins. J Am Dent Assoc 1986;112:829–833.

165. Leinfelder KF. Using a composite resin as a posterior restorative material. J Am Dent Assoc 1991;122:65–70.

166. Letzel H. Survival rates and reasons for failure of posterior composite restorations in multicentre clinical trial. J Dent 1989;17:S10–S17.

166a. Letzel H, van't Hof MA, Vrijhoef MMA, et al. A controlled clinical study of amalgam restorations: survival, failures, and causes of failure. Dent Mater 1989;5:115–121.

167. Levy MP, Feigal RJ. Intermediate bonding agents increase clinical success of occlusal sealants on newly-erupted molars. J Dent Res 1996;75:179.

168. Li J, Nicander I, von Beetzen M, Sundstrom F. Influence of paste temperature at curing on conversion rate and bending strength of light-cured dental composites. J Oral Rehabil 1996;23:298–301.

169. Lumley PJ, Fisher FJ. Tunnel restorations: a long-term pilot study over a minimum of five years. J Dent 1995;23:213–215.

170. Lussi A, Gygax M. Iatrogenic damage to adjacent teeth during classical approximal box preparation. J Dent 1998;26: 435–441.

171. Lutz F, Krejci I, Barbakow F. Chewing pressure vs. wear of composites and opposing enamel cusps. J Dent Res 1992;71: 1525–1529.

172. Lutz F, Krejci I, Barbakow F. Restoration quality in relation to wedge-mediated light channeling. Quintessence Int 1992; 23:763–767.

173. Lutz F, Krejci I, Luescher B, Oldenburg TR. Improved proximal margin adaptation of Class II composite resin restorations by use of light-reflecting wedges. Quintessence Int 1986; 17:659–664.

174. Lutz F, Krejci I, Oldenburg TR. Elimination of polymerization stresses at the margins of posterior composite resin restorations: a new restorative technique. Quintessence Int 1986;17:777.

175. Lutz F, Krejci I, Barbakow F. Quality and durability of marginal adaptation in bonded composite restorations. Dent Mater 1991;7:107–113.

176. Lutz F, Phillips RW, Roulet JF, Setcos JC. In vivo and in vitro wear of potential posterior composites. J Dent Res 1984;63: 914–920.

177. MacGregor KM, Cobb DS, Vargas MA. Physical properties of condensable versus conventional composites [abstract 411]. J Dent Res 1999;78:157.

178. Mair LH. Wear patterns in two amalgams and three posterior composites after 5 years' clinical service. J Dent 1995;23: 107–112.

179. Mair LH. Ten-year clinical assessment of three posterior resin composites and two amalgams. Quintessence Int 1998;29: 483–490.

180. Mair LH, Vowles RW, Cunningham J, Williams DF. The clinical wear of three posterior composites. Br Dent J 1990; 169:355–360.

181. Martens LC, Beyls HMF, De Craene LG, D'Hauwers RFM. Reattachment of original fragment after vertical crown fracture of a permanent central incisor. J Pedod 1989;13:53–62.

182. Martin FE, Bryant RW. Acid-etching of enamel cavity walls. Aust Dent J 1984;29:308–314.

183. Marzouk MA, Ross JA. Cervical enamel crazings associated with occluso-proximal composite restorations in posterior teeth. Am J Dent 1989;2:333–327.

184. Mazer RB, Leinfelder KF, Russell CM. Degradation of microfilled posterior composite. Dent Mater 1992;8(3):185–189.

185. Mehl A, Hickel R, Kunzelmann K-H. Physical properties and gap formation of light-cured composites with and without 'softstart-polymerization'. J Dent 1997;25:321–330.

186. Mertz-Fairhurst EJ, Curtis JW Jr, Ergle JW, et al. Ultraconservative and cariostatic sealed restorations: results at year 10 . J Am Dent Assoc 1998;129:55–66.

187. Mertz-Fairhurst EJ, Fairhurst CW, Williams JE, et al. A comparative clinical study of two pit and fissure sealants: 7-year results in Augusta, GA. J Am Dent Assoc 1984;109:252–255.

188. Miller MB, Castellanos ER, Vargas MA, Denehy GE. Effect of restorative materials on microleakage of Class II composites. J Esthet Dent 1996;8:107–113.

189. Mitchem JC. The use and abuse of aesthetic materials in posterior teeth. Int Dent J 1988;38:119–125.

190. Mitchem JC, Gronas DG. In vivo evaluation of the wear of restorative resin. J Am Dent Assoc 1982;104:335.

191. Moon PC, Chang YH. Effect of DBA layer thickness on composite resin shrinkage stress [abstract 1375]. J Dent Res 1992;71:275.

192. Morin DL, Delong R, Douglas WH. Cusp reinforcement by the acid-etch technique. J Dent Res 1984;63:1075–1078.

193. Munechika T, Suzuki K, Nishiyama M, et al. A comparison of the tensile bond strengths of composite resins to longitudinal and transverse sections of enamel prisms in human teeth. J Dent Res 1984;63:1079.

194. Murchison DF, Charlton DG, Moore WS. Comparative radiopacity of flowable resin composites. Quintessence Int 1999;30:179–184.

195. Nordbo H, Leirskar J, von der Fehr FR. Saucer-shaped cavity preparations for posterior approximal resin composite restorations: observations up to 10 years. Quintessence Int 1998; 29:5–11.

196. Opdam NJ, Feilzer AJ, Roeters JJ, Smale I. Class I occlusal composite resin restorations: in vivo post-operative sensitivity, wall adaptation, and microleakage. Am J Dent 1998;11: 229–234.

197. Opdam NJM, Roeters FJ, Feilzer AJ, Smale I. A radiographic and scanning electron microscopic study of approximal margins of Class II resin composite restorations placed in vivo. J Dent 1998;26:319–327.

198. Opdam NJ, Roeters JJ, Kuijs R, Burgersdijk RC. Necessity of bevels for box only Class II composite restorations. J Prosthet Dent 1998;80(3):274–279.

199. Opdam NJM, Roeters JJM, Burgersdijk RCW. Microleakage of Class II box-type composite restorations. Am J Dent 1998;11:160–164.

200. Opdam NJM, Roeters JJM, Peters TCRB, et al. Consistency of resin composites for posterior use. Dent Mater 1996;12:350–354.

201. Opdam NJM, Roeters JJM, Peters TCRB, et al. Cavity wall adaptation and voids in adhesive Class I resin composite restorations. Dent Mater 1996;12:230–235.

202. Opdam NJM, Roeters FJM, Verdonschot EH. Adaptation and radiographic evaluation of four adhesive systems. J Dent 1997;25:391–397.

202a.Osborne JW, Norman RD, Gale EN. A 14-year clinical assessment of 12 amalgam alloys. Quintessence Int 1991;22: 857–864.

203. Pallesen U, Qvist V. Clinical evaluation of three posterior composite resins: 10-year report [abstract 30]. J Dent Res 1995;74:404.

204. Papa J, Cain C, Messer HH. Efficacy of tunnel restorations in the removal of caries. Quintessence Int 1993;24:715–719.

205. Papa J, Cain C, Messer HH, Wilson PR. Tunnel restorations versus Class II restorations for small proximal lesions: a comparison of tooth strengths. Quintessence Int 1993;24:93–98.

206. Papa J, Wilson PR, Tyas MJ. Tunnel restorations: a review. Quintessence Int 1992;4:4–9.

207. Pearson GJ, Hegarty SM. Cusp movement of molar teeth with composite filling materials in conventional and modified MOD cavities. Br Dent J 1989;166:162–165.

208. Penning C, van Amerongen JP. Microleakage of extended and nonextended Class I composite resin and sealant restorations. J Prosthet Dent 1990;64:131–134.

209. Pereira AC, Basting RT, Pinelli C, et al. Retention and caries prevention of Vitremer and Ketac-bond used as occlusal sealants. Am J Dent 1999;12:62–64.

210. Pilebro CE, van Dijken JWV, Stenberg R. Durability of tunnel restorations in general practice: a three-year multicenter study. Acta Odontol Scand 1999;57:35–39.

211. Pilo R, Oelgiesser D, Cardash HS. A survey of output intensity and potential for depth of cure among light-curing units in clinical use. J Dent 1999;27:235–241.

212. Pires JAF, Cvitko E, Denehy GE, Swift EJ. Effects of curing tip distance on light intensity and composite resin microhardness. Quintessence Int 1993;24:517–521.

213. Podshadley AG, Gullett CE, Binkley TK. Interface strength of incremental placement of visible light-cured composites. J Am Dent Assoc 1985;110:932–934.

214. Prati C. Early marginal microleakage in Class II resin composite restorations. Dent Mater 1989;5:392–398.

215. Pratten DH, Johnson GH. An evaluation of finishing instruments for an anterior and a posterior composite. J Prosthet Dent 1988;60:154.

216. Puppala R, Hegde A, Munshi AK. Laser and light cured composite resin restorations: in-vitro comparison of isotope and dye penetrations. J Clin Pediatr Dent 1996;20:213–218.

217. Qvist V, Johannessen L, Brunn M. Progression of approximal caries in relation to iatrogenic preparation damage. J Dent Res 1992;71(7):1370–1373.

218. Qvist V, Qvist J, Mjor IA. Placement and longevity of tooth-colored restorations in Denmark. Acta Odontol Scand 1990; 48:305–311.

219. Qvist V, Strom C. 11-year assessment of Class-III resin restorations completed with two restorative procedures. Acta Odontol Scand 1993;51:253–262.

220. Rashid R, Ricks J, Monaghan P. Strengths of condensable composite resins with flowable liners [abstract 403]. J Dent Res 1999;78:156.

221. Reeh ES, Messer HH, Douglas WH. Reduction in tooth stiffness as a result of endodontic and restorative procedures. J Endod 1989;15:512–516.

222. Reid JS, Saunders WP, Chen YY. The effect of bonding agent and fissure sealant on microleakage of composite resin restorations. Quintessence Int 1991;22:295–298.

223. Retief DH, Mandras RS, Russell CM. Shear bond strength required to prevent microleakage at the dentin/restoration interface. Am J Dent 1994;7:43–46.

224. Robbins JW, Cooley RL. Microleakage of Ketac silver in the tunnel preparation. Oper Dent 1988;13:8–11.

225. Robbins JW, Summitt JB. Longevity of complex amalgam restorations. Oper Dent 1988;13:54–57.

226. Romcke RG, Lewis DW, Maze BD, Vickerson RA. Retention and maintenance of fissure sealants over 10 years. J Can Dent Assoc 1990;56:235–237.

226a. Roulet JF. Benefits and disadvantages of tooth-colored alternatives to amalgam. J Dent 1997;25:459–473.

227. Rowe AHR. A five year study of the clinical performance of a posterior composite resin restorative material. J Dent 1989;17:S6–S9.

228. Ruddell DE, Thompson JY, Stamatiades PJ, et al. Mechanical properties and wear behavior of condensable composites [abstract 407]. J Dent Res 1999;78:156.

229. Rueggeberg FA, Caughman WF, Curtis JW Jr, Davis HC. Factors affecting cure at depths within light-activated resin composites. Am J Dent 1993;6:91–95.

230. Rueggeberg FA, Jordan DM. Effect of light-tip distance on polymerization of resin composite. Int J Prosthodont 1993;6:364–370.

231. Russell RR, Mazer RB. Microleakage of Class II restorations using a flowable composite as a liner [abstract 203]. J Dent Res 1998;77:131.

232. Sato Y, Fusayama T. Removal of dentin by fuchsin staining. Dent Res 1976;55:678–683.

233. Schwartz R, Murchison D, Hermesch C, et al. Three year clinical evaluation of three dentin treatments [abstract 1188]. J Dent Res 1997;76:162.

234. Segura A, Donly KJ. In vitro posterior composite polymerization recovery following hygroscopic expansion. J Oral Rehabil 1993;20:495–499.

235. Shahdad SA, Kennedy JG. Bond strength of repaired anterior composite resins: an in vitro study. J Dent 1998;26:685–694.

236. Shanthala BM, Munshi AK. Laser vs visible-light cured composite resin: an in vitro shear bond study. J Clin Pediatr Dent 1995;19:121–125.

237. Shapira J, Eidelman E. Six-year clinical evaluation of fissure sealants placed after mechanical preparation: a matched pair study. Pediatr Dent 1986;8:204–205.

238. Shapira J, Fuks A, Chosack A, et al. A comparative clinical study of autopolymerized and light-polymerized fissure sealants: five-year results. Pediatr Dent 1990;12:168–169.

239. Simonsen RJ. Preventive resin restorations (I). Quintessence Int 1978;9:69–76.

240. Simonsen RJ. Preventive resin restorations (II). Quintessence Int 1978;9:95–102.

241. Simonsen RJ, Stallard RE. Sealant-restorations utilizing a diluted filled composite resin: one year results. Quintessence Int 1977;8(6):77–84.

241a. Smales RJ, Webster DA, Leppard PI. Survival predictions of four types of dental restorative materials. J Dent 1991;19:278–282.

241b. Smales RJ, Webster DA, Leppard PI. Survival predictions of amalgam restorations. J Dent 1991;19:272–277.

242. Smales RJ, Wong KC. 2-year clinical performance of a resin-modified glass ionomer sealant. Am J Dent 1999;12:59–61.

243. Söderholm KJ, Zigan M, Ragan M, et al. Hydrolytic degradation of dental composites. J Dent Res 1984;63:1248–1254.

244. Sorensen JA, Dixit NV, White SN, Avera SP. In vitro microleakage of dentin adhesives. J Am Dent Assoc 1991;4:213–218.

245. Stadtler P. A 3-year clinical study of a hybrid composite resin as fissure sealant and as restorative material for Class I restorations. Quintessence Int 1992;23:759–762.

246. Stamplia LL, Nicholls JI, Brudvik JS, Jones DW. Fracture resistance of teeth with resin-bonded restorations. J Prosthet Dent 1986;55:694–698.

247. Stangel I, Barolet RY. Clinical evaluation of two posterior composite resins: two-year results. J Oral Rehabil 1990;17:257–268.

248. Strand GV, Nordbo H, Tveit AB, et al. A 3-year clinical study of tunnel restorations. Eur J Oral Sci 1996;104:384–389.

249. Strand GV, Tveit AB. Effectiveness of caries removal by the partial tunnel preparation. Scand J Dent Res 1993;101:270–273.

250. Strand GV, Tveit AB, Espelid I. Variations among operators in the performance of tunnel preparations in vitro. Scand J Dent Res 1994;102:151–155.

251. Suliman AA, Boyer DB, Lakes RS. Cusp movement in premolars resulting from composite polymerization shrinkage. Dent Mater 1993;9:6–10.

252. Summitt JB, Della Bona A, Burgess JO. The strength of Class II composite resin restorations as affected by preparation design. Quintessence Int 1994;25:251–257.

253. Suzuki S. In vitro wear of condensable resin composite restoratives [abstract 2734]. J Dent Res 1999;78:447.

254. Svanberg M. Class II amalgam restorations, glass-ionomer tunnel restorations, and caries development on adjacent tooth surfaces: a 3-year clinical study. Caries Res 1992;26:315–318.

255. Svanberg M, Krasse B, Ornerfeldt HO. Mutans streptococci in interproximal plaque from amalgam and glass ionomer restorations. Caries Res 1990;24:133–136.

256. Svanberg M, Mjor IA, Orstavik D. Mutans streptococci in plaque from margins of amalgam, composite, and glass-ionomer restorations. J Dent Res 1990;69:861–864.

257. Swift EJ, Triolo PT, Barkmeier WW, Bird JL. Effect of low-viscosity resins on the performance of dental adhesives. Am J Dent 1996;9:100–104.

258. Symons AL, Chu C-Y, Meyers IA. The effect of fissure morphology and pretreatment of the enamel surface on penetration and adhesion of fissure sealants. J Oral Rehabil 1996;23:791–798.

259. Tabassian M, Moon PC. Filler particle characterization in flowable and condensible composite resins [abstract 3022]. J Dent Res 1999;78:483.

260. Tarle Z, Meniga A, Ristic M, et al. The effect of the photo-polymerization method on the quality of composite resin samples. J Oral Rehabil 1998;25:436–442.

261. Tay FR, Gwinnett AJ, Pang KM, Wei SHY. Variability in microleakage observed in a total-etch wet-bonding technique under different handling conditions. J Dent Res 1995;74:1168–1178.

262. Tjan AHL, Bergh BH, Lidner C. Effect of various incremental techniques on the marginal adaptation of Class II composite resin restorations. J Prosthet Dent 1992;67:62–66.

263. Tjan AHL, Tan DE. Microleakage at gingival margins of Class V composite resin restorations rebonded with various low-viscosity resin systems. Quintessence Int 1991;22:565–573.

264. Tolidis K, Setcos JC. Initial degree of polymerization shrinkage exhibited by flowable composite resins [abstract 3015]. J Dent Res 1999;78:482.

265. Torstenson B, Brannstrom M. A new method for sealing composite resin contraction gaps in lined cavities. J Am Dent Assoc 1985;64:450–453.

266. Toyooka J, Taira M, Wakasa K, et al. Radiopacity of 12 visible-light-cured dental composite resins. J Oral Rehabil 1993;20:615–622.

267. Tulunoglu O, Bodur H, Uctasli M, Alacam A. The effect of bonding agents on the microleakage and bond strength of sealant in primary teeth. J Oral Rehabil 1999;26:436–441.

268. Tveit AB, Espelid I. Radiographic diagnosis of caries and marginal defects in connection with radiopaque composite fillings. Dent Mater 1986;2:159–162.

269. Tyas MJ. Colour stability of composite resins: a clinical comparison. Aust Dent J 1992;37(2):88–90.

270. Tyas MJ. Clinical evaluation of five adhesive systems. Am J Dent 1994;7:77–80.

271. Ulvestad H. Clinical trials with fissure sealant materials in Scandanavia. In Silverstone LM, Dogon IL. Proceedings of an International Symposium on The Acid Etch Technique. St Paul, MN: North Central Publishing, 1975:165–174.

272. Uno S, Asmussen E. Marginal adaptation of a restorative resin polymerized at reduced rate. Scand J Dent Res 1991;99:440–444.

273. Unterbrink GL, Muessner R. Influence of light intensity on two restorative systems. J Dent 1995;23:183–189.

274. van Dijken JW, Horstedt P, Waern R. Directed polymerization shrinkage versus a horizontal incremental filling technique: interfacial adaptation in vivo in Class II cavities. Am J Dent 1998;11:165–172.

275. Vandewalle KS, Munro GA, Gureckis KM. Esthetic occlusal composite resin restorations. J Esthet Dent 1994;6:73–76.

276. Venhoven BA, DeGee AJ, Davidson C. Polymerization contraction and conversion of light-curing BisGMA-based methacrylate resins. Biomaterials 1993;14:871–874.

277. Versluis A, Douglas WH, Sakaguchi RL. Thermal expansion coefficient of dental composites measured with strain gauges. Dent Mater 1996;12:290–294.

278. Versluis A, Tantbirojn D, Douglas WH. Do dental composites always shrink toward the light? J Dent Res 1998;77:1435–1445.

279. von Beetzen M, Li J, Nicander I, Sundstrom F. Microhardness and porosity of Class 2 light-cured composite restorations cured with a transparent cone attached to the light-curing wand. Oper Dent 1993;18:103–109.

280. Walshaw PR, McComb D. Microleakage in Class 2 resin composites with low-modulus, intermediate materials [abstract 204]. J Dent Res 1998;77:131.

281. Wang J-C, Charbeneau GT, Gregory WA, Dennison JB. Quantitative evaluation of approximal contacts in Class 2 composite resin restorations: a clinical study. Oper Dent 1989;14:193–202.

282. Warren JA, Clark NP. Posterior composite resin: current trends in restorative techniques, part II. Insertion, finishing, and polishing. Gen Dent 1987;35:497–499.

283. Warren JA, Clark NP. Posterior composite resin: current trends in restorative techniques, part I. Pre-preparation considerations, preparation, dentin treatment, etching/bonding. Gen Dent 1987;35:368–372.

284. Watanabe I, Nakabayashi N. Bonding durability of photocured phenyl-P in TEGDMA to smear layer-retained bovine dentin. Quintessence Int 1993;24:335–342.

285. Welbury RR, Walls AWG, Murray JJ, McCabe JF. The management of occlusal caries in permanent molars. A 5-year clinical trial comparing a minimal composite with an amalgam restoration. Br Dent J 1990;169:361–366.

286. Wendt LK, Koch G. Fissure sealant in permanent first molars after 10 years. Swed Dent J 1988;12:181–185.

287. Wendt SL Jr, Leinfelder KR. Clinical evaluation of a posterior resin composite: 3-year results. Am J Dent 1994;7:207–211.

288. Wieczkowski F, Joynt RB, Klockowski R, Davis EL. Effects of incremental versus bulk fill technique on resistance to cuspal fracture of teeth restored with posterior composites. J Prosthet Dent 1988;60:283–287.

289. Wilder AD, May KN, Bayne SC, et al. 17-year clinical evaluation of UV-cured composite resins in posterior teeth [abstract 2180]. J Dent Res 1996;75:290.

290. Wilder AD, May KN, Leinfelder KF. Three-year clinical study of UV-cured composite resins in posterior teeth. J Prosthet Dent 1983;50:26–30.

291. Wilkie R, Lidums A, Smales R. Class II glass ionomer cermet tunnel, resin sandwich and amalgam restorations over 2 years. Am J Dent 1993;6:181–184.

292. Willems G, Lambrechts P, Braem M, Vanherle G. Composite resins of the 21st century. Quintessence Int 1993;24:641–658.

293. Willems G, Lambrechts P, Braem M, Vanherle G. Three-year follow-up of five posterior composites: in vivo wear. J Dent 1993;21:74–78.

294. Willems G, Lambrechts P, Lesaffre E, et al. Three-year follow-up of five posterior composites: SEM study of differential wear. J Dent 1993;21:79–86.

295. Williams PT, Johnson LN. Composite resin restoratives revisited. J Can Dent Assoc 1993;59:538–543.

296. Wilson EG, Mandradjieff M, Brindock T. Controversies in posterior composite resin restorations. Dent Clin North Am 1990;34:27–44.

297. Wilson HJ. Resin-based restoratives. Braz Dent J 1988;164:326–330.

298. Wilson NHF, Wilson MA, Wastell DG, Smith GA. Performance of Occlusin in butt-joint and bevel-edged preparations: five-year results. Dent Mater 1991;7:92–98.

299. Wu W, Cobb EN. A silver staining technique for investigating wear of restorative dental composites. J Biomed Mater Res 1981;15:343–348.

300. Wu W, Toth EE, Ellison JA. Subsurface damage layer of in vivo worn dental composite restorations. J Dent Res 1984;63:675–680.

301. Zenkner J, Baratieri LN, Monteiro SJ, et al. Clinical and radiographic evaluation of cement tunnel restorations on primary molars. Quintessence Int 1993;24:783–791.

302. Zickert I, Emilson C-G, Krasse B. Correlation of level and duration of streptococcus mutans infection with incidence of dental caries. Infect Immun 1983;39:982–985.

Amalgam Restorations

James B. Summitt/John W. Osborne

The word *amalgam* means an alloy of mercury with another metal or metals.[168] This type of alloying is called *amalgamation*.[5] In dentistry, before these metals are combined with mercury to make dental amalgam, they are known as dental amalgam alloys. Prior to the development of high-copper amalgam alloys, dental amalgam alloys contained at least 65 wt% silver, 29 wt% tin, and less than 6 wt% copper. The high-copper amalgam alloys[76,96] contain between 12 wt% and 30 wt% copper and at least 40 wt% silver.[39] This higher level of copper has resulted in the elimination of the highly corrodible and weak gamma 2 (tin-mercury) phase that existed in the low-copper dental amalgams.[65,106,111]

Zinc is added to amalgam to enhance its mechanical properties,[144] reduce marginal fracture,[120,123] and prolong the service of the restoration.[90,123] When moisture is incorporated during condensation of a zinc-containing low-copper amalgam, delayed expansion will occur.[145] Zinc-containing high-copper amalgams do not exhibit the phenomenon of delayed expansion,[122,127,172] but isolation to prevent any moisture contamination is important for both zinc-containing and zinc-free amalgam restorations.[122] Contamination of dental amalgam with moisture will create porosity in the restoration, which will decrease strength and increase both corrosion and creep.[122,172]

Amalgam is made by mixing mercury with a powder of amalgam alloy. This process is called *trituration*.[130] The powder may be of the lathe-cut variety (Fig 11-1a), which is made by milling an ingot of the alloy, or of the spherical type (Fig 11-1b), which is made by atomizing liquid alloy.[43] The spherical particles usually are not true spheres but take on various rounded shapes. Some dental amalgam alloys contain only lathe-cut particles, called filings; others contain only spheres, and some contain both spheres and filings. Those containing only filings are called *conventional* or *lathe-cut amalgam alloys*, those containing only spheres are called *spherical alloys*, and those containing both filings and spheres are called *admixtures*[39] (Fig 11-1c).

Dental amalgam continues to be the most-used restorative material.[89,165] It has served as a dental restorative for more than 175 years; it was used as early as 1820 in Europe, and, by the mid-1830s, it was in use in the United States.[13,109] At times, its use has been controversial.[109] The most recent controversy is related to amalgam's release of mercury. There is considerable evidence of the safety of dental amalgam.[1,16,71,82,119] To date, there is no confirmed evidence to indicate that the mercury in dental amalgam is related to any disease.[3,6,21,95] Research reveals that no toxic effect has been linked to the level of mercury released from amalgam, even when amalgam restorations are removed.[113,142] Several agencies, including the World Health Organization,[170] the US Public Health Service,[164] the National Institutes of Health,[116] and the Swedish Medical Research Council[14] have reaffirmed their positions that there are no data to compel a change in the current use of dental amalgam.[13,37]

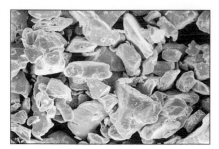

Fig 11-1a Lathe-cut amalgam alloy particles.

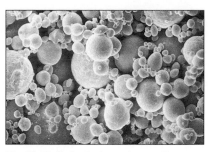

Fig 11-1b Spherical amalgam alloy particles.

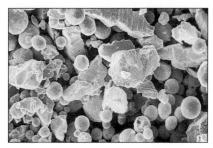

Fig 11-1c Admixed amalgam alloy particles.

Any component of amalgam or any other restorative material can elicit an allergic reaction, but hypersensitivity to mercury is extremely rare. Of those who have a true allergy to mercury, fewer than 1% demonstrate clinically observable reactions to mercury in dental amalgam restorations.[109]

 ## Advantages and Disadvantages

Dental amalgam has many advantages as a restorative material. It is strong, durable, and relatively easy to use. It wears at a rate similar to that of tooth structure. Its ability to corrode results in a reduction of microleakage at its interface with tooth structure.[65] Of the long-term restorative materials, dental amalgam is the least time-consuming to place and has the lowest cost.

Dental amalgam also has disadvantages. It is not tooth-colored, and it does not, on its own, bond to tooth structure, although amalgam bonding systems are proving to be able to provide a mechanical attachment of amalgam to enamel and dentin.[115] Amalgam contains mercury, which must be handled properly or the vapor can create a safety hazard for the dental staff. Nevertheless, because a tooth-colored dental restorative material that has the advantages of dental amalgam has yet to be developed, it is still the primary posterior restorative material, with more than 150 million amalgam restorations placed in the United States each year.

Amalgam, when placed properly in well-designed tooth preparations, will serve well for long periods of time.[90,112,125] Many studies have demonstrated the excellent longevity potential of dental amalgam.[112,123,139,150] This chapter addresses Class 1 and 2 preparations and placement techniques for dental amalgam. Also described are complex restorations involving the replacement of cusps with dental amalgam.

Resistance Form

One of G.V. Black's steps in tooth preparation is obtaining resistance form. There are two considerations in resistance form when a tooth is being prepared to receive an amalgam restoration. First, resistance form should be developed for the restoration; the restoration must be of adequate thickness and have a marginal design that will allow it to bear the forces of mastication without fracture or deformation. In that regard, the restoration must have adequate occlusogingival depth to resist fracture in function or parafunction (bruxing or clenching). Second, the remaining tooth structure must be left in such a state that it, too, will resist the forces of mastication. As much sound tooth structure as possible must be maintained. If adequate resistance form cannot be maintained in the tooth to resist masticatory forces, the weak portion of the occlusal surface should be cut away and restored with amalgam or another strong restorative material.[126]

To maximize resistance form for tooth structure, minimum sound tooth structure should be removed when teeth are prepared for Class 1 or Class 2 amalgam restorations. Several studies[12,17,87,121,166] have demonstrated that, as an amalgam restoration becomes wider faciolingually, the tooth is more subject to fracture and the integrity of the restoration is less likely to be maintained. An increase in the depth of the occlusal portion of an amalgam preparation has also been linked to a decrease in resistance to fracture of the tooth.[17] Class 2 restorations that are confined to the marginal ridge areas (proximal slot restorations) may minimize the severity of tooth fracture compared to Class 2 restorations that extend through occlusal grooves.[30,53] Based on this knowledge, the following goals should guide the preparation and restoration of teeth: *(1)* removal of pathosis (carious tooth structure), *(2)* preservation of the integrity of the tooth and periodontium, and *(3)* maximization of the life of the restored tooth.[125,159]

The Class 1 Preparation

Indications

Occlusal Caries

The indication for an initial Class 1 amalgam restoration is carious tooth structure in the occlusal surface (or in facial or lingual pits in posterior teeth) detected clinically and with bite-wing radiographs. The objectives of treatment are to eliminate caries lesions, to remove any enamel that has been undermined by the caries process, to preserve as much sound tooth structure as possible, and to create a strong restoration that mimics the original sound tooth structure and allows little or no marginal leakage.

For the purpose of this chapter, it is necessary to review the definitions of the terms *groove*, *fissure*, and *pit*.[58] A groove, or a developmental groove, is a linear channel on the surface of a tooth, usually at the junction of dental lobes (cusps or ridges). A fissure is a developmental linear cleft, the result of incomplete fusion of the enamel of adjoining dental lobes. A pit is a pinpoint fissure or the junction of several fissures.

The presence of deep fissures alone does not justify placement of a restoration. When there is concern that a deep fissure may become carious at its base, it should be sealed with a resin fissure sealant or flowable resin composite material. In a tooth that has been diagnosed as having localized fissure caries lesions, the carious tooth structure should be removed and a restoration placed. Remaining fissures that are considered to be susceptible to caries should then be sealed with a resin sealant (Figs 11-2a to 11-2f).

If deep fissures that are to be sealed exhibit enamel demineralization or heavy stains, they may benefit from being prepared with a small bur to a width and depth of approximately 0.4 mm before they are acid etched and sealed with a resin fissure sealant[40,85,148] (Figs 11-3a to 11-3d). Alternatively, these fissures may be opened or cleaned with an air-abrasive instru-

ment or an air-polishing prophylaxis unit[20,42,56,62,167] (Figs 11-4a to 11-4d).

Traditionally, in a Class 1 amalgam preparation, occlusal fissures, or at least those in the developmental grooves, have been included in the preparation, even when caries has not extended throughout the fissures. The justification for this has been that carious dentin, although not evident visually or radiographically, may be lurking at the base of one of those fissures. There is strong evidence that carious dentin inadvertently left at the base of a sealed fissure does not progress[67–69,83,161] and that the sealing of fissures associated with occlusal amalgam restorations is an extremely effective treatment modality.[60,77,107,108] Therefore, the routine extension of cavity preparations through fissures not known to be carious can no longer be justified. Additionally, extension of cavity preparations through grooves in which there are no fissures is contraindicated.

Defective Restorations and Recurrent Caries

Another indication for a Class 1 restoration is the replacement of a restoration that is defective beyond repair or associated with recurrent caries. A recurrent caries lesion is one that occurs adjacent to an existing restoration. Optimally, the margins of a restoration are sealed or leakproof. In reality, most restorations exhibit some leakage at their margins, although it is minimal in most cases. When the leakage becomes greater, usually because of a defective restoration or flexure of tooth structure, plaque can form in the space between the tooth and the restoration, which can lead to caries initiation. There is some evidence that cleaning, etching, and sealing leaky amalgam margins with a resin sealant can prolong the life of a restoration.[31]

Outline Form

When an occlusal restoration must be placed because of initial caries lesions, two guidelines should be applied in establishing the outline form: *(1)* carious tooth structure should be eliminated, and *(2)* margins should be placed on sound tooth structure. The enamel at the margin of the preparation should be supported by sound dentin. Any enamel that has been undermined by the removal of carious dentin should be removed. If a noncarious fissure is evident in the wall of a preparation, the preparation should not be extended solely to include the fissure; the fissure should, instead, be sealed after the amalgam has been placed.

Figs 11-2a to 11-2f Amalgam should be used as a restorative material only in areas where actual carious tooth structure has been removed; remaining noncarious fissures and amalgam restoration margins are etched and sealed with resin fissure sealant.

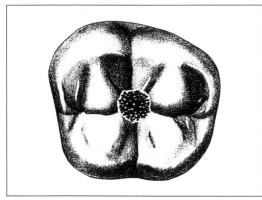

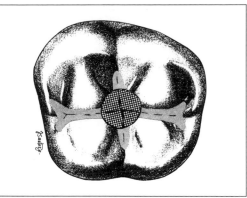

Fig 11-2a This drawing shows the extent of carious dentin as if it could be seen through the occlusal enamel.

Fig 11-2b An amalgam restoration has been placed in the area where carious dentin and unsupported enamel were removed; the remaining fissures were sealed.

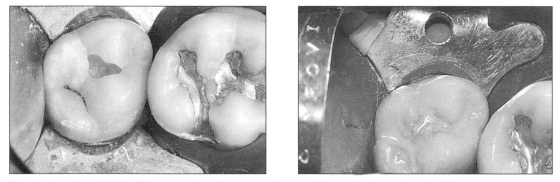

Figs 11-2c and 11-2d Maxillary second molar preparation, sealed restoration, and sealed fissures.

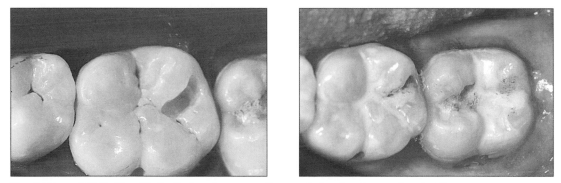

Figs 11-2e and 11-2f Mandibular first molar preparation, sealed restoration, and sealed fissures.

Figs 11-3a to 11-3d Fissures can be opened with a small round bur for sealing.

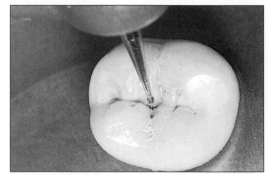

Fig 11-3a A No. 1/16 bur (0.3-mm diameter), 1/8 bur (0.4-mm diameter), or a 1/4 bur (0.5-mm diameter) is used to open the fissures.

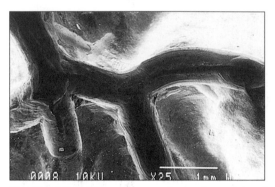

Fig 11-3b The fissure system of a mandibular second molar is shown pretreatment.

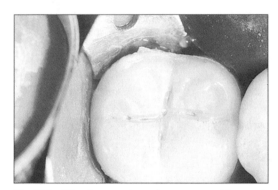

Fig 11-3c The fissures have been opened for sealing.

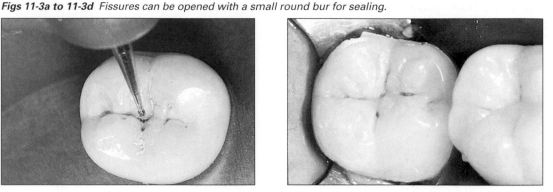

Fig 11-3d Scanning electron photomicrograph of fissures prepared with a small round bur.

If there is no cavitation in the area of the lesion, a bur such as a No. 56, 245, 329, or 330 is used to cut through enamel to gain access to the carious dentin. The preparation is widened to give access to all carious dentin and to remove any enamel not supported by sound dentin. The preparation should be widened only enough to obtain enamel margins supported by sound dentin.

Although the outline form should not contain sharp angles, sound tooth structure should not be removed simply to obtain wide, smooth curves in the outline form. The outline form should be smooth to facilitate the uncovering of the margins during carving of amalgam. That is, the margins of the preparation should not be jagged or rough, because it is difficult for the dentist to know whether a restoration margin appears to be irregular because the enamel margin is rough or because amalgam extends past the margins onto the surface of the tooth (overextended amalgam or amalgam flash).

When replacing a defective restoration or a restoration associated with a recurrent caries lesion, the outline form will be determined by several factors. First, the outline form of the old restoration will have a major influence. Also, the outline form may have to be extended because of additional pathosis. Finally, the resistance form for the tooth structure or restoration may have to be improved, and that will affect the outline form.

Resistance and Retention Form

To provide retention form for the amalgam, opposing walls of Class 1 occlusal restorations should be parallel to each other or should converge occlusally. Enamel rods in most areas of the occlusal surface are directed roughly parallel to the long axis of the tooth,[54] a factor that should be considered when the angulation of the margin of the amalgam preparation

Figs 11-4a to 11-4d Fissures can be opened with an air-abrasion unit (KCP 2000).

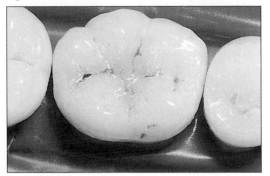

Fig 11-4a The fissure system of a mandibular molar is shown prior to air abrasion.

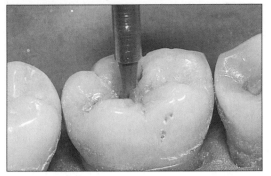

Fig 11-4b Fifty-micron alumina powder is projected into the fissure.

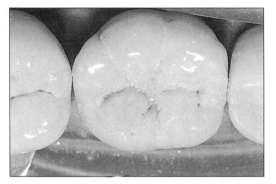

Fig 11-4c The fissures are shown after air abrasion.

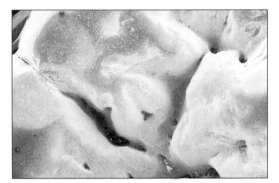

Fig 11-4d Scanning electron photomicrograph of fissures opened with air abrasion.

is designed. To enhance their ability to resist fracture, enamel margins should be prepared at a 90-degree or more obtuse angle; enamel margins of less than 90 degrees are much more subject to fracture (Fig 11-5).

For resistance form in the amalgam restoration, amalgam margins should be approximately 90 degrees. Although many amalgam restorations will have amalgam margins that are significantly less than 90 degrees on the occlusal surface, very acute amalgam margins are much more subject to fracture (Fig 11-6). Marginal fracture will usually cause marginal gaps, or ditches, between the amalgam and the enamel.

If the faciolingual width of the preparation exceeds one third the distance between the tips of the facial and lingual cusps (intercuspal distance), the remaining cusps themselves should be carefully evaluated. Even in narrower preparations, cusps should be evaluated for cracks that could lead to fracture, and the functional loading to which they will be exposed should be assessed. If a cusp is too weak to with-

stand function (Figs 11-7a to 11-7c), it should be reduced for coverage with amalgam or attached in some way to the amalgam to provide cuspal reinforcement (described in the section on complex amalgam restorations).

Occlusal amalgam restorations should have an occlusogingival thickness of at least 1.5 mm, and preferably 2.0 mm, to resist fracture during function (resistance form for the restoration). When carious dentin and the overlying enamel are removed, the preparation will be at least that depth and usually deeper.

Figure 11-8a shows a diagram of a cross section of the crown of a posterior tooth with carious dentin at the base of the fissure. Figure 11-8b shows a cross section of the amalgam restoration that is indicated because of that caries lesion. Figure 11-9 shows the outline form of several occlusal amalgam restorations; the outline form was determined by the extent of the demineralized dentin at the base of the fissures. Again, fissures not known to be carious, in a surface

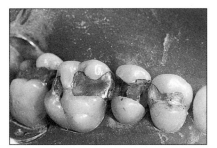

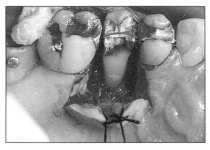

Fig 11-5 An acute cavosurface margin of enamel has the potential for fracture; a 90-degree enamel margin on the occlusal surface will withstand occlusion.

Fig 11-6 The left margin exhibits an acute "fin" of amalgam, which has a greater propensity for fracture, depending on the load applied to it during mastication. The right marginal configuration allows nearly a 90-degree angle for amalgam, imparting greater strength.

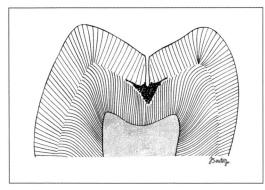

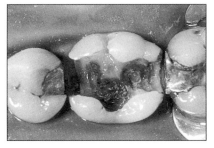

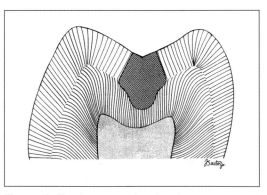

Fig 11-7a The mesio-occlusodistal preparation in the premolar, after removal of a defective restoration, is greater than one third the intercuspal distance; therefore, the cusps should be protected by reduction and coverage with a restoration, or they should be cross splinted (see Fig 11-40).

Fig 11-7b The mesio-occlusodistal preparation in the molar leaves cusps much too thin to resist occlusal loading; they must be reduced and protected with a complete occlusal coverage restoration.

Fig 11-7c The lingual cusp of the maxillary premolar, which was not protected or reinforced during restoration, has fractured.

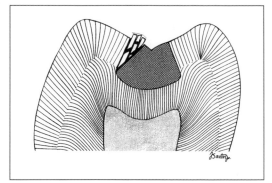

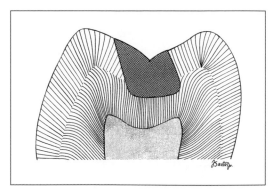

Fig 11-8a Fissure caries in this tooth involves demineralization of the enamel at the depth of the fissure, spread of the caries lesion along the dentinoenamel junction, and penetration of the lesion into dentin.

Fig 11-8b Tooth preparation involves removal of the carious dentin and of the enamel not supported by sound dentin. Only the diseased dentin is removed; additional dentin is not removed simply to create a flat pulpal floor for the preparation.

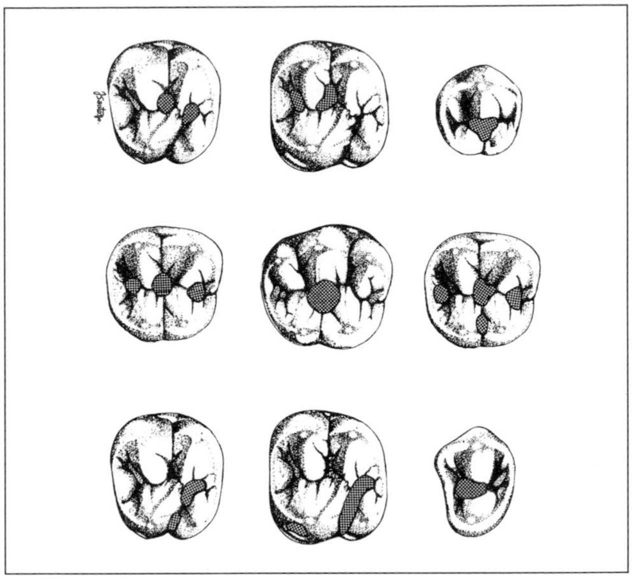

Fig 11-9 Outline form of various Class 1 preparations. The extent of carious demineralization is the determinant of outline form, so outline form will vary in every situation involving caries. Fissures not known to be carious should be sealed with a resin fissure sealant; fissures may be opened with a small bur to a depth of approximately 0.5 mm prior to sealing to ensure sound enamel for bonding.

receiving an amalgam restoration due to fissure caries, should be sealed with a resin fissure sealant.

If an occlusal carious lesion encroaches on the enamel of the proximal surface so that, when the carious dentin is removed, the proximal enamel has no dentinal support, consideration should be given to converting the Class 1 preparation to a Class 2 preparation. An important part of this consideration should be the determination of the forces to which the marginal ridge will be exposed. If there is direct occlusal contact between the opposing tooth and the weakened marginal ridge, the marginal ridge should be removed and restored with amalgam.

The Class 2 Preparation

Indications

An initial Class 2 restoration is usually placed because a carious lesion is present on a proximal surface of a molar or premolar. Proximal carious lesions can sometimes be diagnosed visually during a clinical examination, but they are usually diagnosed with bite-wing radiographs. The depth of the penetration of demineralization in enamel and dentin is actually greater than it appears to be in a bite-wing radiograph.

A carious lesion that appears radiographically to have penetrated about two thirds of the way through the proximal enamel has actually penetrated the dentinoenamel junction (DEJ). However, even if the lesion has slightly penetrated the DEJ, the tooth still has the potential for remineralization if the etiologic conditions are changed.[2,4] Each patient must be individually evaluated for improved oral hygiene, alteration of diet, and reduction in cariogenic bacteria before the decision is made to surgically remove a minimally deep carious lesion. In most cases, a restorative procedure should not be undertaken to treat a proximal carious lesion unless there is radiographic evidence of spread of the lesion at the DEJ and at least slight penetration in dentin toward the pulp.[4]

If a minimally deep dentinal carious lesion, initiated through demineralization of enamel in a proximal surface, necessitates a restoration, it may be treated by what is referred to as a *tunnel restoration*. One clinical study compared the longevity of glass-ionomer and cermet tunnel restorations to small Class 2 slot (defined below) amalgam restorations. That clinical trial, however, demonstrated a relatively high rate of failure for tunnel restorations after 3 years of service, with no failures of the slot amalgam restorations.[93] Because the tunnel restoration does not usually involve the use of dental amalgam, it is discussed in the chapter on direct posterior esthetic restorations (Chapter 10).

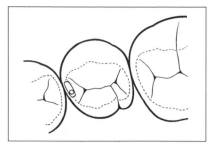

Fig 11-10a For a Class 2 preparation to treat an initial proximal surface caries lesion, an initial cut is made through the marginal ridge with a narrow bur to penetrate to carious dentin; then the slot is widened faciolingually.

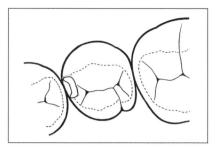

Fig 11-10b The mesial and distal aspects of the proximal enamel plate are thinned to facilitate its fracture and removal.

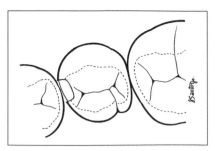

Fig 11-10c The final preparation outline will be determined after all carious tooth structure is removed. It should provide for at least minimal separation of margins from the adjacent tooth.

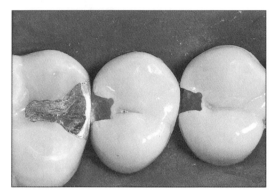

Fig 11-11 In the disto-occlusal slot preparations in the maxillary first and second premolars, the preparations have been opened facially and lingually so that contact is just broken to allow for carving and burnishing.

Outline Form

As with Class 1 restorations, Class 2 restorations that leave as much sound tooth structure as possible will contribute to resistance form for the tooth. Tooth preparation necessitated by a carious lesion on a proximal surface should, when possible, avoid extension of the occlusal outline more than is necessary to allow access to the proximal lesion, to remove demineralized enamel and dentin, and to remove enamel not supported by sound dentin. If an occlusal caries lesion is present, it should be treated with a separate occlusal restoration. If the preparation necessitated by the occlusal caries lesion is in close proximity to the occlusal outline of the proximal preparation, so that there is minimal or no sound tooth structure separating the

two preparations, they should be joined. As when Class 1 occlusal restorations are placed, fissures not known to be carious but believed to be susceptible to caries should be sealed with a resin fissure sealant.[108] Fissures that contact the outline of a Class 1 or Class 2 preparation should be sealed. Retention form for the proximal restoration should be attained within the proximal preparation; the preparation should not be extended further into a sound occlusal surface to provide retention of the proximal restoration, because this will weaken the tooth's resistance to fracture.

Access to the proximal carious lesion is usually made by preparation through the marginal ridge. Creating a slot cut with a small bur, in the center (mesiodistally) of the crest of the marginal ridge and occlusal to the carious lesion (Fig 11-10a), begins the proximal preparation. The slot is deepened gingivally until the bur "falls" into the carious lesion. The preparation is widened facially and lingually to eliminate all demineralized tooth structure at the DEJ and to remove enamel that is not supported by sound dentin. Demineralized enamel should usually also be removed. However, if demineralization is superficial (less than halfway through the enamel), and there is evidence that the patient will reduce his or her caries risk status, consideration should be given to stopping the extension of the preparation short of removing some superficial demineralized enamel. After the amalgam restoration has been placed, the demineralized enamel can be treated with fluoride to enhance remineralization, or it can be acid etched and coated with light-cured resin for at least short-term protection from further demineralization.[57] Alternatively, the demineralized enamel can be removed with a round bur or hand instrument; then the sound enamel walls of the dished-out area can be etched and the area can be restored to contour with bonded resin composite.

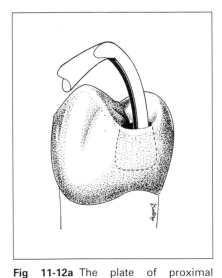

Fig 11-12a The plate of proximal enamel should be fractured with a hand instrument to prevent damage to the adjacent tooth by a bur. The instrument is placed in the slot.

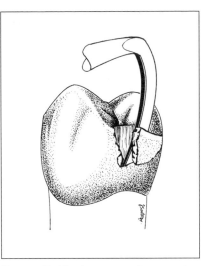

Fig 11-12b The instrument is rotated to fracture the plate.

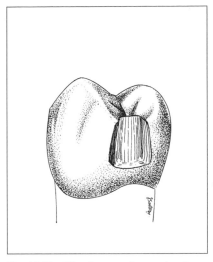

Fig 11-12c The fractured margins have been planed with a gingival margin trimmer or hatchet.

The Class 2 restoration necessitated only because of a proximal carious lesion and having an occlusal outline limited to the marginal ridge area will be referred to in this chapter as a slot restoration. If it involves the distal surface with access from the occlusal surface, it will be called a disto-occlusal (DO) slot restoration (Fig 11-11).

When the proximal slot restoration is prepared, a shell of enamel should be left between the preparation and the adjacent tooth (Figs 11-10b and 11-12a to 11-12c). This will prevent accidental nicking, scarring, or other damage to the adjacent tooth. One study[137] found that proximal surfaces of adjacent teeth were damaged during Class 2 preparation 69% of the time and that these damaged surfaces were almost three times as likely to become carious as were undamaged surfaces. Special care to avoid damage to the adjacent tooth is warranted. Any nicking or scarring of an adjacent tooth should be polished before the restoration is placed.

The proximal surface margins of a Class 2 amalgam preparation should not usually be in contact with the adjacent tooth (Fig 11-10c). Breaking contact slightly will allow the amalgam at those margins to be carved and burnished (with a very thin carver, such as the interproximal carver) during the restoration placement procedure. If, however, to eliminate contact with the adjacent tooth, a significant amount of sound enamel that is supported by sound dentin would have to be cut away, consideration should be given to allowing contact to remain or to using proximal surface stripping with abrasive strips (Figs 11-13a to 11-13c) to avoid widening the preparation simply to break contact.

During removal of carious dentin, the demineralized dentin in the periphery of the preparation (at or near the DEJ) should be removed and the outline form should be extended to ensure that the enamel at the margins of the preparation is supported by sound dentin. Carious dentin should be removed with the largest round bur that will fit into the area. After the periphery of the preparation is clear of demineralized tooth structure, the carious dentin near the pulp should be removed. The bur should be rotated very slowly in a low-speed handpiece; the rotation should be so slow that the individual blades of the bur can be seen as it rotates. The blades of the slowly rotating bur are like multiple spoon excavator blades, but the depth that a blade can penetrate into the carious dentin is limited by the edge angle of the bur and by the depth of each bur blade toward the center of the bur, so the bur will remove only a limited depth of carious dentin during each rotation. During removal of deep carious dentin, this procedure is less likely to result in a pulpal exposure than is the use of a spoon excavator.

315

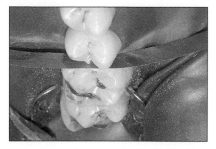
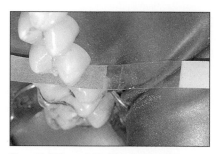
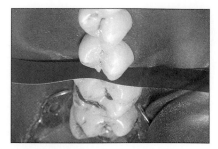

Fig 11-13a A metal-backed abrasive strip is used to provide minimal separation between the proximal cavosurface margins of a Class 2 preparation and the adjacent tooth. The tooth with the preparation or (as in this case) the adjacent tooth surface may be stripped in this way.

Figs 11-13b and 11-13c Strips with successively finer abrasives should be used to polish the abraded surface after separation is obtained.

Resistance and Retention Form

After the shape of the preparation is roughed out with a bur, hand instruments, such as a gingival margin trimmer (11-80-8-14 or 11-95-8-14), may be used to fracture away the shell of enamel, to shape the facial, lingual, and gingival walls and margins, and to scrape away any fragile enamel from the margins (Figs 11-14a to 11-14e). The facial and lingual walls of a Class 2 slot preparation should converge slightly toward the occlusal surface to provide retention form for the restoration (Fig 11-15).

To provide resistance form for the Class 2 amalgam restoration, the proximal preparation should have a mesiodistal dimension of about 1.5 mm or more. If there is sound dentin supporting occlusal enamel in the fossa adjacent to the marginal ridge, that dentin and enamel should be left intact. If the caries lesion extends from the proximal DEJ deeper into dentin, the demineralized dentin should be removed completely, especially in the areas near the DEJ, and sound dentin should be left in place.

The gingival floor of the proximal preparation may be flat and approximately perpendicular to the long axis of the tooth, or it may be curved faciolingually, as determined by the extent and configuration of the carious lesion that necessitated the restoration. The location of the gingival floor, therefore, should be determined by the gingival extent of the carious lesion and/or by the level necessary to provide separation of the gingival margin from the adjacent tooth. The gingival wall, like the facial and lingual walls of the proximal preparation, should form an angle of ap-

proximately 90 degrees with the surface of the tooth. This provides strength to both the amalgam and enamel and prevents enamel not supported by sound dentin from being left at the margins of the restoration.

Convergence toward the occlusal surface of the facial and lingual walls of the proximal slot preparation gives retention form to the restoration to keep it from dislodging occlusally. Although, with initial proximal surface caries lesions, it is not often necessary to extend the Class 2 preparation into occlusal grooves, the operator will frequently need to replace an existing restoration that was prepared with an occlusal extension. If the restoration is extended into occlusal grooves, this extension will provide resistance to displacement of the restoration proximally (that is, toward the adjacent tooth). To provide enough resistance, however, the extension into the occlusal surface must have a faciolingual dimension of at least one fourth the distance between the facial and lingual cusp tips[157] (intercuspal distance), and the facial and lingual margins of the occlusal extension must be approximately parallel to each other in a mesiodistal direction (Fig 11-16a).

Undercuts

If the extension into the occlusal surface is narrower, or if there is no extension into the occlusal grooves, as with the proximal slot restoration, retentive undercuts (retention grooves or points) must be cut into the dentin of the facial and lingual walls of the proximal box (Fig 11-16b). Use of a No. ¼ (ISO 005) round bur, with a head diameter of 0.5 mm,[155,157,158] or a No. ⅛ (ISO 004) round bur, with a head diameter of 0.4

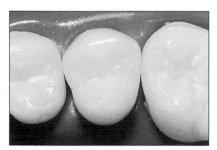

Fig 11-14a A disto-occlusal amalgam preparation will be made because an initial caries lesion is present.

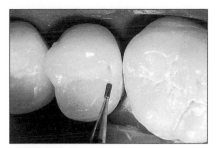

Fig 11-14b A small bur is used to cut a slot, beginning at the crest of the marginal ridge and extending gingivally to "fall" into carious tooth structure. A thin plate of enamel separates the bur from the adjacent tooth to prevent damage to the adjacent tooth.

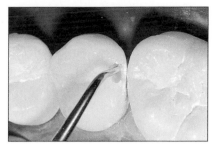

Fig 11-14c A gingival margin trimmer is placed into the slot created by the bur and rotated to apply pressure to the thin plate of proximal enamel.

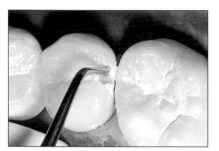

Fig 11-14d The thin plate is fractured.

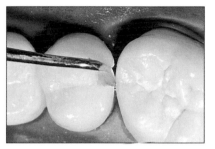

Fig 11-14e The walls and margins are planed with the margin trimmer to smooth them and to eliminate any remaining fragile enamel.

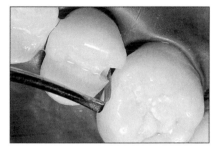

Fig 11-14f There is enough separation of the margins from the adjacent tooth to allow access to a thin carver (IPC) to carve and burnish the margins.

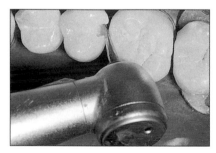

Fig 11-14g Retention grooves are placed with a No. ⅛ or ¼ bur.

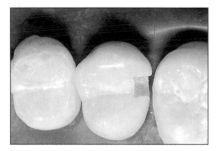

Fig 11-14h The preparation is completed.

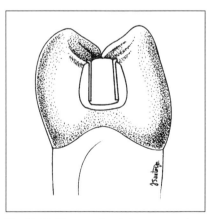

Fig 11-15 The proximal slot preparation, or the proximal box of a Class 2 preparation, should have walls that meet the proximal surface of the tooth at 90 degrees and converge occlusally to provide resistance and retention form.

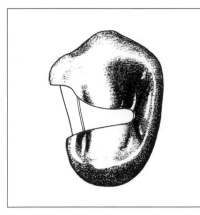

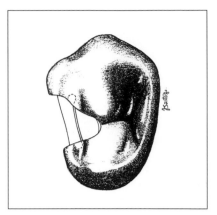

Fig 11-16a Although extension of a Class 2 preparation into occlusal grooves is not usually necessitated by caries, if such an extension is already present from a previous restoration of the tooth, it will provide some resistance form for the proximal portion.

Fig 11-16b An extension without parallel cavosurface margins, however, will not provide the resistance form needed to prevent displacement of the proximal amalgam during mastication, so retention grooves *(dotted lines)* should be added.

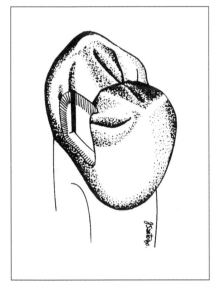

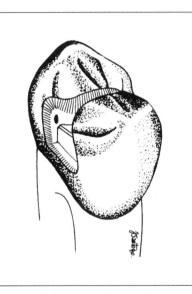

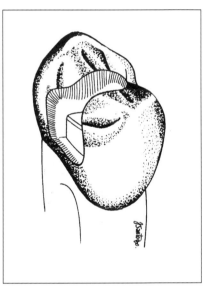

Fig 11-17a In a proximal slot or proximal box–only preparation, retention grooves should be long and very distinct.

Fig 11-17b In preparations with narrow occlusal extensions, short (0.5- to 1.0-mm) retention grooves or points are placed in facial and lingual walls just gingival to the occlusal DEJ.

Fig 11-17c When the occlusal extension is wide (1.5 mm or more faciolingually) and has parallel walls, retention points or grooves are not necessary.

mm, is recommended for preparation of retention grooves and points for Class 2 amalgam restorations (see Fig 11-14g). For a proximal slot restoration, retentive undercuts should be very distinct (at least 0.5 mm deep) and should oppose each other to form a dovetail effect in the dentin. Long grooves, extending from the gingival floor to the occlusal surface, are recommended for a proximal slot restoration[152,158] (Fig 11-17a). If the occlusal extension is narrow, short reten-

tion grooves, or retentive points, should be prepared in the dentin of the facial and lingual walls to supplement the resistance form provided by the occlusal extension[155] (Fig 11-17b). If there is a bulky extension of amalgam into the occlusal surface of the tooth, retentive undercuts should not be necessary[157] (Fig 11-17c). For preparing any retentive undercuts with a bur, it is advisable to use a handpiece at low speed, without water spray, and to use magnification to enable visual-

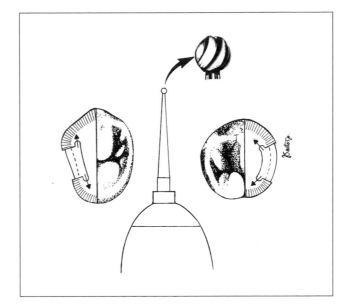

Fig 11-18 Location and direction of retentive undercuts (retention grooves) for the proximal portion of a Class 2 restoration. The illustrated grooves are approximately 0.5 mm wide and 0.5 mm deep (No. ¼ bur head is shown) and are directed approximately parallel to the DEJ (and the external surface of the tooth). *(left)* For a fairly flat surface, such as the proximal surface of a maxillary premolar, the grooves are directed almost in the facial and lingual directions. *(right)* For a convex proximal surface, such as in a mandibular premolar, their direction is considerably vectored.

Figs 11-19a and 11-19b *Proximal slot restorations placed by Dr Miles Markley; photographed in 1992.*

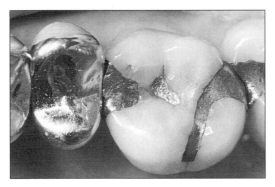

Fig 11-19a The MO slot restoration in the maxillary first molar has served for more than 58 years.

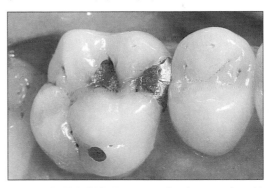

Fig 11-19b This MO slot restoration is more than 20 years old.

ization, because the location and direction of the undercuts are critical to the success of the restoration.

Retentive undercuts in the dentin of the facial and lingual walls should be completely in dentin and not at the DEJ; this obviates the removal of the dentinal support for the proximal enamel adjacent to the restoration. The undercuts should not, however, be placed so far away from the DEJ that the pulp chamber could be penetrated. A good rule is to place retentive undercuts so that there is approximately 0.25 to 0.5 mm of dentin between the groove and the DEJ and so that the groove is approximately 0.5 mm deep and 0.5 mm wide. Again, the 0.5-mm diameter of the No. ¼ round bur, or the 0.4-mm diameter of the No. ⅛ bur, is ideal as a gauge of dimension. So that retentive undercuts do not penetrate through the dentin to

the DEJ when they are placed in the facial and lingual walls, they should be cut to be parallel faciolingually to the DEJ and to the external surface of the tooth (Fig 11-18).

When retentive undercuts are necessary, they must be actual undercuts in the facial and lingual dentin that oppose each other (Fig 11-18). This is especially important in proximal slot restorations, in which the undercuts are the only feature that will prevent dislodgment of the restoration proximally. Without correctly located, distinct retention grooves, a proximal slot restoration is doomed to failure. When well designed, the proximal slot restoration can last indefinitely. Figures 11-19a and 11-19b show two Class 2 slot amalgam restorations; one has been in function for more than 58 years and the other for more than 20 years.

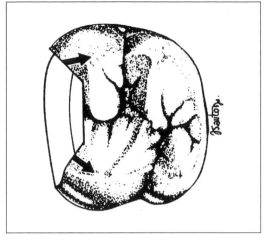

Fig 11-20a For a proximal box that is so wide that retentive undercuts, if placed parallel to the adjacent DEJ, would not oppose each other to provide any undercut retention, undercuts (retention grooves) should not be placed.

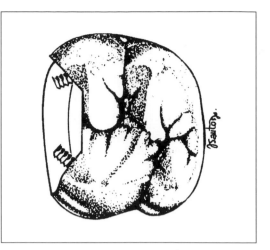

Fig 11-20b Instead, other types of resistance and retention, such as these horizontal self-threading pins, should be employed.

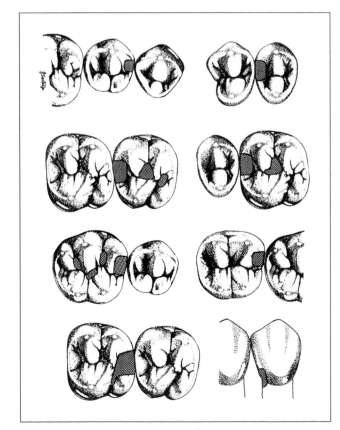

Fig 11-21 Typical outline forms of Class 2 restorations placed to treat initial caries lesions. Because outline form is determined by the pathosis present and the morphology and position of the tooth, there are an infinite number of variations. The bottom right-hand restoration represents a facial slot or keyhole restoration to treat root caries, or caries at the cervical line.

Mechanical Retention

If a proximal box or slot is so wide that retentive undercuts will not oppose each other (Fig 11-20a), another type of retention and resistance method, such as amalgam bonding or a self-threading pin, placed horizontally or vertically, should be used (Fig 11-20b). Amalgam bonding and the use of pins are discussed later in this chapter.

Because the outline form of Class 2 amalgam restorations is always determined by the pathologic problem being treated, there are an infinite number of variations in occlusal outline form. Figure 11-21 illustrates the outline form of some typical Class 2 restorations that would be placed to treat initial carious lesions.

Facial and Lingual Access

Most Class 2 amalgam restorations have occlusal access, as already discussed. If a proximal caries lesion is at or apical to the cementoenamel junction, however, it is often more conservative to use facial, and occasionally lingual, access.[8] The preparation for a Class 2 amalgam restoration with facial or lingual access, sometimes referred to as a *keyhole preparation* or *facial* or *lingual slot preparation*, is similar to a slot preparation with occlusal access. The entire preparation is apical to the proximal contact. The location and configuration of the caries and the access preparation determine the outline form of the keyhole preparation (Fig 11-21, bottom right). Its margins, which are usually on cementum or dentin, should be at approximately 90 degrees to the external surface of the tooth. Groove retention, similar to that recommended for a proximal slot preparation with occlusal access, is indicated and can usually be placed with a No. ¼ or No. ⅛ bur; occasionally, grooves must be placed with a hand instrument, such as a gingival margin trimmer.

Replacement of Restorations with Occlusal Extensions

Patients commonly will have existing Class 2 amalgam restorations that have extensions of the preparation through occlusal fissures and even through nonfissured grooves. Although this preparation outline form should not currently be advocated, existing restorations of this type will need to be replaced from time to time. Therefore, some design concepts to promote their longevity must be discussed. First, the narrower (faciolingually) the extension through the occlusal surface, the less marginal breakdown will occur[12,121] (Fig 11-22). Second, the junction of the proximal portion and the occlusal extension of the Class 2 amalgam preparation must have adequate depth occlusogingivally (1.5 to 2.0 mm) or the proximal portion must have distinct and effective undercuts in the dentin of the facial and lingual walls.[158] The occlusal outline form at the junction of the proximal and occlusal components should not be sharp or jagged, but sound cuspal enamel should not be sacrificed to make the junction smooth.

Complex Preparations

Historically, the term *complex amalgam restoration* referred to one that involved three or more surfaces of a tooth. The term has been redefined in recent years[139] to refer to an amalgam restoration that replaces one or more cusps.

When a metal cuspal-coverage restoration is indicated, a gold casting is considered the restoration of choice. Gold has wear characteristics similar to those of enamel and has the ability to maintain a stable occlusion. However, for various reasons, a gold casting cannot always be chosen as the definitive restoration. In these situations, amalgam is an excellent alternative restorative material.

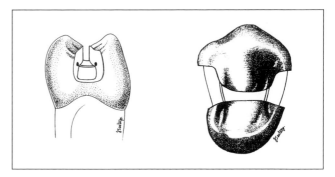

Fig 11-22 When extension through occlusal fissures or grooves cannot be avoided, such as when an old, defective amalgam restoration is being replaced, the faciolingual width of the occlusal portion of the preparation should be kept as narrow as possible to maintain tooth strength. *(left)* Proximal view; *(right)* occlusal view of mesio-occlusodistal preparation.

The efficacy of the amalgam cuspal-coverage restoration has been shown in both laboratory and clinical studies.[91,139,150,153] The key to the successful placement of cuspal-coverage restorations is a thorough understanding of the underlying engineering principles. Preparations for amalgam restorations have traditionally been designed to provide adequate retention form. Retention has been defined as prevention of dislodgment of the restoration along the path of insertion (with tensile forces). Resistance is defined as prevention of dislodgment or fracture by oblique or compressive forces. Although retention form is important in the complex amalgam restoration, more emphasis should be placed on the resistance of both the restoration and the remaining tooth structure. Retention and resistance form can be obtained through the use of metal threaded pins, non-pin mechanical features, and amalgam bonding, all of which will be described.

Cuspal-Coverage Preparations

Often, individuals seek treatment because of a fractured cusp or cusps in posterior teeth. If the treatment option agreed on for the tooth is a complex amalgam restoration, the tooth preparation will usually include removal of any existing amalgam restoration, removal of any carious tooth structure and fragile enamel and/or dentin, and preparation of margins to provide a cavosurface angle of approximately 90 degrees in all areas. In addition, weak cusps that have not fractured

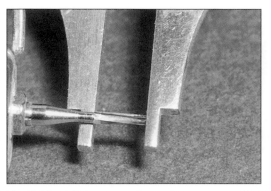

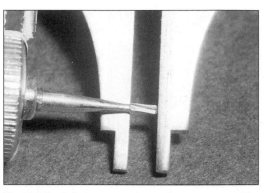

Fig 11-26a A Boley gauge is used to measure a No. 56 bur head (4.0 mm in this case).

Fig 11-26b A Boley gauge is used to measure a No. 330 bur head (2.0 mm in this case). A handy instrument for measuring bur head length is the periodontal probe.

Figs 11-27a to 11-27c Preoperative registration of the height of cusps to be reduced and restored with amalgam.

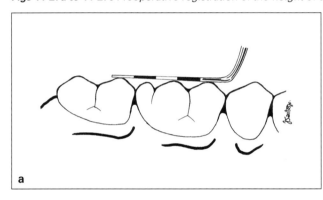

a

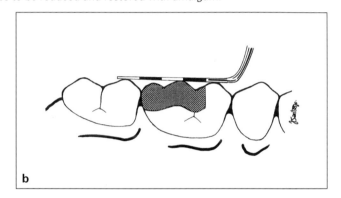

b

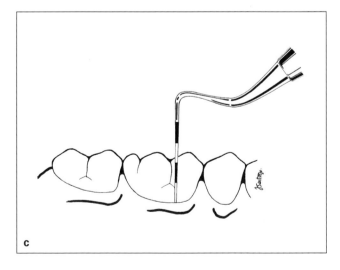

c

Fig 11-27a The midfacial and distofacial cusps are to be reduced for coverage. A periodontal probe is placed along the facial cusp tips of the tooth to be restored and the adjacent teeth, and the relationships of the cusp tips to the probe are remembered or drawn.

Fig 11-27b The amalgam cusp tips of the carved restoration are seen to have a similar relationship to the probe.

Fig 11-27c If there are no adjacent teeth or cusp tips to guide the height of amalgam cusp tips, the distance from a landmark (such as the cervical line) may be measured with a periodontal probe.

Figs 11-28a and 11-28b Scanning electron micrographs of self-threading pins. (Courtesy of Dr John O. Burgess.)

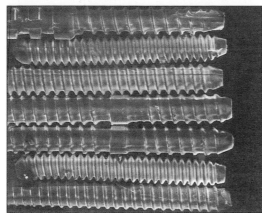

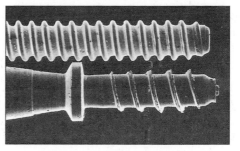

Fig 11-28b *(top)* Coltène/Whaledent TMS Minim pin and *(bottom)* Max pin (with threads more widely separated to allow for greater thickness of dentinal threads).

Fig 11-28a *(top to bottom)* Brasseler PPS (titanium alloy); Denovo Denlok (stainless steel); Vivadent Filpin (titanium); Coltène/Whaledent TMS (Thread Mate System) Link Plus (titanium alloy); Coltène/Whaledent TMS Link Plus (stainless steel); Coltène/Whaledent TMS Minim (stainless steel); Fairfax Dental Stabilok (stainless steel).

A time-saver in practice is to take note of cuspal height and cusp tip location, or even to make a drawing, prior to cuspal reduction, so that cusps may be built and carved back to their original height prior to removal of the rubber dam (Figs 11-27a to 11-27c).

Resistance and Retention Methods

For amalgam restorations that do not replace cusps, or at least large portions of cusps, the walls of the preparation provide retention and resistance form. Retention form is provided by convergent walls and undercuts placed in dentin. When a large amount of cuspal tooth structure is lost or removed, the walls, or portions of them, which provide resistance and retention for the amalgam, are lost. For this reason, it is necessary to add features to the preparation that will provide adequate resistance and retention for the restoration. Several methods of obtaining resistance and retention for complex amalgam restorations are discussed.

Pins

Although pins were first described in the 19th century,[49,73] Markley popularized the concept of cemented stainless steel pins.[99-101] Later, stainless steel pins, which were malleted into slightly undersized

channels in dentin (friction-locked pins),[61] and threaded stainless steel pins, which were screwed into channels in dentin,[59] were developed. Laboratory studies have since investigated the properties of these three types of pins (cemented, friction-locked, and self-threading), and, because of these studies, the self-threading pins are the only ones that are currently popular (Figs 11-28a and 11-28b). In a study by Dilts and coworkers,[46] self-threading pins were found to be more retentive in dentin than cemented or friction-locked pins. The authors also recommended a depth in dentin of 2.0 to 3.0 mm as optimum for self-threading pins. Moffa and others[114] found that a pin length of approximately 2.0 mm into amalgam provides optimum retention. The relationship between retention and the diameter of the pin has also been investigated. As would be expected, larger-diameter pins are more retentive.[46,47,114]

Self-threading pins are manufactured in a variety of configurations. Some are self-shearing and some have heads. Figure 11-28a shows several pins from various manufacturers. In one study of self-threading pins,[28] pins manufactured by Coltène/Whaledent and Brasseler demonstrated superior resistance and retention.

Most currently marketed pins have the metal threads separated to provide thicker, bulkier dentinal threads. When a pin is pulled from a pin channel, it is the dentinal threads that shear and not the metal

Figs 11-29a and 11-29b Color-coded pin channel (twist) drills and pins of various diameters and lengths (Coltène/Whaledent TMS).

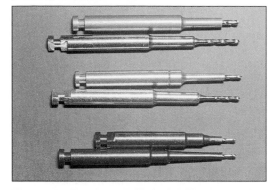

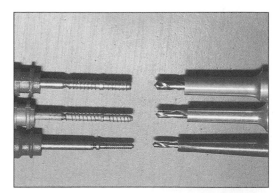

Fig 11-29a Pin channel (Kodex) drills: *(top to bottom)* Regular (gold, 0.027-inch [0.675-mm] diameter, 2.0- and 5.0-mm lengths); Minim (silver, 0.021-inch [0.525-mm] diameter, 2.0- and 5.0-mm lengths); Minikin (red, 0.017-inch [0.425-mm] diameter, 1.5-mm length).

Fig 11-29b Pins with corresponding pin channel drills: *(top to bottom)* Regular (0.031-inch diameter) gold-plated stainless steel Link Plus pin with Regular (0.027-inch diameter) pin channel drill (2.0-mm depth-limiting); Minim (0.024-inch diameter) titanium alloy Link Plus pin with Minim (0.021-inch diameter) pin channel drill (2.0-mm depth-limiting); Minikin (0.019-inch diameter) titanium alloy Link Series pin with Minikin (0.017-inch diameter) pin channel drill (1.5-mm depth-limiting).

threads. The pin design with wider dentinal threads is retained well in dentin (Fig 11-28b). Another feature of many of the currently available pins is a shoulder stop. The purpose of this feature is to prevent the end of the pin from putting stress on the dentin at the end of the pin channel; the PPS pin (Brasseler) and the Max pin (Coltène/Whaledent) have an effective shoulder stop incorporated into their design. A shoulder is a part of the design of the Link Plus pin (Coltène/Whaledent), but its diameter is similar to that of the threads, so it does not provide an effective stop.[102] Although a definite shoulder stop is theoretically beneficial, there is no evidence of problems associated with pins that lack effective shoulder stops.

Coltène/Whaledent pins and pin channel drills in Regular, Minim, and Minikin sizes are shown in Figs 11-29a and 11-29b; a smaller size (Minuta, 0.0135-mm diameter twist drill; 0.015-mm diameter pin) is available, but we have been unable to find a practical use for it. The gold-plated stainless steel TMS Regular and Minim pins (see Figs 11-34b and 11-34c) are also available as self-shearing pins, and in double-shear (two pins in one) form as well as single-shear form. All TMS Link and Link Plus (with shoulder) pins are self-shearing; Link Plus Regular and Minim pins are also available in the two-in-one form. The Link and Link Plus pins are available in either gold-plated stainless steel or titanium alloy; these may be inserted manually or with any low-speed, latch-type hand-

piece. The bulk TMS pins are available only in gold-plated stainless steel and are usually inserted manually. Selection among these pins should be based on operator preference; they all have performed well in laboratory studies.

Number to use. It is difficult to develop a guideline that would determine the appropriate number of pins for all situations. Although it has been demonstrated that as the size and number of pins increase, the amount of resistance form imparted by the pins increases,[25] the number of pins used will vary with the size of pin, the amount of remaining tooth structure, other mechanical resistance features used, the use of amalgam bonding systems, and the expected functional requirements of the final restoration.

Channel preparation. A rubber dam should be in place when pin channels are prepared and when pins are placed to protect the patient from aspiration and to prevent contamination by saliva in case there is pulpal perforation during pin channel preparation.

Because the tips of pin channel drills tend to move when the rotating tip is placed against dentin, it is usually helpful to place an indentation or starting point in the dentin at the desired location for the initiation of the pin channel. The starting point may be placed with a small bur, such as a No. 1/4 or No. 1/8 bur.

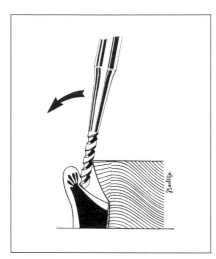

Fig 11-30a To align the twist drill with the side of the tooth when the external tooth surface is obscured, the drill is placed in the sulcus so that the drill is touching the preparation margin; the drill is then rotated *(arrow)*.

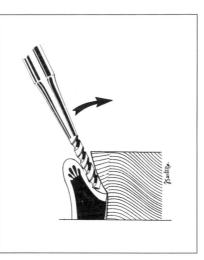

Fig 11-30b With that movement, the tip contacts the external surface and the portion of the drill that was in contact with the margin is rotated slightly away from it; then the length of the drill is rotated *(arrow)*.

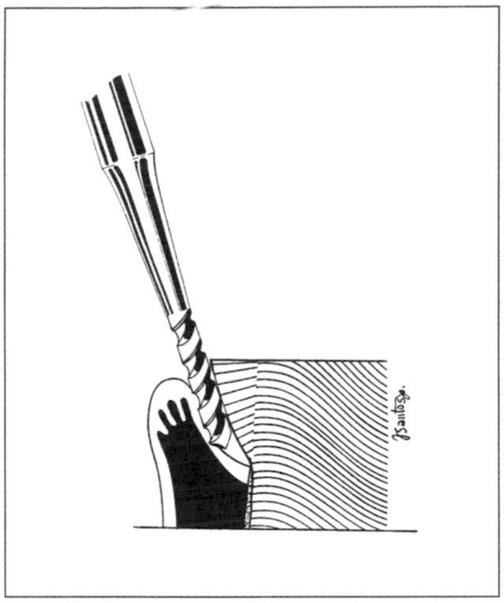

Fig 11-30c With that rotation, the drill returns just to touch the margin. It is now aligned parallel to the external surface.

Various lengths and diameters of twist drills are available for preparation of pin channels (Figs 11-29a and 11-29b). The most popular twist drills have depth-limiting shoulders, which ensure that the optimum pin channel depth is not exceeded. To avoid perforation of either the pulp or the external surface of the tooth, location of the pin channel is critical. The channel should usually be prepared parallel to the nearest external tooth surface. Before channel preparation is initiated, approximately 2.0 mm of the end of the twist drill should be placed against the external surface of the tooth. If that much of the side of the tooth is exposed above the rubber dam, alignment is facilitated. Frequently, however, adjacent soft tissue under the dam obscures visualization of the tooth surface in the area adjacent to the desired pin location. For alignment, the twist drill is placed against the external tooth surface, and the angulation of the drill is changed until the drill separates from the margin of the preparation; it is then rotated back until it just contacts the margin (Figs 11-30a to 11-30c).

Pin channels should be initiated at least 0.5 mm from the DEJ if the nearby preparation margin is coronal to the cementoenamel junction; a 1.0-mm distance from the DEJ is preferable.[46] If the nearby margin is apical to the cementoenamel junction, there should be at least 1.0 mm of dentin between the channel and the external surface of the tooth.

The most common location for pins is at the line angles of the tooth because of the greater thickness of dentin between the external surface and the pulp and the decreased risk of perforation. The risk of perforation is especially increased in furcation areas. Figure 11-31 illustrates the preferable locations for pins.[64] Areas to be avoided in posterior teeth include proximal areas and tooth structure that lies over furcations or concavities in the root. Wherever the pin is to be located, the external surface of the tooth should be assessed and the pin channel drill aligned parallel to it (Figs 11-32a to 11-32c).

Pins should be located so that the channels enter the dentin at approximately 90 degrees to the prepared dentin surface. If a depth-limiting twist drill is used, the drill will not be able to achieve optimum pin channel depth if the surface of dentin adjacent to the entrance of the channel is at an angle to the drill. In addition, a pin should not be located immediately adjacent to a wall of the preparation; there should be access to condense amalgam around the full circumference of the pin. If a pin is located an optimal distance from the DEJ and a dentinal wall is adjacent to the pin, a "cove" may be cut in the dentin to provide adequate space for amalgam (Fig 11-33).

To provide maximum cutting efficiency, the twist drill must be sharp so that it will be efficient at low speeds. A twist drill loses cutting efficiency with ex-

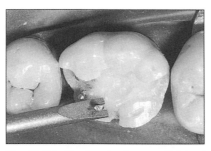

Fig 11-37a To bend pins, a Coltène/Whaledent pin bender can be used.

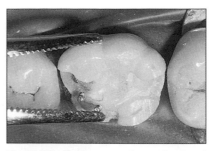

Fig 11-37b If a hemostat is used to bend a pin, the jaw of the hemostat should contact the pin at its tip, and very controlled pressure should be used in bending the pin.

Figs 11-38a to 11-38c Shortening a pin. A light, brushing stroke and air or water coolant should be used while a pin is cut.

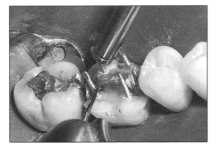

Fig 11-38a When a No. 169L tapered fissure bur is used to approach the pin at approximately 90 degrees, no stabilization is necessary.

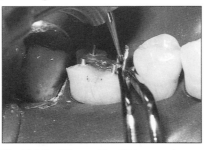

Fig 11-38b When a No. 35 inverted cone bur is approaching the pin obliquely, the pin is stabilized to prevent it from being unscrewed from the pin channel.

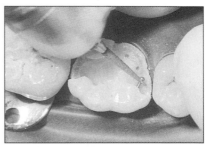

Fig 11-38c This needle-shaped diamond is approaching the pin at approximately 90 degrees.

with either a fissure bur or a diamond in a high-speed handpiece. Both the bur and the diamond should be used with air or water coolant to prevent the pin, and therefore the surrounding tooth structure, from being overheated during the operation. If a bur is used, it must be sharp. If the bur can approach perpendicularly to the pin, the pin does not require stabilization during the cutting process (Fig 11-38a). If the bur approaches from an oblique angle, the clockwise rotation of the bur can cause counterclockwise rotation of the pin so that it is unscrewed. Therefore, if the pin cannot be approached perpendicularly by the bur, it should be grasped with cotton forceps or a hemostat to stabilize it during the cutting process (Fig 11-38b), or, minimally, an instrument should be pressed against the pin during the process to dampen vibration from the bur, which tends to initiate the unscrewing. A long, narrow diamond is preferred by many operators for cutting pins, because it causes less vibration and is less likely to "catch" in the metal of the pin to initiate reverse rotation (Fig 11-38c).

Horizontal Pins

Studies[26,86] have demonstrated the efficacy of using pins oriented horizontally, that is, inserted into the dentin of a vertical wall of a preparation (Figs 11-39a and 11-39b). Burgess[26] found two horizontal self-threading pins (Coltène/Whaledent TMS Minim and Minikin) placed into a free-standing facial cusp of a maxillary premolar to be effective in reinforcing the cusp (Fig 11-39a). Other investigators[86] have found that horizontal pins, used to cross splint cusps of maxillary premolars, reinforce and strengthen the cusps (Fig 11-40).

Adequate dentin must be present for horizontal pins to be employed. When the channels for horizontal pins are prepared, they should be initiated in dentin 0.5 to 1.0 mm from the DEJ. They should be directed approximately parallel to the adjacent DEJ (and external surface of the tooth). But, because of their horizontal orientation, such pin channels, prepared only 1.5 to 2.0 mm deep, will often contact enamel. When the twist drill, in its progress through

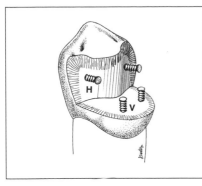

Fig 11-39a Horizontal pins (H) are used to attach the wall of a cusp to the amalgam restoration. Vertical pins (V) attach the restoration to the radicular portion of the tooth.

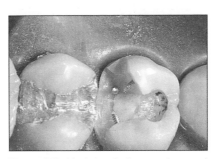

Fig 11-39b Horizontal pins can be used in conjunction with vertical pins. In this clinical situation, a proximal box had to be extended significantly facially to eliminate caries and unsupported enamel.

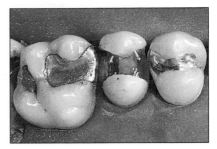

Fig 11-40 Horizontal pins are used to cross splint the cusps of a maxillary premolar.

dentin, seems to stop its penetration short of reaching its depth-limiting shoulder, it is probably because it has reached enamel. Further deepening of the channel should not be attempted; even 1.0 mm of depth will impart some retention for a pin, and attempts to deepen the channel into enamel will result in an enlarged dentinal channel and increased potential for enamel fracture.

Horizontal pins should be positioned fairly near to the occlusal surface in the dentin of a vertical wall, 0.5 mm to 1.0 mm gingival to the occlusal DEJ, so that their mechanical advantage is enhanced for reinforcement of the cusp. A horizontal pin should be oriented so that it will not be near the anticipated surface of the amalgam and so that amalgam may be condensed around the entire circumference of the pin.

Perforation During Pin Channel Preparation

Perforations during pin channel preparation should be avoided through careful design and placement of the channel. However, if a perforation does occur, it is important to determine what has been perforated, the external surface of the tooth or the pulp chamber. When the pulp chamber of a vital tooth has been perforated, the channel should be covered with calcium hydroxide, and another pin channel should be placed in a new location. Alternatively, a different type of resistance feature should be used. A perforation of the external surface of the tooth may be more problematic. If the perforation is located above the epithelial attachment, the channel should be filled with amalgam. If the pin is inserted and the tip protruding on the external surface is cut even with the surface

and polished, the pin will not totally obturate the perforation, and leakage will occur.[35] If the perforation occurs below the epithelial attachment, the channel may be obturated with gutta-percha and zinc oxide–eugenol sealer or with amalgam.

Non-Pin Mechanical Resistance and Retention Features

Birtcil and Venton[15] suggested that more attention be directed toward using the available tooth structure to provide retention and resistance form in complex amalgam restorations. They recommended parallelism in all walls of the preparation, proximal box form, retention grooves in the proximal line angles, box form in buccal and lingual groove areas of molars, dovetails, rectangular boxes in areas other than proximal surfaces, and reduction of undermined cusps for coverage with amalgam. In recent years, several additional non-pin resistance and retention features have been described and investigated. These include the circumferential slot, the amalgapin, and the peripheral shelf.

Circumferential slots. Outhwaite and others,[128] who introduced the circumferential slot prepared with a No. 33 ½ inverted cone bur (Fig 11-41), compared it to four pins (TMS Minim) and found no significant differences between the resistance provided by the two techniques. They also reported that the pin restorations had a greater tendency to slip on their bases before failure, whereas slippage did not occur with circumferential slots. However, slot-retained restorations are more sensitive to displacement during matrix removal than are pin-retained restorations.

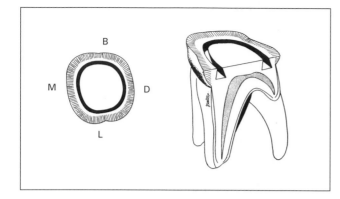

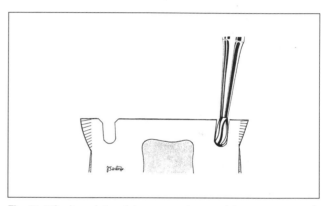

Fig 11-41 A circumferential slot is prepared with a small, inverted cone bur, such as a No. 33½.

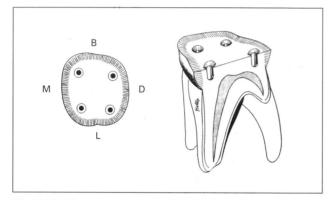

Fig 11-42a The entrances to amalgapin channels are beveled.

Fig 11-42b A variety of burs may be used to prepare amalgapin channels. A bur with a diameter of 0.8 to 1.0 mm, for example, the No. 330 bur, is desirable.

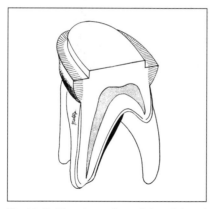

Fig 11-43 The circumferential peripheral shelf has been prepared with a 2.0-mm axial depth and a 1.0-mm cervical depth. For a flat preparation such as this, a peripheral shelf would not be adequate without other forms of resistance.

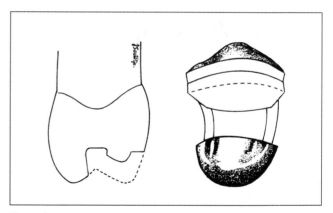

Fig 11-44 A more typical clinical use of a peripheral shelf is for resistance form for the amalgam-covered facial cusp of a premolar. *(left)* Cross-sectional view; *(right)* occlusal view.

Amalgapins. Seng and others[146] tested circular chambers that they cut vertically into dentin to provide resistance and retention form for the restoration; they called these features *amalgam inserts*. Preparations for the inserts were made with a No. 35 inverted cone bur and were approximately 1.4 mm in diameter and depth. In their study, amalgam inserts provided resistance to displacement similar to that provided by self-threading pins. Shavell[149] described a variation of the amalgam insert, which he termed the *amalgapin* (Figs 11-42a and 11-42b). The amalgapin channel described by Shavell was prepared with a No. 1157 or No. 1156 bur and had a depth of 3.0 mm. The margin of the channel entrance was beveled to decrease stress concentration in the amalgam. Laboratory studies of the amalgapin[41,140] have demonstrated that the resistance to displacement provided by amalgapins is similar to that provided by pins. It has been demonstrated[140] that a depth of 1.5 to 2.0 mm is adequate for amalgapins and that an amalgapin with a diameter of 0.8 mm provides resistance similar to that of an amalgapin with a diameter of 1.0 mm. In addition to the burs advocated by Shavell (No. 1156 and No. 1157), others with similar diameters (such as the No. 330 and No. 56) also function well in creating amalgapin channels.[140]

Peripheral shelves. Peripheral shelves provide another form of resistance for complex amalgam restorations (Figs 11-43 and 11-44). A narrow (1.0 mm axially and 1.0 mm cervically) shelf did not perform well in tests for resistance form.[138,154] A wider shelf (2.0 mm axially and 1.0 mm cervically) (Fig 11-43) provided significantly more resistance form. Typically, peripheral shelves, like circumferential slots, are not used circumferentially, but are used only in areas of the preparation where they are needed (Fig 11-44).

Efficacy of Resistance and Retention Methods

For the most part, the resistance form provided by various resistance and retention methods has been tested in flattened molars, as described by Buikema and others,[25] with 4.0-mm-high restorations retained by given resistance features. These teeth were mounted at a 45-degree angle and were loaded in compression; the mean loads at the time of failure were calculated. Although this method of testing is not as enlightening as long-term clinical tests, it probably provides a good indicator of how well a resistance feature will perform in a clinical situation. It has been shown, however, that if these standard resistance-test restorations are loaded at a 90-degree angle instead of a 45-degree angle, the stainless steel pins provide significantly more resistance than amalgam inserts.[88,160] Few forces in the mouth are directed at a 90-degree angle to the long axis of the tooth, however, and few restorations are placed on preparations that are totally flat, without any walls or irregularities in the dentin.

One of the most telling studies pertaining to resistance form for complex amalgam restorations was reported by Plasmans and coworkers.[133] This group created preparations for complex amalgam restorations that combined the use of boxes, shelves, and amalgapins as resistance and retention features. They then loaded specimens at 45 degrees, as in most previous studies of resistance form, but they loaded half of the restorations from one side and half from the other. Their finding was, generally, that more load was required to cause failure of a restoration when the resistance and retention features (walls of shelves, boxes, and amalgapin channels) that opposed the direction of the load were increased.

It is important to distribute mechanical resistance features into all areas of the preparation and not to cluster them in any area.[32,133,160] Figures 11-45a to 11-45d show a restoration that originally replaced two missing cusps of a mandibular molar. The probable cause of failure was that the resistance features (pins) were clustered on the lingual aspect of the cavity preparation. In function, there was nothing to attach the facial aspect of the restoration to the tooth. If two of the four vertical pins had been placed in the facial portion of the preparation (Fig 11-45e), or if two horizontal pins had been placed in the facial cusps (Figs 11-45f and 11-45g), the restoration would, in all likelihood, have had adequate resistance to withstand its load in function.

When the technical requirements for placement of vertical pins can be met, vertical pins provide excellent retention and resistance form. However, risks are involved with pin placement: crazing of tooth structure, perforation into the pulp or periodontium, and weakening of the amalgam restoration over pins.[27] Additionally, the use of both vertical and horizontal pins may be limited by inadequate access; in these cases, alternative resistance and retention methods should be employed. When a cusp has been reduced, and increased resistance form is needed, an amalgapin or a segment of a peripheral shelf or circumferential slot may be indicated.

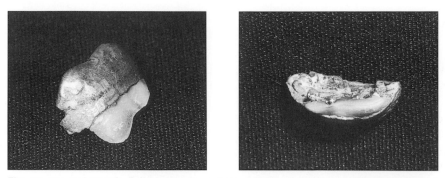

Figs 11-45a and 11-45b Failed complex amalgam restoration that replaced the lingual cusps of a mandibular molar. Note the fin of cervical tooth structure that fractured.

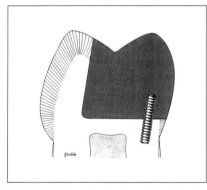

Fig 11-45c The dentin lingual to the pin was the only tooth structure that was opposing a lingually directed load on the restoration.

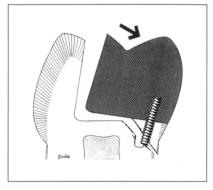

Fig 11-45d A load pushing the restoration lingually caused failure. Failure can be attributed to a lack of distribution of resistance and retention features.

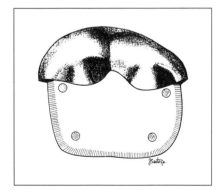

Fig 11-45e Alternatively, had two of the four pins been placed vertically in the facial aspect of the preparation, this could have reduced the likelihood of failure.

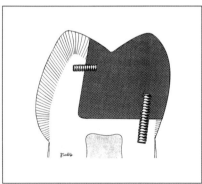

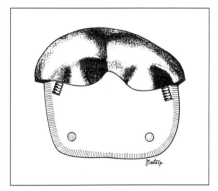

Figs 11-45f and 11-45g Had two of the four pins been located horizontally, failure would likely have been averted.

Amalgam Bonding

The use of adhesive resins to increase the retention, resistance, and marginal seal of amalgam restorations has gained much popularity. A few clinical studies have demonstrated effectiveness for several years of service.[7,94,147,151,153] Three-year results were reported for one clinical study[153] in which 30 bonded (Amalgambond Plus with HPA powder, Parkell) and 30 pin-retained (TMS pins) amalgam restorations were compared; each restoration replaced at least one cusp. At 3 years, 92% of the restorations were available for evaluation. Of the bonded restorations, all were still fully functional and the teeth vital. In the pin-retained group, there was an 11% failure rate. Failure modes included the need for endodontic therapy (two teeth) and a fractured cusp adjacent to the restoration (one tooth). In another clinical study of complex amalgam restorations,[7] all bonded and pin-retained restorations were classified as successful at 2 years.

Although clinical research data in several studies[7,91,151,153] support the efficacy of bonding as the sole provider of resistance and retention, the service time in these studies remains short. Amalgam bonding procedures may replace mechanical resistance and retention features some time in the future, but, because of the relatively short duration of current clinical studies, it would be prudent until then to use bonding resin in conjunction with mechanical features. Several in vitro studies have demonstrated the effect of using pins in combination with amalgam bonding.[29,74,75,92] In one of those studies,[29] the mean resistance provided by a filled amalgam bonding material combined with self-threading pins was approximately equal to the sum of the mean resistance produced by pins alone and the mean resistance produced by amalgam bonding alone. So, for large restorations, a combination of amalgam bonding systems with mechanical resistance features is recommended. This recommendation may change as additional longevity evidence accumulates.

For use of bonding resins in amalgam restorations, current research suggests the improved efficacy of filled resins compared with unfilled or minimally filled resins.[44,92,141,156] The method of incorporation of the filler varies from manufacturer to manufacturer. One system (Amalgambond Plus, Parkell) uses very fine methyl methacrylate powder, added to the liquid resin, as the filler.[110] Another system (All-Bond 2 and Liner F, Bisco) uses a filled flowable resin composite

liner to provide the filled resin. With both types of system, the amalgam is condensed into the filled resin while the resin is in a viscous liquid form. Microscopic "fingers" of resin are incorporated into the amalgam at the interface. When hardened, these provide the attachment of amalgam to resin. Because light cannot penetrate to the resin underlying amalgam restorations, it is important to use a self-curing or chemically activated bonding resin. The bonding resin of an amalgam bonding system will be supplied in two parts that are to be mixed. Either chemically cured resins or dual-cured (chemical and light initiation) resins may be effective. The attachment of resin to tooth structure when amalgam bonding systems are used is accomplished as with other dental bonding systems, as described in Chapter 8.

There is ample evidence of decreased leakage of fluids when an amalgam bonding system is used compared with noncoated or varnish-coated amalgam cavity walls.[10,11,33,48,84,162] Many dentists have reported that amalgam bonding systems have reduced the incidence of postoperative tooth sensitivity, but research has not supported these observations. Clinical studies[24,81] comparing postoperative sensitivity in bonded and nonbonded restorations have reported no significant difference.

For reinforcing cusps in posterior teeth weakened by significant pathosis or large restorations, there is in vitro evidence that amalgam bonding can result in some strengthening of teeth.[19,50,118,131] However, some of this effect may be lost with time.[18,66,143] At present, it is still advisable to reduce severely weakened cusps for replacement and protection with a strong restorative material.[27] The use of amalgam for this purpose is described in this chapter. Other types of occlusal-coverage restorations are described in several other chapters.

Amalgam bonding should not be used as the sole means of retaining an amalgam restoration but may be effective for supplementing mechanical resistance features in large, complex amalgam restorations, especially those replacing cusps. It should not be relied on to reinforce severely weakened cusps; such cusps should be reduced and restored with amalgam, or should be protected by another type of restoration that provides cuspal coverage. A filled amalgam bonding system should be used. Amalgam bonding should be used when an improved initial seal is needed, such as after a direct or indirect pulp capping procedure in the tooth being restored.

Figs 11-47a to 11-47j *Tofflemire matrix system.*

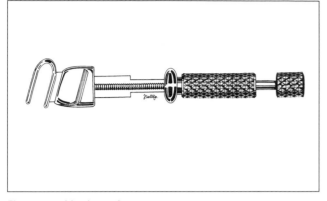

Fig 11-47a Matrix retainer.

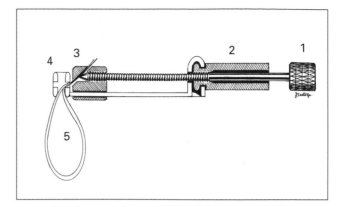

Fig 11-47b Parts of the assembly: (1) set-screw; (2) rotating spindle; (3) slide; (4) head; (5) band.

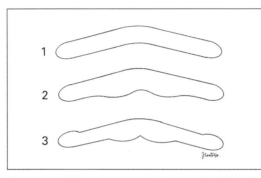

Fig 11-47c Three common shapes of Tofflemire matrix flat bands (No. 1 is also called a Universal band; No. 2 and No. 3 are also called MOD bands).

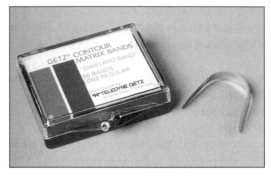

Fig 11-47d Precontoured Dixieland Bands.

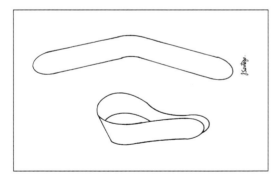

Fig 11-47e The matrix band is folded for insertion into the retainer.

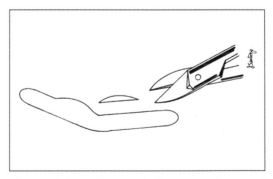

Fig 11-47f One of the projections of a No. 2 or 3 band may be cut if there is only one deep proximal area of the preparation.

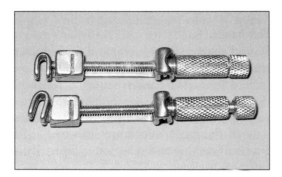

Fig 11-47g Two types of Tofflemire retainer: *(top)* straight; *(bottom)* contra-angled.

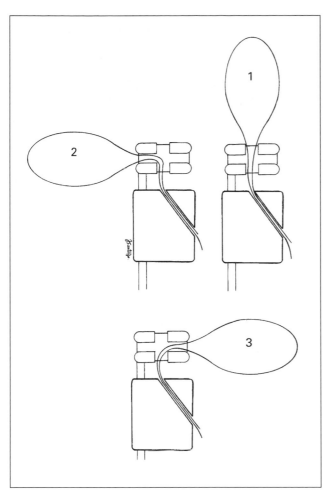

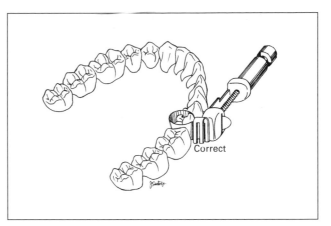

Fig 11-47i The matrix must be assembled with the slots in the head directed gingivally.

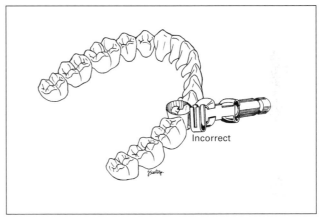

Fig 11-47h The loop of the band may extend from the head of the retainer in one of three directions: (1) straight; (2) left; (3) right.

Fig 11-47j The slots in the head of the matrix should not be directed occlusally.

By far the most frequently used shape is the No. 1, or Universal, band. The No. 2 band (so-called MOD band) has two extensions projecting at its gingival edge to allow matrix application in teeth with very deep gingival margins in the proximal aspects of the tooth. In most cases, there will be only one deep area, so one of the extensions is usually cut off with scissors (Fig 11-47f). The No. 3 band also has projections for deeper gingival margins, but the band is narrower than the No. 2 band. The No. 3 band is ordinarily considered suitable for premolars and the No. 2 band for molars, but the size that best suits the situation should be used.

Because these bands are flat, they should be contoured so that they will impart physiologic contours to the restorations. A flat band may be contoured before it is placed in the retainer. The band is laid on a paper pad, or other compressible surface, and the

area to be contoured is heavily rubbed with an ovoid burnisher, a beavertail burnisher, the convex back of the blade of a spoon excavator, or a convex side of the cotton forceps. A band may also be contoured after it has been applied to the tooth. The area to be contoured is rubbed with the back of the blade of the spoon excavator or other thin, convex instrument (Fig 11-48a). Contact with the adjacent tooth should be more than a pinpoint touch (Fig 11-48b).

Precontoured bands. Precontoured Tofflemire matrix bands are also available. One such band is the Dixieland Band (Teledyne Getz) developed by Dr Wilmer Eames (Fig 11-47d). When these bands are removed from interproximal contacts, the contour must be considered, and the band must be rotated in such a way that the trailing edge does not break or alter the shape of the marginal ridge as the band is being removed.

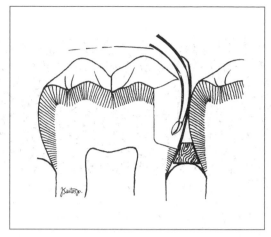

Fig 11-48a The convex side of a spoon excavator is used to impart a convex contour to the matrix band.

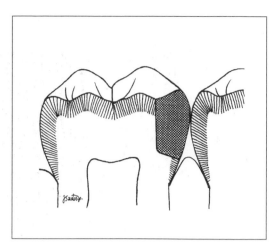

Fig 11-48b This will help to achieve a contact area, as opposed to a pinpoint contact, with the adjacent tooth.

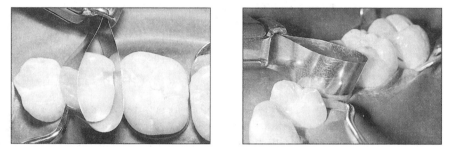

Figs 11-49a and 11-49b The blade of a plastic filling instrument has been placed into the gingival embrasure and is being slightly rotated (torqued) to provide enough separation to allow the matrix band to slip through the contact.

Placement

Assembly. When the matrix retainer and band are assembled, the two ends of the matrix band must be even as they protrude from the diagonal slot of the slide. The loop can extend from the retainer in three different ways: straight, to the left, or to the right (see Fig 11-47h). The straight assembly is for restorations near the front of the mouth where the rubber dam–covered cheek will not get in the way if the retainer protrudes perpendicularly from the line of teeth. The right and left assemblies allow the retainer to be aligned parallel or tangent to the line of teeth in more posterior areas. The band should be placed in the retainer so that the loop extends from the appropriate side of the retainer and the set-screw knob is directed toward the front of the mouth. Because of the shape of the Tofflemire matrix band, when it is placed in the retainer, one opening of the

loop has a greater diameter than the other (see Fig 11-47e). In other words, the loop will be shaped somewhat like a funnel. The wider opening is oriented toward the occlusal aspect. The short knob of the set-screw is tightened so that the matrix band is held securely.

Application. The matrix is applied to the tooth to be restored. The matrix band will slide easily through the interproximal contact area when the preparation has opened the contact. It will often slide through an intact contact as well (for example, the mesial contact when there is a disto-occlusal preparation). If it will not slide through the intact contact, a bladed plastic filling instrument (such as the No. 1-2, Figs 11-49a and 11-49b) may be used to open the contact slightly to allow the band through. For this slight tooth separation, the blade of the instrument is placed in the gingival embrasure (gingival to the contact), moved

Figs 11-50a to 11-50d Wooden interproximal wedges.

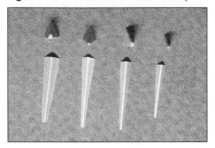

Fig 11-50a Wizard wedges have a triangular shape.

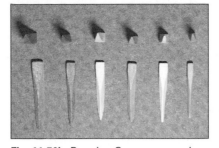

Fig 11-50b Premier Sycamore wedges are shaped to impart a more physiologic contour to the matrix. There is a larger selection of sizes, and they are color coded for easy selection.

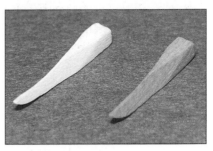

Fig 11-50c Note the anatomic shape of the Premier Sycamore wedges. The snow-sled point helps to prevent catching of the rubber dam during insertion.

occlusally until it is stopped by the contact, and torqued very slightly. At the same time, the matrix band is slipped through the contact. When the matrix is around the tooth, it should be tightened snugly, but not too tightly because a very tight matrix will deform the tooth.[9,135,136]

Wedging. Wooden wedges may be placed from either the facial or the lingual aspect. A wedge should usually be inserted from the side with the widest embrasure. For example, between the first and second premolars, the largest embrasure is usually the lingual embrasure. The wedge should be tightly inserted to enable development of an adequate contact despite the thickness of the matrix material.

Wedges are available in a variety of shapes and sizes. Figure 11-50a shows Wizard wedges (Teledyne-Water Pik), which are triangular and available in four sizes. Figures 11-50b and 11-50c show Sycamore wedges (Premier), which are shaped to aid the establishment of physiologic proximal contours. The Premier wedges, with seven color-coded sizes, are recommended for amalgam restorations.

The matrix band must extend gingival to the gingival margin of the proximal box of a Class 2 restoration, and the wedge must be positioned so that its base is also gingival to the gingival margin. If the wedge cannot be placed so that its base is gingival to the preparation margin, a concavity will be created in the matrix just occlusal to the gingival margin, and this concavity will be transferred to the amalgam. Occasionally, the gingival papilla will need to be surgically reflected from the interproximal area to allow the wedge to be positioned apical to the gingival margin. Another option is to use a rigid bladed instrument to hold the matrix against the gingival margin

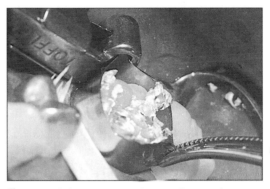

Fig 11-50d A custom-made wooden wedge may also be used. This one was made from a tongue blade.

during condensation. Custom wedges may be made for special situations; the wedge in Fig 11-50d was fabricated from a wooden tongue blade.

Contouring. The band should be burnished and contoured to impart the desired proximal contours to the restoration. This can be accomplished with the back (convex side) of a spoon excavator (Fig 11-48a). The wedged matrix should be in solid contact with the adjacent tooth in the desired contact area. It should be possible to feel the convexity of the proximal surface of the adjacent tooth with an instrument through the matrix as the matrix is burnished.

Removal

In a multiple surface restoration, amalgam is condensed in the preparation after matrix placement. Amalgam condensation is discussed in the next section.

When restoration with a Tofflemire matrix has been completed, first the slide and then the set-screw is loosened. A finger or thumb is placed on the loop of the matrix band to keep it in place and the retainer is pulled occlusally to remove it. The distal end of the matrix is grasped and pulled occlusally and lingually (if the free ends are on the facial aspect) and out of the distal contact of the tooth. The mesial end is then grasped and pulled facially and occlusally until the band is out of the contact. The matrix band can be grasped with fingers, cotton forceps, or a hemostat. There are a few tricks that may help the dentist remove the Tofflemire matrix without breaking the marginal ridge:

1. As the matrix edge is coming out of the contact, the matrix can be tipped so that the edge will not "flip" the newly carved marginal ridge and break it.
2. A condenser can be held against the marginal ridge to support it and prevent it from breaking as the matrix is removed.
3. The movement of the band should be primarily to the facial or lingual aspect as the band slips occlusally out of the contact.
4. The band may be cut close to the teeth on the lingual aspect and then pulled facially from the contact.

The matrix band should be used only once and then discarded.

Other Matrix Systems

Many matrix systems other than Tofflemire matrices are available (Figs 11-51 to 11-55). Each has its own advantages and disadvantages. In addition, stainless steel matrix material may be spot welded to provide a custom matrix for any situation. One commercial system (Denovo) has prewelded bands in various sizes (Figs 11-51a and 11-51b). To remove spot-welded matrices, a small bur in a high-speed handpiece is used to cut through the welds and allow the two ends of the matrix to separate for removal. The absence of a matrix retainer in the Denovo system is a distinct advantage.

T-bands have long been used in dentistry and provide a very simple and inexpensive matrix system (Fig 11-52). The AutoMatrix system (Caulk/Dentsply) has a built-in matrix retainer that is much smaller than the Tofflemire matrix retainer, which is an advantage (Figs 11-53a and 11-53b). The Palodent matrix (Darway) system provides small, precontoured matrices that are placed, wedged, and held in place by a flexible metal Bitine ring. A major advantage of this system is that,

for a restoration involving only one proximal surface, there is no need for the matrix to be placed in the other contact (Figs 11-54a to 11-54c). The Omni-Matrix (Innovadent) is basically a disposable Tofflemire retainer and band that is preassembled and has a head that moves from side to side (Fig 11-55). Because there is no assembly time, this system takes less time to use than a Tofflemire matrix, but it is more expensive.

Reinforcing Matrices with Modeling Compound

Among the desirable qualities of a matrix are rigidity and maintenance of the shape established by the operator. When a Class 2 preparation has only proximal boxes that are adjacent to other teeth, and when the preparation does not, to any significant degree, extend to facial and lingual surfaces, the stainless steel matrix is usually well supported by the adjacent tooth or teeth. In these cases, no reinforcement is necessary. In larger restorations that involve surfaces not supported by adjacent teeth, it is often desirable to reinforce or support the matrix in some way in these areas to maintain the rigidity and shape of the matrix.

Occasionally, a single unsupported area of a matrix may be reinforced during condensation by the operator, who places a finger or holds an instrument against the matrix in a facial or lingual area. For large unsupported areas, however, modeling compound may be used (Figs 11-56a to 11-56j).

There are various ways of applying compound to support a metal matrix. Probably the most simple is to employ a stick of compound (Fig 11-56a). Approximately 1.0 inch of one end of the compound stick is heated over an alcohol burner. The stick is moved back and forth, while being rotated, over the tip of the flame (Fig 11-56b). After 5 to 10 seconds, the stick is removed from the flame and held for a few seconds until the heat has diffused to the center of the stick, as indicated by its starting to droop or sag (Fig 11-56c). At that point, the 1.0-inch end is soft enough to carry to the matrix and press into place with a dampened, gloved finger (Fig 11-56d). If adhesion of the compound to the matrix and adjacent teeth is desired, the softened end of the stick should be passed through the flame again before it is carried to the mouth; this will provide a tacky surface that will impart some adhesion.

After the compound is pressed into place (Fig 11-56e), it is cooled and hardened with air from the three-way syringe. The matrix may be recontoured after compound application. A warmed instrument is

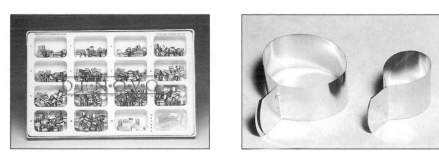

Figs 11-51a and 11-51b Denovo matrix system.

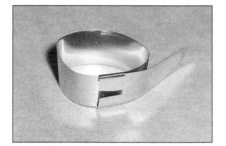

Figs 11-52 T-band matrix.

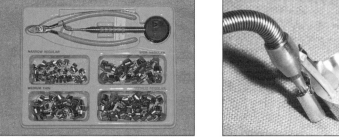

Figs 11-53a and 11-53b AutoMatrix system. Note the cable-drive wrench for adjusting the size of the loop.

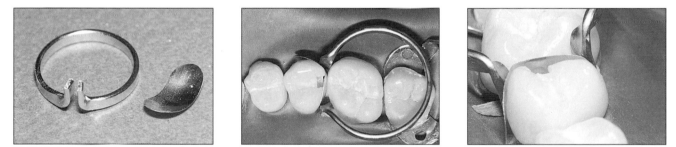

Figs 11-54a to 11-54c Palodent matrix system. Note the metal ring for holding the ends of the matrix snugly against the facial and lingual enamel. It will also provide some tooth separation.

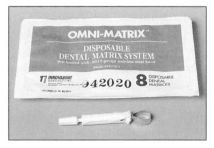

Fig 11-55 The Omni-Matrix is basically a preassembled Tofflemire retainer and band that is intended for one-time use and then disposal.

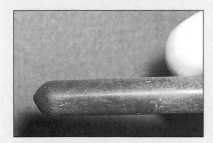

Fig 11-56a Modeling compound can be used to support a matrix.

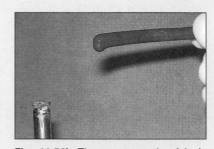

Fig 11-56b The compound stick is heated over an alcohol flame, then removed from the flame to allow warmth to diffuse to the core of the stick.

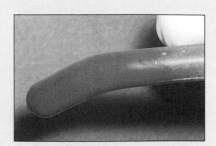

Fig 11-56c When the warmed tip of the compound stick begins to droop, softness is through and through, and the compound is ready for use.

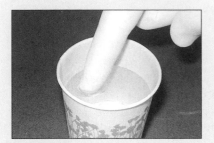

Fig 11-56d A finger is dampened in water to prevent the glove from sticking to the softened compound.

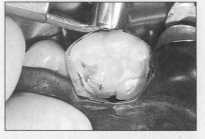

Fig 11-56e The compound has been pressed into place. It will be cooled with air to reharden it.

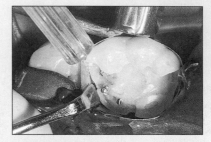

Fig 11-56f The matrix may be recontoured after application of the compound. A warmed instrument is used to soften the compound and reshape the matrix.

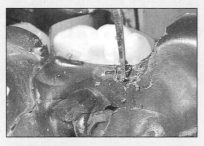

Fig 11-56g Any compound extending past the edge of the matrix should be trimmed to prevent chipping during amalgam condensation.

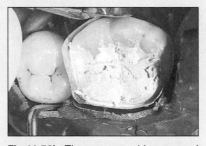

Fig 11-56h The compound is removed after amalgam condensation and initial carving.

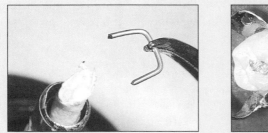

Figs 11-56i and 11-56j Staples can be used to hold compound segments in place.

used inside the matrix to soften the compound and exert pressure on the matrix to give it the shape that will allow the restoration contours and shape to be similar to the original shape of the tooth (Fig 11-56f). Again, the compound should be cooled with air after reshaping with a warmed instrument. If modeling compound extends occlusal to the occlusal edge of the matrix band, it should be trimmed back with a sharp instrument (Fig 11-56g) or pieces of compound could chip off during amalgam condensation and contaminate the amalgam.

If condensation forces dislodge the compound, matrix reinforcement will be lost; steps should be taken, therefore, to assure that the compound does not dislodge. While it is soft, a portion of it may be pushed onto the cusps of an adjacent tooth to provide retention, or, when compound is present on both the facial and lingual aspects, a staple-shaped piece of metal, made from a paper clip or other wire, may be warmed in the flame (Fig 11-56i) and placed to hold the facial and lingual segments of compound together (Fig 11-56j). When it is time to remove the staple, the tips of a hemostat are warmed in the flame, the staple is grasped, and the heat is allowed to diffuse into the compound surrounding the staple so that it is softened. The compound can usually be pried away from the adjacent teeth and matrix with an instrument such as a Hollenback carver or enamel hatchet (Fig 11-56h). After the compound is removed, the matrix may be removed as previously described.

Matrices for Bonded Amalgam Restorations

If a hydrophilic resin or bonding system is used to coat the walls of the preparation, the material should be applied before the matrix is placed, or care should be taken to prevent or minimize resin application to the matrix. If resin is applied to the matrix, it may cause the matrix to stick to the amalgam. This sticking can lead to fracture of the amalgam during removal of the matrix. Attachment of the matrix to the amalgam is most significant when amalgam bonding materials are used. Because amalgam must be inserted immediately after placement of the adhesive, the bonding material cannot be placed before matrix application; the best solution at present is to avoid, as much as possible, getting the bonding material on the matrix. A very small applicator should be used to apply the resin to the preparation walls so that it may be kept away from the matrix. It is advisable to try to stop the resin approximately 1 mm short of the cavo-

surface margins that are adjacent to the margins. Unless the set of the material is too advanced by the time the amalgam is placed, it will be pushed to the margin in a thin coat as the amalgam is condensed.

Because matrices that resist the bonding materials are not yet available, the application of a very thin coat of wax, with a wax pencil or crayon or with a piece of inlay wax or boxing wax, may be helpful. The wax is rubbed onto the inner surface of the matrix band, and excess is rubbed off with a gloved finger.

Placement of Amalgam

The technique for amalgam placement is basically the same regardless of the type or classification of the preparation. Amalgam is mixed (triturated), carried to the cavity preparation, and condensed into the preparation so that voids are eliminated and all areas of the preparation are filled. The amalgam is then carved to reproduce the portion of the tooth that is missing.

Spherical alloys produce an amalgam that requires a lower mercury-alloy ratio and less condensation force. However, the direction of the condensing force is extremely important for spherical amalgams. They do not adapt to the cavity walls as well as lathe-cut or admixture amalgams.[97] Spherical amalgams are said to be less condensable, and lateral condensation is even more important when spherical amalgams are used than when conventional or admixture amalgams are used. It is also somewhat more difficult to obtain good interproximal contacts in Class 2 amalgam restorations with spherical amalgams than with lathe-cut amalgams or admixtures. It has been demonstrated, however, that spherical amalgams are less sensitive to variations in condensation pressure than the amalgams containing nonspherical particles.[22] In addition, the spherical materials generally have a shorter working time and demonstrate a faster set than the admixtures.

Trituration

The trituration process includes the combining or mixing of liquid mercury with dry amalgam alloy powder. Electric amalgam mixers (also called amalgamators and amalgam triturators) are used for the trituration process (Figs 11-57a to 11-57c). The objective is to re-

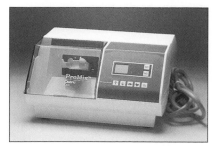

Fig 11-57a Pro-Mix amalgamator (Caulk/Dentsply).

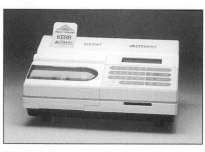

Fig 11-57b Automix amalgamator (Kerr/Sybron).

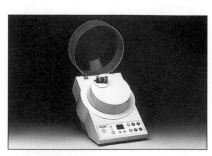

Fig 11-57c RotoMix centrifugal capsule mixer (ESPE).

move the oxide coating and wet each particle of alloy with mercury.[111] This begins the reaction that will produce a solid mass. Although amalgam alloy pellets and bottled mercury are still available separately, the use of precapsulated amalgam alloy, that is, a weighed, standardized amount of amalgam powder and mercury sealed into a capsule, is strongly recommended. The precapsulated products are not only ready for trituration, but they provide more consistent mixes of amalgam and virtually eliminate the possibility of mercury spills in the dental office.

The duration and speed of trituration should be just enough to coat all alloy particles with mercury, produce the amalgam matrix, and provide a plastic mix. Excessive trituration should be avoided because it generates heat and creates excess matrix in the microstructure of the resulting set material. In addition, an overtriturated mix of amalgam will set prematurely after trituration, and this will prevent adequate condensation and adaptation to the walls of the preparation, resulting in a weakened product. A mix of amalgam that is too plastic due to excess mercury, or, as is more frequently the case, is not plastic enough, must be discarded. A good mix of amalgam is plastic enough to condense well. If the mix is too hard, brittle, or hot, reduction of the mixing time and/or the mixing speed is indicated.

Condensation

Condensation is the process of compressing and directing the dental amalgam into the tooth preparation with amalgam-condensing instruments (called condensers or pluggers) until the preparation is completely filled, and then overfilled, with a dense mass of amalgam. Proper condensation of the amalgam promotes adaptation of the amalgam to the walls of the preparation,

and it compacts the material, eliminating voids and reducing the amount of residual mercury in the restoration. Both voids and increased residual mercury have been associated with a weakened amalgam product, so effective condensation continues trituration[124] and increases the strength[22,124] and serviceability[90] of the restoration.

Adequate condensation technique requires that a significant amount of force be applied to the condenser.[23] The force should be 2 to 5 kg (5 to 10 lbs) for a condensable amalgam (admixture or conventional); the condensation force required for spherical amalgams will be considerably less,[22,124] because heavy forces tend to push the spherical particles to the side and "punch through" the amalgam mass. The size of the condenser nib (end) determines the amount of pressure actually transferred from the operator's hand to the amalgam mass; the larger the nib, the less force per unit area (pressure) is applied to the mass for a given force from the operator's hand. In other words, when a larger-faced condenser is used, the operator must exert more force on the condenser to deliver adequate condensation pressure. Larger condensers should be used for spherical amalgam, rather than for admixtures, to allow adequate force to be applied without displacement of the spherical amalgam to the side.

When amalgam bonding systems are used, amalgam must be condensed into the bonding resin on all walls of the preparation before filling of the preparation is begun.

Adequate condensation force will cause a slight movement of the patient's mandible or head, and often this movement will need to be stabilized by the dentist or assistant. A secure finger rest will enable the operator to perform more controlled, forceful strokes, using arm as well as finger pressure. The condensers are held with the pen grasp or a modification.

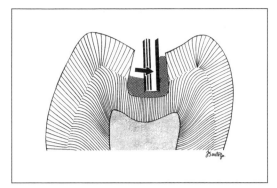

Fig 11-58a Lateral condensation, toward all walls, and toward the adjacent tooth in a Class 2 restoration, will improve adaptation to walls and ensure a contact area with the adjacent tooth.

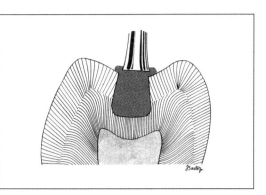

Fig 11-58b Overfill should be condensed with a large condenser.

Many operators use a finger or thumb of the hand that is not holding the condenser to apply additional condensation force. It has been demonstrated that dentists tend to use less condensation pressure during the later stages of amalgam placement; investigators[23] have emphasized the need for maintaining condensation pressures for both admixed and spherical amalgams throughout the condensation process.

After the preparation has been made ready to receive the amalgam, the amalgam alloy and mercury should be mixed or triturated to give a plastic and moldable mass of amalgam. For most restorations, an amalgam carrier is valuable for delivering the amalgam to the preparation (see Fig 6-35). For small restorations and for placing amalgam in proximal box preparations, care must be exercised to ensure increments of amalgam are small enough. If increments are too large, the condensing force cannot be adequate to adapt the amalgam material at the deepest area of the preparation. For very large complex amalgam preparations, the entire mix may be carried to the preparation, or the mix may be divided in half and one half at a time carried to the preparation with cotton forceps. No matter how the amalgam is carried, it should be spread in the preparation so that the increment is thin for optimum condensation. Each portion of amalgam carried to the preparation should result in an increment thickness of 1.0 mm or thinner to ensure maximum condensation effectiveness.

Condensers that fit into all areas of the preparation should be used. Flat-faced, round condensers are generally considered to allow maximum condensation pressure. Convex-ended condensers are also available, as are flat-ended condensers with diamond, rectangular, and triangular shapes. When spherical amalgams are used, the largest condenser that will fit into the area of the preparation where the amalgam is being condensed should be used. For all amalgams, a large condenser should be used for the overfilling of the preparation.

Amalgam must be condensed into the preparation as soon as trituration is completed. One increment of amalgam should not be allowed to set significantly before the next increment is added. Amalgam should be condensed both vertically and horizontally or laterally (toward the walls of the preparation). This will promote a close adaptation of the amalgam to the walls as well as to the floor of the preparation. Lateral condensation, whether or not an amalgam bonding system is being used, can be achieved in more than one way. One is to alter the direction of the face (end) of the condenser so that the face is pushed toward the walls. Another method is to place the condenser into the preparation vertically, then to move it laterally toward the walls so that the side of the condenser condenses the amalgam against the walls (Fig 11-58a). Lateral condensation is especially important for spherical amalgams because, paradoxically, it is more difficult to adapt these materials to cavity walls.

When amalgam is condensed, mercury tends to be brought to the surface, creating a mercury-rich amalgam on the surface. To reduce the amount of mercury left in the restoration (residual mercury), the preparation is overfilled (Fig 11-58b) and the mercury-rich excess is carved off. The lower the residual mercury in the carved restoration, the greater its strength[130] and the better the expected longevity of the restoration.

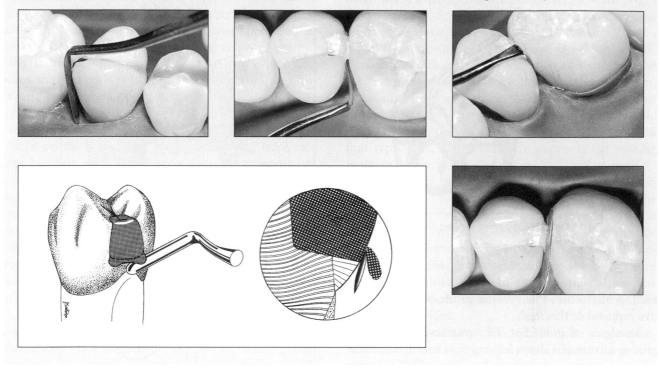

Fig 11-61 An interproximal carver is used to remove flash and to contour and burnish the amalgam in interproximal areas.

Adjusting the Occlusion

When the carving appears to be correct, the dam is removed, and the occlusion is checked. This is accomplished with articulating ribbon, which marks the points of contact when the mandibular and maxillary teeth are brought together (Figs 11-62a and 11-62b). It is wise not to ask the patient to close, because, if the amalgam has not been carved adequately, it will be "high" in occlusion so that it contacts first, prior to any other tooth contact. The masseter muscles are very strong, and when the proprioceptive innervation relates to the patient's brain that there is something between the maxillary and mandibular teeth, it is reflex action for the patient to attempt to masticate it. In the case of a high amalgam restoration, disaster can result; the amalgam will usually be fractured, and the operator will have to remove the remaining amalgam and begin again.

It is best, therefore, for the dentist to perform the tapping of the teeth by grasping the patient's chin, having the patient close to very near contact, and then, by hand, manipulating the mandible so that mandibular and maxillary teeth arc tapped together in centric occlusion (maximum intercuspation). The dentist's arm, no matter how strong, will be unable to impart nearly as much force in mandibular closure as the masseter muscles are capable of achieving. An alternative to this tapping by the dentist is to instruct the patient to "very, very gently, tap the back teeth together."

The amalgam must be carved until contacts on the restoration occur simultaneously with other centric contacts on that tooth and adjacent teeth. These can be seen as marks made by articulating ribbon, but they should also be felt by the dentist with 0.0005-inch (12-μm) thick shimstock (Artus) (Figs 11-63a and 11-63b). To do this, the patient should be instructed to close in centric occlusion ("bite the back teeth together") while shimstock is in place on the tooth being restored. With the teeth in centric occlusion, the shimstock should be held securely in place. The same test should be performed with the shimstock on adjacent teeth, and it should again be held securely (assuming that those teeth held shimstock prior to the restorative procedure). If the adjacent teeth do not hold the shimstock, the newly placed restoration is probably in hyperocclusion and needs additional carving.

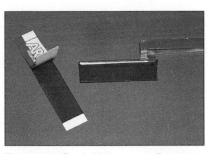

Fig 11-62a For initial gross adjustment, a piece of articulating paper with a thickness of 20 µm (0.0008-inch) or more is useful. When articulating paper forceps are used, the total length of the piece of articulating tape or paper should be supported by the forceps.

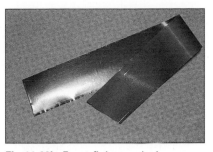

Fig 11-62b For refining occlusion, especially in complex amalgam restorations, an articulating tape with a thickness of 15 µm (0.0006-inch) or less is advantageous.

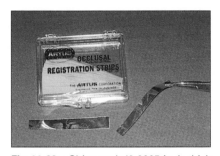

Fig 11-63a Shimstock (0.0005-inch thick Mylar) is supplied in books with paper separators between pieces of silver-colored shimstock. It may be held in the fingers or with a hemostat (as shown at lower right).

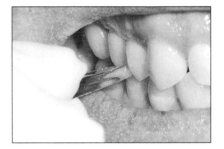

Fig 11-63b Shimstock is used to "feel" contacts between maxillary and mandibular teeth.

When the restoration is correct in centric occlusion, it must be checked to ensure that no interferences are caused by the restoration in eccentric movements. This may also be evaluated with the use of the shimstock. Two colors of articulating ribbon (preferably ribbons that do not easily cause smudge marks), one color for lateral and protrusive excursions, and the other to mark centric occlusion, are used. To eliminate eccentric contacts in the amalgam, the amalgam marked with the color used to register the excursions should be carved, and the amalgam marked with the centric marks should be left alone. For complex amalgam restorations, it should be ensured that the restoration does not cause interference in the slide between centric relation and centric occlusion (or maximum intercuspation).

Postcarve Burnishing

Postcarve burnishing is the light rubbing of the surface of a carved amalgam restoration with a burnisher, such as the PKT3. Heavy forces should not be used, and postcarve burnishing should be avoided near the margins of restorations of fast-setting amalgam.[169] The purpose of postcarve burnishing is to smooth the surface of the restoration.

After completion of carving and postcarve burnishing, if the carving time was short and the amalgam is still fairly soft, the surface may be wiped over with a dry or water-damp cotton ball or cotton roll to provide additional smoothing. If the set of the amalgam is advanced, so that the cotton will not smooth the

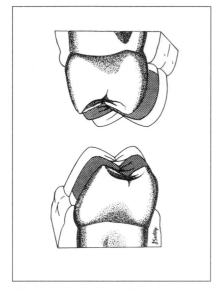

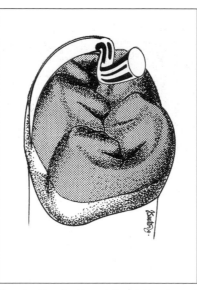

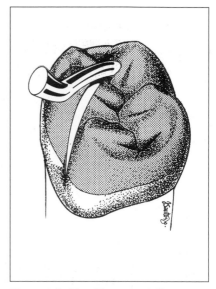

Fig 11-64 Facial and lingual contours are noted by looking down the line of teeth in a quadrant. The contour of the restoration must harmonize with natural tooth contours in the quadrant.

Fig 11-65a A No. 14L sickle-shaped carver will carve a very convex surface if it approaches the surface to be carved at just less than a 90-degree angle.

Fig 11-65b The No. 14L sickle-shaped carver will carve a surface with less convexity if it is rotated so that it approaches the surface at an angle of much less than 90 degrees.

surface, a rubber prophylaxis cup with damp flour of pumice or prophylaxis paste will smooth the amalgam (see the section on finishing and polishing, page 359). If the cup is used, it should be rotating at a very low speed and should be kept moving at all times; if the cup is allowed to rotate in one place, it will groove the recently carved amalgam.

Placement of Amalgam in Complex Preparations

Several special considerations for placing complex amalgam restorations, such as the possible need for reinforcement of matrices with compound, have already been discussed. Following are some other considerations that may help the operator to successfully place complex amalgam restorations:

1. Visualize the finished product, and shape the matrix to allow for that product.
2. In addition to visualizing the height of the cusp tips before making the tooth preparation and building cusps back to that height, make a mental picture of facial and lingual contours before cutting away natural tooth structure so that you can reproduce the natural contours in amalgam as closely as pos-

sible. Note the contours by viewing down the line of teeth from the facial and/or lingual aspect. Make sure that the final contours harmonize with the contours of other teeth in the quadrant (Fig 11-64; see also Fig 11-66ee).
3. Place larger increments of amalgam, for instance, the entire two-spill (600-mg) mix, when replacing the entire occlusal surface of a molar, or a half mix for less extensive restorations.
4. Consider the use of carvers that contribute to proper contours, such as the No. 14L carver, which simplifies the carving of convex axial contours (Figs 11-65a and 11-65b).
5. Because carving of large amalgam restorations involves the carving of more surface area, consider sharpening the carvers during the procedure to allow more efficient carving.
6. Smooth the carved amalgam with a slurry of flour of pumice or with a prophylaxis paste.

A series showing the insertion of a complex amalgam restoration, beginning with matrix application and ending just before rubber dam removal, is shown in Figs 11-66a to 11-66ee. Several amalgam preparations and restorations are shown in Figs 11-67 to 11-79.

Figs 11-66a to 11-66ee Condensation and carving of a complex amalgam restoration.

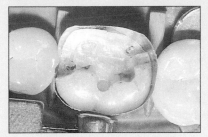

Fig 11-66a A Tofflemire matrix is placed and shaped to provide desired contours.

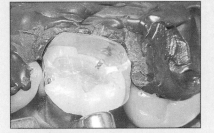

Fig 11-66b The matrix is stabilized with modeling compound.

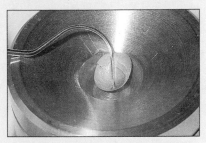

Fig 11-66c A two-spill mix of amalgam is halved.

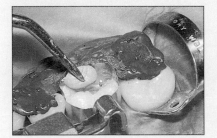

Fig 11-66d Half of the mix of amalgam is carried to the preparation.

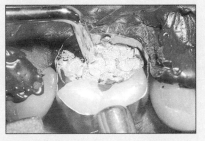

Fig 11-66e Amalgam is spread over the entire preparation floor and condensed.

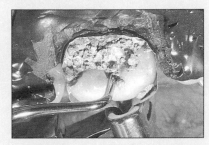

Fig 11-66f A small condenser is used to condense amalgam into the amalgapin channel.

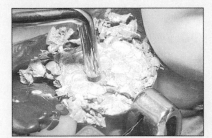

Fig 11-66g Amalgam increments are added in 1.0-mm thicknesses until the preparation is overfilled.

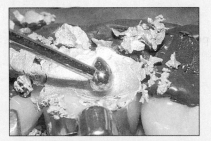

Fig 11-66h Amalgam shaping is begun with a large ovoid burnisher used to pinch excess amalgam off against the enamel (precarved burnishing).

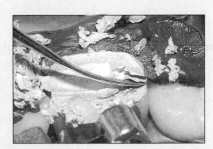

Fig 11-66i Marginal ridge shaping is begun by reducing amalgam in the area to the approximate desired height of the marginal ridge.

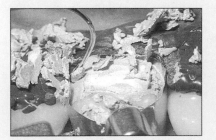

Fig 11-66j The occlusal embrasure is formed with an explorer tip.

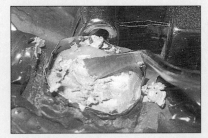
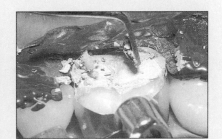

Figs 11-66k and 11-66l A chisel-shaped carver (Walls No. 3) is used to begin shaping cusps and grooves while the matrix is still in place.

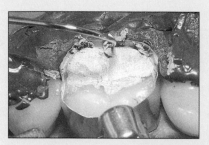 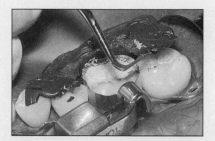

Fig 11-66m An explorer tip is used to begin shaping the lingual contour inside the matrix.

Fig 11-66n The compound and matrix are removed.

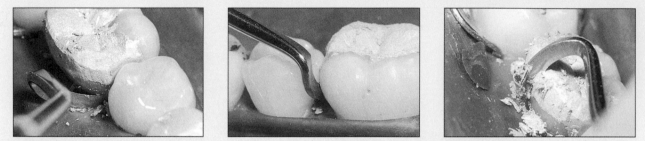

Figs 11-66o to 11-66q A sickle-shaped carver (No.14L) is used to remove gingival flash, shape proximal surfaces, and shape lingual contour.

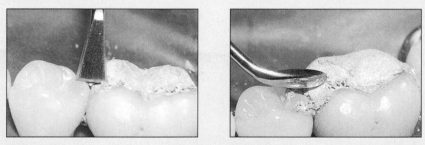

Figs 11-66r and 11-66s The marginal ridges are adjusted to height by resting the carver (Walls No. 3) on the adjacent marginal ridges.

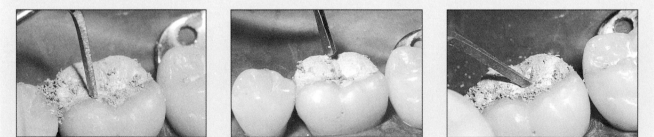

Figs 11-66t to 11-66v The occlusal anatomy is refined with a hoe.

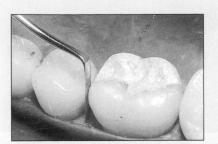

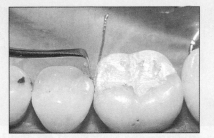

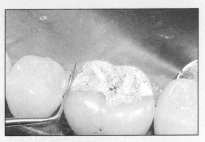

Figs 11-66w and 11-66x The proximal contours and contact position are refined with a very thin interproximal carver.

Fig 11-66y The occlusal embrasure is refined with an interproximal carver, which is rested on the adjacent enamel to guide the marginal ridge contour.

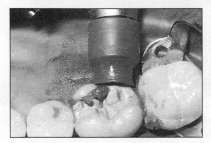

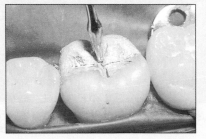

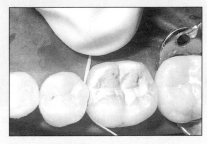

Fig 11-66z The surface is smoothed with a medium-grit prophylaxis paste in a rubber cup.

Fig 11-66aa The bases of the grooves are smoothed with a burnisher (PKT 3).

Fig 11-66bb The proximal contours are "felt" with floss to ensure smoothness and to clear any amalgam carvings from the contact.

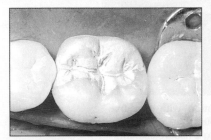

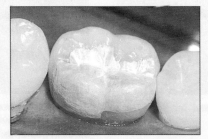

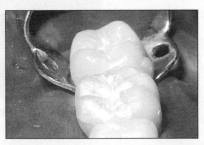

Figs 11-66cc to 11-66ee Carving is completed. Note that the lingual contour harmonizes with the contours of the adjacent teeth. The rubber dam is then removed, the occlusion is refined, and the surface is resmoothed with pumice or a prophylaxis paste.

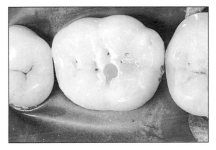

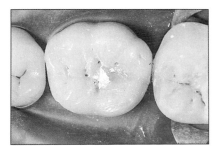

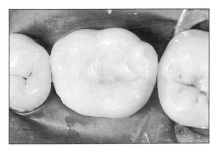

Fig 11-67a A small area of carious dentin and overlying unsupported enamel has been removed to complete the occlusal amalgam preparation.

Fig 11-67b The preparation is filled with amalgam.

Fig 11-67c The remaining occlusal fissures were opened with a No. ¼ bur to a depth of 0.5 mm, etched, and sealed with resin fissure sealant.

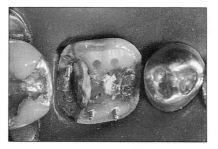

Fig 11-76a Complex amalgam preparation with pins, boxes, amalgapins, and a shelf.

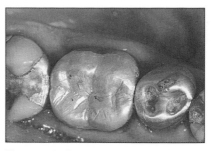

Fig 11-76b Complex amalgam restoration.

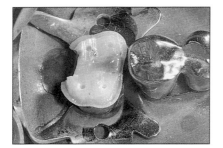

Fig 11-77a Complex amalgam preparation with boxes, amalgapins, and a shelf.

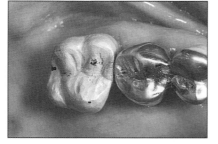

Fig 11-77b Complex amalgam restoration.

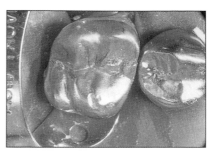

Fig 11-77c Restoration at 3 years.

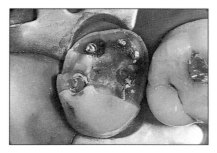

Fig 11-78a Complex amalgam preparation, which used horizontal and vertical pins.

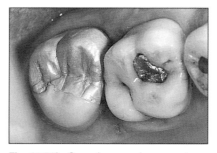

Fig 11-78b Complex amalgam restoration.

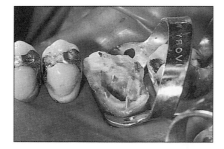

Fig 11-79a Complex amalgam preparation for a severely broken-down, endodontically treated molar, utilizing the chamber plus horizontal and vertical pins.

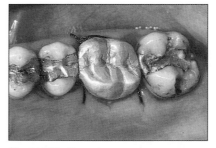

Fig 11-79b Complex amalgam restoration.

Figs 11-81a and 11-81b Abrasive disks, manufactured for polishing resin composite restorations, are also useful for polishing amalgam.

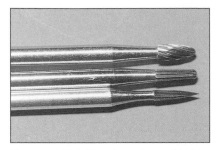

Fig 11-80 Finishing burs for a friction-grip handpiece: *(top to bottom)* No. 7404 (bud or egg shaped), No. 7803 (bullet shaped), No. 7901 (needle shaped).

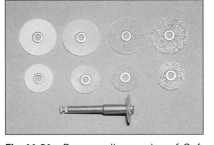

Fig 11-81a Brown-yellow series of Sof-Lex disks and the pop-on mandrel (3M). Also available is the thicker, but more flexible, black-blue series of Sof-Lex disks.

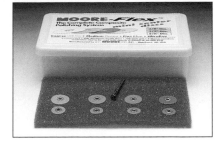

Fig 11-81b Moore-Flex disks (EC Moore) are similar to the Sof-Lex disks.

Finishing and Polishing Amalgam Restorations

Finishing of an amalgam restoration includes evaluating the restoration for problems and correcting those, ensuring that the margins are even and that the contours and occlusion are correct, and smoothing the restoration. Polishing is defined as smoothing the surface to a point of high gloss or luster. It has been demonstrated that polishing a high-copper amalgam restoration does not enhance its clinical performance,[104] but finishing is an important part of restoration placement. Finishing is usually accomplished at the placement appointment, but it may be refined at succeeding appointments.

Despite the lack of evidence that longevity is increased or performance improved when an amalgam restoration is polished, a high luster is often more comfortable to the patient's tongue than an unpolished surface, so polishing is sometimes desirable. There are no contraindications to polishing a restoration, but care must be taken not to create excessive heat during the polishing procedure. Excessive heat generation may be injurious to the pulp of a vital tooth.

After placement of a restoration, its surface should be rubbed with a burnisher or with dry or damp cotton until it is smooth. For amalgam with a more advanced set, a rubber cup with wet pumice or a prophylaxis paste may be used to smooth the restoration. Polishing of an amalgam restoration should be accomplished at a succeeding appointment, or at least

several hours after placement of the restoration. If an amalgam is adequately smoothed at the placement appointment, imparting a high luster is usually a very simple and quick procedure.[51] If the restoration is not made smooth at placement, more time is required for polishing.

If, at the time of polishing, the restoration surface is not smooth, it should be smoothed. Gross smoothing of set amalgam can be accomplished with sharp amalgam carvers and finishing burs (Fig 11-80). For polishing convex surfaces (facial, lingual, and proximal), a series of progressively finer disks may be used (Figs 11-81a and 11-81b). Alternatives for smoothing and polishing convex surfaces are the abrasive-impregnated rubber cups, first the coarser cups, and then the finer cups (Figs 11-82a and 11-82b). Abrasive-impregnated rubber points are useful for smoothing and polishing concave surfaces such as the occlusal surface. It is especially important that rubber polishers and abrasive disks are used with an abundance of air coolant and intermittent contact with the amalgam to prevent excessive generation of heat.

Although the disks and rubber polishers are more convenient, a less expensive, time-tested alternative method is the use of a prophylaxis cup, first with pumice in a water carrier as the "prepolishing" step, and then with tin oxide in a water or alcohol carrier for a high shine. One study[51] showed the pumice and tin oxide polishing procedure to be faster, but the investigator concluded that the impregnated points and cups are more desirable because they do not produce splatter.

Figs 11-82a and 11-82b *Abrasive-impregnated rubber cups and points.*

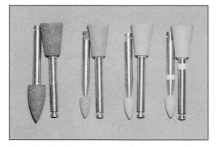

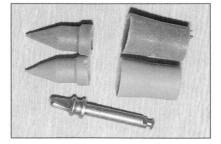

Fig 11-82a Brasseler cups and points: *(left to right)* coarsest (black), prepolish (brown), high shine (gray), and super high shine (yellow band).

Fig 11-82b Min-Identoflex polishers (Centrix): brown (prepolish) point and cup; green (final polish) point and cup. These polishers snap onto the mandrel shown.

A highly polished amalgam restoration is often more pleasing to the dentist than to the patient. A high polish can make a posterior amalgam restoration more noticeable, and this can be esthetically unpleasing to the patient. If this should occur, air abrasion with 50-µm aluminum oxide (Microetcher, Danville Engineering) or abrasion with pumice and a prophylaxis cup may be used to eliminate the high shine without making the restoration noticeably rough to the patient's tongue.

Repair of Amalgam Restorations

When an amalgam restoration has a defective area but the remainder of the restoration is adequate, a repair procedure may be the most appropriate treatment. For instance, if a cusp that was left in place adjacent to an amalgam restoration has fractured but the remaining amalgam restoration is serviceable, it might be appropriate to simply build a new cusp with amalgam. Or, if an amalgam fracture has occurred in the mesial box portion of a mesio-occlusodistal restoration, but the remaining disto-occlusal portion involves a very gingivally deep distal margin, the most conservative and simplest treatment might be to replace only the mesio-occlusal portion of the restoration.

Attachment of new amalgam to old can be achieved, but the attachment strength is only 30% to 60% of unrepaired amalgam.[45,67,78] Additional mechanical retention or amalgam bonding should be considered.

References

1. Ahlquist M, Bergtsson C, Furnes B. Number of amalgam fillings in relation to cardiovascular disease, diabetes, cancer, and early death in Swedish women. Community Dent Oral Epidemiol 1988;16:227–231.

2. Anderson MH, Bales DJ, Omnell KA. Modern management of dental caries: the cutting edge is not the dental bur. J Am Dent Assoc 1993;124:37–44.

3. Anneroth G, Ericson T, Johnsson I, et al. Comprehensive medical examination of a group of patients with alleged adverse effects from dental amalgams. Acta Odontol Scand 1992;50:101–111.

4. Anusavice KJ. Treatment regimens in preventive and restorative dentistry. J Am Dent Assoc 1995;126:727–743.

5. Anusavice KJ. Phillips' Science of Dental Materials, ed 10. Philadelphia: Saunders, 1996.

6. Bagedahl-Strindlund M, Ilie M, Furhoff A-K, et al. A multidisciplinary clinical study of patents suffering from illness associated with mercury released from dental restorations: psychiatric aspects. Acta Psychiatr Scand 1997;96:475–482.

7. Belcher MA, Stewart GP. Two-year clinical evaluation of an amalgam adhesive. J Am Dent Assoc 1997;128:309–314.

8. Battock RD, Rhoades J, Lund MR. Management of proximal caries on the roots of posterior teeth. Oper Dent 1979;4:108–112.

9. Bell JG. An elementary study of deformation of molar teeth during amalgam restorative procedures. Aust Dent J 1977;22:177–181.

10. Ben-Amar A, Liberman R, Judes H, Nordenberg D. Long-term use of dentine adhesive as an interfacial sealer under Class II amalgam restorations. J Oral Rehabil 1990;17:37–42.

11. Berry FA, Tjan AHL. Microleakage of amalgam restorations lined with dentin adhesives. Am J Dent 1994;7:333–336.

12. Berry TG, Laswell HR, Osborne JW, Gale EN. Width of isthmus and marginal failure of restorations of amalgam. Oper Dent 1981;6:55–58.

13. Berry TG, Nicholson J, Troendle K. Almost two centuries with amalgam: where are we today? J Am Dent Assoc 1994;125:392–399.

14. Bergman B, Bostrom H. Larsson KS, Loe H (eds). Potential Biological Consequences of Mercury Released from Dental Amalgam. A State of the Art Conference in Stockholm, April 1992. Stockholm: Swedish Medical Research Council, 1992.

15. Birtcil RF, Venton EA. Extracoronal amalgam restorations utilizing available tooth structure for retention. J Prosthet Dent 1976;35:171–178.

16. Björkman L, Pedersen NA, Lichtenstein P. Physical and mental health related to dental amalgam fillings in Swedish twins. Community Dent Oral Epidemiol 1996;24:260–267.

17. Blaser PK, Lund MR, Cochran MA, Potter RH. Effects of designs of Class 2 preparations on resistance of teeth to fracture. Oper Dent 1983;8:6–10.

18. Bonilla E, White SN. Fatigue of resin-bonded amalgam restorations. Oper Dent 1996;21:122–126.

19. Boyer DB, Roth L. Fracture resistance of teeth with bonded amalgams. Am J Dent 1994;7:91–94.

20. Brocklehurst PR, Joshi RI, Northeast SE. The effect of air-polishing occlusal surfaces on the penetration of fissures by a sealant. Int J Paediatr Dent 1992;2:157–162.

21. Bratel J, Haraldson T, Ottosson J-O. Potential side effects of dental amalgam restorations: no relation between mercury levels in the body and mental disorders. Eur J Oral Sci 1997; 105:244–250.

22. Brown IH, Miller DR. Alloy particle shape and sensitivity of high-copper amalgams to manipulative variables. Am J Dent 1993;6:248–254.

23. Brown IH, Maiolo C, Miller DR. Variation in condensation pressure during clinical packing of amalgam restorations. Am J Dent 1993;6:255–259.

24. Browning WD, Johnson WW, Gregory PN. Postoperative pain following bonded amalgam restorations. Oper Dent 1997;22: 66–71.

25. Buikema DJ, Mayhew RB, Voss JE, Bales DJ. Pins and their relation to cavity resistance form for amalgam. Quintessence Int 1985;16:187–190.

26. Burgess JO. Horizontal pins: a study of tooth reinforcement. J Prosthet Dent 1985;53:317–322.

27. Burgess JO, Hartsfield C, Jordan T. Strength of amalgam with varying amalgam thickness covering the pins [abstract 549]. J Dent Res 1990;69:177.

28. Burgess JO, Summitt JB. Retention and resistance provided by nine self-threading pins. Oper Dent 1991;16:55–60.

29. Burgess JO, Alvarez AN, Summitt JB. Fracture resistance of complex amalgams. Oper Dent 1997;22:128–132.

30. Caron GA, Murchison DF, Broom JC, Cohen RB. Resistance to fracture of teeth with various preparations for amalgam [abstract 208]. J Dent Res 1994;73:127.

31. Cassin AM, Pearson GJ, Picton DCA. Fissure sealants as a means of prolonging longevity of amalgam restorations—an in-vitro feasibility study. Clin Mater 1991;7:203–207.

32. Certosimo AJ, House RC, Anderson MH. The effect of cross-sectional area on transverse strength of amalgapin-retained restorations. Oper Dent 1991;18:70–76.

33. Charlton DG, Moore BK, Swartz ML. In vitro evaluation of the use of resin liners to reduce microleakage and improve retention of amalgam restorations. Oper Dent 1992;17:112–119.

34. Charlton DG, Murchison DF, Moor BK. Incorporation of adhesive liners in amalgam: effect on compressive strength and creep. Am J Dent 1991;4(4):184–188.

35. Collins JF, Antonson DE. Treatment of external pin perforations. J Acad Gen Dent 1987;35:200–202.

36. Cooley RL, Marshall TD, Young JM, Huddleston AM. Effect of sterilization on the strength and cutting efficiency of twist drills. Quintessence Int 1990;21:919–923.

37. Corbin SB, Kohn WG. The benefits and risks of dental amalgam: current findings reviewed. J Am Dent Assoc 1994;125: 381–388.

38. Cox CF, Suzuki S. Re-evaluating pulp protection: calcium hydroxide liners vs. cohesive hybridization. J Am Dent Assoc 1994;125:823–830.

39. Craig RG. Restorative Dental Materials, ed 9. St Louis: Mosby-Year Book, 1993.

40. Dachi SF, Stigers RW. Reduction of pulpal inflammation and thermal sensitivity in amalgam-restored teeth treated with copal varnish. J Am Dent Assoc 1967;74:1281–1285.

41. Davis SP, Summitt JB, Mayhew RB, Hawley RJ. Self-threading pins and amalgapins compared in resistance form for complex amalgam restorations. Oper Dent 1983;8:88–93.

42. DeCraene LGP, Martens LC, Dermaut LR, Surmont PAS. A clinical evaluation of a light-cured fissure sealant (Helioseal). J Dent Child 1989;56:97–102.

43. Demaree NC, Taylor DF. Properties of dental amalgams made from spherical alloy particles. J Dent Res 1962;41:890–896.

44. Diefenderfer KE, Reinhardt JW. Shear bond strengths of ten adhesive resin/amalgam combinations. Oper Dent 1997;22: 50–56.

45. Diefenderfer KE, Reinhardt JW, Brown SB. Surface treatment effects on amalgam repair strength. Am J Dent 1997;10:9–14.

46. Dilts WE, Welk DA, Stovall J. Retentive properties of pin materials in pin-retained silver amalgam restorations. J Am Dent Assoc 1968;77:1085.

47. Dilts WE, Duncanson MG, Collard EW, Parmley LE. Retention of self-threading pins. J Can Dent Assoc 1981;47:119–120.

48. Dutton FB, Summitt JB, Chan DCN, Garcia-Godoy F. Effect of a resin lining and rebonding on the marginal leakage of amalgam restorations. J Dent 1993;21:52–56.

49. Dwinelle WH. Crystalline gold, its varieties, properties, and use. Am J Dent Sci 1855;5:249–297.

50. Eakle WS, Staninec M, Lacy AM. Effect of bonded amalgam on the fracture resistance of teeth. J Prosthet Dent 1992;68: 257–260.

51. Eames WB. A clinical view of dental amalgam. Dent Clin North Am 1976;20:385–395.

52. Edgren BN, Denehy GE. Microleakage of amalgam restorations using Amalgambond and Copalite. Am J Dent 1992;5: 296–298.

53. El-Mowafy OM. Fracture strength and fracture patterns of maxillary premolars with approximal slot cavities. Oper Dent 1993;18:160–166.

54. Fernandes DP, Chevitarese O. The orientation and direction of rods in dental enamel. J Prosthet Dent 1991;65:793–800.

55. Fitchie JG, Reeves GW, Scarbrough AR, Hembree JH. Microleakage of a new cavity varnish with a high-copper spherical amalgam alloy. Oper Dent 1990;15:136–140.

56. Garcia-Godoy F, Medlock JW. An SEM study of the effects of air-polishing on fissure surfaces. Quintessence Int 1988;19: 465–467.

57. Garcia-Godoy F, Summitt J, Donly K, Buikema D. Resistance to further demineralization of white spot lesions by sealing [abstract 1643]. J Dent Res 1993;72:309.

58. Glossary of Operative Dentistry Terms, ed 1. Washington DC: Academy of Operative Dentistry, 1983.

59. Going RE. Pin-retained amalgam. J Am Dent Assoc 1966;73: 619–624.

60. Going RE, Loesche WJ, Grainger DA, Syed SA. The viability of microorganisms in carious lesions five years after covering with a fissure sealant. J Am Dent Assoc 1978;97:455–462.

61. Goldstein PM. Retention pins are friction-locked without use of cement. J Am Dent Assoc 1966;73:1103–1106.

62. Goldstein RE, Parkins FM. Using air-abrasive technology to diagnose and restore pit and fissure caries. J Am Dent Assoc 1995;126:761–766.

63. Gordan VV, Mjor IA, Hucke RD, Smith GE. Effect of different liner treatment on postoperative sensitivity of amalgam restorations. Quintessence Int 1999;30:55–59.

64. Gourley JW. Favorable locations for pins in molars. Oper Dent 1980;5:2.

65. Guthrom CE, Johnson LD, Lawless KR. Corrosion of dental amalgam and its phases. J Dent Res 1983;62:1372–1381.

66. Gwinnett AJ, Yu S. Effect of long-term water storage on dentin bonding. Am J Dent 1995;8:109–111.

67. Hadavi F, Hey JH, Czech D, Ambrose ER. Tensile bond strength of repaired amalgam. J Prosthet Dent 1992;67:313-317.

68. Handelman SL, Washburn F, Wopperer P. Two-year report of sealant effect on bacteria in dental caries. J Am Dent Assoc 1976;93:967–970.

69. Handelman SL, Leverett DH, Iker HP. Longitudinal radiographic evaluation of the progress of caries under sealants. J Pedod 1985;9:119–126.

70. Hazen SP, Osborne JW. Relationship of operative dentistry to periodontal health. Dent Clin North Am 1967; Mar 245–254.

71. Henningsson M, Sundbom E. Defensive characteristics in individuals with amalgam illness as measured by the percept-genetic method. Defense Mechanism Test. Acta Odontol Scand 1996;54:176–181.

72. Hovgaard O, Larsen MJ, Fejerskov O. Tooth hypersensitivity in relation to the quality of restorations [abstract 1667]. J Dent Res 1991;70:474.

73. How WS. Bright metal screw posts and copper amalgam. Dent Cosmos 1839;31:237–238.

74. Imbery TA, Burgess JO, Batzer RC. Comparing the resistance of dentin bonding agents and pins in amalgam restorations. J Am Dent Assoc 1995;126:753–758.

75. Imbery TA, Hilton TJ, Reagan SE. Retention of complex amalgam restorations using self-threading pins, amalgapins, and Amalgambond. Am J Dent 1995;8:117–121.

76. Innes DBK, Youdelis WV. Dispersion strengthened amalgam. J Can Dent Assoc 1963;29:587–593.

77. Jensen ME, Handelman SL. Effect of an autopolymerizing sealant on viability of microflora in occlusal dental caries. Scand J Dent Res 1980;88:382–388.

78. Jessip JP, Vandervalle KS, Hermesch CB, Buikema DS. Effects of surface treatments on amalgam repair. Oper Dent 1998;23:15–20.

79. Kanai S. Structure studies of amalgam. II. Effect of burnishing on the margins of occlusal amalgam fillings. Acta Odontol Scand 1966;24:47–53.

80. Karamursel-Ulukapi I, Lussi A, Stich H, Hotz P. Comparison of the sealing ability of four cavity varnishes: an in vitro study. Dent Mater 1991;7:84–87.

81. Kennington B, Davis RD, Murchison DF. Short-term clinical evaluation of post-operative sensitivity with bonded amalgams. Am J Dent 1998;11:177–180.

82. Kingman A, Albertini T, Brown LJ. Mercury concentration in urine and whole blood associated with amalgam exposure in a US military population. J Dent Res 1998;77:461–471.

83. Kline J, Boyer D. Comparison of bonding amalgam and composite to enamel and dentin [abstract 741]. J Dent Res 1995;74:104.

84. Korale ME, Meiers JC. Microleakage of dentin bonding systems used with spherical and admixed amalgams. Am J Dent 1996;9:249–252.

85. Kramer PF, Zelante F, Simionato MRL. The immediate and long-term effects of invasive and noninvasive pit and fissure sealing techniques on the microflora in occlusal fissures of human dentin. Pediatr Dent 1993;16:108–112.

86. Lambert RL, Robinson FB, Lindemuth JS. Coronal reinforcement with cross-splinted pin-amalgam restorations. J Prosthet Dent 1985;54:346–349.

87. Larson TD, Douglas WH, Geisfeld RE. Effect of prepared cavities on the strength of teeth. Oper Dent 1981;6:2-5.

88. Leach CD, Martinoff JT, Lee CV. A second look at the amalgapin technique. J Calif Dent Assoc 1983;11:43–49.

89. Leinfelder KF. Dental amalgam alloys. Curr Opin Dent 1991;1:214–217.

90. Letzel H, van't Hof MA, Marshall GW, Marshall SJ. The influence of amalgam alloy on the survival of amalgam restorations: a secondary analysis of multiple controlled trials. J Dent Res 1997;76:1787–1798.

91. Liberman R, Judes H, Cohen E, Eli I. Restoration of posterior pulpless teeth: amalgam overlay versus cast gold onlay restorations. J Prosthet Dent 1987;57:540–543.

92. Lo CS, Millstein PL, Nathanson D. In vitro shear strength of bonded amalgam cores with and without pins. J Prosthet Dent 1995;74:385–391.

93. Lumley PJ, Fisher FJ. Tunnel restorations: a long-term pilot study over a minimum of five years. J Dent 1995;23:213-215.

94. Mach Z, Ruzickova T, Staninec M, Setcos JC. Bonded amalgam restorations: three year clinical results [abstract 3106]. J Dent Res 1998;77(special issue B):1020.

95. Mackert JR, Berglund A. Mercury exposure from dental amalgam fillings: absorbed dose and the potential for adverse health effects. Crit Rev Oral Biol Med 1997;8:411–436.

96. Mahler DB. Discovery! The high-copper dental amalgam alloys. J Dent Res 1997;76:537–541.

97. Mahler DB. The amalgam-tooth interface. Oper Dent 1996;21:230–236.

98. Manders CA, Garcia-Godoy F, Barnwell GM. Effect of a copal varnish, ZOE or glass ionomer cement bases on microleakage of amalgam restorations. Am J Dent 1990;3:63–66.

99. Markley MR. Pin reinforcement and retention of amalgam foundations. J Am Dent Assoc 1958;56:675–679.

100. Markley MR. Pin-retained and pin-reinforced amalgam. J Am Dent Assoc 1966;73:1295–1300.

101. Markley MR. Pin retained and reinforced restorations and foundations. Dent Clin North Am 1967;3:229–244.

102. Marshall TD, Porter KH, Re GJ. In vitro evaluation of the shoulder stop in a self-threading pin. J Prosthet Dent 1986;56:428–430.

103. Marshall TD, Cooley RL. Evaluation of the Max titanium alloy retentive pins. Am J Dent 1989;2:349–353.

104. Mayhew RB, Schmeltzer LD, Pierson WP. Effect of polishing on the marginal integrity of high-copper amalgams. Oper Dent 1986;11:8–13.

105. McComb D, Ben-Amar A, Brown J. Sealing efficacy of therapeutic varnishes used with silver amalgam restorations. Oper Dent 1990;15:122–128.

106. Marek M, Okabe T, Butts MB, Fairhurst CW. Corrosion of the (Cu-Sn) phase in dental amalgam. J Biomed Mater Res 1983;17:921–29.

107. Mertz-Fairhurst E, Smith CD, Williams JE, et al. Cariostatic and ultraconservative sealed restorations: six-year results. Quintessence Int 1992;23:827–838.

108. Mertz-Fairhurst E, Curtis JW, Ergle JW, et al. Ultraconservative and cariostatic sealed restorations: results at year 10. J Am Dent Assoc 1998;129:55–66.

109. Miller A, Okabe T, DePaola DP, Cole JS. Amalgam and mercury toxicity: an update. Tex Dent J 1991;108:25–29.

110. Miller B, Chan DC, Cardenas HL, Summitt JB. Powder additive effect on shear bond strengths of bonded amalgam (abstract 1346). J Dent Res 1998;77(special issue A):274.

111. Mitchell RJ, Okabe T. Setting reactions in dental amalgam part 1. Crit Rev Oral Biol Med 1996;7:12–22.

112. Mjör IA, Jokstad A, Qvist V. Longevity of posterior restorations. Int Dent J 1990;40:11–17.

113. Molin M, Bergman B, Marklund SL, et al. Mercury, selenium, and glutathione peroxidase before and after amalgam removal in man. Acta Odontol Scand 1990;48:189–202.

114. Moffa JP, Razzano MR, Doyle MG. Pins—A comparison of their retentive properties. J Am Dent Assoc 1969;78:529.

115. Nakabayashi N, Watanabe A, Gendusa NJ. Dentin adhesion of "modified" 4-META/MMA-TBB resin: function of HEMA. Dent Mater 1992;8:259–264.

116. National Institutes of Health. Technology Assessment Conference. Effects and Side-Effects of Dental Restorative Materials. Bethesda, MD: US Department of Health and Human Services, 1991.

117. Newitter DA, Gwinnett AJ, Caputo L. The dulling of twist drills during pin channel placement. Am J Dent 1989;2:81–85.

118. Oliveira JP, Cochran MA, Moore BK. Influence of bonded amalgam restorations on the fracture strength of teeth. Oper Dent 1996;21:111–115.

119. Osborne JW, Albino JE. Psychological and medical effects of intake of mercury from dental amalgams. Am J Dent 1999;12:151-156.

120. Osborne JW, Berry TG. Zinc containing high copper amalgam: a three-year clinical evaluation. Am J Dent 1992;5:43–45.

121. Osborne JW, Gale EN. Relationship of restoration width, tooth position, and alloy to fracture at the margins of 13- to 14-year-old amalgams. J Dent Res 1990;69:1599–1601.

122. Osborne JW, Howell ML. Effects of water contamination on certain properties of high copper amalgams. Am J Dent 1994;7:337–341.

123. Osborne JW, Norman RD. 13-year clinical assessment of 10 amalgam alloys. Dent Mater 1990;6:189–194.

124. Osborne JW, Phillips RW, Norman RD, Swartz ML. Influence of certain manipulative variables upon the static creep of amalgam. J Dent Res 1977;56:616–621.

125. Osborne JW, Norman RD, Gale EN. A 14-year clinical assessment of 12 amalgam alloys. Quintessence Int 1991;22:857–864.

126. Osborne JW, Summitt JB. Extension for prevention: is it relevant today? Am J Dent 1998;11:189–196.

127. Osborne JW. Expansion of contaminated dental amalgams assessed by photoelastic resin [abstract 2556]. J Dent Res 1998;77(special issue B):951.

128. Outhwaite WC, Garman TA, Pashley DH. Pin vs. slot retention in extensive amalgam restorations. J Prosthet Dent 1979;41:396–400.

129. Panopoulos P, Mejare B, Edwall L. Effects of ammonia and organic acids on the intradental sensory nerve activity. Acta Odontol Scand 1983;41:209–215.

130. Pashley EL, Galloway SE, Pashley DH. Protective effects of cavity liners on dentin. Oper Dent 1990;15:11–17.

131. Pilo R, Brosh T, Chweidan H. Cusp reinforcement by bonding of amalgam restorations. J Dent 1998;26:467–472.

132. Piperno S, Barouch E, Hirsch SM, Kaim JM. Thermal discomfort of teeth related to presence or absence of cement bases under amalgam restorations. Oper Dent 1982;7:92–96.

133. Plasmans PJJM, Kusters ST, Thissen AMG, et al. Effects of preparation design on the resistance for extensive amalgam restorations. Oper Dent 1987;12:42–47.

134. Podshadley AG, Chambers MS. A new instrument for placement of self-threading retention pins. J Prosthet Dent 1994;71:429.

135. Powell GL, Nicholls JI, Shurtz DE. Deformation of human teeth under the action of an amalgam matrix band. Oper Dent 1977;2:64–69.

136. Powell GL, Nicholls JI, Molvar MP. Influence of matrix bands, dehydration, and amalgam condensation on deformation of teeth. Oper Dent 1980;5:95–101.

137. Qvist V, Johannessen L, Bruun M. Progression of approximal caries in relation of iatrogenic preparation damage. J Dent Res 1992;71:1370–1373.

138. Reagan SE, Gray SE, Hilton TJ. Fracture resistance of complex amalgam restorations with peripheral shelves used as resistance features. Am J Dent 1993;6:225–228.

139. Robbins JW, Summitt JB. Longevity of complex amalgam restorations. Oper Dent 1988;13:54–57.

140. Roddy WC, Blank LW, Rupp NW, Pelleu GB. Channel depth and diameter effects on transverse strength of amalgapin-retained restorations. Oper Dent 1987;12:2–9.

141. Ruzickova T, Staninec M, Marshall GW. SEM analysis of resin-amalgam adhesion after debonding [abstract 2289]. J Dent Res 1994;73(special issue):388.

142. Sandborgh-Englund G, Elunder CG, Langworth S, et al. Mercury in biological fluids after amalgam removal. J Dent Res 1998;77:615–626.

143. Santos AC, Meiers JC. Fracture resistance of premolars with MOD amalgam restorations lined with Amalgambond. Oper Dent 1994;19:2–6.

144. Sarkar NK, Park JR. Mechanism of improved corrosion resistance of Zn-containing dental amalgams. J Dent Res 1988;67:1312–1316.

145. Schoonover IC, Souder W, Beall JR. Excessive expansion of dental amalgam. J Am Dent Assoc 1942;29:1825–1832.

146. Seng GF, Rupell OL, Nance GL, Pompura JP. Placement of retentive amalgam inserts in tooth structure for supplemental retention. J Acad Gen Dent 1980;28:62 66.

147. Setcos JC, Staninec M, Wilson NHF. Clinical evaluation of bonded amalgam restorations over two years [abstract 2589]. J Dent Res 1998;77(special issue B):955.

148. Shapira J, Eidelman E. The influence of mechanical preparation of enamel prior to etching on the retention of sealants: three-year follow-up. J Pedod 1984;8:272–277.

149. Shavell HM. The amalgapin technique for complex amalgam restorations. J Calif Dent Assoc 1980;8:48–55.

150. Smales RJ. Longevity of cusp-covered amalgams: survivals after 15 years. Oper Dent 1991;16:17–20.

151. Staninec M, Marshall GW, Lowe A, Ruzickova T. Clinical research on bonded amalgam restorations, part 1: SEM study of in vivo bonded amalgam restorations. Gen Dent 1997;45(4):356–362.

152. Sturdevant JR, Taylor DF, Leonard RH, et al. Conservative preparation designs for Class II amalgam restorations. Dent Mater 1987;3:144–148.

153. Summitt J, Burgess J, Berry T, et al. Three year evaluation of Amalgambond Plus and pin-retained restorations [abstract 2716]. J Dent Res 1999;78: (special issue):445.

154. Summitt JB, Burgess JO, Kaiser DA, et al. Resistance form provided to complex amalgam restorations by pins, amalgapins, peripheral shelves, and combinations. Am J Dent 1991;4:268–272.

155. Summitt JB, Howell ML, Burgess JO, et al. Effect of grooves on resistance form of conservative Class 2 amalgams. Oper Dent 1992;17:50–56.

156. Summitt JB, Miller B, Buikema DJ, Chan DCN. Shear bond strength of Amalgambond Plus cold and at room temperature [abstract 1345]. J Dent Res 1998;77(special issue A):274.

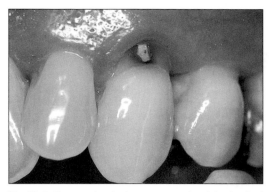

Fig 12-1 Root caries lesion on a tooth with gingival recession.

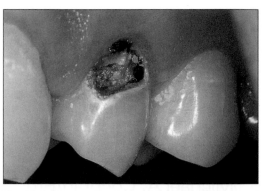

Fig 12-2 Root caries lesion undermining coronal enamel.

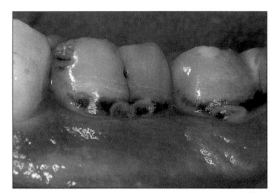

Fig 12-3 Active root caries lesion extending laterally.

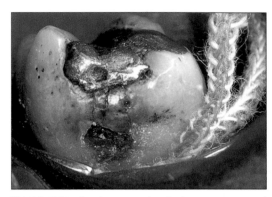

Fig 12-4 Proximal root caries lesion on a second molar.

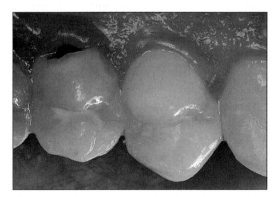

Fig 12-5 Carious lesion on the lingual aspect of a second premolar.

more inactive).[11,13,37,112] While there has been some relation shown between color, texture, and dominant microorganism, the data have been conflicting and the link remains tenuous.[75]

Caries activity may occur on any exposed root surface, but initial lesions on the facial and proximal surfaces are most common.[62] Some studies have sug-

gested that 50% to 75% of root caries lesions begin proximally (Fig 12-4).[44,122] Lingual/palatal locations are seen much less frequently as isolated lesions (Fig 12-5). In the mandible, molars appear to be the most susceptible to root caries followed by premolars, canines, and incisors, while in the maxilla the order is reversed.[62,69,70] It is common for many of these lesions to be obscured by plaque, food debris, and calculus, so accurate diagnosis is best accomplished after thorough debridement and prophylaxis.

Histochemistry, Histopathology, and Microbiology

The caries process on root surfaces is very similar to that in coronal caries. Plaque bacteria capable of metabolizing dietary carbohydrates into acids produce a drop in pH that initiates demineralization tooth structure. Root surfaces are more vulnerable to chemical

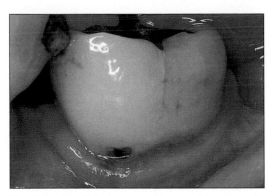

Fig 12-6a Small lesion in a 45-year-old patient. At this stage, with cavitation, a restoration should be placed to prevent circumferential spread, and a preventive regimen should be initiated.

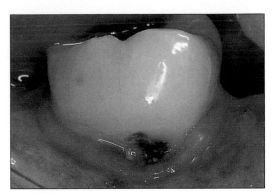

Fig 12-6b Larger lesion in the same patient.

dissolution than enamel surfaces.[87] The drop in pH necessary for demineralization in cementum and dentin (pH 6.2 to 6.7) is less than that required for enamel (pH 5.4 to 5.5).[5,53] This means that, given the proper environment, both the initiation and progression of root surface caries will occur more rapidly in dentin than in an enamel surface. In addition, acid challenges can occur more readily and may continue for an extended period of time.[34] Any alteration in the delicate balance between the rates of demineralization and remineralization can result in the initiation of the caries process.[94,129]

While we tend to think of root surfaces as being covered with cementum, some studies[98] suggest that the cementum and enamel are not confluent in as many as 30% of teeth. For patients receiving periodontal therapy, the cementum on accessible root surfaces is often partially removed during scaling and root planing procedures. Therefore, root caries commonly begins on a dentin interface. Regardless of the surface, the creation of an acid environment by cariogenic bacteria initiates the caries process. Cemental clefts can form due to physical and chemical changes, allowing infiltration of bacteria into the dentinal tubules. Surface dissolution continues, followed by further demineralization and destruction of the collagen matrix.[57] Early microcavitation enlarges and produces the characteristic circumferential spreading seen with these lesions (Figs 12-6a and 12-6b).

Some lesions become arrested. As demineralization progresses, there is a reactive sclerosing of the tubules and crystal formation, resulting in hypermineralization of the dentinal tubules. This sclerosis is believed to be a result of the pulp's reaction to the stimulus of the caries process. The sclerotic appearance of many advanced le-

sions is probably related to the differences in mineral content found between the peritubular and intertubular dentin.[125] Various preventive regimens can lead to the arrest of root surface lesions. Arrested lesions frequently appear very dark and are hard on tactile examination.

Many studies attempting to determine the causative agent of root caries have used selective culture techniques that focus on the identification of a limited number of bacterial species.[12,120] Unfortunately, this type of culturing often excludes some species that are directly or indirectly related. Studies of the predominant cultivable microflora, while more time and labor intensive, appear to be more useful in delineating the group of oral bacteria associated with the root caries process.[106,129]

Currently, no specific microorganisms have been conclusively proven to cause root surface caries. Early studies[59,109,112] pointed to *Actinomyces viscosus* as a prime suspect. More recent studies, however, have questioned the dominant role of *Actinomyces* while emphasizing the importance of *Streptococcus mutans* and *Lactobacillus*.[10,11,14,32,41,66,75,101,121] Lynch[75] and Zambon and Kasprzak[129] point out that, based on extensive research, *S mutans* and *Lactobacillus* spp both fulfill the criteria for implicating bacteria in the etiology of a mixed infection. They also suggest that virulence factors of specific species probably play an important role in both the formation and progress of root surface lesions. It is likely that root caries is a continuous, destructive process involving a succession of bacterial populations that vary depending on the condition of the substrate and the depth of the lesion.[106,121] Modern molecular biology techniques, involving ribosomal RNA sequencing and DNA and RNA probes, may offer solutions to defining both species and virulence factors associated with root caries lesions.

Prevalence and Incidence

Because root caries can be initiated only when root surfaces are exposed to the oral environment, the population presumed to be most at risk is older adults. However, younger patients with periodontal problems are susceptible as well. One epidemiologic study in Great Britain[115] found gingival recession in 60% of the population between 25 and 34 years of age. In addition, the most recent National Health and Nutrition Examination Survey for the United States reported gingival recession in all age groups 18 years and older.[15] It should also be noted that root surface exposure does not mean that caries activity is inevitable.

The actual prevalence of root caries is difficult to assess.[18] Interpretation of data from prevalence and incidence studies is complicated due to differences in diagnostic criteria, treatment decisions, and lack of homogeneity of the observed populations.[21] Numerous studies have reported the prevalence of root caries and its relationship with increasing age,[6,7,9,62,73] while international surveys have estimated that the disease affects 60% to 90% of adults.[37,49,64,71,74,80] In addition, it has been suggested that approximately 1 in 9 root surfaces is at risk of becoming carious.[62] The extent of root caries appears to have a negative correlation with the number of teeth present. Because more mandibular teeth are retained in older individuals, these teeth have a higher incidence of root caries than do maxillary teeth.[52,62,73,111] Other studies[42,43,49,62,61,127] suggest that approximately 15% to 20% of all teeth with gingival recession are affected by root caries, and the mean number of teeth affected per person is about 2.8.[64,87] It has also been stated that if root caries prevalence is based on the presence of active, restored, and arrested lesions, virtually every dentate American over age 65 years is at risk.[38]

Incidence data have been derived primarily from studies conducted on selected populations such as the chronically ill or nursing home residents. These studies[7,56,70,100,104,123] vary in duration from 1 to 8 years and report root caries/root restoration experience ranging from 19% to 69% depending on the population observed. Two studies on noninstitutionalized adults over 65 years of age have reported similar incidences of root caries, 44%[46] and 37%.[69] The attack rates (mean surfaces per mouth) calculated for exposed root surfaces in the latter two studies ranged from 3.8[69] to 5.4[46] over a 3-year period.

Despite the variability of available data, there is general agreement that the prevalence of root caries will increase in the dentate older population. The prevalence of untreated caries, in general, has been found to be constant with age.[80,115] Statistically, however, as the number of teeth decreases with age, the ratio of caries per tooth at risk increases, and root caries is a component of this. Thus, the ongoing loss of teeth with age is likely to produce an underestimation of the prevalence of root caries.[9] In the United States, it has been predicted that the dentate population over 65 years of age will reach 85% or higher by 2020.[9]

Risk Factors and Assessment

The risk factors associated with root caries are provided below (see box). It is of critical importance that clinicians identify persons at risk early in the root caries process, ideally before the disease is clinically apparent. Early detection permits preventive and chemotherapeutic intervention to potentially enhance treatment outcome.

Because exposure of the root surface to the oral environment is a prerequisite for root surface caries, any patient with attachment loss, gingival recession,

---

Risk Factors for Root Caries

Exposure of root surfaces
  Attachment loss
  Gingival recession
  Periodontal pocketing
Inadequate oral hygiene
  Low priority to patient
  Physical impairment
  Cognitive impairment
Cariogenic diet
Diminished salivary flow and/or buffering capacity
  Chronic medical conditions
  Medications
  Surgical/radiation therapy
  Physiologic aging
Previous caries/restorations
Lack of access to and/or interest in dental services
  Low socioeconomic status
  Low educational level
Removable prosthesis
Advanced age
Eight or more missing teeth
Male gender
Smoking, alcoholism, drug use
Possibly ethnicity

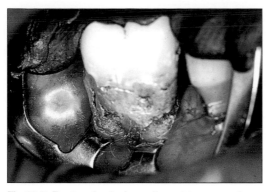

Fig 12-7 Root caries lesion adjacent to an amalgam margin.

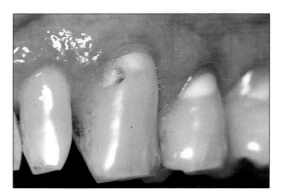

Fig 12-8 Caries lesion adjacent to a resin restoration in a xerostomic patient. Glass-ionomer restorations in the same patient did not exhibit recurrent caries lesions for the duration of the 5-year study.[79]

and/or periodontal pocketing is at risk for initiation of the disease process.[31] Patients in this category who are frequently overlooked are patients with cervical and proximal restorations that terminate on cemental surfaces. Even though the root surface may not be readily visible, the need for and placement of these restorations has met the primary risk criteria.

All normal risk factors for caries development are applicable to root caries, including inadequate oral hygiene, cariogenic diet, and poor utilization of routine dental services. Past caries/restorative experience has also been shown to have a strong correlation and generally indicates the presence of conditions/behaviors that support caries activity (Fig 12-7).[8,60,69,72,76,97,105] Unfortunately, the effect of these conditions may be magnified in the root caries process as well as impacted by the myriad changes associated with aging and related health problems and treatments.

In relation to caries activity, salivary flow rate is considered the most important of the nonmicrobial salivary parameters[22] since the cariostatic activity or efficacy of other salivary parameters is dependent on the flow rate.[113] Unstimulated flow rate has been shown to have a greater effect on salivary clearance time than stimulated flow[67,68] and is more affected by conditions producing hypofunction of the salivary glands.[27] A loss or significant reduction of unstimulated salivary flow results in xerostomia, or "dry mouth," and is positively correlated with a number of adverse oral conditions, including rapidly progressive dental caries and periodontal disease (Fig 12-8).[47,99] While there is debate as to the amount of saliva necessary to maintain oral health, an unstimulated flow rate of less than 0.2 mL/min is considered to be below normal.[27,47]

Xerostomia can be caused by a variety of factors,[4,5,47] including radiation therapy of the head and neck, immunosuppressive therapy, radioactive iodine therapy, autoimmune diseases, HIV infection, and a myriad of commonly prescribed medications (see box).

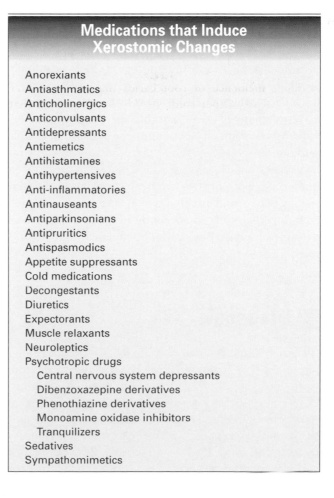

Medications that Induce Xerostomic Changes

Anorexiants
Antiasthmatics
Anticholinergics
Anticonvulsants
Antidepressants
Antiemetics
Antihistamines
Antihypertensives
Anti-inflammatories
Antinauseants
Antiparkinsonians
Antipruritics
Antispasmodics
Appetite suppressants
Cold medications
Decongestants
Diuretics
Expectorants
Muscle relaxants
Neuroleptics
Psychotropic drugs
    Central nervous system depressants
    Dibenzoxazepine derivatives
    Phenothiazine derivatives
    Monoamine oxidase inhibitors
    Tranquilizers
Sedatives
Sympathomimetics

Basic management of xerostomic patients involves finding ways to reduce their oral dryness. If functioning salivary gland tissue is present, stimulation of natural flow is preferable to saliva substitutes. Pilocarpine (MGI Pharma) can be an extremely effective salivary gland stimulant.[39] However, it has numerous side effects, contraindications, and drug interactions that make consultation with the patient's primary care physician mandatory before suggesting its use. Oral moisturizers are sometimes the only option for relieving the symptoms of xerostomia. These saliva substitutes can be used on a regular basis, but some commercial products have been found to have a pH below the demineralization point of enamel[47] and should be avoided.

The use of removable partial dentures has also been noted as a risk factor in this disease.[107] The position of retentive clasps and lingual/palatal connectors can contribute to retention of food debris and gingival recession. While initial design may have been appropriate, prolonged wear and alterations of the clasps can produce physical stripping of the gingiva and abrasion of the tooth surface.

Other factors that contribute to the potential for root caries include previous caries and restorative experience. Studies have indicated that individuals who have coronal caries are 2 to 3.5 times more likely to develop root caries.[45,93] Root caries is generally more prevalent and severe among males than females.[80] Smoking has also been implicated as a risk factor in both periodontal disease[116] and root caries.[102] Ethnicity is a relatively new variable in caries studies because of the difficulty in obtaining appropriate sample population sizes.[96,103] While there have been some indications that Asians[95,96] and blacks[29,69] exhibit a higher incidence of root caries, these data are not consistent between available studies, and the trends may be associated with socioeconomic factors, behavioral variables, and/or past caries experience and not directly related to race.

Diagnosis

Although clinicians detect root caries lesions by judging changes in color (yellow, brown, black), texture (soft, hard), and surface contour (regular, irregular), examination strategies should focus on patients at risk for root caries. Therefore, the first step in diagnosis of root caries is early identification of contributory factors and oral hygiene practices. Because plaque and debris often severely limit the visibility of root surfaces, a thorough dental prophylaxis should precede any clinical examination of patients at risk for root caries. Gentle tissue displacement with an air syringe and retraction with hand instruments can offer a better view of subgingival and interproximal areas, while the use of transillumination and/or lighted mirrors as well as intraoral cameras can also enhance visibility and improve diagnostic capability.

Lynch[75] found texture to be the best predictor of microbiologic activity in root caries lesions. Tactile exploration should be done carefully with only moderate pressure since the root surface is inherently softer than enamel. The gradient in tactile sensation between sound and carious cementum/dentin is much less than that between sound and carious enamel.[65] Active lesions may or may not display obvious cavitation and are generally described as "tacky" or "leathery" to tactile exploration while offering some resistance to removal of the explorer tip. One study demonstrated that an alteration in the explorer tip (producing a 30-degree angle at the tip of the explorer) increased the ability of the operator to detect root caries lesions.[85]

Radiographs can be useful in identifying early proximal root lesions, but can occasionally be prone to misinterpretation because of cervical "burnout" artifacts. Vertical bite-wing radiographs permit better evaluation of the proximal root surfaces in persons with significant loss of attachment.[58]

Future diagnostic tools and techniques, such as dye-enhanced laser fluorescence (DELF) and quantitative laser fluorescence (QLF), have shown promise in in vitro[3,40] and in vivo[2,23,24] studies in enamel. This type of diagnostic aid should eventually be helpful in differentiating between active and inactive lesions by finding a correlation between lesion severity and degree of mineral loss. Clarification is needed since the current system of classification of root caries is generally considered unsatisfactory.[118]

Preventive and Chemotherapeutic Strategies

Clinical observations suggest that root caries lesions can be arrested, obviating restorative therapy.[26,33] The majority of evidence relating to demineralization and remineralization in root caries lesions comes from in vitro research.[35,51] However, in vivo[88,106] and in situ[89,90,92] studies have demonstrated success in pre-

Treatment Protocol for Patients at Risk for Root Caries

Eliminate active infection

For cavitated lesions (both coronal and root surface), treat restoratively

Seal deep, retentive pits and fissures

Implement preventive measures

Increase patient awareness of potential problems

Survey diet; recommend modifications as necessary

Instruct on prophylaxis and oral hygiene

Provide periodontal therapy as needed

Evaluate salivary flow rate

Provide in-office fluoride

- Gels: 1.23% acidulated phosphate fluoride or 2% neutral sodium fluoride; 4-minute tray technique, 4 applications over 2 to 4 weeks
- Varnishes: Duraflor (Pharmascience), Duraphat (Colgate), Fluor Protector (Vivadent); isolate each quadrant with cotton rolls, apply to teeth, repeat in 3 to 6 months

Home fluoride: fluoride-containing dentifrices, gels, rinses (prefer at least 3 fluoride exposures daily)

- Xylitol chewing gum: chew 2 pieces for 5 minutes, 3 times daily (preferably within 5 minutes after each meal)

Prescribe antibacterial mouth rinses (after active carious lesions are eliminated)

- Chlorhexidine gluconate (0.12%): rinse with ½ ounce for 30 seconds, morning and night for 2 weeks

Examine at 3-month recall

Monitor and reinforce preventive measures

Monitor sealant retention

Perform bacterial testing (*Streptococcus mutans* test)

- If scores are 0 or 1, continue home fluoride administration and recall in 3 months
- If scores are 2 or 3, repeat program

Possible reasons for persistently high *S mutans* levels

- Patient maintaining high refined carbohydrate diet
- Lack of patient compliance with program
- Undetected carious lesions still present
- Possible inoculation from another individual (eg, spouse)

---

venting and/or arresting root caries through plaque removal, diet modification, and topical fluoride application.

Plaque removal alone has been shown to play an important role in arresting active root caries.[33] In situ studies have confirmed that both plaque thickness and acidogenic response to sucrose exposure are significantly reduced when lesions become inactive.[90,91] A 0.12% chlorhexidine rinse (Peridex, Zila; Periogard, Colgate) can also be used in treating root caries cases. While chlorhexidine has been used primarily as an antimicrobial treatment for gingivitis and periodontal disease, it is very effective in eliminating cariogenic bacteria.

Topical fluoride is accepted as an appropriate chemotherapeutic agent in the management of root caries. Prevention/arrest of root surface lesions has been demonstrated in both in situ and clinical studies using fluoridated water,[16,54,110] fluoride gels,[13] fluoride mouth rinses,[114] fluoride dentifrices,[56] fluoride varnishes,[33] fluoride chewing gums,[25] and intraoral fluoride-releasing devices.[25,81] A synergistic, beneficial effect of argon laser irradiation and acidulated phosphate fluoride (APF) gels on root lesions in vitro has also been demonstrated.[50] However, the optimum delivery system of fluoride for protection against root caries has yet to be determined.[35]

A large number of studies have shown the benefits of substituting dietary polyols for sucrose in chewable dietary items. Xylitol, a 5-carbon sugar alcohol, has been under investigation since the early 1970s and has been found to be a safe and effective dietary supplement in humans (approved by the FDA in 1963 for special dietary purposes). Xylitol is not metabolized by *S mutans* and has been shown to have an anticariogenic effect,[86,117] decrease plaque formation,[55] increase plaque pH,[1] and enhance remineralization.[126] Extensive research over the past 25 years has demonstrated that a 5- to 10-g daily consumption of xylitol in the form of gum can result in a 30% to 85% reduction in dental caries.[77,78]

The use of calcium phosphate has also been investigated as a mechanism for arresting root caries,[20] and many new preventive strategies are on the horizon. The goal of the dental practitioner should be to initiate preventive and remineralization therapies that will inhibit or eliminate the disease process before tissue destruction occurs. The excavation of actively carious tooth structure and placement of restorative materials is, at best, a repair of the damages inflicted by the disease process and does not address the control of the disease itself. An effective preventive/remineralization regimen for the treatment of patients at risk for root caries is outlined above (see box).

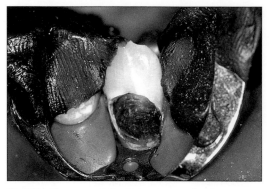

Fig 12-9 Because of the importance of a dry operating field, unobstructed access, and good visibility for treatment of root caries lesions, isolation is key to long-term success.

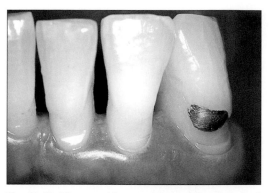

Fig 12-10 Direct gold restoration performing well 43 years after placement.

Restorative Treatment

Clearly, many root caries lesions do not need restorative treatment. Accessible, shallow lesions can be made caries free and easy to clean through caries debridement with hand instruments, finishing burs, and/or polishing disks.[13,124] Arrested lesions with a hard to leathery surface are often amenable to treatment with topical fluorides in combination with a chlorhexidine rinse.[11]

When root caries has progressed such that restoration of lost structure is necessary, the dentist faces difficulties that differ considerably from those posed by many coronal lesions. The challenges to the restorative dentist include impaired visibility, difficult access, moisture control, pulpal proximity, and the nature of the dentin substrate itself. These factors tend to compromise the ideal restoration, which should conserve remaining tooth structure and provide long-term integrity of marginal seal. There is general agreement today that, when possible, adhesive fluoride-releasing restorative materials are preferred.[17]

Isolation is the key to long-term success in root surface restorations. Inability to obtain a dry operating field, unobstructed access, and visibility frequently results in a compromised restoration. The use of rubber dam and retractors, retraction cord, and/or surgical exposure will usually satisfy the necessary criteria. At times, the isolation may take more time than the actual preparation and restoration to obtain a satisfactory result (Fig 12-9).

Preparation design for cervical lesions and the properties of dental materials are described in other chapters. Preparation should involve removal of demineralized tooth structure with only minimal removal of sound tooth tissue for access and retention.

Direct Filling Gold

When properly placed and maintained in the right oral environment, gold foil restorations provide unequaled durability and longevity (Fig 12-10). Unfortunately, due to their perceived technique sensitivity and placement time, they are offered by a diminishing number of practitioners. Cavity preparation for direct gold placement requires removal of sound tooth structure for mechanical retention, and gold offers no chemotherapeutic benefit. However, these restorations are extremely well tolerated by supporting tissues and have demonstrated excellent longevity. For the xerostomic patient, this would not be the restorative material of choice because of cost, lack of chemotherapeutic effect, and likelihood of failure.

Silver Amalgam

Amalgam has the longest clinical history of the direct restorative materials with the exception of the direct filling golds. It has excellent wear characteristics, increasing marginal seal over time, and some bacteriostatic properties (Fig 12-11). Amalgam is relatively easy to place and is less sensitive to variations in handling than many other materials. Like direct gold, amalgam must be mechanically retained and does not offer significant chemotherapeutic benefit. With the

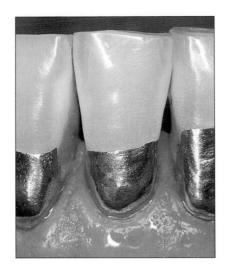

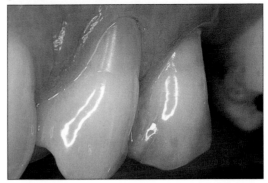

Fig 12-11 Eighteen-year-old amalgam restorations in mandibular incisors.

Fig 12-12 Resin composites placed with a fourth-generation bonding system.

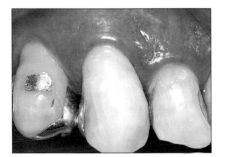

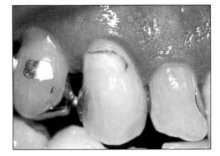

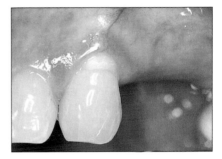

Fig 12-13a A resin composite restoration immediately after placement.

Fig 12-13b The same restoration 18 months later showing leakage at the restoration-cementum interface.

Fig 12-14 A Ketac-Fil (ESPE) conventional glass-ionomer restoration placed 10 years earlier.

introduction of adhesive fluoride-releasing materials and the current demand for tooth-colored restorations, the use of amalgam in cervical lesions has declined. While not recommended for use in xerostomic patients, it may still be the material of choice when isolation is a problem.

Resin Composite

With the advent of relatively reliable dentin bonding systems, resin composite materials, including compomers (polyacid-modified resins) and flowable composites, have become extremely popular with dental practitioners (Fig 12-12). Unfortunately, all of these materials exhibit a degree of polymerization shrinkage that can severely stress the adhesive interface provided by dentin bonding systems. When this is combined with the difference in coefficient of thermal expansion between these materials and tooth struc-

ture, the result is often a loss of marginal seal and microleakage (Figs 12-13a and 12-13b). Fluoride release is less than that of glass ionomer, and these materials do not currently offer any fluoride uptake. They are primarily indicated in root caries situations where esthetics is of major importance. Microfilled or hybrid resin composites appear to offer advantages over compomers and flowable composites.

Glass-Ionomer Cement/ Resin-Modified Glass-Ionomer Cement

Glass-ionomer cement is the material of choice for most root caries lesions (see Chapter 13). The material offers adhesive bonding, long-term fluoride release, and the ability to "recharge" or take up fluoride when exposed to an external source (eg, topical application, mouth rinse). Clinical studies have demonstrated successful 10-year longevity[79] (Fig 12-14) as well as reasonable success in xerostomic patients.[48]

Conclusion

Dental caries is a bacterial infectious disease associated with diet[119] and should be treated as such. Extensive research has moved our concept of caries from the early "worm theory" to a better understanding of the multifactorial, chronic nature of the disease. For this reason, modern dentistry has experienced a paradigm shift, with a move from complete reliance on the traditional surgical (restorative) approach to an acceptance of the fact that treatment of dental caries is not complete until the infection and contributing factors are controlled. This concept should guide the management of both coronal and root surface caries.

References

1. Aguirre-Zero O, Zero DT, Proskin HM. Effect of chewing xylitol chewing gum on salivary flow rate and the acidogenic potential of dental plaque. Caries Res 1993;27:55–59.

2. Al-Khateeb S, Angma-Mansson B, DeJosselin E. In vivo quantification of changes in caries lesions in orthodontic patients [abstract]. J Dent Res 1996;75:127.

3. Ando M, Analoui M, Schemehorn BR. Comparison of lesion analysis by microradiography and confocal microscopy [abstract 209]. J Dent Res 1995;74:48.

4. Astroth JD. Caring for the elderly adult: how to prevent, manage root surface caries. Dent Teamwork 1996;9:15–19.

5. Atkinson JC, Wu AJ. Salivary gland dysfunction: causes, symptoms, treatment. J Am Dent Assoc 1994;125:409–416.

6. Banting DW, Ellen RP, Fillery ED. Prevalence of root surface caries among institutional older persons. Community Dent Oral Epidemiol 1980;8:84–88.

7. Banting DW, Ellen RP, Fillery ED. A longitudinal study of root caries: baseline and incidence data. J Dent Res 1985;64:1141–1144.

8. Beck JD, Kohout F, Hunt RJ. Identification of high caries risk adults: attitudes, social factors and diseases. Int Dent J 1988;38:231–238.

9. Beck JD. The epidemiology of root caries: North American studies. Adv Dent Res 1993;7:42–51.

10. Beighton D, Hellyer PH, Lynch EJ, Heath MR. Salivary levels of mutans streptococci, lactobacilli, yeasts, and root caries prevalence in non-institutionalized elderly dental patients. Community Dent Oral Epidemiol 1991;219:302–307.

11. Beighton D, Lynch E, Heath MR. A microbiological study of primary root-caries lesions with different treatment needs. J Dent Res 1993;72:623–629.

12. Beighton D, Lynch E. Comparison of selected microflora of plaque and underlying carious dentine associated with primary root caries lesions. Caries Res 1995;29:154.

13. Billings RJ, Brown LR, Kaster AG. Contemporary treatment strategies for root surface dental caries. Gerodontology 1985;1:20–27.

14. Brown LR, Billings RJ, Kaster AG. Quantitative comparisons of potentially cariogenic microorganisms cultured from non-carious and carious root and coronal tooth surfaces. Infect Immun 1986;51:765–770.

15. Brown LJ, Brunelle JA, Kingman A. Periodontal status in the United States, 1988-1991: Prevalence, extent, and demographic variation. J Dent Res 1996;75(special issue):672–683.

16. Brustman B. Impact of exposure to fluoride adequate water on root surface caries in the elderly. Gerodontics 1986;2:203–207.

17. Burgess JO. Dental materials for the restoration of root surface caries. Am J Dent 1995;8:342–351.

18. Burt BA, Ismail AI, Edlund SA. Root caries in an optimally fluoridated and high-fluoride community. J Dent Res 1986;65:1154–1158.

19. Christensen GJ. A new challenge—root caries in mature people. J Am Dent Assoc 1996;127:379–380.

20. Chow LC, Takagi S. Remineralization of root lesions with concentrated calcium and phosphate solutions. Den Mater J 1995;14:131–136.

21. Clarkson JE. Epidemiology of root caries. Am J Dent 1995;8:329–334.

22. Dawes C. A mathematical model of salivary clearance of sugar from the oral cavity. Caries Res 1983;17:321–324.

23. de Josselin de Jong E, Sundstrom F, Angmar-Mansson B, Ten Bosch JJ. QLF-vision: reproducibility of in vivo quantification of enamel mineral loss [abstract]. J Dent Res 1994;73:200.

24. de Josselin de Jong E, Sundstrom F, Westerling H, et al. A new method for in vivo quantification of changes in initial enamel caries with laser fluorescence. Caries Res 1995;29:2–7.

25. De Los Santos R, Lin YT, Corpron RE, et al. In situ remineralization of root surface lesions using a fluoride chewing gum or a fluoride releasing device. Caries Res 1994;28:441–446.

26. De Paola PF. Caries in our aging populations: what are we learning? In: Bowen WH, Tabak LA (eds). Cariology for the Nineties. Rochester: University of Rochester Press; 1993:25–35.

27. Dodds M, Suddick R. Caries risk assessment for determination of focus and intensity of prevention in a dental school clinic. J Dent Educ 1995;59:945–956.

28. Douglass CW, Furino A. Balancing dental service requirements and supplies: epidemiologic and demographic evidence. J Am Dent Assoc 1990;121:587–592.

29. Drake CW, Hunt RJ, Beck JD, Koch GG. Eighteen-month coronal caries incidence in North Carolina older adults. J Public Health Dent 1994;54:24–30.

30. Drury TF, Brown LJ, Zion GR. Tooth retention and tooth loss in the permanent dentition of adults: 1988–1991. J Dent Res 1996;75(special issue):684–695.

31. El-Hadary ME, Ramadan AE, Kamar AA, Nour ZM. A study of the incidence of and distribution of root surface caries and its relation to periodontal disease. Egypt Dent J 1975;21:43–52.

32. Emilson CG, Klock B, Sanford CB. Microbial flora associated with presence of root surface caries in periodontally treated patients. Scand J Dent Res 1988;96:40–49.

33. Emilson CG, Ravald N, Birkhed D. Effects of a 12-month prophylactic programme on selected oral bacterial populations on root surfaces with active and inactive carious lesions. Caries Res 1993;27:195–200.

34. Erickson RL. Root surface treatment with glass ionomers and resin composites. Am J Dent 1994:7:279.

35. Featherstone JDB. Fluoride, remineralization and root caries. Am J Dent 1994;7:271–274.

36. Fedele DJ, Sheets CG. Issues in the treatment of root caries in older adults. J Esthet Dent 1998;10:243–252.

37. Fejerskov O, Luan WM, Nyvad B, et al. Active and inactive root surface caries lesions in a selected group of 60-90 year old Danes. Caries Res 1991;25:385–391.

38. Fejerskov O. Recent advancements in the treatment of root surface caries. Int Dent J 1994;44:139.

39. Ferguson M. Pilocarpine and other cholinergic drugs in the management of salivary gland dysfunction. Oral Surg Oral Med Oral Path 1993;75:186–191.

40. Ferreira AG, Analoui M, Ando M. Using dye enhanced QLF for analyzing incipient lesions [abstract 1446]. J Dent Res 1995;74:192.

41. Fure S, Romaniec M, Emilson CG, Krasse B. Proportions of *Streptococcus mutans*, lactobacilli and *Actinomyces* spp in root surface plaque. Scand J Dent Res 1987;95:119–123.

42. Fure S, Zickert I. Prevalence of root surface caries in 55, 65, and 75 year old Swedish individuals. Community Dent Oral Epidemiol 1990;18:100–105.

43. Gustavsen F, Clive JM, Tveit AF. Root caries prevalence in a Norwegian adult dental population. Gerodontics 1988;18:100–105.

44. Hals E, Selvig KA. Correlated electron probe microanalysis and microradiography of carious and normal dental cementum. Caries Res 1977;11:62–75.

45. Hand JS, Hunt RJ, Beck JD. Incidence of coronal and root caries in an older adult. J Public Health Dent 1988;48:14–19.

46. Hand JS, Hunt RJ, Beck JD. Coronal and root caries in older Iowans: 36 month incidence. Gerodontics 1988;4:136–139.

47. Haveman CW, Redding SW. Dental management and treatment of xerostomic patients. Texas Dent J 1998;115:43–56.

48. Haveman CW, Burgess JO, Summitt JB. A clinical comparison of restorative materials for caries in xerostomic patients [abstract 1441]. J Dent Res 1999;78:286.

49. Hellyer PH, Beighton D, Heath MR, Lynch EJ. Root caries in older people attending a general dental practice in East Sussex. Br Dent J 1990;169:201–206.

50. Hicks MJ, Westerman GH, Flaitz CM, et al. Effects of argon laser irradiation and acidulated phosphate fluoride on root caries. Am J Dent 1995;8:10–14.

51. Hicks MJ, Flaitz CM, Garcia-Godoy F. Root-surface caries formation: effect of in vitro APF treatment. J Am Dent Assoc 1998;129:449–453.

52. Hix JO, O'Leary TJ. The relationship between cemental caries, oral hygiene status and fermentable carbohydrate levels. J Periodontol 1976;47:398–404.

53. Hoppenbrouwers PMM, Driessens FCM, Borggreven JMPM. The mineral solubility of human tooth roots. Arch Oral Biol 1987;32:219.

54. Hunt RJ, Eldredge JB, Beck JD. Effect of residence in a fluoridated community on the incidence of coronal and root caries in an older adult population. J Public Health Dent 1989;49:138–141.

55. Isotupa KP, Gunn S, Chen CY, et al. Effect of polyol gums on dental plaque in orthodontic patients. Am J Orthod Dentofac Orthop 1995;107:497–504.

56. Jensen ME, Kohout F. The effect of a fluoride dentifrice on root and coronal caries in an older adult population. J Am Dent Assoc 1988;117:829–832.

57. Johansen E. Electron microscopic and chemical studies of carious lesions with reference to the organic phase of affected tissues. Ann NY Acad Sci 1965;131:776–785.

58. Jones JA. Root caries: prevention and chemotherapy. Am J Dent 1995;8:352–357.

59. Jordan HV, Hammond BF. Filamentous bacteria isolated from human root caries. Arch Oral Biol 1972;17:1333–1342.

60. Joshi A, Papas AS, Giunta J. Root caries incidence and associated risk factors in middle-aged and older adults. Gerodontology 1993;10:83–89.

61. Kalsbeek H, Truin GJ, Burgersdijk R, van't Hof M. Tooth loss and dental caries in Dutch adults. Community Dent Oral Epidemiol 1991;19:201–204.

62. Katz RV, Hazen SP, Chilton NW, Mumma RD Jr. Prevalence and intraoral distribution of root caries in an adult population. Caries Res 1982;16:265–271.

63. Katz RV. Development of an index for the prevalence of root caries. J Dent Res 1984;63:814–818.

64. Katz RV. Root caries—is it the problem of the future? J Can Dent Assoc 1985;51:511–514.

65. Katz RV. The clinical diagnosis of root caries: issues for the clinician and researcher. Am J Dent 1995;8:335–341.

66. Keltjens HM, Schaeken MJ, van der Hoeven JS, Hendrilos JC. Microflora of plaque from sound and carious root surfaces. Caries Res 1987;21:193–199.

67. Lagerlöf F, Dawes R, Dawes C. Salivary clearance of sugar and its effects on pH changes by *Streptococcus mitior* in an artificial mouth. J Dent Res 1984;63:1266–1270.

68. Lagerlöf F, Dawes C. The effect of swallowing frequency on oral sugar clearance and pH changes by *Streptococcus mitior* in vivo after sucrose ingestion. J Dent Res 1985;64:1229–1232.

69. Lawrence HP, Hunt RJ, Beck JD. Three-year root caries incidence and risk modeling in older adults in North Carolina. J Public Health Dent 1995;55:69–78.

70. Leske GS, Ripa LW. Three-year root caries increments: an analysis of teeth and surfaces at risk. Gerodontology 1989;8:17–21.

71. Locker D, Slade GD, Leake JL. Prevalence of and factors associated with root decay in older adults in Canada. J Dent Res 1989;68:768–772.

72. Locker D. Incidence of root caries in an older Canadian population. Community Dent Oral Epidemiol 1996;24:403–407.

73. Lohse W, Carter H, Brunelle J. The prevalence of root surface caries in a military population. Mil Med 1977;142:700–703.

74. Luan WM, Boelum V, Chen X. Dental caries in adult and elderly Chinese. J Dent Res 1989;68:1771–1776.

75. Lynch E. Relationship between clinical criteria and microflora of primary root caries. In: Stookey GK (ed). Early Detection of Dental Caries. Cincinnati, OH: Sidney Printing Works, 1996:195–242.

76. MacEntee MI, Clark DC, Glick N. Predictors of caries in old age. Gerodontology 1993;10:90–97.

77. Mäkinen KK, Bennett CA, Hujoel PP, et al. Xylitol chewing gums and caries rates: a 40-month cohort study. J Dent Res 1995;74:1904–1913.

78. Mäkinen KK, Mäkinen PL, Pape HR Jr. Stabilisation of rampant caries: polyol gums and arrest of dentine caries in two long-term cohort studies in young subjects. Int Dent J 1995;45(suppl 1):93–107.

79. Matis BA, Cochran MA, Carlson TJ. Longevity of glass-ionomer restorative materials: results of a 10-year evaluation. Quintessence Int 1996;27:373–382.

80. Miller AJ, Brunell JA, Carlos JD, et al. Oral Health of United States Adults (NIH Publication no. 87-2868). Bethesda, MD: US Department of Health and Human Services, 1987.

81. Mirth DB, Shern RJ, Emilson CG, et al. Clinical evaluation of an intraoral device for controlled release of fluoride. J Am Dent Assoc 1982;105:791–797.

82. Mjör IA. Placement and replacement of restorations. Oper Dent 1981;6:49–54.

83. Mjör IA. Frequency of secondary caries at various anatomical locations. Oper Dent 1985;10:88–92.

84. National Institutes of Health. Technology Assessment Conference. Effects and side effects of dental restorative materials. Bethesda, MD: US Department of Health and Human Services, 1991.

85. Newitter DA, Katz RV, Clive JM. Detection of root caries: sensitivity and specificity of a modified explorer. Gerodontics 1985;1:65–67.

86. Nuuja T, Meurman JH, Torkko H. Xylitol and the bactericidal effect of chlorhexidine and fluoride on *Streptococcus mutans* and *Streptococcus sanguis*. Acta Odontol Scand 1993; 51:109–114.

87. Nyvad B, Fejerskov O. Root surface caries: clinical, histopathological and microbiological features and clinical implications. Int Dent J 1982;32:312–326.

88. Nyvad B, Fejerskov O. Active root-surface caries converted into inactive caries as a response to oral hygiene. Scand J Dent Res 1986;94:281–284.

89. Nyvad B, ten Cate JM, Fejerskov O. Microradiography of experimental root-surface caries in man. Caries Res 1989;23: 218–224.

90. Nyvad B, Larsen MJ. Effect of daily plaque removal on Stephan pH response of active root caries lesions in situ. Caries Res 1992;26:227–228.

91. Nyvad B, Fejerskov O. Effect of tooth cleaning on microbial invasion of experimental root surface caries [abstract 78]. Caries Res 1993;27:229.

92. Nyvad B, ten Cate JM, Fejerskov O. Arrest of root surface caries in situ. J Dent Res 1997;76:1845–1853.

93. Pappas A, Koski A, Guinta J. Prevalence and intraoral distribution of coronal and root caries in middle-aged and older adults. Caries Res 1992;26:459–465.

94. Park KK, Zitterbart PA, Christen AG. Preventive management of root caries: state of the art. Indiana Dent Assoc J 1987;66: 11–19.

95. Persson RE, Persson GR, Powell LV, Kiyak HA. Periodontal effects of a biobehavioral prevention program. J Clin Periodontol 1999;25:322–329.

96. Powell LV, Leroux BG, Persson RE, Kiyak HA. Factors associated with caries incidence in an elderly population. Community Dent Oral Epidemiol 1998;26:170–176.

97. Powell LV, Mancl LA, Senft GD. Exploration of prediction models for caries risk assessment of the geriatric population. Community Dent Oral Epidemiol 1991;19:291–295.

98. Ramsey DJ, Ripa LW. Enamel prism orientation and enamel cementum relationship in the cervical region of premolars. Br Dent J 1969;126:165–167.

99. Ravald N, Hamp SE. Prediction of root surface caries in patients treated for advanced periodontal disease. J Clin Periodontol 1981;8:400–414.

100. Ravald N, Hamp SE, Birkhed D. Long-term evaluation of root surface caries in periodontally treated patients. J Clin Periodontol 1986;13:758–767.

101. Ravald N, Birkhed D. Factors associated with active and inactive root caries in patients with periodontal disease. Caries Res 1991;25:377–384.

102. Ravald N, Birkhed D. Prediction of root caries in periodontally treated patients maintained with different fluoride programmes. Caries Res 1992;26:450–458.

103. Ravald N, Birkhed D, Hamp SE. Root caries susceptibility in periodontally treated patients. Results after 12 years. J Clin Periodontol 1993;20:124–129.

104. Ripa LW, Leske GS, Forte F. Effect of a 0.05% neutral NaF mouthrinse on coronal and root caries of adults. Gerodontology 1987;6:131–136.

105. Scheinin A, Pienihakkinen K, Tiekso J, Holmberg S. Multifactorial modeling for root caries prediction. Community Dent Oral Epidemiol 1992;20:35–37.

106. Schupbach P, Osterwalder V, Guggenheim B. Human root caries: microbiota of a limited number of root caries lesions. Caries Res 1996;30:52–64.

107. Shay K. Management of the institutionalized geriatric dental patient. J Prosthet Dent 1994;72:510.

108. Shay K. Root caries in the elderly: an update for the next century. Indiana Dent Assoc J 1997–98;37–43.

109. Socransky SS, Hubersak C, Propas D. Introduction of periodontal destruction in gnotobiotic rats by a human oral strain of *Actimomyces naeslundii*. Arch Oral Biol 1970;15:993–995.

110. Stamm JW, Banting DW, Imrey PB. Adult root caries survey of two similar communities with contrasting natural water fluoride levels. J Am Dent Assoc 1990;120:143–149.

111. Sumney DL, Jordan HV, Englander HR. The prevalence of root surface caries in selected populations. J Periodontol 1973;44:500–504.

112. Syed SA, Loesche WJ, Pape HL Jr, Grenier E. Predominant cultivable flora isolated from human root surface caries plaque. Infect Immun 1975;11:727–731.

113. Tenovuo J. Salivary parameters of relevance in assessing caries activity in individuals and populations. Community Dent Oral Epidemiol 1997;25:82–86.

114. Teranaka T, Koulourides T. Effect of 100 ppm fluoride mouthrinse on experimental root caries in human. Caries Res 1987;21:326–332.

115. Todd JE, Lader D. Adult Dental Health 1988. United Kingdom. London: HMSO, 1991:114.

116. Tonetti MS. Cigarette smoking and periodontal diseases: etiology and management of disease. Ann Periodontol 1998; 3:88–101.

117. Trahan L. Xylitol: a review of its action on mutans streptococci and dental plaque—its clinical significance. Int Dent J 1995;45(suppl 1):77–92.

118. van der Veen MH, Tsuda H, Arends J, ten Bosch JJ. Evaluation of sodium fluorescein for quantitative diagnosis of root caries. J Dent Res 1996;75:588–593.

119. van Houte J, Jordan HV, Laraway R, et al. Association of the microbial flora of dental plaque and saliva with human root surface caries. J Dent Res 1990;69:1463–1468.

120. van Houte J, Lopman J, Kent R. The predominant cultivable flora of sound and carious human root surfaces. J Dent Res 1994;73:727–734.

121. van Strijp AJ, van Steenbergen TJ, Ten Cate JM. Bacterial colonization of mineralized and completely demineralized dentine in situ. Caries Res 1997;31:349–355.

122. Wag BJ. Root surface caries: a review. Community Dent Health 1984;1:11–20.

123. Wallace MC, Retief DH, Bradley EL. Incidence of root caries in older adults [abstract 272]. J Dent Res 1988;67:147.

124. Wallace MC, Retief DH, Bradley EL. The 48-month increment of root caries in an urban population of older adults participating in a preventive dental program. J Public Health Dent 1993;43:133–137.

125. Weber DF. Human dentin sclerosis: a microradiographic survey. Arch Oral Biol 1974;19:163–169.

126. Wennerholm K, Arends J, Birkhed D, et al. Effect of xylitol and sorbitol in chewing-gums on mutans streptococci, plaque pH and mineral loss of enamel. Caries Res 1994;28:48–54.

127. Whelton HP, Holland TJ, O'Mullane DM. The prevalence of root surface caries amongst Irish adults. Gerodontology 1993;10:72–75.

128. Winn DM, Brunelle JA, Selwitz RH, et al. Coronal and root caries in dentition of adults in the United States: 1988-1991. J Dent Res 1996;75(special issue):642–651.

129. Zambon J, Kasprzak SA. Microbiology and histopathology of human root caries. Am J Dent 1995;6:323–328.

chapter

13 Fluoride-Releasing Materials

John O. Burgess

Fluorides are an important adjunct in the prevention of caries. In addition to professionally applied fluorides and fluoride-containing dentifrices, fluorides may be introduced into the oral environment with fluoride-releasing restorative materials. This chapter discusses fluoride-releasing materials, their effectiveness in inhibiting recurrent caries, and their clinical longevity. The caries process and other methods of caries management are discussed in Chapter 4. Root caries and its prevention and treatment are discussed in Chapter 12.

Caries is a dynamic process in which mineral is removed during times of high acid production by bacterial plaque (demineralization) and replaced during periods of neutral pH (remineralization). Remineralization is the process by which mineral is deposited into tooth structure from salivary calcium and phosphate during periods of neutral pH. The remineralization process is facilitated by fluoride and can arrest carious demineralization by the formation of a hard outer surface.

Dentinal caries is similar to enamel caries, except that dentin demineralization begins at a higher pH (6.4 compared to 5.5) and proceeds about twice as rapidly since dentin has only half the mineral content. Low fluoride levels are insufficient to initiate dentin remineralization but are adequate to facilitate enamel remineralization.[68] In enamel, at fluoride levels around 3 parts per million (ppm), the balance of mineral uptake and loss is shifted from net demineralization to net remineralization.[36] Because dentin composes most root structure and because root surface caries lesions require significantly greater amounts of fluoride than enamel caries lesions to promote remineralization, restorative materials that release fluoride are often recommended for root surfaces.

The Fluoride-Releasing Materials Continuum

The first popular fluoride-releasing tooth-colored restorative material was silicate cement. Although this material had no bonding properties and did not survive well in the oral environment, recurrent caries lesions associated with silicate cement restorations were rare. This anticaries effect was eventually associated with fluoride release by the material. Most current fluoride-releasing materials have the goal of inhibiting recurrent caries, especially in patients at high risk for developing new lesions.

Fluoride-releasing materials may be classified into four categories[4,5,8] based on similarities in physical, mechanical, and setting properties (Fig 13-1 and Table 13-1). Fluoride-releasing resin composites are on one end of the continuum and conventional glass ionomers on the other. Compomers appear near the

377

Table 13-1 Mechanical properties of the materials continuum[60]

	Material class			
	Glass ionomer	Resin-modified glass ionomer	Compomer	Fluoride-releasing composite
Flexural strength (MPa)	15–25	35–70	60–94	85–97
Compressive strength (MPa)	170–200*	180–210	190–250	230–270
Diametral tensile strength (MPa)	22–25	35–40	45–47	40–60
Shear bond strength (MPa)	3–7	7–16	14–22	24–28
Fluoride release	High	High	Moderate	Low
Fluoride recharge	High	High	Moderate	Low

*Ultimate compressive strength. Glass ionomers may achieve this after several weeks' storage prior to testing; early strengths are significantly lower.

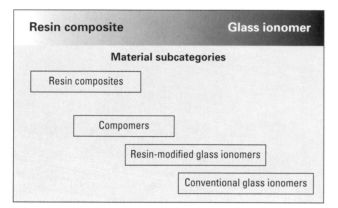

Fig 13-1 The fluoride-releasing materials continuum. Locations on the continuum are characterized by both compositional variants and available cure mechanisms.

resin composite end, and resin-modified glass ionomers are positioned nearer to the conventional glass ionomers.

Resin composites (Table 13-1) have better mechanical properties, no inherent adhesive properties, greater thermal expansion coefficients, and better wear resistance compared with other materials in the continuum, but they have the least fluoride release. Glass ionomers have inherent adhesive properties, release comparatively high amounts of fluoride, and have thermal expansion coefficients similar to tooth structure, but their mechanical properties and wear resistance are poor. Resin-modified glass ionomers contain elements of glass ionomers and light-cured resins. These materials have properties similar to glass ionomers and, like glass ionomers, should not be used for restorations in occlusal load–bearing areas. Although compomers are blends of resin composite and glass ionomer, they incorporate more resin than resin-

modified glass ionomers, and their physical and mechanical properties are more closely related to fluoride-releasing resin composites. Compomers require a bonding system and acid etching of tooth structure to achieve a clinically usable bond. They release more fluoride than resin composites but less than glass ionomers and are more abrasion resistant than conventional or resin-modified glass ionomers.

The early glass-ionomer restorative materials, called glass-ionomer cements, were rough, had less than optimum esthetic qualities, and had to be protected from hydration and dehydration with a varnish or light-cured resin, applied to the surface immediately after placement. Finishing was delayed for 24 hours with the earlier materials; this delay was later shortened, through modification of the material, to 7 minutes. The unmodified glass-ionomer materials are rarely used today.

Fluoride Release

Fluoride released from glass-ionomer restorations has been collected in whole saliva in vivo.[32] It is incorporated into bacteria[3] and inhibits bacterial acid production.[64] Fluoride released from glass ionomer and silicate cement is incorporated into tooth structure.[30] Those increased fluoride levels in teeth have been measured with a microbiopsy technique[61] and an electron probe.[24] The fluoride in plaque on teeth adjacent or several teeth distant to teeth restored with glass ionomer is not increased, however. Protection provided by fluoride-releasing materials is probably confined to tooth structure immediately adjacent to the restoration. One study demonstrated that fluoride released from restorative materials has an effective zone of about 1 mm from the restoration's margin.[67]

In vivo research by Hatibovic-Kofman and Koch[32] and by Hattab et al[34] found significant increases in fluoride in saliva following placement of glass-ionomer restorations. In one study,[32] salivary fluoride concentrations remained elevated even 1 year after placement of glass-ionomer restorations (0.3 ppm after placement, 0.04 ppm 1 year later). In another study,[34] four subjects wore maxillary appliances with four glass-ionomer (Ketac-Fil, ESPE) restorations every night. The unstimulated salivary fluoride content was measured before insertion of the device and after overnight wear. In all subjects, fluoride release increased after wearing the appliance.

Perrin et al[59] measured the fluoride release from four glass-ionomer cements and reported that the greatest release occurred on the first day, decreasing sharply the second day, and gradually diminishing over 3 weeks to a low-level, long-term release. After 1 year, all specimens were still releasing fluoride with daily concentrations of at least 0.5 ppm. Other studies have also shown a "burst" of fluoride release, with high early release for 1 to 2 days, followed by a rapid decline.[2,9,10,18,23,25,27,28,45,46,49,74]

Manufacturers of some glass-ionomer materials recommend placing an adhesive or protective surface coating on the glass-ionomer restoration as a final step after finishing. Although this may improve esthetics of the restoration, the coating decreases fluoride release or uptake until abrasion removes the coating. McKnight-Hanes and Whitford[45] and Burkett et al[9] reported that varnishing glass-ionomer samples decreased fluoride release by 61% to 76%.

Cranfield et al,[10] in a comprehensive study of fluoride-releasing materials, reported that fluoride release is influenced by specimen shape, with specimens with larger surface areas releasing more fluoride. They also reported that pH influenced fluoride release. Lower pH mediums produced higher fluoride release, probably due to erosion of the glass-ionomer surface.

Fluoride released from a restoration can be incorporated into tooth structure in the walls of a restoration. If a resin adhesive is used to "bond" the fluoride-releasing material to tooth structure, fluoride is prevented from moving into the walls of the preparation by the resin. In addition to evaluating fluoride release at the restoration surface, the McKnight-Hanes and Whitford[45] and Burkett et al[9] studies demonstrated that applying adhesive to the prepared cavity effectively prevented fluoride uptake to the tooth structure in the walls of the preparation.

Fluoride Recharging

Perhaps the most important variable in fluoride release is not the amount of fluoride released from the material initially after placement, since this declines rapidly with time, but the ability of the material to be recharged with fluoride from external sources. Forsten evaluated fluoride release[27] and uptake[26] by glass ionomers, examining whether glass-ionomer materials could not only release fluoride, but also take up fluoride from a fluoride-rich environment—in essence he measured their recharge capability. He reported that, after an initial high rate of fluoride release, a constant level of release occurred at about 3 weeks and that topical fluoride applications could recharge glass-ionomer restorations. Forsten[26] also reported a constant release rate of approximately 0.5 µg/mL to 1.0 µg/mL for all glass ionomers except cermets (glass ionomers containing silver particles) during the second year. Other investigators[11,15,33] have also reported the recharge phenomenon when fluoride solutions are used.

Compomers and resin-modified glass ionomers can be recharged as well.[75] Resin-modified glass ionomers (Photac-Fil, ESPE; Vitremer, 3M; and Fuji II LC, GC) and conventional glass ionomers (Fuji IX, GC America; and Ketac-Molar, ESPE) demonstrated the greatest fluoride recharge capacity. Fluoride-releasing resin composites such as Heliomolar (Ivoclar) and Tetric-Ceram (Ivoclar) released no additional fluoride after being exposed to the fluoride-rich solution. The compomers, Dyract AP (Dentsply) and Compoglass (Ivoclar), had a recharge capacity intermediate between resin-modified glass ionomers and resin composites. For those materials demonstrating recharge capability, the fluoride release remained at increased levels for only 1 day. This recharge capability may be due to the microporosities present in glass ionomers and resin-modified glass ionomers.

It would appear that glass-ionomer restorative materials are fluoride reservoirs; once the fluoride is depleted, it may be replenished from other fluoride sources such as toothpastes, mouth rinses, or topical fluoride solutions. The release after recharge is short, and recharge must be accomplished daily to maintain an elevated level.

The pH of the topical fluoride[6,16,20] used to recharge glass-ionomer restorations is important. Studies have reported that acidic topical fluoride solutions found in acidulated phosphate fluoride solutions and other acidified fluoride preparations cause degra-

ionomer restorations. It clearly demonstrates the effectiveness of fluoride-releasing materials in noncompliant patients.

The results of this study were supported by a recent report by Haveman et al[35] using a similar population. In this study, conventional glass-ionomer (Ketac-Fil), resin-modified glass-ionomer (Vitremer), and amalgam (Tytin, Kerr) Class 5 restorations were used to treat caries in xerostomic patients. At the 2-year recall, the percentage of Ketac-Fil restorations with recurrent caries was 30%; with Vitremer restorations, 21%; and with Tytin restorations, 53%. Restorations with fluoride-releasing materials had significantly fewer recurrent carious lesions than those with non–fluoride-releasing materials. Both studies suggest that fluoride-releasing materials are effective in reducing recurrent caries. However, recurrent caries were produced in both studies, demonstrating quite clearly that the remineralizing effects of fluoride released from restorations can be overwhelmed if the acid challenge is great enough.

Not all studies on recurrent caries inhibition demonstrate a clear benefit from fluoride release, however. Tyas[69] found no significant difference in recurrent caries in teeth restored with resin composite (Silux, 3M) or glass ionomer (Fuji II) in a population at low risk for caries. In two other clinical studies[47,48] involving almost 7,000 restorations, recurrent caries developed within 10 years for amalgam restorations, 8 years for resin composite restorations, and 5 years for glass-ionomer restorations. In fact, recurrent caries led to the replacement of almost half of the glass-ionomer restorations. In these populations, fluoride released from glass-ionomer restorations did not provide protection against primary or recurrent caries. It must be pointed out, however, that these were retrospective studies in which glass ionomer was used for patients at high risk for caries. In other words, the populations compared were not comparable. These studies reinforce the conclusion that fluoride-releasing materials do not prevent recurrent caries but should be viewed as one part of a complete program to reduce caries incidence.

How Much Fluoride Is Enough?

The question remains, however: how much fluoride release from restorative materials is enough to inhibit recurrent or secondary caries? DeSchepper et al[14] reported that all antibacterial activity from glass ionomers was lost when the pH of the glass-ionomer liquid was adjusted to 5. Other studies have found that a minimum inhibitory concentration of 100 to 200 µg/mL of sodium fluoride is required to inhibit the growth of oral streptococci[19] while concentrations up to 30-fold were necessary to be bactericidal. Naturally occurring fluoride at concentrations as high as 21 µg/mL does not produce any obvious effects on the composition of supragingival plaque. No glass ionomer maintains its acidity longer than 48 hours. Because fluoride-releasing materials release reduced amounts of fluoride and other ions, with time, bacteria and plaque accumulate on glass-ionomer restorations. Therefore, the direct bactericidal effect of fluoride released from restorative materials is very limited and is due to the combination of fluoride and acidity. Although the fluoride levels in bacteria associated with glass-ionomer restorations are elevated, the effect of fluoride on reducing bacterial acid production, bacteria metabolism, and division has yet to be clarified.

High levels of fluoride release produce remineralization of enamel and dentin. One study[17] has demonstrated that enamel demineralization decreased as fluoride release from a resin composite restorative material increased. By extrapolating data, the authors concluded that a resin composite releasing 200 to 300 µg/cm^2 of fluoride over a 1-month period would completely inhibit secondary caries. Unfortunately, this is approximately 40 to 50 times more fluoride than the release rate of current fluoride-releasing resin composites.

The remineralization of dentin is more complex than that of enamel. Active dentinal caries destroys collagen matrix as well as demineralizing apatite crystals. Remineralization of dentin may be affected by the remaining mineral, the remaining collagen, or the ultrastructure of the dentin. Collagen matrix devoid of mineral does not support remineralization.[71] The difficulty in protecting root surfaces with fluoride-releasing resin composite may be due to the higher concentrations of fluoride needed to remineralize root surfaces compared to enamel surfaces. Wefel[71] reported that demineralized dentin, with its exposed organic matrix, did not act as a suitable matrix for remineralization, but that remineralization did occur on any remaining apatite crystals. It seems clear that increased fluoride is required to remineralize dentin and that the degree of remineralization that can occur in dentin may be controlled by the amount of remaining mineral content.

Eichmiller and Marjenhoff[18] authored an excellent review of fluoride-releasing materials and noted that caries inhibition and remineralization potential have been shown in vitro by all fluoride-releasing materials when release rates were approximately 1 µg/mL. Resin-modified and conventional glass ionomers have similar fluoride release and recharge rates.[12]

Based on the previous studies, it is recommended that materials with a long-term fluoride release rate of at least 2 to 3 µg/mL/day be used. With present materials, this rate of release can be maintained only by use of supplemental fluorides via fluoride recharge.

Clinical Considerations for Fluoride-Releasing Materials

Although the recurrent caries inhibition effects of fluoride-releasing materials are evident, their clinical effectiveness has been questioned based on the durability of the material. Even in primary teeth, these materials should be used selectively, and the time that the material will be expected to survive (how long the tooth will remain in the oral cavity) should be evaluated against its wear effectiveness. One report[60] describes the wear resistance of a compomer (Dyract, Dentsply) and shows that this material has lower wear resistance than resin composite. At 1 year in a clinical evaluation of 91 Dyract restorations in conservative Class 1 and 2 restorations in primary teeth, the mean wear of Dyract was 190 µm, compared to approximately 10 µm with a wear-resistant resin composite. Another study,[38] measuring marginal adaptation of Class 2 restorations in the permanent dentition, reported that compomers showed such poor adaptation after 6 months of clinical wear that they should not be used as definitive restorations in load-bearing areas. Although the absolute numbers may vary, the typical compomer undergoes greater wear than the typical resin composite. Therefore, compomers should not be used in Class 1 or 2 load-bearing areas in the permanent dentition.

Three recent studies[1,37,40] have reported the clinical success of Dyract as a Class 5 restorative material in noncarious cervical lesions. In these studies, Dyract was clinically acceptable at the end of 3 years[37] and was superior to resin-modified glass ionomers.[1,40] Compomers continue to improve as new versions are introduced. However, much clinical testing is necessary to document their clinical performance before they can be endorsed.

For treating carious lesions, especially in the patient with high caries risk, resin-modified glass ionomers and fluoride-releasing resin composites have the greatest potential for success. Resin-modified glass ionomers are recommended as the esthetic restorative material of choice in the Class 5 situation for patients with high caries risk, especially those with diminished salivary flow, due to their high fluoride release and fluoride recharge capability. Because resin-modified glass ionomers have poorer wear resistance than fluoride-releasing resin composites, a resin composite should be used for restoration in load-bearing areas. The open sandwich technique for treating caries in the high-risk patient was successful at the 3-year recall in a report of a recent clinical trial[7] in which Class 2 composite restorations were placed in patients with moderate to high caries risk. The open sandwich restorations placed Vitremer resin-modified glass ionomer in the gingival portion of the proximal box and covered that material with Z100 (3M) resin composite. The sandwich technique in Class 2 restorations combines the wear resistance of a posterior resin composite with the fluoride release and recharge potential of resin-modified glass ionomers or compomers. In this technique, the fluoride-releasing material is placed into the proximal box of a preparation when the gingival margin extends to cementum or dentin. The resin-modified glass ionomer or compomer is cured, and resin composite is used to restore the occlusal surface for adequate wear resistance. Because enamel can be remineralized with fluoride released from fluoride-releasing resin composite,[17] occlusal load–bearing areas should be restored with resin composite. Proximal areas should be restored with materials that have maximum fluoride release and recharge potential, such as a resin-modified glass ionomer. Conventional glass ionomers are less successful in the sandwich technique.[72]

As materials continue to proliferate, it becomes increasingly difficult to choose the appropriate material for a particular clinical situation. Fluoride-releasing materials are no exception, and clinicians need guidelines to select and use these materials. There is modest but growing evidence from clinical trials that fluoride-releasing materials, especially glass ionomers, reduce the occurrence of recurrent caries. There is also evidence of a dose-response relationship between fluoride release and decreasing caries. While higher fluoride-releasing materials have greater caries protecting effects, these materials are not panaceas. The physical limitations of glass ionomers and compomers and their poor wear resistance contribute markedly to restoration failure. Evidence suggests that resin-modified glass-ionomer materials may provide an improved combination of physical integrity and caries inhibition.

References

1. Abdalla AI, Alhadainy HA, Garcia-Godoy F. Clinical evaluation of glass ionomers and compomers in Class 5 carious lesions. Am J Dent 1997;10:18–20.

2. Alvarez AN, Burgess JO, Chan DCN. Short term fluoride release of six ionomers—recharged, coated and abraded [abstract 260]. J Dent Res 1994;73:134.

3. Benelli EM, Serra MC, Rodrigues AL Jr, Cury JA. In situ anticariogenic potential of glass ionomer cement. Caries Res 1993;27:280–284.

4. Burgess J, Norling B, Summitt JB. Advances in glass ionomer material. Esthet Dent Update 1993;4:54–58.

5. Burgess JO, Norling B, Ong J, Rawls R. Directly placed esthetic restorative materials. Compend Cont Dent Ed 1996;17:731–748.

6. Burgess JO, Cardenas HL. Surface roughness of topical fluoride treated glass ionomers [abstract 775]. J Dent Res 1995;74:108.

7. Burgess JO, Summitt JB, Robbins JW, et al. Clinical evaluation of base, sandwich and bonded Class 2 resin composite restorations [abstract 304]. J Dent Res 1999;78:531.

8. Burgess JO, Norling BK, Summitt JB. Resin ionomer restorative materials: the new generation. J Esthetic Dent 1994;6:207–215.

9. Burkett L, Burgess JO, Chan DCN, Norling BK. Fluoride release of glass ionomers coated and not coated with adhesive [abstract 1242]. J Dent Res 1993;72:258.

10. Cranfield M, Kuhn A, Winter GB. Factors relating to the rate of fluoride-ion release from glass-ionomer cement. J Dent 1982;10:333–341.

11. Damen JJM, Buijs MJ, ten Cate JM. Uptake and release of fluoride by saliva-coated glass ionomer cement. Caries Res 1996;30:454–457.

12. de Araujo FB, García-Godoy F, Cury JA, Conceição EN. Fluoride release from fluoride-containing materials. Oper Dent 1996;21:185–190.

13. DeSchepper ED, Thrasher MR, Thurmond BA. Antibacterial effects of light-cured liners. Am J Dent 1989;2:74–76.

14. DeSchepper ED, White RR, von der Lehr W. Antibacterial effects of glass ionomers. Amer J Dent 1989;2:51–6.

15. Diaz-Arnold AM, Holmes DC, Wistrom DW, Swift EJ. Short-term fluoride release/uptake of glass ionomer restoratives. Dent Mater 1995;11:96–101.

16. Diaz-Arnold AM, Wistrom DW, Swift EJ. Topical fluoride and glass ionomer microhardness. Am J Dent 1995;8:134–136.

17. Dijkman GEHM, Arends J. Long-term fluoride release of visible light-activated composites in vitro: a correlation with in situ demineralization data. Caries Res 1993;27:117–123.

18. Eichmiller FC, Marjenhoff WA. Fluoride-releasing dental restorative materials. Oper Dent 1998;23:218–228.

19. Ekstrand J, Fejerskov O, Silverstone LM. Fluoride in Dentistry. Copenhagen: Munksgaard, 1988:76.

20. El-Badrawy WA, McComb D. Effect of home-use fluoride gels on resin-modified glass-ionomer cements. Oper Dent 1998;23:2–9.

21. Forss H, Jokinen J, Spets-Happonen S, et al. Fluoride and mutans streptococci in plaque growing on glass ionomer and composite. Caries Res 1991;25:454–458.

22. Forss H, Nase L, Seppa L. Fluoride and caries associated microflora in plaque on old GIC fillings [abstract 2468]. J Dent Res 1994;73:410.

23. Forsten L, Paunio IK. Fluoride release by silicate cements and resin composites. Scand J Dent Res 1972;80:515–519.

24. Forsten L, Rytomaa I, Anttila A, Keinonen J. Fluoride uptake from restorative dental materials by human enamel. Scand J Dent Res 1976;84:391–395.

25. Forsten L. Fluoride release of glass ionomers. J Esthet Dent 1994;6:216–222.

26. Forsten L. Fluoride release and uptake by glass ionomers. Scand J Dent Res 1991;99:241–245.

27. Forsten L. Short- and long-term fluoride release from glass ionomers and other fluoride-containing filling materials in vitro. Scand J Dent Res 1990;98:179–185.

28. Forsten L. Fluoride release from a glass ionomer cement. Scand J Dent Res 1977;85:503–504.

29. Fricker JP, McLachlan MD. Clinical studies of glass ionomer cements—part 2, a two year clinical study comparing glass ionomer cement with zinc phosphate cement. Aust Orthod J 1987;10:12–14.

30. Halgren A, Oliveby A, Twetman S. Fluoride concentration in plaque adjacent to orthodontic appliances retained with glass ionomer cement. Caries Res 1993;27:51–54.

31. Hals E, Norderval IT. Histopathology of experimental in vivo caries around silicate fillings. Acta Odont Scand 1973;31:357–367.

32. Hatibovic-Kofman S, Koch G. Fluoride release from glass ionomer cement in vivo and in vitro. Swed Dent J 1991;15:253–258.

33. Hatibovic-Kofman S, Koch G, Elkstrand J. Glass ionomer materials as a re-chargeable F-release system [abstract 260]. J Dent Res 1994;73:134.

34. Hattab FN, el-Mowafy OM, Salem NS, el-Badrawy WA. An in vivo study on the release of fluoride from glass-ionomer cement. Quintessence Int 1991;22:221–224.

35. Haveman C, Burgess J, Summitt JB. A clinical comparison of restorative materials for caries in xerostomic patients [abstract 1441]. J Dent Res 1999;78:286.

36. Jacobson APM, Strang R, Stephen KW. Effect of low fluoride levels in de/remineralising solutions of a pH-cycling model. Caries Res 1991;25;230–231.

37. Jedynakiewicz NM, Martin N, Fletcher JM. A three year evaluation of a compomer restorative [abstract 1189]. J Dent Res 1997;76:162.

38. Kersten S, Besek MJ, Lutz F. Marginal adaptation in class II compomer restorations in vivo [abstract 2286]. J Dent Res 1999;78:391.

39. Kvam E, Broch J, Nissen-Meyer IH. Comparison between a zinc phosphate cement and a glass ionomer cement for cementation of orthodontic bands. Eur J Orthod 1983;5:307–313.

40. Loher C, Kunzelman RH, Hickel R. Clinical evaluation of glass ionomer cements (LC), compomer and composite restorations in Class V cavities—two year results [abstract 1190]. J Dent Res 1997;76:162.

41. Loyola-Rodriguez JP, Garcia-Godoy F, Lindquist R. Growth inhibition of glass ionomer cements on mutans streptococci. Pediatr Dent 1994;16:346–349.

42. Lundstrom F, Krasse B. Streptococcus mutans and lactobacillus frequency in orthodontic patients: the effect of chlorhexidine treatments. Eur J Orthod 1987;2:27–39.

43. Marcusson A, Norevall L, Persson M. White spot reduction when using glass ionomer cement for bonding in orthodontics: a longitudinal and comparative study. Eur J Orthod 1997;19:233–242.

44. McComb D, Ericson D. Antimicrobial action of new proprietary lining cements. J Dent Res 1987;66:1025–1028.

45. McKnight-Hanes C, Whitford GM. Fluoride release from three glass ionomer materials and the effects of varnishing with or without finishing. Caries Res 1992;26:345–350.

46. Mitra SB. In vitro fluoride release from a light-cured glass-ionomer liner/base. J Dent Res 1991;70:75–78.

47. Mjör IA, Jokstadt A. Five-year study of Class II restorations in permanent teeth using amalgam, glass polyalkenoate (ionomer) cermet and resin-based composite materials. J Dent 1993;21:338–343.

48. Mjör IA. Glass-ionomer cement restorations and secondary caries: a preliminary report. Quintessence Int 1996;27:171–174.

49. Momoi Y, McCabe JF. Fluoride release from light-activated glass ionomer restorative cements. Dent Mater 1993;9:151–154.

50. Niessen LC, Gibson G. Oral health for a lifetime: preventive strategies for the older adult. Quintessence Int 1997;28:626–630.

51. Norman RD, Mehra RV, Swartz ML, Phillips RW. Effects of restorative materials on plaque composition. J Dent Res 1972;51:1596–1601.

52. Norman RD, Phillips RW, Swartz ML. Fluoride uptake by enamel from certain dental materials. J Dent Res 1960;39:11–16.

53. Norman RD, Platt JR, Phillips RW, Swartz ML. Additional studies on fluoride uptake by enamel from certain dental materials. J Dent Res 1961;40:529–537.

54. Norris DS, McInnes-Ledoux P, Schwaninger B, Weinberg R. Retention of orthodontic bands with new fluoride-releasing cements. Am J Orthod 1986;89:206–211.

55. O'Reilly MM, Featherstone JDB. Demineralization and remineralization around orthodontic appliances: an in vivo study. Am J Orthod Dentofac Orthop 1987;92:33–40.

56. Ogaard B, Rölla G, Arends J, ten Cate JM. Orthodontic appliances and enamel demineralization. Part 2. Prevention and treatment of lesions. Am J Orthod Dentofac Orthop 1988;94:123–128.

57. Ortendahl T, Thilander B, Svanberg M. Mutans streptococci and incipient caries adjacent to glass ionomer cement or resin-based composite in orthodontics. Am J Orthod Dentofac Orthop 1997;112:271–274.

58. Palenik CJ, Behnen MJ, Setcos JC, Miller CH. Inhibition of microbial adherence and growth by various glass ionomers in vitro. Dent Mater 1992;8:16–20.

59. Perrin C, Persin M, Sarrazin J. A comparison of fluoride release from four glass ionomer cements. Quintessence Int 1994;25:603–608.

60. Peters TCRB, Roeters JJM, Frankenmolen FWA. Clinical evaluation of Dyract in primary molars: 1-year results. Am J Dent 1996;9:83–87.

61. Phillips RW, Swartz ML. Effect of certain restorative materials on solubility of enamel. J Am Dent Assoc 1957;54:623–636.

62. Rezk-Lega F, Øgaard B, Rölla G. Availability of fluoride from glass-ionomer luting cements in human saliva. Scand J Dent Res 1991;99:60–63.

63. Seeholzer HW, Dasch W. Bonding with a glass ionomer cement. J Clin Orthod 1986;22:165–169.

64. Seppä L, Korhonen A, Nuutinen A. Inhibitory effect on S. mutans by fluoride-treated conventional and resin-reinforced glass ionomer cements. Eur J Oral Sci 1995;103:182–185.

65. Stirrups DR. A comparative clinical trial of a glass ionomer and a zinc phosphate cement for securing orthodontic bands. Br J Orthod 1991;18:15–20.

66. Svanberg M, Mjor IA, Orstavik D. Mutans streptococci in plaque from margins of amalgam, composite, and glass-ionomer restorations. J Dent Res 1990;69:861–864.

67. Tantbirojn D, Douglas WH, Versluis A. Inhibitive effect of a resin-modified glass ionomer cement on remote artificial caries. Caries Res 1997;31:275–280.

68. ten Cate JM, Buijs MJ, Damen JJM. PH-cycling of enamel and dentin lesions in the presence of low concentrations of fluoride. Eur J Oral Sci 1995:103;362–367.

69. Tyas MJ. Cariostatic effect of glass ionomer cement: a five year study. Aust Dent J 1991;36:236–239.

70. van Dijken JW, Kalfas S, Litra V, Oliveby A. Fluoride and mutans streptococci levels in plaque on aged restorations of resin-modified glass ionomer cement, compomer and resin composite. Caries Res 1997;31:379–383.

71. Wefel JS. Root caries histopathology and chemistry. Am J Dent 1994;7:261–265.

72. Welbury RR, Murray JJ. A clinical trial of the glass ionomer cement–composite resin "sandwich" technique in class II cavities in permanent premolar and molar teeth. Quintessence Int 1990;21:507–512.

73. Wood RE, Maxymiw WG, McComb D. A clinical comparison of glass ionomer (polyalkenoate) and silver amalgam restorations in the treatment of Class 5 caries in xerostomic head and neck cancer patients. Oper Dent 1993;18:94–102.

74. Woolford MJ, Grieve AR. Release of fluoride from glass polyalkenoate (ionomer) cement subjected to radiant heat. J Dent 1995;23:233–237.

75. Xu X, Burgess JO, Turpin-Mair JS. Fluoride release and recharge of fluoride-releasing restorative materials [abstract 431]. J Dent Res 1999;78:159.

14

Class 5 Restorations

Clifford B. Starr

Class 5 lesions are those carious and noncarious defects found in the gingival third of facial and lingual tooth surfaces. They require special attention, treatment planning, and restorative techniques because of differences from other defects affecting teeth. Class 5 carious lesions are produced by bacterial plaque attaching to the surface of teeth and producing demineralization as described in Chapter 4. But the etiology of noncarious Class 5 lesions, estimated to occur in 31% to 56%[15,45,60] of the population, is both unclear and controversial.[6,28] Certainly erosion and abrasion play a part in the formation of some Class 5, or cervical, lesions, but the role of occlusion, and the formation of defects called abfraction lesions, is less clear. Because of the location of Class 5 lesions, access for restorative treatment is often troublesome, moisture control can be exceedingly difficult to obtain and maintain, and soft tissue surgical approaches may be required. Due to the physical properties of tooth structure and restorative materials, long-term retention of the restoration presents a unique challenge. In some cases, noncarious cervical lesions may be left untreated. Some lesions can be treated without cavity preparation, and others require preparation to obtain adequate retention of the restoration (Fig 14-1).

Etiology of Noncarious Cervical Lesions

Erosion has been defined as loss of tooth structure due to chemical action.[30,43,45] Thus erosion of facial or lingual cervical tooth structure may create lesions.

This can be prominent in patients with oral habits such as constant citrus ingestion, continuous exposure to airborne acids or chlorinated swimming pool water, or gastrointestinal problems that produce repeated exposure of teeth to gastric acids.[37,41,45,60] In these cases, the oral lesions generally present a rounded, cupped-out defect initially confined to the enamel (Fig 14-2). If left untreated, the loss of tooth structure due to the chemical attack will accelerate once dentin has been reached, and a deeper pattern of destruction, still generally rounded, will be seen.

Abrasion is defined as loss of tooth structure by mechanical or frictional forces.[30,43,45] These lesions are commonly caused by excessive toothbrushing, but repeated and excessive forces by other materials and appliances, such as dental floss, toothpicks, or removable appliances, may also produce defects. The lesions commonly caused by brushing appear as V-shaped notches in teeth and often occur in teeth that are facially prominent in the arch. These lesions can progress rapidly if they occur at the cementoenamel junction, because the enamel is thin and the mechanical forces can wear the dentin and cementum away quickly (Fig 14-3).

Abfraction is defined as loss of tooth structure due to flexural forces.[30] It is a theory proposed to explain the development of some V-shaped notches in teeth[12,43] (Fig 14-4). The theory states that as teeth flex under occlusal load, stresses are transmitted to the cervical area causing cervical enamel rods to fracture and dislodge (Fig 14-5). Over time, with increased flexural movements, a V-shaped notch develops, and the tooth becomes weaker as tooth structure is lost and the tooth flexure increases. However, if

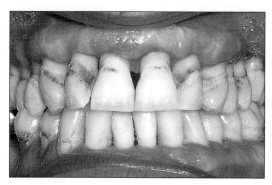

Fig 14-1a Numerous stained Class 5 carious lesions.

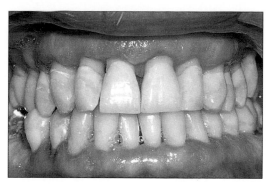

Fig 14-1b The teeth have been restored to meet the patient's esthetic demands.

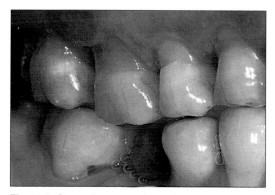

Fig 14-2 Cupped, saucer-shaped noncarious cervical lesions consistent with erosion.

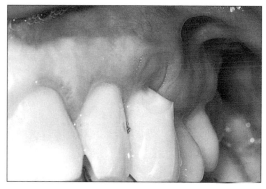

Fig 14-3 A moderately deep, V-shaped cervical notch in a maxillary canine.

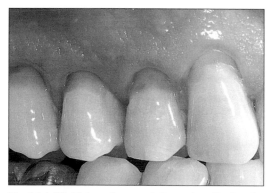

Fig 14-4 Multiple adjacent defects that fit the description of abfraction lesions.

Fig 14-5 The abfraction theory holds that tooth flexure causes loosening of enamel rods, which initiates the cervical lesions.

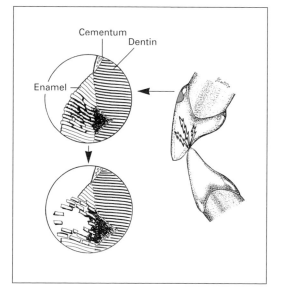

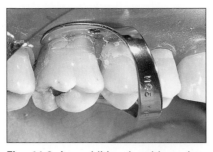

Fig 14-6 An additional rubber dam clamp is sometimes helpful to retract the rubber dam and soft tissue.

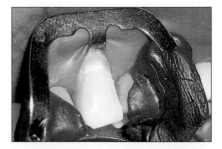

Fig 14-7a A No. 212SA clamp stabilized with modeling compound.

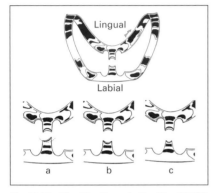

Fig 14-7b Modifications to the No. 212SA clamp are sometimes necessary for proper adaptation to the tooth.

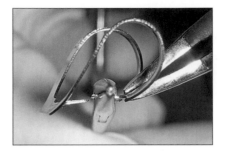

Fig 14-7c With two sets of pliers, the lingual jaw of the No. 212SA clamp is bent incisally/occlusally so that it rests on lingual tooth structure, avoiding damage to gingival tissues.

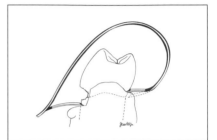

Fig 14-7d Modified (solid line) and unmodified (dotted line) No. 212SA clamp.

abfraction were a common cause of these noncarious cervical lesions, one would expect to find many lingual V-shaped cervical notches in teeth with lingual wear facets associated with group function occlusion, but these are not commonly observed. The abfraction theory also cannot explain the formation of V-shaped notches in Class 5 restorative materials.

While there is not yet strong evidence that abfraction causes the initiation and progression of noncarious cervical lesions, an association between increased loss of Class 5 restorations and wear facets has been determined.[34,57] Patients with heavy occlusal loads and clinical evidence of bruxism have a higher occurrence of Class 5 restoration loss than patients with mutually protected occlusion without wear facets.[34,57]

Access and Isolation

When cervical lesions occur supragingivally, access to the area for preparation and restoration is often easily obtained. But if the lesion has progressed to or below the free gingival margin, isolation for complete caries removal, tooth preparation, restoration placement, and finishing can be difficult. If a restoration is placed without obtaining complete access to sound tooth structure on all margins, carious tooth structure may remain and the restoration may fail. Even in noncarious lesions, inability to gain sufficient access to the gingival margin may result in a poor restoration-tooth interface, increased microleakage, and premature loss of the restoration.

Nonsurgical Retraction

While a rubber dam is the ideal method of field isolation and moisture control for all direct placement restorations, many Class 5 lesions can be adequately treated using cotton rolls, retraction cord, and other materials to isolate the lesion and absorb moisture. If the lesion extends to or below the gingival margin, a rubber dam is useful to retract the tissue. Often a rubber dam retracting clamp placed directly on the tooth to be restored will provide additional gingival retrac-

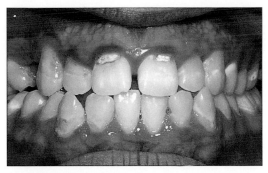

Fig 14-8a Carious Class 5 lesions on teeth 8 and 9 requiring surgical access.

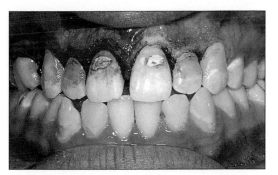

Fig 14-8b A gingivectomy exposes the full extent of the clinical crowns and provides access to the lesions.

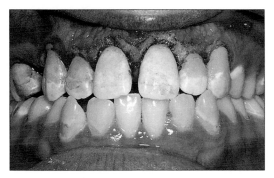

Fig 14-8c Teeth 8 and 9 after placement of restorations.

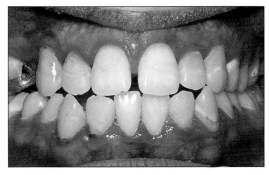

Fig 14-8d Restorations and soft tissue after 2 weeks of healing.

tion (Fig 14-6). A No. 212SA clamp is effective for this purpose (Fig 14-7a), but modifications to the clamp may be necessary to provide adequate retraction (Figs 14-7b to 14-7d).

The clamp must be stabilized to keep it from moving and possibly damaging the restoration or the tooth surface during the operative procedure. Modeling compound is the traditional stabilizing material used (see Fig 7-24), but expired resin composite can often be light cured quickly into place. If lesions in two adjacent teeth are to be treated, modified No. 212SA clamps can be used to provide field isolation (see Fig 14-10d and Figs 7-21c and 7-21d).

Surgical Retraction

Gingivoplasty

When the rubber dam clamp is not able to provide complete visualization and access to the entire lesion, a surgical approach must be used. First, the width of attached gingiva is determined by subtracting the probing depth from the width of keratinized tissue. If an adequate amount of attached, keratinized gingiva will remain after surgery, a gingivoplasty may be useful in providing access as long as the lesion to be treated will be fully exposed and the biologic width will not be violated[50,61,68] (Figs 14-8a to 14-8d). If gingivoplasty would result in less than 3 mm of attached gingiva adjacent to the restoration, an apically positioned flap or graft procedure may be necessary to preserve or increase the zone of attached gingiva.[50]

Miniflap

As described in Chapter 7, the use of miniflaps can often provide sufficient access to subgingival lesions.[61,68,75] Small vertical incisions, not including the papillae, are made mesial and distal to the lesion (Figs 14-9a to 14-9e; see also Fig 7-47). It is essential that the entire lesion be exposed, including all demineralized tooth structure. The incisions should not be extended past the mucogingival junction. This will allow the small flap of keratinized tissue to be reflected and replaced to the same position after completion of the restoration; sutures are usually not necessary. If the flap extends past the mucogingival junction, sutures will be required after the restorative procedure has been completed.

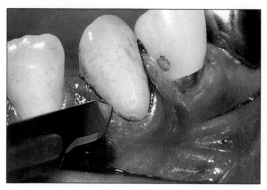

Fig 14-9a Position of scalpel for making miniflap incision.

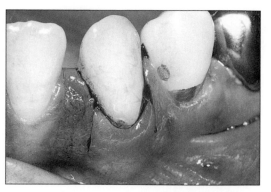

Fig 14-9b Mesial and distal miniflap incisions.

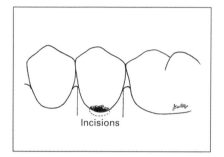

Fig 14-9c Short vertical incisions are made within the keratinized tissue at the line angles of the tooth. This allows additional tissue retraction with minimal trauma to the tissue or attachment apparatus.

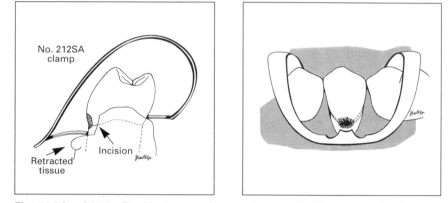

Figs 14-9d and 14-9e The No. 212SA retracting clamp and rubber dam are in place.

Conventional Flap Surgery

On occasion, the miniflap provides insufficient access, and a larger mucoperiosteal flap is required for the cervical restorations.[20,32,46,61,68] If restorations on two adjacent teeth are to be placed simultaneously, a miniflap cannot be used and a mucoperiosteal flap is needed to provide sufficient restorative access (Fig 14-10). If the measurement is less than 3 mm from the crest of the gingiva to the crest of alveolar bone (biologic width), surgical crown lengthening with ostectomy must be performed to provide sufficient access to the lesion and to reestablish dimension for a healthy connective tissue and junctional epithelial attachment[50] (Figs 14-11a and 14-11b). A mucoperiosteal flap should be reflected and ostectomy performed to provide the necessary 3-mm dimension. In some cases, repositioning the envelope flap to its original location will provide the optimal result for esthetics and function. In other cases, the flap will need to

be apically positioned. It is important to remember that the flap will not reattach to the newly placed restoration. If the margin of the flap is placed 3 mm occlusal or incisal to the gingival margin of the restoration, the tooth will immediately have a 3-mm pocket adjacent to the restoration. After healing, a 3-mm pocket will remain, or the gingival margin will recede until it reaches a stable position.

Timing of Surgery

It is often advantageous to have periodontal surgical procedures accomplished before tooth restoration. At least 6 weeks must elapse after surgery to obtain maturation of the altered periodontium.[50] In esthetic areas, a longer healing period is often required to allow the gingival margin to heal to its stable position before restoration placement. In some cases, a combined surgical-restorative procedure provides better access to the restorative site, since the soft tissue flap is

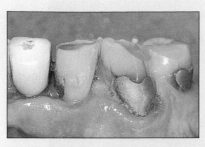

Fig 14-10a Defective Class 5 restorations in teeth 21 and 22 with subgingival margins.

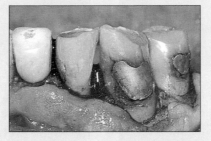

Fig 14-10b An envelope flap is reflected, revealing larger defects than were originally evident.

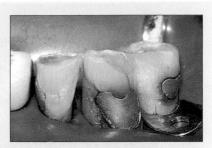

Fig 14-10c The rubber dam provides good control of bleeding and moisture but insufficient isolation of tooth 22.

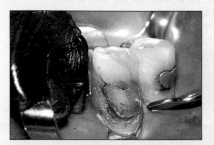

Fig 14-10d A modified No. 212SA clamp or a Schultz clamp, stabilized with modeling compound, provides additional retraction and isolation.

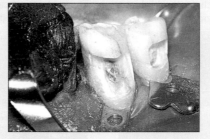

Fig 14-10e The final preparations.

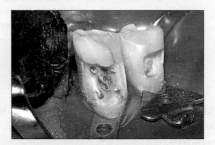

Fig 14-10f Pins were placed in tooth 22 for additional retention.

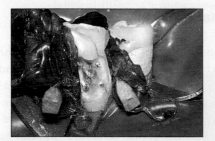

Fig 14-10g A custom matrix, stabilized with wedges and compound, provides lateral walls and support for amalgam placement.

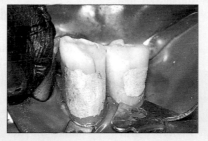

Fig 14-10h The completed restorations.

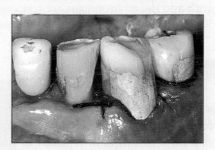

Fig 14-10i The envelope flap is returned to place and sutured.

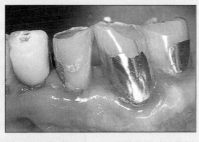

Fig 14-10j The final, polished restorations after 2 weeks of soft tissue healing.

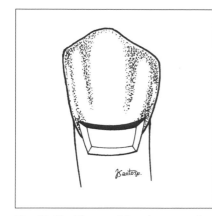

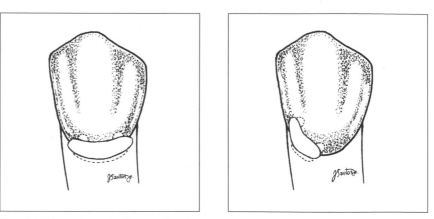

Fig 14-13a The traditional preparation for a Class 5 direct gold restoration had a trapezoidal outline form.

Figs 14-13b and 14-13c The outline form currently recommended for all restorative materials includes removal of carious tooth structure and unsupported enamel and the addition of undercuts. The amount of undercut retention will be reduced or eliminated when adhesive techniques are used.

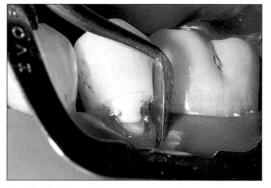

Fig 14-14 A hand instrument may be used as a matrix for Class 5 amalgam restorations.

removed. Caries-disclosing agents have been shown to be useful in helping clinicians distinguish between demineralized and sound tooth structure.[4,10,39,67]

Amalgam

Amalgam preparations will be the same whether the lesion requiring the placement of the restoration is carious or noncarious. The preparation should be extended only enough to provide removal of caries and unsupported enamel (Figs 14-13a to 14-13c). There is no need to make sharp internal line angles, nor to remove sound dentin for actual depth greater than 1 mm. The cavosurface margins should be as close to 90 degrees as possible. Cavosurface bevels are contraindicated with amalgam because of its low edge strength. With this design, the walls of the Class 5 preparation often diverge because of the curvature of the tooth surface. For

nonbonded amalgam restorations, grooves should be placed in the dentin of both the occlusal and gingival walls to help retain the amalgam. In large preparations, pins or other retentive devices may also be beneficial. Alternatively, amalgam bonding systems may be effective for retaining amalgam restorations.[9,16,24,29,53,65,66]

If the mesial and distal walls are flared so that the amalgam has no lateral walls to confine it for condensation, a custom matrix may be used to facilitate restoration placement and condensation. The simplest method for a facial Class 5 amalgam restoration is to use a hand instrument (Fig 14-14). If the preparation wraps well into the proximal areas, this method may not suffice. Another simple method utilizes a Tofflemire matrix band cut to a length that wraps around the lingual aspect of the tooth and extends slightly facial to the interproximal contacts (see Fig 14-10g). Interproximal wedges are placed to support and stabilize the matrix, and modeling compound may be softened and pressed interproximally if further support is needed.

After the amalgam has been carved to proper contours, a smoother surface may be attained with burnishing then smoothing with a rubber cup and a fine abrasive paste. Although polishing has been shown to have no long-term benefit,[49] a smooth surface tends to be less plaque retentive.

Bonded Tooth-Colored Restorations

When adhesive restorative materials are used, unsupported enamel should be removed to prevent the potential fracture of weakened enamel margins during or after restoration placement. Many techniques and materials have been developed in an attempt to obtain long-term retention for esthetic materials placed in cervical locations. Polymerization shrinkage can cause resin composite to pull away from the tooth restoration interface, leaving an open margin and pathway for microleakage to occur.[18] For moderate-sized to large restorations, incremental resin composite placement is recommended to decrease the effects of polymerization shrinkage[3,44,47,51,73] (Fig 14-15).

If the margins of the restoration will be completely within enamel, the retention of bonded restorations should be predictably successful. One study supports beveling the gingival margin as long as it remains entirely in enamel,[33] and this remains prudent to provide an optimum area for enamel bonding. However, with the excellent capability of current bonding systems to attach composite to dentin as well as enamel, beveling of enamel margins may be necessary only when it would improve esthetic blending of the resin with the tooth structure.

Frequently, the lesion extends onto the root surface, where no enamel is available for bonding. If bonded restorations are placed with no mechanical, undercut retention and the bonding system is relied on to provide all retention, the opportunity for microleakage at the gingival margin increases. Beveling the gingival margin that ends on cementum may increase microleakage.[54] This microleakage can result in the initiation of caries under the restoration, sensitivity, discoloration, or loss of the restoration. It is this microleakage that has spurred the development of new materials and techniques for Class 5 restorations.

Although abfraction as an etiologic agent remains controversial, the role tooth flexure plays in the premature loss of cervical restorations is well supported.[34,51,57] As lateral forces are placed on the buccal or lingual cusp of the tooth, the cusp may deflect. These forces may result in dislodgment of a Class 5 restoration with insufficient retention. If the restoration is retained, the flexural forces at the gingival margin may increase leakage at that site. Cusp flexure can be even greater if there is a Class 2 restoration in the tooth,[5] causing greater flexure in the cervical area. To decrease the need for mechanical retention, very effective adhesive materials have been developed.

An often overlooked treatment that may be important to successful restoration longevity is occlusal adjustment to reduce eccentric loading of the tooth with the Class 5 restoration.[44] This could decrease the dislodging forces placed on the cervical restoration and enhance its longevity.

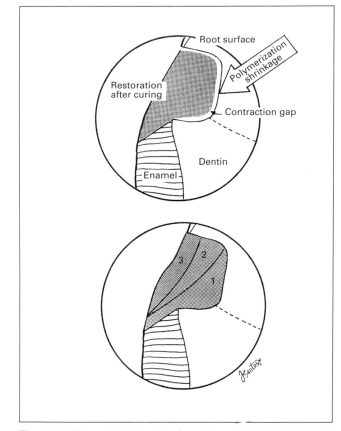

Fig 14-15 If the gingival margin is on the root surface, the resin composite should be placed in at least two increments to compensate for polymerization shrinkage.

Resin Composite

The extent and depth of the lesion should determine the outline and depth of the preparation for resin composite, whether the lesion is carious or noncarious. Although high rates of retention for Class 5 resin composite restorations have been reported using several of the more recent resin bonding systems, mechanical undercuts will enhance retention.[22,44,51,58] A groove made with a No. ¼ or ⅛ bur in the dentin of the gingival wall has resulted in decreased gap formation at the gingival margin when the preparation extends to the root surface (Fig 14-16).[3,77] Unless a bevel would remove all or most of the enamel in any area of the preparation, enamel margins should be beveled to increase surface area for bonding and to enhance esthetics. In many noncarious cervical lesions, the enamel is already beveled, and additional beveling is not necessary.

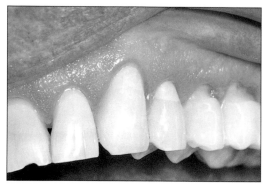

Fig 14-18a Multiple adjacent Class 5 lesions in teeth 11 to 15.

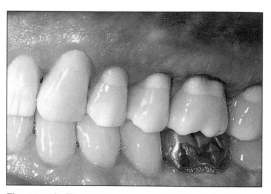

Fig 14-18b The teeth were restored with conventional glass ionomer, which is opaque and relatively unesthetic.

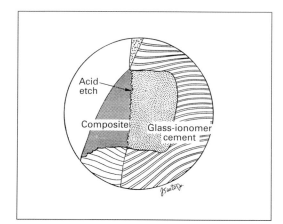

Fig 14-19 The sandwich technique combines a glass-ionomer base with a veneer of resin composite.

of fluoride-releasing materials, fall between resin composites and resin-modified glass-ionomer materials, but are much more like resin composites. They require acid etching of both enamel and dentin and the use of a dentin bonding system. Although most of their physical properties are inferior to conventional resin composites,[26,53] in one study their abrasion resistance was similar to that of hybrid composites.[27] Compomers are indicated for use in low-stress areas and are considered more flexible and less susceptible to dislodgment in Class 5 situations. One clinical study has strongly supported this contention by reporting a 100% retention rate after 3 years.[23]

Dentinal Sensitivity

Dentinal sensitivity, a problem reported to affect approximately one in seven persons,[42] is often associated with gingival recession and noncarious cervical lesions.[57] Sensitivity is caused by exposure of dentinal tubules that communicate between the pulp and the oral cavity; the degree of sensitivity is influenced by the number and size of the open tubules.[2,55] The hydrodynamic theory[13] is the most widely accepted explanation of dentinal sensitivity. Changes in the direction of fluid movement within open dentinal tubules are perceived as pain by mechanoreceptors near the pulp. Tactile, thermal, or osmotic stimuli can induce changes in fluid flow and elicit a pain response.

Dentinal hypersensitivity secondary to gingival recession is best treated surgically with root coverage procedures such as connective tissue grafts.[36,52] However, periodontal surgery is not always a treatment option. Therefore, other methods of treating dentin hypersensitivity may be necessary. Treatment or prevention of hypersensitivity is usually accomplished by the use of some method to occlude the open tubules.[35,56,74] Dentin adhesives provide at least short-term relief.[21,76] Oxalate solutions, used alone or in combination with electrophoresis, are reported to be successful.[35,56] Stannous fluorides have also been used with positive results.[71,72] Potassium nitrate, available in dentifrices or as a gel for application in the dental office, is also reported to be an effective desensitizing agent.[40,71] It is thought to act directly on nerve membranes to reduce sensory nerve activity,[40] rather than causing occlusion of the tubules.[35]

References

1. Abdalla AI, Al Hadnainy HA. Clinical evaluation of hybrid ionomer restoratives in Class 5 abrasion lesions: two-year results. Quintessence Int 1997;28:255–258.

2. Absi EG, Addy M, Adams D. Dentin hypersensivity. A study of the patency of dentinal tubules in sensitive and non-sensitive cervical dentin. J Clin Periodontol 1987;14:280–284.

3. Albers, H. Tooth Colored Restorations, ed 8. Santa Rosa, CA: Alto Books, 1996:8c1–8c6.

4. Anderson MH, Charbeneau GT. A comparison of digital and optical criteria for detecting carious dentin. J Prosthet Dent 1985;53:643–646.

5. Assif D, Marshak B, Pilo R. Cuspal flexure associated with amalgam restorations. J Prosthet Dent 1990;60:258–262.

6. Bader JD, Levitch LC, Shugars DA, et al. How dentists classified and treated noncarious cervical lesions. J Am Dent Assoc 1993;124:46–54.

7. Baum LG, Phillips RW, Lund MR. Textbook of Operative Dentistry, ed 3. Philadelphia: Saunders, 1995:210–212, 262.

8. Bayne SC, Thompson JY, Swift EJ Jr, et al. A characterization of first-generation flowable composites. J Am Dent Assoc 1998;129:567–577.

9. Belcher MA, Stewart GP. Two year clinical evaluation of an amalgam adhesive. J Am Dent Assoc 1997;128:309–314.

10. Boston DW, Graver HT. Histological study of an acid red caries-disclosing dye. Oper Dent 1989;14:186–192.

11. Brackett WW, Gilpatrick RO, Browning WD, Gregory PN. Two-year clinical performance of a resin modified glass ionomer restorative material. Oper Dent 1999;24:9–13.

12. Braem M, Lambrechts P, Vanherle G. Stress induced cervical lesions. J Prosthet Dent 1992;67:718–722.

13. Brannstrom M. The hydrodynamics of the dentinal tubule and of pulp fluid. A discussion of its significance in relation to dentinal sensitivity. Caries Res 1976;1:310–322.

14. Browning WD, Dennison JB. A survey of failure modes in resin composite restorations. Oper Dent 1996;21:160–166.

15. Browning WD, Brackett WW, Gilpatrick RO. Retention of microfilled and hybrid resin-based composite in noncarious Class 5 lesions: a double blind, randomized clinical trial. Oper Dent 1999;24:26–30.

16. Burgess JO, Summitt JB, Osborne JW, et al. One-year evaluation of Amalgabond Plus and pin-retained amalgam restorations [abstract 428]. J Dent Res 1997;76(special issue):67.

17. Burgess J, Norling B, Summitt J. Resin ionomer restorative materials: the new generation. J Esthet Dent 1994;6:207–215.

18. Carvalho RM, Pereira JC, Yoshiyama M, Pashley DH. A review of polymerization contraction: the influence of stress development versus stress relief. Oper Dent 1996;21:17–24.

19. Crispin BJ. Contemporary Esthetic Dentistry: Practice Fundamentals. Chicago: Quintessence, 1994:112.

20. Cuenin M, Clem B. Periodontal and restorative treatment of the Class 5 lesion. Gen Dent 1993;41:252–254.

21. Dall, Orologio GD, Malferrari S. Desensitizing effects of Gluma and Gluma 2000 on hypersensitive dentin. Am J Dent 1993;6:283–286.

22. Duke ES, Robbins JW, Snyder DS. Clinical evaluation of a dentin adhesive system: 3 year results. Quintessence Int 1991; 22:889–895.

23. Elderton RJ, Vowles RW, Bell CJ, Marshall KJ. Three year retention of cervical compomer restorations in non-undercut cavities [abstract 1185]. J Dent Res 1997;76:162.

24. Evans DB, Neme AML. Shear bond strength of composite resin and amalgam adhesive systems to dentin. Am J Dent 1999;12:19–25.

25. Farah JW. Fluoride releasing restorative materials. Dental Advisor 1998;15(10):4–5.

26. Farah JW. Compomers. Dental Advisor 1998;15(8):1–5.

27. Frazier KB, Rueggeberg FA, Mettenburg DJ. Comparison of wear-resistance of Class 5 restorative materials. J Esthet Dent 1998;10:309–314.

28. Gallien GS, Kaplan I, Owens BM. A review of noncarious dental cervical lesions. Compend Contin Educ Dent 1994;15: 1366–1374.

29. Gorucu J, Tiritoglu M, Ozgunaltay G. Effects of preparation designs and adhesive systems on retention of class II amalgam restorations. J Prosthet Dent 1997;78:250–254.

30. Grippo JO. Abfractions: a new classification of hard tissue lesions of teeth. J Esthet Dent 1991;3:14–19.

31. Grippo JO. Non carious cervical lesions: the decision to ignore or restore. J Esthet Dent 1992;4:55–64.

32. Hagge MS, Rector TM. Review of periodontal considerations and surgical retraction techniques for operative dentistry. Oper Dent 1993;18:179–186.

33. Hall LHS, Cochran MA, Swartz ML. Class 5 resin composite restorations: margin configuration and distance from the CEJ. Oper Dent 1993;18:246–250.

34. Heymann HO, Sturdevant JR, Bayne S, et al. Examining tooth flexure effects. J Am Dent Assoc 1991;122:41–47.

35. Hodosh M, Hodosh SH, Hodosh AJ. About dentinal hypersensitivity. Compend Contin Educ Dent 1994;15:658–667.

36. Ito K, Murai S. Adjacent gingival recession treated with expanded polytetrafluoroethylene membranes: a report of two cases. J Periodontol 1996;67:443–450.

37. Jarvinen V, Meurman JH, Hyvaarien H. Dental erosion and upper gastrointestinal disorders. Oral Surg Oral Med Oral Pathol 1988;65:298–303.

38. Jensen ME, Chan DCN. Polymerization shrinkage and microleakage. In Vanherle G, Smith DC, eds. Posterior Resin Composite Dental Restorative Materials. Utrecht, The Netherlands: Szulc, 1985:243–262.

39. Kidd EAM, Joyston-Bechal S, Smith MM, et al. The use of a caries detector dye in cavity preparation. Br Dent J 1989; 167:132–134.

40. Kim SA. Hypersensitive teeth: desensitization of pulpal sensory nerves. J Endod 1986;12:482–485.

41. Knewitz JL, Drisko CL. Anorexia nervosa and bulimia: a review. Compend Contin Educ Dent 1988;9:244–247.

42. Krauser JT. Hypersensitive teeth. Part 1. Etiology. J Prosthet Dent 1986;56:153–156.

43. Lee WC, Eakle WS. Possible role of tensile stress in the etiology of cervical erosive lesions in teeth. J Prosthet Dent 1984; 52:374–380.

44. Leinfelder KF. Restoration of abfracted lesions. Compend Contin Educ Dent 1994;15:1396–1400.

45. Levitch LC, Bader JD, Shugars DA, Heymann HO. Non-carious cervical lesions. J Dent 1994;22:195–207.

46. Lundergan W, Hughes WR Jr. Crown lengthening: a surgical flap approach. Compend Contin Educ Dent 1996;17:833–842.

47. Lutz F, Krejci I, Oldenburg TR. Elimination of polymerization stresses at the margins of posterior resin composite restorations: a new restorative technique. Quintessence Int 1986;17: 777–784.

48. Matis BA, Cochran M, Carlson T. Longevity of glass ionomer restorative materials: results of a 10-year evaluation. Quintessence Int 1996;27:373–382.

399

49. Mayhew RB, Schmeltzer LD, Pierson WP. Effect of polishing on the marginal integrity of high copper amalgam. Oper Dent 1986;11:8–13.

50. Maynard JG, Wilson RDK. Physiologic dimensions of the periodontium significant to the restorative dentist. J Periodontol 1979;50:170–174.

51. McCoy RB, Anderson MH, Lepe X, Johnson GH. Clinical success of Class 5 composite resin restorations without mechanical retention. J Am Dent Assoc 1998;129:593–599.

52. Nevins M, Mellonig JT. Periodontal Therapy: Clinical Approaches and Evidence of Success, Volume I. Chicago: Quintessence, 1998:339.

53. Oliveira JP, Cochran MA, Moore BK. Influence of bonded amalgam restorations on the fracture strength of teeth. Oper Dent 1996;21:110–115.

54. Owens BM, Halter TK, Brown DM. Microleakage of tooth colored restorations with a beveled gingival margin. Quintessence Int 1998;29:356–361.

55. Pashley DH. Mechanisms of dentin sensitivity. Dent Clin North Am 1990;34:449–493.

56. Pashley DH, Muzzin K. Clinical Management of Dentin Hypersensitivity. Philadelphia: Lippincott, 1990.

57. Powell LV, Johnson GH, Gordon GE. Factors associated with clinical success of cervical abrasion/erosion restorations. Oper Dent 1995;20:7–13.

58. Powell LV, Johnson GH, Gordon GE. Clinical evaluation of Class 5 abrasion/erosion restorations [abstract 1514]. J Dent Res 1992;71:705.

59. Powell LV, Gordon GE, Johnson GH. Sensitivity of restored Class 5 abrasion/erosion lesions. J Am Dent Assoc 1990; 121:694–696.

60. Poynter ME, Wright PS. Tooth wear and some factors influencing its severity. Rest Dent 1990;6:8–11.

61. Reagan SE. Periodontal access techniques for restorative dentistry. Gen Dent 1989; 37:117–121.

62. Robbins J, Duke E, Schwartz R, Trevino D. Clinical evaluation of a glass ionomer restorative in cervical abrasions [abstract 171]. J Dent Res 1996;75:39.

63. Schwartz JL, Anderson MH, Pelleu GB Jr. Reducing microleakage with the glass ionomer/resin sandwich technique. Oper Dent 1990;15:186–192.

64. Smith EDK, Martin FE. Microleakage of glass ionomer/composite resin restorations: a laboratory study. The influence of glass ionomer cement. Austr Dent J 1992;37:23–30.

65. Staninec M, Eakle WS, Silverstein S, et al. Bonded amalgam sealants: two-year clinical results. J Am Dent Assoc 1998; 129:323–329.

66. Staninec M, Marshall GW, Lowe A, Ruzickova T. Clinical research on bonded amalgam restorations. Gen Dent 1997;45: 356–362.

67. Starr CB, Langenderfer WR. Use of a caries disclosing agent to improve dental residents' ability to detect caries. Oper Dent 1993;18:110–114.

68. Starr CB. Management of periodontal tissues for restorative dentistry. J Esthet Dent 1991;3:195–208.

69. Sturdevant CM, Robeson TM, Heymann HO, Sturdevant JR. The Art and Science of Operative Dentistry, ed 3. St Louis: Mosby, 1995:486–499.

70. Suzuki M, Jordan RE. Glass ionomer-composite sandwich technique. J Am Dent Assoc 1990;120:55–57.

71. Tarbet WJ, Silverman G, Fratarcangelo PA, Kanapka JA. Home treatment for dentinal hypersensitivity: a comparative study. J Am Dent Assoc 1982;105:227–230.

72. Thrash WJ, Dodds MWJ, Jones DL. The effect of stannous fluoride on dentinal hypersensitivity. Int Dent J 1994;44: 107–118.

73. Tjan AHL, Bergh BH, Lidner C. Effect of various incremental techniques on marginal adaptation of Class II resin composite restorations. J Prosthet Dent 1992;67:62–66.

73a. Trevino D, Duke E, Robbins J, Summitt J. Clinical evaluation of Scotchbond Multi-Purpose adhesive system in cervical abrasions [abstract 3037]. J Dent Res 1996;75(special issue):397.

74. Trowbridge HO, Silver DR. A review of current approaches to in-office management of tooth hypersensitivity. Dent Clin North Am 1990;34:561–581.

75. Vandewalle KS, Vigil G. Guidelines for the restoration of Class 5 lesions. Gen Dent 1997;45:254–260.

76. Watanabe T, Sano M, Itoh K, Wakumoto S. The effects of primers on the sensitivity of dentin. Dent Mater 1991;7: 148–150.

77. White SN, MacEntee MI, Cho G. Restorative treatment for geriatric root caries. J Calif Dent Assoc 1994;22:55–60.

78. Yau L, Perry R. Three body wear of light-cured flowable composites [abstract 3276]. J Dent Res 1997;76(special issue A):423.

15 Natural Tooth Bleaching

Van B. Haywood/Thomas G. Berry

Bleaching has been used to achieve a lighter and more desirable tooth color for over a century. Dental journals in the last half of the 19th century frequently contained articles on the efficacy of bleaching teeth.[75,97] The safety of the procedure was well investigated and the chemistry understood. Although the process was thought to be time-consuming and relapse was considered a consistent problem, bleaching was well accepted.[20,83,91] By the mid-1800s, the bleaching agent of choice for nonvital teeth was chloride of lime.[36] Around that time, Truman[83] introduced chlorine from a calcium hydroxide and acetic acid solution for bleaching nonvital teeth; this was supplied commercially as a liquid chloride of soda. Other agents used in the 1800s for nonvital tooth bleaching included aluminum chloride,[54] oxalic acid,[15,97] Pyrozone (etherperoxide) (McKesson and Robbins),[6] hydrogen dioxide (hydrogen peroxide or perhydrol),[82] sodium peroxide,[82] sodium hypophosphate,[55] chloride of lime,[12,55] and cyanide of potassium. The active ingredient common to all of these was as an oxidizing agent, which acted either directly or indirectly on the organic portion of the tooth. Sulfurous acid, in contrast, achieved results as a reducing agent.[80] Generally, the most effective yet safe bleaching agents were direct oxidizers or an indirect oxidizer such as a chlorine derivative.[40,91] However, the choice of bleaching agent depended primarily on the stain being removed. Iron stains were removed with oxalic acid, silver and copper stains with chlorine, and iodine stains with ammonia.[7,81,122] The metallic stains (such as from amalgam) were considered the most resistant to bleaching. Concern about the effect of some of these bleaching agents on the teeth, tissues, and health of the patient was raised because some agents used, such as cyanide of potassium, were very poisonous.[12] Other bleaching agents were caustic.

The early emphasis was on bleaching nonvital teeth. However, as early as the 1890s, a 3% solution of Pyrozone was used safely as a mouthwash by both children and adults. It reduced caries and whitened the teeth.[8] A 5% solution proved to be safe and effective, but a 25% solution was caustic, causing tissue burns.[8] By 1910, the current technique, using hydrogen peroxide activated by heat or light, was well established. Over the next few decades, the bleaching agents varied. By the 1940s, hydrogen peroxide and ether were used for vital teeth,[120] while, by the late 1950s, etherperoxide (Pyrozone) and sodium perborate were used for nonvital teeth.[101,121]

The current home bleaching technique, employing a custom-fit tray containing 10% carbamide peroxide solution, was first used by Klusmier in the late 1960s.[65] However, the profession did not embrace the concept until it was described in a 1989 article,[66] the publication of which coincided with the market introduction of carbamide peroxide as a bleaching agent.[50,58] This ushered in the current technique for at-home bleaching.

Types and Nature of Stains/Discolorations

Many types of color problems affect the appearance of the teeth. Because the cause of these problems varies, the speed with which they may be removed also varies. Discolorations may be *extrinsic* or *intrinsic*. Extrinsic stains are located on the surface of the tooth and are most easily removed by external cleaning. Intrinsic stains are located within the tooth and are accessible only by bleaching. Some extrinsic stains that remain on the tooth for a long time become intrinsic. Extrinsic color changes may be due to poor oral hygiene, ingestion of chromatogenic foods and drinks, and tobacco use. Intrinsic color changes may be caused by aging, ingestion of chromatogenic foods and drink, tobacco usage, microcracks in the enamel, tetracycline medication, excessive fluoride ingestion, severe jaundice in infancy, porphyria, dental caries, restorations, and the thinning of the enamel layer. Other, but less frequent, medical situations and conditions may also cause the loss of a desirable tooth color.

The causes of staining need to be carefully assessed to better predict the rate and degree to which bleaching will improve tooth color, since some stains are more responsive to the process.[66,79] For instance, the yellow discoloration of aging responds quickly to bleaching in most cases, whereas a blue-gray tetracycline stain is tenacious.[62] In general, tetracycline-stained teeth are the slowest to respond to bleaching; brown-fluoresced teeth are moderately responsive; and teeth discolored by age, genetics, smoking, or coffee are the fastest to respond.[62,70] White spots are not removed by bleaching, but may be less noticeable when the remainder of the tooth is lighter. By recognizing the likely cause of the stain, the dentist can better tell the patient the rate at which the teeth may lighten in color and the limits on the amount of improvement that can be expected.

Discoloration from drug ingestion may occur either before the tooth is fully formed or later. Tetracycline is incorporated into the dentin sometime during tooth calcification (Fig 15-1), probably through chelation with calcium, forming tetracycline orthophosphate.[95] There are several variations of tetracycline, and each derivative produces a different color in the tooth. Some teeth may be "banded" from the ingestion of different derivatives of tetracycline. When the teeth are exposed to sunlight, they become darker, with a distinct gray/blue-gray tinge. The teeth not exposed to the sunlight (eg, molars) do not darken to the same degree but remain more yellow in color. Tetracycline has also been reported to discolor fully formed, erupted permanent teeth. This discoloration is most often associated with minocycline, a drug commonly used in the treatment of acne. The primary route of deposition is thought to be in the secondary dentin, although some reports suggest a staining similar to iron deposition. Other antibiotics may also interact with calcium, iron, or other elements to form insoluble complexes that stain teeth.[25]

Excessive fluoride in drinking water, greater than 1 to 2 parts per million (ppm), can cause metabolic alteration in the ameloblasts, resulting in a defective matrix and improper calcification of teeth.[14,33] An affected tooth shows a hypomineralized, porous subsurface enamel and a well-mineralized surface layer. These teeth have a glazed surface and may be very white except for areas of yellow, brown (Fig 15-2), or even black shading.

Some systemic conditions can cause tooth discoloration. Severe jaundice leads to staining by bilirubin. Erythroblastosis fetalis may also stain the teeth by the destruction of red blood cells. Porphyria, a rare condition, manifests with purplish-brown teeth.

Aging is a common cause of discoloration. Over time, the underlying dentin tends to darken from the formation of secondary dentin, which is darker and more opaque than the original dentin. This occurs while the overlying enamel is thinning, a combination that often produces distinctly darker teeth.

Dental caries produces varying stains during its process. Examples of caries-induced discolorations include an opaque white "halo," a grayish tinge, or a brown-to-black stain. These stains arise from the bacterial degradation of food debris. Metallic restorations, most notably dental amalgam, may cause a distinct staining of the tooth in addition to the shadow they may cast through adjacent enamel walls.

Current Bleaching Modalities

Mode of Action

The bleaching process is designed to enable the oxidizing agent to reach sites within the enamel and dentin to allow a chemical reaction to occur. No matter the bleaching technique or specific bleaching action, the intention is to deliver the active ingredient to the discolored segments of the tooth to dislodge or decolor the chromatic particles.

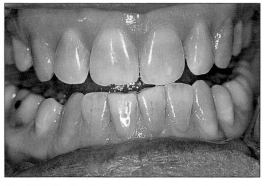

Fig 15-1 Teeth demonstrating moderate, grayish tetracycline stain.

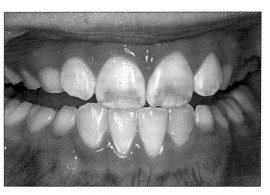

Fig 15-2 Fluorosis stain produces brownish areas surrounded by whiter areas.

Hydrogen peroxide diffuses through the organic matrix of the enamel and dentin because of its low molecular weight.[16,17,27,63] One current theory of whitening is that the free radicals attack organic molecules to achieve stability; this releases other radicals. These radicals can react with other unsaturated bonds, disrupting the electron conjugation and providing a change in the absorption energy of the organic molecules in the enamel. The simpler molecules formed reflect less light so the tooth appears lighter in shade.[47] In the early stages of this process, bleaching opens the more highly pigmented carbon-ring compounds and converts them to chains that are lighter in color. The carbon double-bond compounds (yellow in color) are converted to hydroxy groups (essentially colorless). The bleaching process continues to the extent that all the original pigment is rendered essentially colorless.[3] At this point, lightening of the teeth reaches a plateau in regard to the speed at which it progresses. The continuation of the bleaching process is not beneficial beyond this point. Further research is needed to determine both what gives the tooth its baseline color and, in turn, the oxidation reaction of bleaching that changes the tooth color.

The chemistry of carbamide peroxide used in at-home bleaching is thought to be a bit different from hydrogen peroxide, although the final stages do involve the reaction of hydrogen peroxide with the compounds within the tooth. When introduced into the mouth, the agent breaks down into urea and hydrogen peroxide, both of which access the internal portions of the tooth in minutes. In addition, bleaching not only removes discoloration from within the tooth, it also alters/brightens the inherent color of the dentin itself.

Types of Bleaching Therapy

Generally, bleaching can be first categorized into treatment for either nonvital teeth or vital teeth. Furthermore, nonvital teeth can be treated in the office or outside of the office. Outside-the-office treatment consists of applying a material inside or outside the tooth that actively lightens the tooth while the patient is away from the office. The in-office technique accomplishes all lightening during treatment in the office.

Vital tooth bleaching also has an in-office technique or an outside-the-office (at-home) technique from which to choose. Inside-the-office techniques include the application of a bleaching material to teeth isolated by a rubber dam and may include activation of the process by heat or light. At-home bleaching uses a different bleaching agent applied in a custom-fit tray that the patient wears at home, usually while sleeping.

Factors Affecting Both the In-Office and At-Home Bleaching Processes

Several factors must be carefully considered before bleaching is begun and then controlled during the process to ensure maximum benefit. The factors include the following.

Surface Cleanliness

All surface debris must be removed to distinguish intrinsic stains from extrinsic staining and to ensure that the agent has maximum contact with the tooth surface. However, bleaching should not be initiated until 2 weeks after cleaning to allow any gingival or tooth sensitivity related to the prophylaxis to abate.

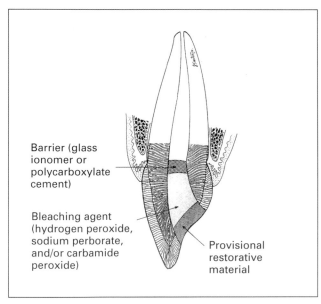

Barrier (glass ionomer or polycarboxylate cement)

Bleaching agent (hydrogen peroxide, sodium perborate, and/or carbamide peroxide)

Provisional restorative material

Fig 15-6 The restorative material blocking the canal at the cementoenamel junction decreases dispersion of the bleaching agent through the root surface.

applied[90,109] and 0% to 6% without heat application.[73,90] Any of several factors may also need to be present for resorption to occur, including: *(1)* deficiency in the cementum, exposing the cervical dentin to the oral cavity (normally affecting approximately 10% of the population); *(2)* injury to the periodontal ligament, triggering an inflammatory response (trauma); and *(3)* infection, sustaining the inflammation.

The cementum deficiencies expose permeable dentin that can allow toxic substances and bacteria from within the chamber and root canals to emerge at the root surface where they may cause an inflammatory process in the periodontal ligament.[44] A 30% solution of hydrogen peroxide is caustic enough to alter the chemical structure of cementum and dentin,[108] decrease their microhardness[88] and resorbability,[110] and enhance transtubular propagation of bacteria.[72] The solution diffuses through the radicular dentinal tubules at an enhanced rate if cementum deficiencies are present[113] and when heat is applied.[112] These data indicate that internal bleaching with 30% hydrogen peroxide is not as safe as originally believed. However, a history of trauma and marked overheating are major factors in resorption, in addition to cementum defects.

Research has been conducted to determine if a protective restorative material can be placed in the cervical portion of the tooth to prevent this problem

(Fig 15-6). Unfortunately, this restorative base reduces the diffusion but does not prevent it[18,109] and does not necessarily protect the tooth against root resorption.[28] However, most of the teeth reported with cervical resorption did not have a base placed over the gutta-percha.

The alternative to hydrogen peroxide is sodium perborate used by itself. The sodium perborate may not be as powerful a bleaching agent. Studies have shown that three applications of sodium perborate mixed with water are as effective as 30% hydrogen peroxide and sodium perborate.[111] One study showed no root resorption after 3 years using sodium perborate, with a 90% esthetic success rate initially and a 49% esthetic success rate after 3 years.[74] A newer technique involves the placement of 10% carbamide peroxide sealed into the chamber. This lower concentration of peroxide also provides a large safety margin.

Another technique, which has limited application, is the practice of preparing the tooth as for the walking bleach technique combined with the at-home tray technique. The pulp chamber is left open, allowing the patient to place 10% carbamide peroxide inside the chamber and, at the same time, apply it externally with the tray. This technique, called "inside-outside bleaching," is very effective. However, it is best suited for patients who are very responsible and capable of applying the solution intraorally. With this technique, a barrier should be placed over the gutta-percha to prevent contamination of the root canal.

The initial esthetic success rate of internal bleaching is limited and may be temporary. Furthermore, external root resorption is a definite, though small, risk with the high concentration of hydrogen peroxide. Even after several applications of sodium perborate mixed with water, the results may not be satisfactory. Satisfactory results, when achieved, usually persist for 1 to 3 years, although they may be permanent. Nevertheless, the safest treatment for internal bleaching remains sodium perborate mixed with water or 10% carbamide peroxide, used after the placement of a protective material in the cervical area.

Vital Bleaching

Vital bleaching may be accomplished by either of two techniques, each with some variations. The in-office technique currently is not as popular as the at-home technique, but it has historically met with success, and there are some definite indications for its use (Figs 15-7a and 15-7b).

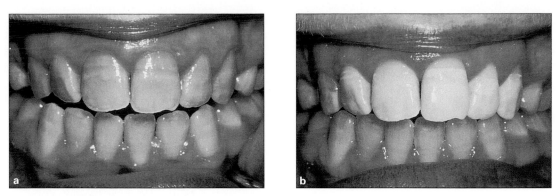

Figs 15-7a and 15-7b In-office bleaching can produce very good results quickly. (Courtesy of Dr Sandra Madison.) (a) Prior to bleaching. (b) After one bleaching session.

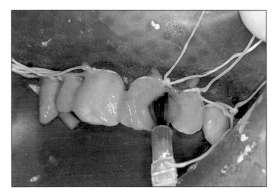

Fig 15-8 The rubber dam protects the soft tissues from the hydrogen peroxide bleach.

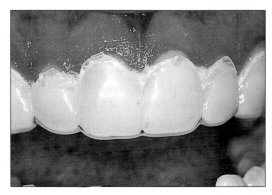

Fig 15-9 A well-adapted tray better confines the carbamide peroxide to the target teeth in the at-home technique.

In-Office Technique

In-office bleaching of vital teeth generally uses a 35% hydrogen peroxide solution placed directly on the teeth and may involve application of light/heat to activate/enhance the peroxide release.[39,51] Because the hydrogen peroxide concentration is so high, soft tissues must be very well protected to prevent injury (Fig 15-8). This technique is intended to quickly produce the bleaching effect with limited need for patient compliance. It is indicated for achieving more rapid results or for patients who may have difficulty following the regimen for the at-home technique. There are several potential disadvantages, however. The fee is usually higher because more chairtime is required, there is a possibility of tissue injury from the more potent agent used, and the results may not be as good as with the slower at-home method.

At-Home Technique

At-home bleaching is the more commonly used bleaching process because it is easy to perform and is usually less expensive for the patient. It uses a custom-fit tray with a 10% solution of carbamide peroxide (Fig 15-9) (approximately equal to a 3.4% solution of hydrogen peroxide). Although the process requires longer contact time compared to the in-office bleaching technique,[57] it is safe, and the results are generally excellent. Manufacturers have offered carbamide peroxide in a variety of concentrations, ranging from 10% to over 20%, but the best combination of safety, limited side effects, and speed of action is obtained with a 10% solution of carbamide peroxide approved by the American Dental Association (ADA). Products carrying the ADA accepted label have passed a rigorous set of safety and efficacy standards. A survey indicated that 90% of the dentists surveyed used a 10% carbamide peroxide for at-home bleaching of vital teeth.[24]

Safety Factors

Safety concerns include: tooth/pulpal problems; periodontal/adjacent oral structures response; and systemic effects.

Tooth and Pulpal Problems

The short-term pulpal response varies from patient to patient and even from tooth to tooth. Although penetration of peroxide through the tooth to the pulp can produce sensitivity, the pulp remains healthy and the sensitivity is completely reversible.[26,117] It is important that the process be carefully monitored to avoid creating great sensitivity in the teeth. The patient should not be anesthetized for an in-office procedure so that he or she will be able to detect early onset of sensitivity. Patients undergoing at-home bleaching must also be informed that there will be minor sensitivity in as many as two of three patients.

If sensitivity occurs, there are a number of approaches that can involve either passive treatment or active treatment. Passive treatment involves shortening the duration of treatment or the frequency of treatment, or interrupting the process for a day or more to allow the teeth to recover. The procedure can then be resumed. Active treatment involves the application of medicaments using the same bleaching tray. Historically, fluoride has been applied for sensitivity. Fluoride acts as a tubule blocker to limit the fluid flow to the pulp. Even fluoride treatment prior to initiating bleaching may reduce sensitivity. A more direct treatment is the application of 3% to 5% potassium nitrate gel in the tray. (Potassium nitrate preparations are available from several bleaching agent manufacturers.) Potassium nitrate penetrates the tooth to the pulp and has a numbing or calming effect on nerve transmission. Potassium nitrate is found in many desensitizing toothpastes, but generally takes 2 weeks to be effective via toothbrushing. However, application of a potassium nitrate preparation in the tray for 30 to 60 minutes before or after bleaching can reduce or eliminate sensitivity in many patients. Often treatment for sensitivity is a combination approach involving alteration of treatment time, frequency of treatment, and medications, including ibuprofen for inflammation, desensitizing toothpaste, and desensitizing medicament applied in the tray.

Questions have been raised about the effect of bleaching on the structure of the tooth itself. Recent studies have shown, with low pH solutions, a detectable loss of calcium from the surface enamel, along with a slight loss in surface hardness to a depth of approximately 25 µm.[124,127] However, this loss has not been shown to be significant because the surface quickly remineralizes after the procedure is completed. In fact, there is less change in the calcium content of the tooth and surface hardness from 6 hours of bleaching with 10% carbamide peroxide than when a carbonated drink is consumed in a 2- to 3-minute period. No noticeable change in the surface luster and topography is seen clinically.

Soft Tissue Response

The more powerful in-office bleaching agents (30% to 35% hydrogen peroxide) can easily produce a tissue burn, turning the tissue white (Fig 15-10).[11,34,92] If the exposure is limited in time and in quantity, it is quickly reversible with no long-term consequences. Rehydration and application of an antiseptic ointment (eg, Orabase B, Colgate Oral Pharmaceutical) quickly return the color to the tissue, reassuring the patient that the problem is not permanent.[9] Nevertheless, it can cause significant temporary discomfort and some alarm when first seen. It is important to protect soft tissues with a rubber dam or other means to avoid tissue burns (Fig 15-11).

Although soft tissue irritation during at-home bleaching has been reported,[119] the irritation is most likely the result of an ill-fitting tray rather than from the agent itself.[89] Reports concerning any harmful effects to soft tissues from hydrogen peroxide indicate that the effects resulted from dosages and exposure times that greatly exceeded those prescribed in any at-home bleaching technique. At-home agents containing 10% carbamide peroxide are not potent enough to produce significant or long-lasting effects on the soft tissues.[130]

Studies have indicated that approximately one third of the patients experienced no detectable side effects after bleaching. The other two thirds experienced only transitory and minor tooth sensitivity and/or tissue irritation of short duration.[24,70] When examined at the cellular level, these effects on the soft tissue are less than or equal to those produced by commonly accepted dental medicaments such as eugenol and endodontic sealers.[131] The toxicity and mutagenicity of hydrogen peroxide are dose related. Concentrations used in the at-home bleaching technique are not sufficient to be of concern. A low dose of hydrogen peroxide over a long time actually allows the cells of the oral tissues to adjust to the dosage even if it is increased beyond the original tolerable dosage. In the long history of these materials involving tissue contact in patients ranging in age from infancy to old age, there has been no demonstrated problem.

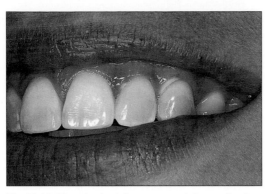

Fig 15-10 The gingival tissue around the canine has been chemically burned by contact with 35% hydrogen peroxide.

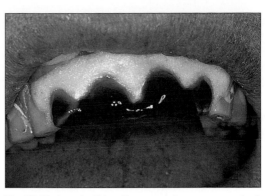

Fig 15-11 A resin "dam" around the target teeth. A 35% hydrogen peroxide bleach has been applied.

Systemic Effects and Responses

There is more concern about possible adverse effects of at-home bleaching agents, although their concentrations are far less potent than those of the in-office bleaches. In-office bleach is carefully controlled and placed on the teeth only, avoiding contact with soft tissues. The patient swallows no solution. Very little, if any, of the agent is absorbed systemically. The at-home bleach, applied in the tray, unavoidably contacts soft tissues in many areas over several hours each day. Additionally, it is likely that the patient swallows small amounts of very dilute hydrogen peroxide during the bleaching procedure.[60] This has not proven to be a problem, however. Although very high concentrations of some forms of peroxide are mutagenic,[1,133] physiologic mechanisms quickly repair any limited damage that might occur.[21] Low levels of hydrogen peroxide do not cause real problems.[129] In fact, hydrogen peroxide has been approved as safe for use as a human food additive with no residues. Carbamide peroxide is also used for the treatment of candidiasis in newborn infants. The conclusion, after decades of use and extensive research, is that the use of hydrogen peroxide in bleaching teeth is safe.[43,104,118,123,125]

Indications for Bleaching

The primary indication for bleaching is patient dissatisfaction with tooth color. While the source of the discoloration affects the degree of success and the rapidity with which it can be eliminated or minimized, it has been shown that even the most persistent discolorations can be lightened if the treatment is sufficiently extended. Bleaching may be done in lieu of bonded resin composite restorations, porcelain veneers, or crowns to improve the tooth color. Patients may be satisfied with the results of bleaching such that more invasive treatment is not needed. Even if laminate veneers are to be placed, the lighter color of the bleached teeth allows lighter and more translucent veneers, enhancing the natural appearance. Other indications include extending the esthetic life of existing crowns that are lighter than the natural teeth by returning the color of the natural teeth to the shade of the crown, or treating single dark teeth that are vital or nonvital.

Contraindications for Bleaching

Although bleaching is a safe and effective aid in improving the appearance of the teeth, not every discolored tooth requires bleaching. Superficial or extrinsic stains may be completely removed by a rubber cup with prophylaxis paste or by light abrasion with a rotary polishing device. The removal of a discolored lesion and/or a dark restoration and placement of a tooth-colored material may well make a marked improvement in the appearance of a tooth. Patients with hypersensitive teeth are generally not good candidates for bleaching. In-office bleaching advocates do not use bleaching for children with large pulps or teeth with cracks. At-home bleaching is generally not indicated for pregnant women or persons allergic to the ingredients in the carbamide peroxide preparations.

There are few contraindications to bleaching. Since there is some evidence that peroxides may enhance the effect of known carcinogens, it may be prudent to have the patient forego tobacco use during the period of the bleaching process.[13,62,102] Although there is no evidence that bleaching is harmful to the fetus or to infants, it has been recommended that pregnant and lactating women do not undergo bleaching because of gingival irritation and total drug ingestion restrictions.[53,61] Patients with existing esthetic restorations must be warned that when bleaching lightens the natural tooth color, restorations may appear relatively dark and unattractive. The need for new restorations lighter in shade should be discussed with the patient.

Some teeth are very sensitive for any one of several reasons. Contraindications cited for in-office bleaching with high concentrations of hydrogen peroxide include teeth with extremely large pulps, exposed root surfaces, or severe enamel loss. In one study, Nathanson and Parra determined that there was no noticeable difference in the sensitivity reported by young patients compared to sensitivity reported by older patients, so larger pulp size may not be a factor.[99] In a study of at-home bleaching with carbamide peroxide, Leonard et al[86] determined that there were no predictors of individuals who would experience sensitivity other than a history of sensitive teeth and more than one bleach application per day. All other delineators, such as pulp size, exposed dentin, cracks, gingival recession, caries, sex or age of the patient, or other physical characteristics, were not predictive of those who would have sensitivity. Because bleaching tends to produce some sensitivity under ordinary circumstances, patients with pre-existing tooth sensitivity must be cautioned that increased sensitivity, albeit transitory, will occur. If this is likely to be a problem, the placement of a desensitizing solution containing fluoride or potassium nitrate can be alternated with the bleaching solution.[22,85] This will increase the time needed to achieve the desired lightness of the teeth.

Patients with a history of temporomandibular disorder (TMD) may not be good candidates for at-home bleaching or may need to wear the tray during the day only. Bruxers also may have to alter wear times for at-home treatment or have several trays fabricated during treatment.

Bleaching does interfere with the bonding process because it results in a very high oxygen concentration in the enamel and dentin, which hinders polymerization of the resin composite.[9,93,126] A delay of 7 to 10 days after bleaching allows dissipation of the excess oxygen from the tooth structure so there is no interference with the polymerization reaction.[10] Waiting 1 to 2 weeks is also important in resin composite bonding to allow the shade of the bleached teeth to stabilize.

Treatment Planning and Patient Education

Projecting the amount of time expected for treatment, as well as integrating the time in the complete treatment plan for bleaching to occur, is important to successful therapy. A basic understanding of the cause of the discoloration is necessary to better predict the course and duration of the treatment as well as the final outcome. Whether to use at-home or in-office bleaching is based on patient preference and on the patient's ability and willingness to comply with the treatment protocol. Patients who are unwilling or unable to comply with the protocol for the at-home technique, or who are eager to finish the bleaching in a very short period of time regardless of the cost, are good candidates for in-office bleaching. Subsequent treatment procedures need to be planned so that the limits of the bleaching treatment are discussed in the total context of solving the patient's other dental problems. The patient should be informed that bleaching should be performed before any esthetic restorative procedures, since the shade of any restoration placed previously will not be altered by bleaching. Therefore, restorations that matched the teeth prior to bleaching will no longer match. The information concerning the decision to bleach or not, as well as the rationale and costs for choosing a particular method, must be recorded to verify that the dentist and patient agree on the procedures and their predicted outcomes.

Shade Selection and Record Collection

A shade guide identifies the existing tooth color to establish the baseline (Fig 15-12). If the shade guide does not have a match for the tooth color, it should be estimated. It is important that the patient agree that the shade tab is the closest match to the current shade of the teeth. This shade should be recorded in the chart with the patient observing the entry. The patient may have difficulty recalling the original shade and, therefore, may be disappointed in the outcome because he or she may not believe that significant change has occurred. The patient should see the shade tab that represents the predicted target shade. The contrast between the tab representing the original shade and one showing the shade to be achieved may lead to more realistic patient expectations, especially if the patient already has light teeth. The best way to

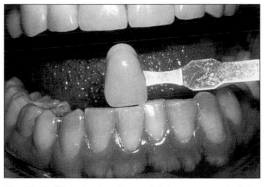

Fig 15-12 The shade tab establishes a record of the existing color.

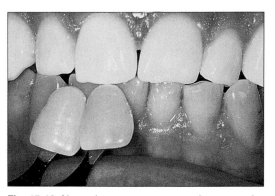

Fig 15-13 Note the strong contrast between the bleached maxillary teeth and the unbleached mandibular teeth (which match the shade tab).

avoid such a problem is to bleach one arch at a time. In addition to minimizing the potential for TMD problems, it preserves one arch for an ongoing comparison of progress. Another reason for treating one arch at a time is that the cost to test the success of the procedure is reduced, making the treatment option more attractive to many patients. If it is deemed a success by the patient, the opposing arch can be bleached for an additional fee (Fig 15-13).

For added documentation, close-up photographs of the patient's teeth and a full face photograph of the patient with a full smile should be kept as part of the patient's record. The photographs may be helpful in treatment planning, in reminding the patient of the original appearance of the teeth, and as a record for a ceramist fabricating any restorations. The photographs should be taken at a consistent magnification and pose. Placing the incisal edges of the teeth in the bleached arch against the incisal edges of the teeth in the unbleached arch enables the best comparison of the before and after shades, emphasizing the effect of bleaching. Impressions for diagnostic casts are necessary if bleaching trays are to be used for the at-home technique.

Patient Education

The patient needs to be well informed about the bleaching procedure. The office/clinic should have information available for each patient explaining the process, precautions, possible side effects, number of applications or appointments, total time required, and the likely results. The dentist should explain to the patient why the particular technique has been chosen. The steps of the procedure and consequences for not following them should be outlined. For the at-home technique, loading and insertion of the bleaching tray should be demonstrated and the length for each wear session outlined. Any questions the patient might have should be answered at the appointment. The patient should sign a consent form that indicates that he or she has been informed about the procedure, its expected outcome, and any potential side effects. The consent form should also list other treatment options for this condition and state that those remain if the bleaching is not successful.

Bleaching Techniques

In-Office Technique for Vital Teeth

In-office bleaching utilizes a much more potent agent (usually a 35% solution of hydrogen peroxide, as opposed to a 10% solution of carbamide peroxide for the at-home technique). This powerful agent (10 times as powerful as a 10% carbamide peroxide) is necessary to produce the rapid improvement expected of an in-office procedure (Figs 15-14a and 15-14b).

The oral/perioral structures must be protected during the procedure. Generally, this is best accomplished with a well-placed, ligated rubber dam, tightly adapted around the cervical areas of the teeth.[52,59] For the single isolated tooth, it may be possible to protect the gingiva with cotton rolls and a "liquid rubber dam" (light-polymerized resin). The light-polymerized

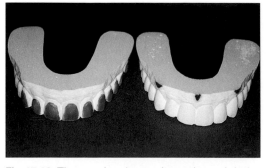

Fig 15-16 The cast has been trimmed to minimize bulk to aid in adapting the tray. Relief areas (for reservoirs) have been added to the cast on the left but not to the one on the right.

sides, until the vestibule is eliminated and a hole appears in the palate. The base of the cast should be as thin as 0.5 inch or trimmed to a horseshoe shape, leaving only the maxillary or mandibular teeth and periodontal tissues remaining with no palatal or tongue section included. The base should be flat, with the central incisors perpendicular to it (Fig 15-16). This makes it easier to adapt the vacuum-formed tray material around the teeth and avoids the development of folds and wrinkles during fabrication. If the palate or tongue section remains, it is helpful to drill a hole through that section so that the vacuum better adapts the tray material in all areas of the cast.

A number of materials have been used in tray fabrication, including materials used in fabricating orthodontic positioners, athletic mouthguards, provisional splints, and antisnoring devices. The original nightguard vital bleaching article[66] proposed a thick, semirigid material. The newer materials that have been developed since that time are thinner and softer, easier to shape and trim, and have reduced gingival and occlusal side effects.

Decisions to be made about tray design include whether to scallop the tray and whether to add reservoirs. Some advocates of at-home bleaching were concerned that the agent would harm gingival tissues over time. They recommended a scalloped tray border positioned 1 mm incisal to the soft tissue to avoid any contact of the tray/bleaching agent with the tissue (Figs 15-17a and 15-17b).[105,114] This practice is not necessary for successful bleaching but may help in seating the tray when using highly viscous materials, to avoid pressure on the teeth and resulting sensitivity, or when gingival tissues are very delicate.[32,115,116]

Scalloping may be indicated for sticky, non–water-soluble materials, as they tend to adhere to the gingiva and may produce localized irritation. However, scalloping may even be counterproductive if a water-soluble material is being applied, as the material is easily removed from the tray by saliva. Additionally, scalloping can be annoying to the tongue or lips, depending on the patient and the teeth-to-tissue relationships. When tissue irritation during an at-home bleaching regimen has been reported, it often resulted from poor adaptation of a rigid tray and usually occurred because moveable structures (tongue, lips, or cheek) rubbed against a rough edge of the tray.[68]

There has been the concern that the inability of the shortened tray to hold the agent against the cervical portion of the tooth could initially produce an uneven bleaching effect by leaving a distinctly darker band at the cervical area. This, however, has not been shown to be the case. If an appropriate material is used and the patient situation does not dictate otherwise, the tray may contact or even cover gingival tissue with no problem. Watery solutions require tissue contact by the tray in order to maintain the bleaching material inside the tray. If tissue contact is preferred, the tray should not extend into tissue undercuts or be tight enough to blanch tissue. Some clinicians do not cover the incisive papilla to avoid pressure on the underlying nerve. Termination of the tray borders should be smooth and not on the top of palatal rugae. Tori, exostoses, or thin areas of tissue, such as over the canine eminence, should not be covered if avoidable.

Another feature of tray design uses spacers placed on the facial surface of the cast to create reservoirs in the tray for bleaching material. Foam liners for the tray have been advocated in an attempt to hold the bleaching agent against the teeth in a more confining way by preventing the flow of the agent to more dependent areas of the tray. Despite manufacturers' claims that inclusion of foam liners gives a more rapid bleaching effect, research has shown that there is no advantage in inserting a foam liner into the tray.[69] Some techniques incorporate a reservoir on the facial intaglio surface of the tray to hold a greater volume of the agent in the target areas of the teeth to enhance the process.[35,41] The theory seems sound, but there is no evidence that the creation of reservoirs actually improves the bleaching process. It is assumed that the solution, whether in greater volume in a reservoir or in lesser volume because of no reservoir, degrades at the same rate. Some clinicians do not advocate placement of reservoirs in the tray.[58,87,119] However, there may be some benefit to having the extra space provided

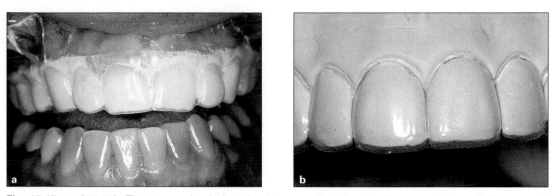

Figs 15-17a and 15-17b The tray can be designed as (a) nonscalloped, extending up onto the soft tissue, or (b) scalloped to the tissue contours around the teeth.

by the reservoirs; it may help in seating the tray and avoiding undue pressure on the teeth, which can cause sensitivity, especially if a very viscous solution is used. Easy seating of the tray avoids pressure on the teeth and tissue discomfort. These reservoir spaces are easy to form using a light-polymerized resin, supplied by manufacturers, which is placed 0.5 to 1.0 mm thick on the facial surfaces of the teeth of the cast, terminating 1.0 mm short of the gingival area and not extending into the embrasures. Other options are the application of fingernail polish, die spacer, or tin foil to the cast. The reservoir design should still allow the edge of the tray to contact the tooth. Spacers should not be placed in areas of occlusion (such as the incisal aspects of mandibular anterior teeth or the lingual aspects of maxillary anterior teeth), since the contact of the opposing teeth will displace the material from the tray.

Patient Instructions for At-Home Bleaching

Patient instructions should address: expectations and course of treatment; technique for applying the bleaching agent; frequency and length of time for wearing the tray; tooth sensitivity/tissue irritation problems; interim appointments; and variations in total fee related to course of treatment.

It is critical that the patient understands the process and can make appropriate adjustments in the protocol (eg, discontinuing tray wear for 1 or 2 days if sensitivity begins to develop). The patient must recognize any developing problems early and inform the dentist. While this is a dentist-supervised procedure, most of the process occurs out of the sight of the dentist, so the patient becomes the progress monitor. The patient should be instructed to place enough of the solution into the tray to cover the facial surfaces of the target teeth, which includes the most posterior tooth visible

when the patient smiles, laughs, or talks. Seating and removing the tray should be demonstrated to ensure that there is no problem and that the patient is able to do so without undue difficulty or harm to the tray or the oral structures. To avoid tissue injury, the tray should be "peeled" from the second molar area rather than being "dug out with fingernails" in the canine region.

Instructions for Tray Wear. The patient should understand that he or she is to wear the tray for 4 or more hours per day/night, but that the specific consecutive 4-hour period is discretionary. Wear of less than 4 hours is a waste of the agent because the agent retains its potency for several hours. One study demonstrated that 60% of the active agent remained after 4 hours.[100] Probably the best option is for the patient to wear the tray during the sleep hours. Although the agent has lost most of its potency after 5 plus hours, compliance is much better when the bleaching treatment becomes part of a regular routine. If sensitivity is not a problem, the patient can even have two wearing periods per day. While this speeds the process, it is also likely to provoke tooth sensitivity, so the patient should be informed of this potential problem. After the loaded tray is seated, the patient should use a wet/damp cloth or finger to wipe the areas adjacent to the borders of the tray to clean away any excess. This is to remove any bleaching agent that has escaped the borders of the tray to prevent swallowing. The patient should be reminded to rinse and gently brush the tray after each session before storing it in a cool environment until the next bleaching session.

The bleaching process varies in the amount of time required. Some readily discernible improvement may occur within 2 to 14 days, or it may take as long as 6

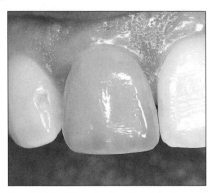

Fig 15-18a The single discolored tooth may require unique tray design.

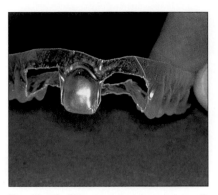

Fig 15-18b The tray is trimmed to fit around the discolored tooth only.

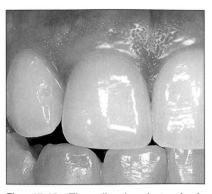

Fig 15-18c The discolored tooth is whitened; other teeth are not affected.

to 12 months.[68] The time depends on the type of discoloration, patient compliance, and whether or not any tooth sensitivity occurs. It may be helpful to recall the patient after 5 to 7 days to check progress. The changes may occur somewhat slowly, albeit steadily, so the patient may forget the original shade. Therefore, the changes may not be readily noticeable to the patient. The patient can be shown the shade tab representing the original color to contrast with the new whiteness of the teeth, or the patient can compare the treated maxillary arch with the untreated mandibular arch. At the interim appointment, tray adjustments may be made if necessary. The protocol can be reviewed to ensure that the patient is following it correctly. Alterations in protocol can be made to eliminate or minimize any problems or to speed the process. Some teeth may respond to bleaching more rapidly than others. More severely discolored and less responsive teeth may need more sessions of bleaching than others.[61,64] When isolated problem teeth exist, one approach is to begin treatment of the problem tooth/teeth before the other teeth (Fig 15-18a to 15-18c). Place the bleaching solution in the area(s) of the tray corresponding to the problem area for a few days before treating all the teeth. The patient should be made aware extra bleaching time for certain teeth may be necessary and that the problem tooth/teeth may become even more of a contrast for a short time because the other teeth whiten more rapidly. Some teeth exhibit a splotchy look as different portions of the tooth respond at different rates. The patient should be encouraged to continue treatment until the remainder of the tooth achieves the same color. The splotchy areas tend to abate on completion of treatment. Considerable whitening of the teeth is routinely predictable (Figs 15-19 to 15-24).

Techniques for Tetracycline-Stained Teeth

Patients whose teeth have been stained by tetracycline ingestion present a great restorative challenge. Tetracycline can be deposited in fetal tooth buds if ingested by an expectant mother in the third trimester of pregnancy or by a child during the tooth-formation years, between ages 3 to 4 months and 7 to 8 years.[96,98] Tetracycline may also be deposited in the teeth in early adult years if it is taken on a long-term basis for skin conditions (acne), especially during the formation of secondary dentin, during growth periods, and after trauma.

Tetracycline has several different analogues (tetracycline, doxycycline, oxytetracycline, minocycline, chlortetracycline, demeclocycline, etc) that may produce several basic colors in the teeth. Colors may include various intensities of gray, blue, brown, and yellow. If seemingly normal yellow teeth are not responsive to the conventional 2 weeks of bleaching treatment, they may, in fact, be tetracycline stained.

Recent research has shown that tetracycline-stained teeth may respond to bleaching treatments but at a rate different from teeth stained by other agents (Figs 15-25 and 15-26).[67] Whereas the normal bleaching time is 2 to 6 weeks, some tetracycline-stained

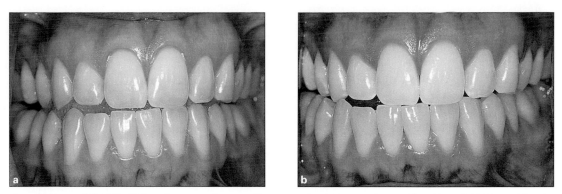

Figs 15-19a and 15-19b Yellow-brown stains usually respond quickly to at-home bleaching. (a) Prior to bleaching. (b) After 1 month.

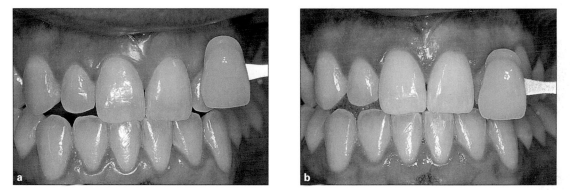

Figs 15-20a and 15-20b Many gray stains respond well to at-home bleaching. (a) Prior to bleaching. (b) Results after 4+ weeks.

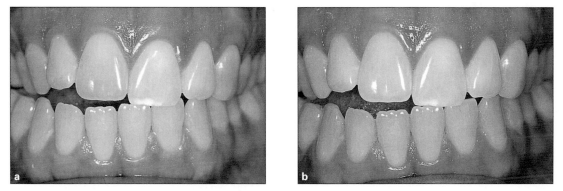

Figs 15-21a and 15-21b White spots become less noticeable when the teeth are whitened. (a) Prior to bleaching. (b) After bleaching. Note that the white spot is unchanged.

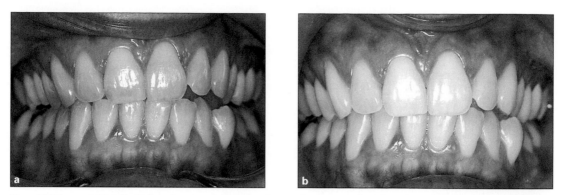

Figs 15-22a and 15-22b Yellow-brown stains can be easily removed with at-home bleaching. (a) Prior to bleaching. (b) After bleaching.

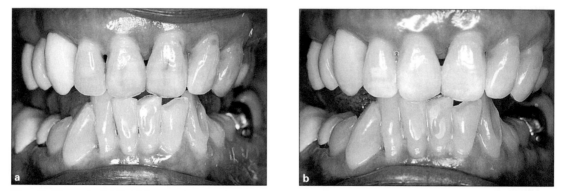

Figs 15-23a and 15-23b Yellow stains can be more readily removed from the coronal portion than from the root of the tooth. (a) Prior to bleaching. (b) After bleaching. The roots retain their yellowish coloration.

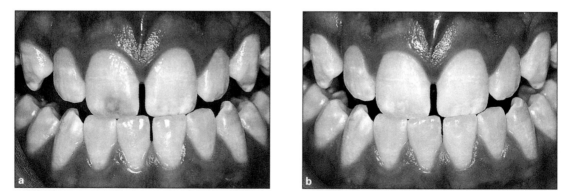

Figs 15-24a and 15-24b Fluorosis stains can be whitened. (a) Prior to bleaching. (b) After bleaching.

Figs 15-25a to 15-25c Tetracycline stains are tenacious; results come much more slowly than with other types of stains.

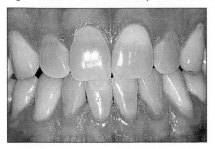

Fig 15-25a Prior to bleaching.

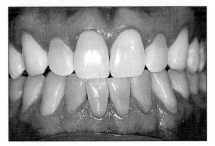

Fig 15-25b Treatment midpoint.

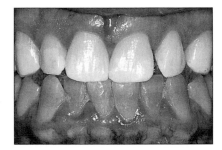

Fig 15-25c After approximately 7 months of at-home bleaching.

Figs 15-26a to 15-26c A generalized tetracycline stain.

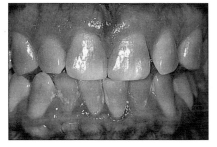

Fig 15-26a Prior to bleaching.

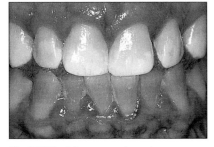

Fig 15-26b After several weeks.

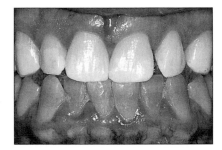

Fig 15-26c After more than 8 months of at-home bleaching.

teeth may require 2 to 12 months of daily treatment to achieve a satisfactory result. Tetracycline-stained teeth do not generally lose all their discoloration, although the tooth color is often much improved. The teeth may retain slightly grayness.

Research on the longevity of color change achieved indicates that most patients will have some degree of lightening and that 8 of 10 patients can expect to retain that lightening for at least 1 year. Even those patients who experience some regression indicate that they were glad they bleached their teeth and would do it again. A follow-up study showed a patient satisfaction rate at 83% 4.5 years after bleaching.[86]

There are several factors to consider when using extended time periods for bleaching tetracycline-stained teeth.[68] First, the location of the stained area has a great impact on the prognosis for success. A tooth generally lightens from the incisal to the gingival area because the tooth gets progressively thicker from incisal to gingival. Teeth heavily stained in the gingival one third have the poorest prognosis for complete lightening. The further toward the incisal edge the stain resides, the better the prognosis. In any

situation, absolute predictions of success are unrealistic. Patients must understand that each discoloration responds differently and that they may not see results in the first few months.

Extended treatment may increase the likelihood of tooth sensitivity. To avoid or mitigate sensitivity, patients may have to titrate their exposure time (from overnight to 1 to 2 hours daily) or exposure frequency (from every night to every second or third night). As with short-term bleaching, the presence of pretreatment sensitivity and the frequency of solution application are the only predictors of possible sensitivity. In extended-treatment situations, sensitivity may be sporadic and subside with no treatment. If it is chronic, patients may wish to apply fluoride or potassium nitrate solutions in the bleaching tray for 30 minutes either as needed or before the application of the bleaching solution. Desensitizing toothpastes containing potassium nitrate, used before the application of the bleaching agent, may also provide some relief or even help prevent sensitivity. A reduction in the concentration of carbamide peroxide may also help.

A practical consideration is the amount of bleaching material necessary for extended treatment and the appropriate fee for service. Practitioners may choose to either have an increased total fee or use the initial fee for their normal bleaching treatment with a monthly fee for each additional month of treatment. Patients can then pay as they go for extended treatment if there is continued, albeit slow, improvement.

Generally, teeth severely stained in gingival areas are candidates for porcelain veneers or crowns; however, it is generally best to attempt bleaching first. Bleaching may achieve adequate results and eliminate the need for veneers, even if the result is not as esthetic as with veneers. The bleaching may have only a limited lightening effect, but it can reduce the amount of opacity necessary in the veneer for masking. Even if there is no change from the bleaching treatment, the patient is aware that the most conservative avenues have been attempted first and is assured that porcelain veneers are the best option remaining.

Dentists and physicians are well aware of the effect of tetracycline ingestion on dental esthetics, although the results of tetracycline absorption in teenagers treated for acne has only recently been reported. Despite this awareness, tetracycline-stained teeth will continue to be seen. Tetracycline is still the drug of choice for outpatient treatment of Rocky Mountain spotted fever and is the most widely prescribed drug for acne. Dentists should consider bleaching a reasonable treatment option for the discoloration resulting from this treatment if the patient is willing to comply with extended treatment and does not expect total elimination of the stain.

Other Considerations

Effect on Restorations

Bleaching has little or no effect on most of the common restorative materials.[78] Perhaps its most significant effect is that it lightens teeth enough that previously placed restorations may appear comparatively dark, leading to the question of replacement. Bleaching has no effect on porcelain. It does encourage the release of mercury from some types of amalgam restorations. The clinical significance of this is not known.[77] The surface of some types of resin composite is roughened slightly, and the hardness may be very slightly increased, but neither is clinically significant.[23,46] Bleaching does affect methacrylate provi-

sional restorative materials, causing them to yellow slightly.[107] Although bleaching releases much oxygen into the tooth, the bond of existing restorations is not weakened. There are no contraindications for bleaching in the presence of existing bonded restorations. However, as previously stated, the oxygen-rich tooth structure does not provide a good surface for bonding new restorations. The oxygen released hinders the polymerization of the resin.[93,126] A delay of a week or more following the bleaching process allows this effect to dissipate so that bonding can effectively be performed.[60] This also allows the tooth shade to stabilize before selection of the restorative material shade. A drying agent, such as acetone, can be used to diminish the oxygen in the outer layers of the tooth if there is concern that oxygen has been retained in the surface.[10]

Alternatives to Bleaching

The alternatives to bleaching are more aggressive in relation to the tooth structure and/or to the gingival tissues. These procedures include microabrasion, macroabrasion, bonded resin composite veneering, porcelain veneers, and porcelain or metal-ceramic restorations. Although all of these are legitimate treatment techniques with proven efficacy, they rely on the removal of tooth structure and/or the addition of material to the tooth, which may result in overcontouring and subsequent tissue insult.

Microabrasion and Macroabrasion

One decision in the esthetic treatment planning for a patient is whether to remove a discoloration by bleaching or by removal of tooth structure. Microabrasion is a process in which the tooth surface is subjected to a combination of an acid and an abrasive (Figs 15-27a to 15-27d).[30,31] The acid removes mineral content, leaving the outer 22 to 27 μm weakened enough that the abrasive, with which the acid is mixed, quickly removes the stained outer surface of the tooth. Although the amount of enamel removed is very limited, this abrasive technique alters the outer surface of the enamel as the undesirable coloration is removed or at least altered. The abrasive, usually suspended in a water-soluble gel containing a low concentration of hydrochloric acid, is applied with a rubber cup or stiff bristle brush for 20 to 30 seconds to acid-conditioned enamel.[29] Superficial discolorations can usually be removed from the enamel surface, but it is not possible to know in advance whether the dis-

Figs 15-27a to 15-27d Microabrasion represents an alternative method of stain removal or modification.

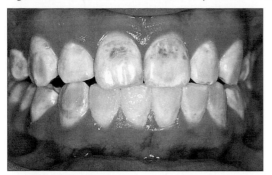

Fig 15-27a Original stains.

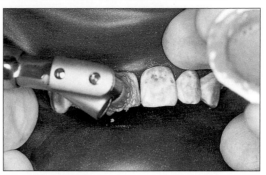

Fig 15-27b Application of acid/abrasive paste.

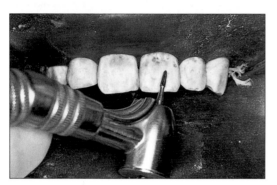

Fig 15-27c Removal of superficial stained enamel.

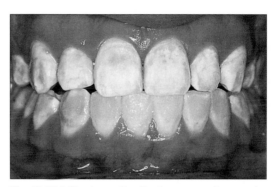

Fig 15-27d Final results. Resin composite can be bonded to conceal remaining discoloration.

coloration is superficial. Should the discoloration extend to the dentin or become more visible, a resin composite restoration will need to be placed to seal the defect and restore contour. The choice of resin composite to place poses a dilemma as to whether the material matches the original tooth color or the color the tooth will be. It is best to bleach first unless the tooth enamel is of a chalky texture. Then when abrasive techniques are initiated, the tooth shade is already established should a resin composite restoration be required. Bleaching has been estimated to remove 80% of brown discolorations. White discolorations are not removed, but may be much less noticeable when the surrounding area of the tooth is lightened. If bleaching is unsuccessful, then the more aggressive techniques can be initiated. The patient should be informed of the treatment options (bleaching, abrasion, bonding) before treatment and should understand the different fees for these procedures.

Another form of abrasion is macroabrasion. In this technique, the abrasion can be achieved by applying a fine diamond or carbide-finishing bur to the enamel at relatively low speeds and very light pressure. The effect is much the same as with the acid/abrasive technique. When using a high-speed handpiece, water should be applied to maintain the coloration of the teeth. As some teeth dehydrate, more subsurface defects may become visible; for these, treatment is not indicated. Air abrasive techniques can also be used quite effectively for microabrasion or macroabrasion. Only fine abrasive particles should be used to avoid over-reduction of the tooth. Over-reduction can be corrected by adding resin composite to the undercontoured areas.

All three techniques (diamond-stone surface alteration, chemical-physical microabrasion, and kinetic-energy preparation [air abrasion]) rely on the selective reduction of the outer surface of the tooth. While they may be very effective in removing a relatively shallow discolored area, they are not intended to eliminate overall discoloration, especially if it involves the underlying dentin. However, they are valuable techniques for treating limited areas and for supplement-

Figs 15-28a to 15-28d Porcelain veneers on tetracycline-stained teeth often do not completely mask the discoloration. Bleaching of exposed enamel surfaces may lighten the teeth as seen through the veneers.

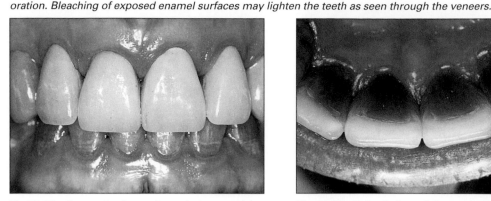

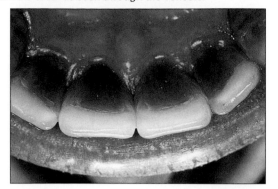

Fig 15-28a Gray stain shows through the porcelain.

Fig 15-28b Palatal view of the teeth. Note the dark shadow of the teeth under the porcelain.

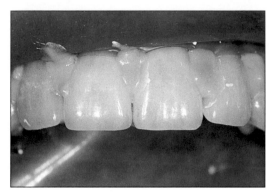

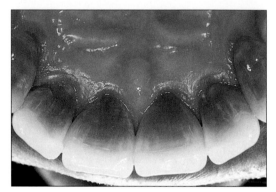

Fig 15-28c Hydrogen peroxide (35%) applied to lingual and proximal surfaces.

Fig 15-28d Teeth lightened after one appointment.

ing tooth bleaching. For patients with a limited demand for an esthetic improvement in the color of the teeth, abrasion alone may satisfy the patient's needs. If abrasion techniques do not completely satisfy the desires, more extravagant procedures may be performed. Abrasive techniques do not interfere with the placement of veneers or crowns.

Bleaching Before and After Placement of Veneers

Discolored teeth may be treated with bonded restorations to cover/disguise the underlying stain. It may be possible to place the material with little or no tooth reduction. The teeth can be first treated with microabrasion or macroabrasion to remove discolored areas and then acid etched. The esthetic material, such as resin composite or porcelain (see Chapter 16), is then bonded to the tooth to provide good color and

form. However, the natural appearance of the veneered surface depends strongly on some light reflecting from the underlying tooth structure. If the tooth structure is stained too darkly, the discoloration will show through the translucent resin composite or ceramic veneer. The only solution is to make the veneering material thicker and less translucent. To avoid overcontouring the tooth/restoration, it is necessary to remove more of the facial and proximal tooth structure to achieve the esthetic and functional objectives. Successful bleaching therapy would eliminate the need for a thicker veneer and more tooth reduction.

Bleaching is possible even for teeth that have already received veneers. Bleaching teeth from the lingual surface can alter the apparent color of the translucent restoration on the facial surface (Figs 15-28 and 15-29), improving esthetics.[71]

Figs 15-29a to 15-29d Another example of bleaching tetracycline-stained teeth that have porcelain veneers.

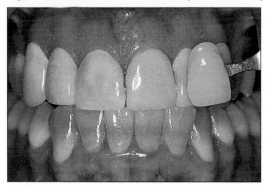

Fig 15-29a Prior to bleaching.

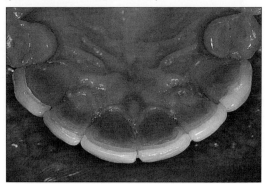

Fig 15-29b Palatal view prior to bleaching. The gray tetracycline stain is obvious.

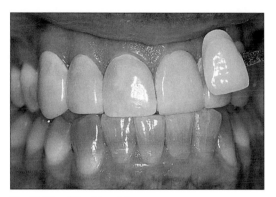

Fig 15-29c After bleaching.

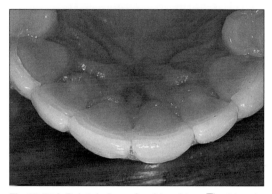

Fig 15-29d Palatal view after bleaching. The bleaching process has lightened the teeth noticeably.

References

1. Abu-Shakra A, Zeiger E. Effects of Salmonella genotypes and testing protocols on H_2O_2-induced mutation. Mutagenesis 1990;5(5):469–473.

2. ADA Council on Scientific Affairs. Laser-assisted bleaching: an update. J Am Dent Assoc 1998;129:1484–1487.

3. Albers H. Lightening natural teeth. ADEPT Report 1991;2(1): 1–24.

4. al-Nazhan S. External root resorption after bleaching: a case report. Oral Surg Oral Med Oral Pathol 1991;72(5):607–609.

5. Anic I, Pavelic B, Matsumoto K. In vitro pulp chamber temperature rises associated with the argon laser polymerization of composite resin. Lasers Surg Med 1996;19(4):438–444.

6. Atkinson CB. Fancies and some facts. Dent Cosmos 1861; 3:57–60.

7. Atkinson WH. Bleaching teeth, when discolored from loss of vitality: means for preventing their discoloration and ulceration. Dent Cosmos 1862;3:74–77.

8. Atkinson CB. Hints, queries, and comments: pyrozone. Dent Cosmos 1893;35:330–332.

9. Barghi N. Making a clinical decision for vital tooth bleaching: at-home or in-office. Compend Contin Educ Dent 1998;19(8): 831–838.

10. Barghi N, Godwin JM. Reducing the adverse effect of bleaching on composite-enamel bond. J Esthet Dent 1994;6(4): 157–161.

11. Barghi N, Morgan J. Bleaching following porcelain veneers: clinical cases. Am J Dent 1997;10(5):254–256.

12. Barker GT. The causes and treatment of discolored teeth. Dent Cosmos 1861;3:305–311.

13. Berry JH. What about whiteners? Safety concerns explored. J Am Dent Assoc 1990;121:222–225.

14. Black GV, McKay FS. Mottled teeth: an endemic developmental imperfection of the enamel of the teeth heretofore unknown in the literature of dentistry. Dent Cosmos 1916;58:129.

15. Bogue EA. Bleaching teeth. Dent Cosmos 1872;14:1–3.

16. Bowles WH, Thompson LR. Vital bleaching: the effect of heat and hydrogen peroxide on pulpal enzymes. J Endod 1986; 12(3):108–112.

17. Bowles WH, Ugwuneri Z. Pulp chamber penetration by hydrogen peroxide following vital bleaching procedures. J Endod 1987;13(8):375–377.

18. Brighton DM, Harrington GW, Nicholls JI. Intracanal isolating barriers as they relate to bleaching. J Endod 1994;20(5):228–232.

19. Brown G. Factors influencing successful bleaching of the discolored root-filled tooth. Oral Surg Oral Med Oral Pathol 1965;20:238–244.

20. Burchard HH. A Textbook of Dental Pathology and Therapeutics. Philadelphia: Lea & Febiger, 1898.

21. Cantoni O, Murray D, Meyn RE. Effect of 3-aminobenzamide on DNA strand-break rejoining and cytotoxicity in CHO cells treated with hydrogen peroxide. Biochim Biophys Acta 1986;867(3):135–143.

22. Carrillo A, Arredondo Trevino MV, Haywood VB. Simultaneous bleaching of vital teeth and an open-chamber non-vital tooth with 10% carbamide peroxide. Quintessence Int 1998;29:643–648.

23. Christensen GJ. Tooth bleaching, home-use products. Clin Res Assoc Newsletter 1989;13(12):1.

24. Christensen GJ. Home-use bleaching survey—1991. Clin Res Assoc Newsletter 1991;15(10):2.

25. Chung HY, Bowles WH. Oxidative changes in minocycline leading to intrinsic dental staining [abstract A1855]. J Dent Res 1989;68(special issue):413.

26. Cohen SC. Human pulpal response to bleaching procedures on vital teeth. J Endod 1979;5(5):134–138.

27. Cooper JS, Bokmeyer TJ, Bowles WH. Penetration of the pulp chamber by carbamide peroxide bleaching agents. J Endod 1992;18(7):315–317.

28. Costas FL, Wong M. Intracoronal isolating barriers: effect of location on root leakage and effectiveness of bleaching agents. J Endod 1991;17(8):365–368.

29. Croll TP. Enamel microabrasion: observations after 10 years. J Am Dent Assoc 1997;128(suppl):45S–50S.

30. Croll TP, Bullock GA. Enamel microabrasion for removal of smooth surface decalcification lesions. J Clin Orthod 1994;28(6):365–370.

31. Croll TP, Segura A, Donly KJ. Enamel microabrasion: new considerations in 1993. Pract Periodont Aesthet Dent 1993;5:19–29.

32. Curtis JW, Dickinson GL, Downey MC, et al. Assessing the effects of 10 percent carbamide peroxide on oral soft tissues. J Am Dent Assoc 1996;127:1218–1223.

33. Dodson DL, Bowles WH. Production of minocyclines pigment by tissue extracts [abstract A1267]. J Dent Res 1991;70(special issue):424.

34. Dorman HL, Bishop JG. Production of experimental edema in dog tongue with dilute hydrogen peroxide. Oral Surg Oral Med Oral Pathol 1970;29(1):38–43.

35. Dunn JR. Dentist-prescribed home bleaching: current status. Compend Contin Educ Dent 1998;19:760–764.

36. Dwinelle WW. Ninth Annual Meeting of American Society of Dental Surgeons, Article X. Am J Dent Sci 1850;1:57–61.

37. Fasanaro TS. Bleaching teeth: history, chemicals, and methods used for common tooth discolorations. J Esthet Dent 1992;4(3):71–78.

38. Feiglin B. A 6-year recall study of clinically chemically bleached teeth. Oral Surg Oral Med Oral Pathol 1987;63:610–613.

39. Feinman RA, Goldstein RE, Garber DA. Bleaching Teeth. Chicago: Quintessence, 1987.

40. Franchi GJ. A practical technique for bleaching discolored crowns of young permanent incisors. J Dent Child 1953;20:68–69.

41. Frazier KB. Nightguard bleaching to lighten a restored, non-vital discolored tooth. Compend Contin Educ Dent 1998;19:810–813. (Published erratum appears in Compend Contin Educ Dent 1998;19:864.)

42. Freccia WF, Peters DD, Lorton L, Bernier WE. An in vitro comparison of nonvital bleaching techniques in the discolored tooth. J Endod 1982;8(2):70–77.

43. Freedman GA. Safety of tooth whitening. Dent Today 1990;9(3):32–33.

44. Friedman S. Internal bleaching: long-term outcomes and complications. J Am Dent Assoc 1997;128(suppl):51S–55S.

45. Friedman S, Rotstein I, Libfeld H, et al. Incidence of external root resorption and esthetic results in 58 bleached pulpless teeth. Endod Dent Traumatol 1988;4(1):23–26.

46. Friend GW, Jones JE, Wamble SH, Covington JS. Carbamide peroxide tooth bleaching: changes to compositie resins after prolonged exposure [abstract A2432]. J Dent Res 1991;70 (special issue):570.

47. Frysh H. Chemistry of bleaching. In Goldstein RE, Garber DA, eds. Complete Dental Bleaching. Chicago: Quintessence, 1995.

48. Frysh H, Bowles WH, Baker F, Rivera-Hidalgo G. Effect of pH on bleaching efficiency [abstract A2248]. J Dent Res 1993;72(special issue):384.

49. Gimlin DR, Schindler WG. The management of postbleaching cervical resorption. J Endod 1990;16(6):292–297.

50. Goldstein FW. New "at-home" bleaching technique introduced. Cosmetic Dent GP 1989;June:6–7.

51. Goldstein RE. Bleaching teeth: new materials—new role. J Am Dent Assoc 1987;115(special issue):44E-52E. (Published erratum appears in J Am Dent Assoc 1988;116:156.)

52. Goldstein RE. In-office bleaching: where we came from, where we are today. J Am Dent Assoc 1997;128 (suppl):11S–15S.

53. Goldstein RE, Garber DA. Complete Dental Bleaching. Chicago: Quintessence, 1995.

54. Harlan AW. Proceedings of the American Dental Association—Twenty-third Annual Session. Dent Cosmos 1884;26:97–98.

55. Harlan AW. The dental pulp, its destruction, and methods of treatment of teeth discolored by its retention in the pulp chamber or canals. Dent Cosmos 1891;31:137–141.

56. Harrington GW, Natkin E. External resorption associated with bleaching of pulpless teeth. J Endod 1979;5(11):344–348.

57. Haywood VB. Nightguard vital bleaching: current information and research. Esthet Dent Update 1990;1(2):20–25.

58. Haywood VB. Overview and status of mouthguard bleaching. J Esthet Dent 1991;3(5):157–161.

59. Haywood VB. Bleaching of vital and nonvital teeth. Curr Opin Dent 1992(2);142–149 .

60. Haywood VB. History, safety, and effectiveness of current bleaching techniques and applications of the nightguard vital bleaching technique. Quintessence Int 1992;23(7):471–488.

61. Haywood VB. Commonly asked questions about nightguard vital bleaching. J Indiana Dent Assoc 1993;72(5):28–33.

62. Haywood VB. Nightguard vital bleaching: information and consent form. Esthet Dent Update 1995;6(5):130–132.

63. Haywood VB. Current concepts: bleaching of vital teeth. Quintessence Int 1997;28:424–425.

64. Haywood VB. Nightguard vital bleaching and in-office bleaching. Contemp Esthet Rest Prac 1998;July/Aug:78–81.

65. Haywood VB, Drake M. Research on whitening teeth makes news. NC Dent Rev 1990;7(2):9.

66. Haywood VB, Heymann HO. Nightguard vital bleaching. Quintessence Int 1989;20:173–176.

67. Haywood VB, Leonard RH. Six- and 12-month color stability after 6 months bleaching tetracycline teeth [abstract 2891]. J Dent Res 1996;75(special issue):379.

68. Haywood VB, Leonard RH, Dickinson GL. Efficacy of six months of nightguard vital bleaching of tetracycline-stained teeth. J Esthet Dent 1997;9(1):13–19.

69. Haywood VB, Leonard RH Jr, Nelson CF. Efficacy of foam liner in 10% carbamide peroxide bleaching technique. Quintessence Int 1993;24(9):663–666.

70. Haywood VB, Leonard RH, Nelson CF, Brunson WD. Effectiveness, side effects and long-term status of nightguard vital bleaching. J Am Dent Assoc 1994;125:1219–1226.

71. Haywood VB, Parker MH. Nightguard vital bleaching beneath existing porcelain veneers: a case report. Quintessence Int 1999;30:743–747.

72. Heling I, Parson A, Rotstein I. Effect of bleaching agents on dentin permeability to Streptococcus faecalis. J Endod 1995;21(11):540–542.

73. Heller D, Skribner J, Lin LM. Effect of intracoronal bleaching on external cervical root resorption. J Endod 1992;18(4):145–148.

74. Holmstrup G, Palm AM, Lambjerg-Hansen H. Bleaching of discoloured root-filled teeth. Endod Dent Traumatol 1988;4(5):197–201.

75. How WS. Esthetic dentistry. Dent Cosmos 1886;28:741–745.

76. Howell RA. The prognosis of bleached root-filled teeth. Int Endod J 1981;14(1):22–26.

77. Hummert TW, Osborne JW, Norling BK, Cardenas HL. Mercury in solution following exposure of various amalgams to carbamide peroxides. Am J Dent 1993;6(6):305–309.

78. Hunsaker KJ, Christensen GJ, Christensen RP. Tooth bleaching and chemicals—influence on teeth and restorations [abstract A1558]. J Dent Res 1990;69(special issue):303.

79. Jordan RE, Boksman L. Conservative vital bleaching treatment of discolored dentition. Compend Contin Educ Dent 1984;5:803–805, 807.

80. Kirk EC. The chemical bleaching of teeth. Dent Cosmos 1889;31:273–283.

81. Kirk EC. An American Textbook of Operative Dentistry, ed 2. Philadelphia: Lea Brothers, 1890:540–560.

82. Kirk EC. Hints, queries, and comments: sodium peroxide. Dent Cosmos 1893;35:1265–1267.

83. Kirk EC. Chemical principles involved in tooth discoloration. Dent Cosmos 1906;48:947–954.

84. Lado EA, Stanley HR, Weisman MI. Cervical resorption in bleached teeth. Oral Surg Oral Med Oral Pathol 1983;55(1):78–80.

85. Leonard RH Jr. Efficacy, longevity, side effects, and patient perceptions of nightguard vital bleaching. Compend Contin Educ Dent 1998;19(8):766–774.

86. Leonard RH, Haywood VB, Eagle JC, et al. Nightguard vital bleaching of tetracycline stained teeth: 54 months post-treatment. J Esthet Dent 1999;11:265–277.

87. Leonard RH Jr, Haywood VB, Phillips C. Risk factors for developing tooth sensitivity and gingival irritation associated with nightguard vital bleaching. Quintessence Int 1997;28:527–534.

88. Lewinstein I, Hirschfeld Z, Stabholz A, Rotstein I. Effect of hydrogen peroxide and sodium perborate on the microhardness of human enamel and dentin. J Endod 1994;20(2):61–63.

89. Li Y. Toxicological considerations of tooth bleaching using peroxide-containing agents. J Am Dent Assoc 1997;128 (suppl):31S–36S.

90. Madison S, Walton R. Cervical root resorption following bleaching of endodontically treated teeth. J Endod 1990;16 (12):570–574.

91. Marshall JS. Principles and Practice of Operative Dentistry. Philadelphia: Lippincott, 1901:464–476.

92. Martin JH, Bishop JG, Guentherman RH, Dorman HL. Cellular response of gingiva to prolonged application of dilute hydrogen peroxide. J Periodontol 1968;39(4):208–210.

93. McGuckin RS, Thurmond BA, Osovitz S. In vitro enamel shear bond strengths following vital bleaching [abstract A892]. J Dent Res 1991;70(special issue):377.

94. Melcer J, Chaumette MT, Zebulon S, et al. Preliminary report on the effect of the CO2 laser beam on the dental pulp of the Macaca mulatta primate and the beagle dog. J Endod 1985;11(1):1–5.

95. Mello HS. The mechanism of tetracycline staining in primary and permanent teeth. J Dent Child 1967;34(6):478.

96. Moffitt JM, Cooley RO, Olsen NH, et al. Prediction of tetracycline-induced tooth discoloration. J Am Dent Assoc 1974;88:547–552.

97. M'Quillen JH. Elongation and discoloration of a superior central incisor. Dent Cosmos 1868;10:225–227.

98. Mull MM. The tetracyclines and the teeth. Dent Abstr 1967;12:346–350.

99. Nathanson D, Parra C. Bleaching vital teeth: a review and clinical study. Compend Contin Educ Dent 1987;8:490–497.

100. Nathoo SA, Richter R, Smith S, Zhang YP. Kinetics of carbamide peroxide degradation in bleaching trays [abstract A2149]. J Dent Res 1996;75(special issue):286.

101. Pearson HH. Bleaching of the discolored pulpless tooth. J Am Dent Assoc 1958;56:64–65.

102. Pieroli DA, Navarro MFL, Coradazzi JL, Consolaro A. Evaluation of carcinogenic potential of bleaching agents in DMBA-induction model [abstract A2149]. J Dent Res 1996;75 (special issue):332.

103. Powell GL, Morton TH, Whisenant BK. Argon laser oral safety parameters for teeth. Lasers Surg Med 1993;13 (5):548–552.

104. Reddy J, Salkin LM. The effect of a urea peroxide rinse on dental plaque and gingivitis. J Periodontol 1976;47 (10):607–610.

105. Reinhardt JW, Eivins SE, Swift EJ Jr, Denehy GE. A clinical study of nightguard vital bleaching. Quintessence Int 1993;24:379–384.

106. Robertson WD, Melfi RC. Pulpal response to vital bleaching procedures. J Endod 1980;6(7):645–649.

107. Robinson FG, Haywood VB, Myers M. Effect of 10 percent carbamide peroxide on color of provisional restoration materials. J Am Dent Assoc 1997;128:727–731.

108. Rotstein I, Dankner E, Goldman A, et al. Histochemical analysis of dental hard tissues following bleaching. J Endod 1996;22(1):23–26.

109. Rotstein I, Friedman S, Mor C, et al. Histological characterization of bleaching-induced external root resorption in dogs. J Endod 1991;17(9):436–441.

110. Rotstein I, Lehr Z, Gedalia I. Effect of bleaching agents on inorganic components of human dentin and cementum. J Endod 1992;18(6):290–293.

111. Rotstein I, Mor C, Friedman S. Prognosis of intracoronal bleaching with sodium perborate preparations in vitro: 1-year study. J Endod 1993;19(1):10–12.

112. Rotstein I, Torek Y, Lewinstein I. Effect of bleaching time and temperature on the radicular penetration of hydrogen peroxide. Endod Dent Traumatol 1991;7(5):196–198.

113. Rotstein I, Torek Y, Misgav R. Effect of cementum defects on radicular penetration of 30% H2O2 during intracoronal bleaching. J Endod 1991;17(5):230–233.

114. Russell CM, Dickinson GL, Johnson MH, et al. Dentist-supervised home bleaching with ten percent carbamide peroxide gel: a six-month study. J Esthet Dent 1996;8(4):177–182.

115. Scherer W, Palat M, Hittelman E, et al. At-home bleaching system: effect on gingival tissue. J Esthet Dent 1992;4(3):86–89.

116. Schulte JR, Morrissette DB, Gasior EJ, Czajewski MV. Clinical changes in the gingiva as a result of at-home bleaching. Compend Contin Educ Dent 1993;14:1362–1372.

117. Seale NS, McIntosh JE, Taylor AN. Pulpal reaction to bleaching of teeth in dogs. J Dent Res 1981;60(5):948–953.

118. Shipman B, Cohen E, Kaslick RS. The effect of a urea peroxide gel on plaque deposits and gingival status. J Periodontol 1971;42(5):283–285.

119. Small BW. Bleaching with 10 percent carbamide peroxide: an 18-month study. Gen Dent 1994;42(2):142–146.

120. Smith MS, McInnes JW. Further studies on methods of removing brown stains from mottled teeth. J Am Dent Assoc 1942;29:571.

121. Spasser JF. A simple bleaching technique using sodium perborate. N Y Dent J 1961;27:332–334.

122. Stillwagen TC. Bleaching teeth. Dent Cosmos 1870; 12:625–627.

123. Stindt DJ, Quenette L. An overview of Gly-Oxide liquid in control and prevention of dental disease. Compend Contin Educ Dent 1989;10:514–519.

124. Swift EJ Jr, Perdigaoa J. Effects of bleaching on teeth and restorations. Compend Contin Educ Dent 1998;19:815–820.

125. Tartakow DJ, Smith RS, Spinelli JA. Urea peroxide solution in the treatment of gingivitis in orthodontics. Am J Orthod 1978;73:560–567.

126. Titley KC, Torneck CD, Smith DC, Adibfar A. Adhesion of composite resin to bleached and unbleached bovine enamel. J Dent Res 1988;67:1523–1528. (Published erratum appears in J Dent Res 1989;68:inside back cover.)

127. Tong LS, Pang MK, Mok NY, et al. The effects of etching, micro-abrasion, and bleaching on surface enamel. J Dent Res 1993;72:67–71.

128. Trotman ER. Dyeing and chemical technology of treatable fibers. In Encyclopedia of Science and Technology, vol 2, ed 6. New York: McGraw-Hill, 1987.

129. White WE Jr, Pruitt KM, Mansson-Rahemtulla B. Peroxidase-thiocyanate-peroxide antibacterial system does not damage DNA. Antimicrob Agents Chemother 1983;23(2):267–272.

130. Woolverton CJ, Haywood VB, Heymann HO. Toxicity of two carbamide peroxide products used in nightguard vital bleaching. Am J Dent 1993;6(6):310–314.

131. Yu D, Powell GL, Higuchi WI, Fox JL. Comparison of three lasers on dental pulp chamber temperature. J Clin Laser Med Surg 1993;11:119–122.

132. Zaragoza VMT. Bleaching teeth: technique. EstoModeo 1984; 9:7–30.

133. Zeigler-Skylakakis K, Andrae U. Mutagenicity of hydrogen peroxide in V79 Chinese hamster cells. Mutat Res 1987;192(1):65–67.

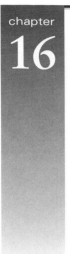

16 Porcelain Veneers

J. William Robbins

The porcelain veneer has gained wide acceptance in recent years as a primary restoration in esthetic dentistry. Since its introduction in the early 1980s, it has undergone an evolution in both techniques and materials. A significant number of long-term clinical studies confirm the excellent durability of the porcelain veneer restoration.[6,12,14,18,24,25,28]

Indications and Limitations

Porcelain veneers may be used to modify a tooth's color, shape, length, or alignment, to close space, and to restore fractured and endodontically treated teeth (see Fig 21-25). The patient should be informed, however, of the possible morbidity associated with a specific indication, as well as the generally accepted limitations. Informed consent should include, but not be limited to, the following possible complications: (1) postoperative sensitivity; (2) marginal discoloration; (3) fracture; (4) debonding; and (5) wear of opposing teeth.

Treatment Planning

The patient's self-image must be considered during the initial patient interview.[15] A key element in the diagnostic phase is a clarification of the patient's expectations. If it can be determined initially that the patient's expectations are unrealistic, future grief may be avoided.

Assessment of the Face

When a treatment plan is being developed that includes restoration of teeth in the esthetic zone, attention must be directed not only to the shape and color of the teeth, but to the shape of the face, the lips, the maxillary and mandibular lip lines, and the skin color. The teeth can be used to accentuate a positive feature or de-emphasize a negative feature. For example, a patient with a narrow face may desire longer and narrower teeth to emphasize the facial shape or shorter, rounded teeth to soften the narrowness of the face.

It is also important to evaluate skin color, especially if there is a possibility that it will change over time. For example, if porcelain veneers are being planned for a white patient with a dark tan, a determination must be made regarding the longevity of the tan prior to shade selection. If the dark tan is transient and skin color will revert to a lighter tone, this will significantly affect the decision on the color of the porcelain veneers. Veneers that appear to be bright and high in value against the tan skin will look more yellow and lower in value as the skin tone becomes lighter. All of these parameters must be consciously considered during the diagnostic phase if consistently excellent results are to be obtained.

Assessment of the Smile

After the facial features have been considered, attention must be directed to the smile and its components. During the initial interview, the dentist should pay

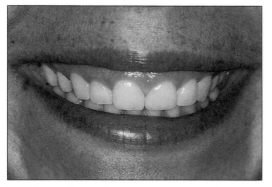

Fig 16-4a Short clinical crowns resulting from excess gingival coverage.

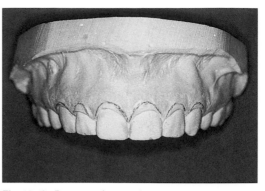

Fig 16-4b Preoperative study cast with lines drawn to aid in the fabrication of a diagnostic composite overlay.

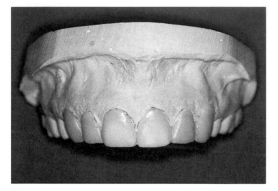

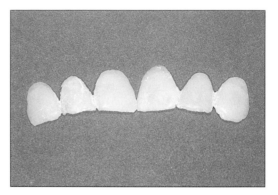

Figs 16-4c and 16-4d Diagnostic composite overlay.

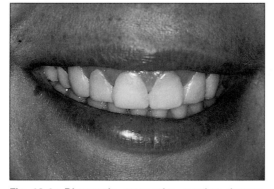

Fig 16-4e Diagnostic composite overlay demonstrating the benefit of crown lengthening of the anterior teeth.

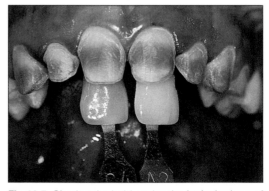

Fig 16-5 Shade tabs held under the incisal edges of the prepared teeth. Preparations of tetracycline-stained teeth are routinely extended interproximally through the contact area. In this patient, more interproximal tooth structure was removed because of existing Class 3 restorations.

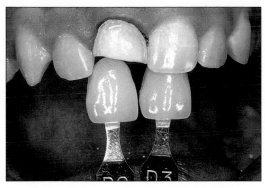

Fig 16-6a Preparation of a single fractured central incisor for a porcelain veneer with shade tabs for laboratory communication.

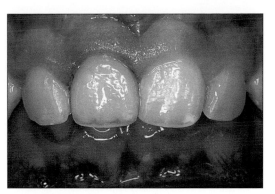

Fig 16-6b Single veneer on the right central incisor immediately after placement. (Porcelain veneer created by Steve McGowan, CDT, Arcus Laboratory.)

Photographs

Preoperative photographs offer another important diagnostic aid. These serve to document the preoperative condition and aid the technician in the fabrication of the veneers. The series should include a full-face smile, a retracted frontal image of maxillary and mandibular teeth in occlusion, a retracted frontal view with a shade tab held directly beneath the incisal edges of the maxillary incisors, a retracted close-up view of the teeth to be veneered, with and without a shade tab, and a postpreparation view of the teeth to be veneered, with a shade tab (Fig 16-5). In addition, other photographs, such as a profile or a view of the intraoral diagnostic mock-up, should be included if they can benefit the laboratory technician.

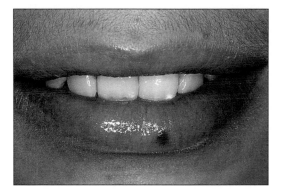

Fig 16-6c Final porcelain veneer restoration of the right central incisor.

Single Veneer

Perhaps the most difficult procedure in esthetic restorative dentistry is to perfectly match a full-coverage restoration to an adjacent natural central incisor. Commonly, the porcelain veneer is the restoration of choice in this situation. If the tooth to be restored is not significantly discolored, the porcelain veneer is an excellent restorative option. The major advantage of the single porcelain veneer restoration is the dentist's ability to increase or decrease the value of the restoration with the bonding resin cement (Figs 16-6a to 16-6c).

Multiple Veneers

When the clinician has the option of veneering multiple anterior teeth, the problem of shade matching is minimized. It is easier to deal in even numbers when veneers are placed on anterior teeth. It is much simpler to veneer two central incisors than to attempt to match a veneer to a natural tooth. Therefore, the chances of obtaining an optimally esthetic result are enhanced when two, four, six, or eight veneers are placed.

An option that is commonly chosen is the placement of six veneers from canine to canine. In Fig 16-7, the anterior teeth are brighter and bolder, while the buccal corridor appears to become darker. This accentuates the anterior teeth and commonly creates the unpleasant illusion that the anterior teeth are larger and longer as well as brighter. This does not usually occur when only the four incisors are veneered (Figs 16-8a and 16-8b). Therefore, when veneers are planned for the incisors, but there is no esthetic or functional requirement for canine veneers, the esthetic result is enhanced when the canines are left unrestored. However, when all six anterior teeth require

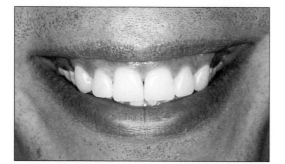

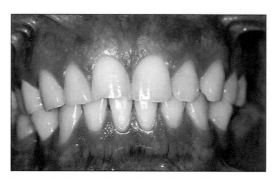

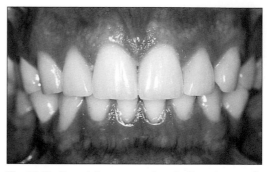

Fig 16-7 Porcelain veneers bonded on all maxillary anterior teeth. Note the apparent separation of anterior and posterior segments of the mouth because of the boldness of the porcelain veneers. (From Robbins.[21])

Fig 16-8a Preoperative view of maxillary central and lateral incisors.

Fig 16-8b Porcelain veneers bonded on the maxillary central and lateral incisors to blend esthetically with the maxillary canines. (Porcelain veneers created by Gilbert Young, CDT, GNS Dental Laboratory.)

veneers, consideration should be given to veneering one or more posterior teeth on each side, depending on the posterior extent of the smile and the maxillary arch form.

Tooth Preparation

The preparation of teeth for porcelain veneers is usually uncomplicated when the basic principles are understood and followed. The amount of tooth structure removed during preparation is determined by the position of the tooth in the arch and the color of the tooth. If the tooth is facioverted, more tooth structure will be removed so that the final restoration will have the correct facial contours. If the tooth is linguoverted, very little preparation is required other than a peripheral finish line. In a routine preparation, the facial enamel is reduced approximately 0.3 to 0.5 mm (Fig 16-9). This can be accomplished with depth

cut burs, which are available from several manufacturers (Fig 16-10). After the depth cuts are made, the enamel is uniformly removed with a round-ended, tapered diamond. However, if the underlying tooth color is dark, the preparation must be deepened to allow for increased porcelain thickness. With darker tetracycline-stained teeth, the preparation should be approximately 0.7 mm deep in the area of the stain.

Anterior Teeth

Gingival Finish Lines

When preparing teeth for porcelain veneers, it is essential to remember that the strongest and most predictable bond is to enamel. The more dentin that is exposed during the preparation, the poorer the bond of the veneer and the poorer the ultimate stress distribution during function.[27] For maxillary porcelain veneers, the gingival margin of the veneer should be routinely placed at the gingival crest or slightly subgingivally. A primary goal of the preparation is to

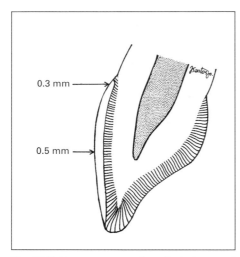

Fig 16-9 Veneer preparation that does not cover the incisal edge of the maxillary anterior tooth.

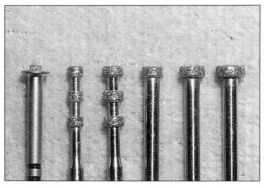

Fig 16-10 Depth cut burs of different designs and depths.

have all margins on sound enamel, because the stress distribution in the veneer is much improved when all margins are bonded to enamel. The amount of exposed dentin in the central portion of the veneer preparation becomes much less important when all of the margins are bonded to enamel.[27] Because the enamel is only approximately 0.3 mm thick 0.5 mm from the cementoenamel junction,[5] it is difficult to obtain adequate preparation depth while preserving the enamel. This commonly results in an overcontoured veneer,[17] which may act as a coetiologic factor in marginal inflammation. Therefore, unless the teeth to be veneered are dark (low value), the gingival preparation should not routinely extend more than minimally into the gingival sulcus.

When mandibular anterior teeth are prepared for porcelain veneers, the considerations are different from those for maxillary teeth. In most patients, the gingival half of the mandibular incisors remains covered by the lower lip at all times, resulting in no esthetic display. In addition, the marginal gingiva of the mandibular anterior teeth is commonly thin, and the gingival sulcus is narrow and shallow, making the placement of gingival retraction cord very difficult. For these reasons, the gingival margin of the preparation for mandibular anterior teeth is ideally placed at least 1.0 mm incisal to the marginal gingiva (see Fig 16-23a).

Interproximal Contact Area

For the purposes of veneer fabrication and placement, it is important that the preparation not be finished in the interproximal contact area. When the margin is stopped in the interproximal contact area, it is difficult to accurately capture the margin in the final impression. Additionally, veneer fabrication is more difficult for the laboratory technician, and bonding and finishing procedures are more difficult for the dentist. For these reasons, the preparation must either stop facial to the interproximal contact area (Fig 16-11a) or extend completely through the contact area to the lingual surface (Fig 16-11b).

The major long-term problem with porcelain veneers is marginal staining.[18,25] This staining is most apparent at the proximal margins. Therefore, the current trend is to extend the preparation through the interproximal contacts from the mesial aspect of the canine to the mesial aspect of the contralateral canine. (There is no esthetic need to extend the preparation through the contact areas on the distal surfaces of the canine teeth.) In this way, any proximal marginal staining is concealed. With dark teeth (eg, tetracycline-stained teeth), it is imperative that the preparation extend completely through the interproximal contact area to the lingual surface (see Fig 16-5). This decreases the risk of a dark shadow appearing around the periphery of the veneers.

Incisal Edge

There is ongoing debate regarding the need to cover the incisal edge of a maxillary tooth with the porcelain veneer. If there is no esthetic requirement to change the incisal shape or length, and there is adequate remaining incisal tooth structure after facial re-

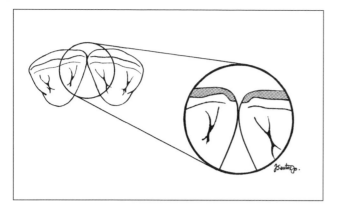

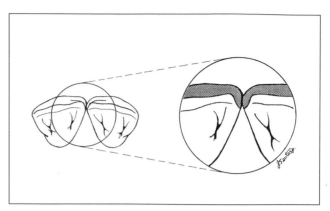

Fig 16-11a Preparation extending slightly facial to the interproximal contact area.

Fig 16-11b Preparation extending completely through the interproximal contact area to the palatal surface.

duction, the incisal margin may be terminated at the facioincisal line angle (see Fig 16-9). This preparation is most commonly indicated for linguoverted teeth. An alternative is the "window preparation" (Fig 16-12). This preparation provides the most protection for the veneer during function; however, it results in a visible composite-veneer interface at the facioincisal margin. This preparation is most commonly indicated for the maxillary canine that has the correct length and incisal edge configuration and has a large lingual wear facet from the gingival margin to the incisal edge. Because it is preferable not to place a veneer margin in a wear facet, the window preparation is appropriate. Neither of these preparations can be used, however, when the tooth is being lengthened incisally with the porcelain veneer.

When the maxillary incisal edge is not reduced during the preparation, the veneer is inevitably thicker, and the incisal edge is too round buccolingually, lacking a more natural, sharp facioincisal line angle. Additionally, veneers that do not cover the incisal edge are significantly more difficult to orient correctly during bonding.

Therefore, the most universally applicable preparation, which allows the technician to incorporate the natural incisal translucency into the veneer, requires incisal edge reduction. If the incisal edge of the maxillary tooth is to be covered with the veneer, there must be room for at least 1.0 mm of porcelain over the incisal edge. However, a 2-mm incisal edge reduction (Fig 16-13) allows the laboratory technician to provide maximum esthetics in the incisal third of the veneer. The incisal edge should be flattened, leaving a butt margin on the lingual surface.[4,16] It is important to round the sharp incisofacial line angle of the preparation to prevent stress concentration in the bonded

veneer. The proximal portion of the preparation should follow the papilla and extend slightly under the interproximal contact to ensure coverage of the tooth in this area (Fig 16-14). This extension is termed the "elbow preparation." If the tooth is not prepared in this manner, the darker, unprepared triangle of natural tooth structure results in less than optimal esthetics.

The incisal edges of mandibular anterior teeth should be routinely covered with porcelain of at least 1.5 to 2.0 mm thickness (Fig 16-15). Incisal edge flattening with a resultant lingual butt margin is also recommended for mandibular anterior teeth. Again, the incisofacial line angle of the preparation must be rounded.

When multiple teeth are being prepared, incisal reduction should be symmetrical (eg, both prepared lateral incisors should be the same length) for more uniform esthetics in the final restorations. After completion of all veneer preparations, the dentist should retract the patient's lips and confirm that the preparations are symmetrical and parallel to the horizon.

Overlapping Teeth

When overlapping teeth are being prepared, the paths of insertion of the veneers must be considered. Where there is significant malalignment of the teeth, it is usually impossible to develop paths of insertion for the veneers without extending the preparations completely through the interproximal contact areas.

Space Closure

Preparation of teeth for space closure presents a unique situation. To obtain smooth lingual contours, the proximal finish lines adjacent to the space must be made more lingual. The wider the space to be closed,

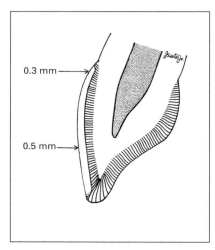

Fig 16-12 Window preparation on a maxillary anterior tooth.

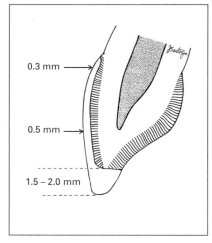

Fig 16-13 Standard veneer preparation for maxillary anterior teeth. Incisal reduction is 1.5 to 2.0 mm.

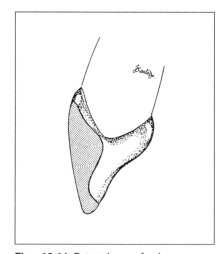

Fig 16-14 Extension of the veneer preparation into the subcontact area for improved esthetics.

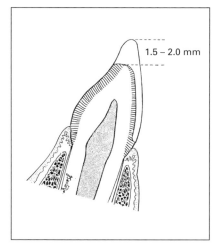

Fig 16-15 Veneer preparation on a mandibular incisor. There is at least 1.5 to 2.0 mm of incisal reduction, and the gingival margin is at least 1.0 mm incisal to the gingival crest.

the more lingually the tooth must be prepared (Figs 16-16a and 16-16b). Also, the proximal margins adjacent to the space must be made subgingivally so that the gingival contours of the veneers minimize the black triangle between the bottom of the interproximal contact area and the tip of the papilla. However, the gingival margin of the veneer should be no closer than 2.5 mm from the crest of the alveolar bone.[13]

Premolars

The considerations for preparing maxillary premolars are similar to those for anterior teeth. The ve-

neer preparation of the maxillary premolar may end on the facial surface of the tooth if the functional and esthetic requirements are met (Fig 16-17). Ideally, the occlusal margin should be placed so that it is not in an occlusal contact area and so that the opposing cusp does not function across it. If the anterior guidance immediately discludes the posterior teeth, the occlusal margin can be placed anywhere on the lingual incline of the buccal cusp, as long as there is no occlusal stop directly on the margin (Fig 16-18). However, when group function occlusion is present, it may be necessary to extend the occlusal margin to the central groove. In this circumstance, occlusal reduction must be adequate to allow for an

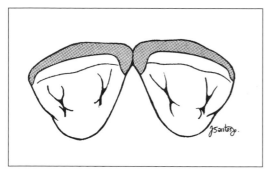

Fig 16-16a Porcelain veneer preparations for closing a small-to-moderate diastema.

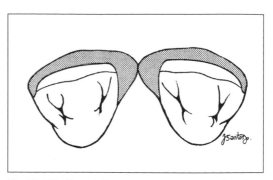

Fig 16-16b Porcelain veneer preparations for closing a large diastema. The preparations extend to the midpalatal surfaces of the central incisors to develop adequate lingual contours.

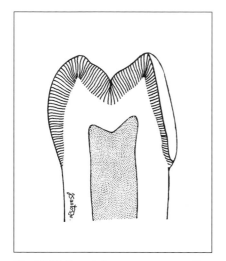

Fig 16-17 Porcelain veneer preparation that does not cover the buccal cusp of the maxillary premolar.

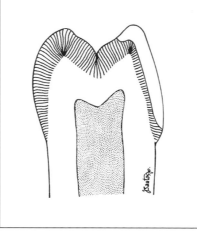

Fig 16-18 Veneer preparation overlapping the buccal cusp. There should be no occlusal stop directly on the veneer margin.

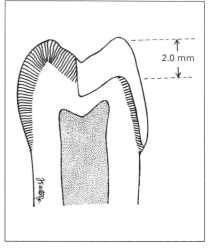

2.0 mm

Fig 16-19 Porcelain veneer preparation that covers the buccal cusp of the maxillary premolar. Note the 2.0 mm of occlusal reduction on the buccal cusp.

onlay of at least a 2-mm thickness over the buccal cusp, blending to the 0.3- to 0.5-mm reduction of the facial surface (Fig 16-19). In mandibular premolars, because the esthetic cusp is also the functional cusp, the tooth must generally be prepared for a porcelain onlay rather than simply for a buccal porcelain veneer (see Chapter 18).

Existing Restorations

Existing resin composite restorations can complicate the veneer preparation. Ideally, no margins should be finished on an existing resin composite restoration. One clinical study reported a significantly higher failure rate for porcelain veneers placed over existing resin composite restorations.[24] The resin composite restoration should be removed during tooth preparation for the veneer, and the missing tooth structure should be replaced as part of the porcelain veneer[2] (Figs 16-20a to 16-20c). Small areas of resin composite can remain centrally in the preparation to serve as an undercut block-out material.

Fractured Incisal Edge

A unique indication for the porcelain veneer is the restoration of the fractured incisal edge of an incisor (Figs 16-21a to 16-21c). Although there are few clinical data to support this use of veneers, the laboratory data[2] are favorable. The limits for the amount of

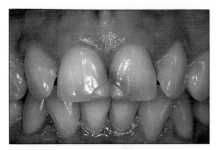

Fig 16-20a Maxillary central incisors with large Class 4 resin composite restorations.

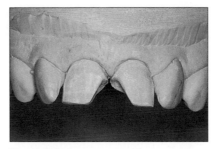

Fig 16-20b Stone cast with preparations of the maxillary central incisors for porcelain veneers. The resin composite is removed, and the missing tooth structure is replaced with the porcelain veneers.

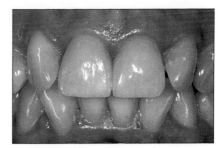

Fig 16-20c Porcelain veneer restorations on maxillary central incisors. (Porcelain veneers created by Steve McGowan, CDT, Arcus Laboratory.)

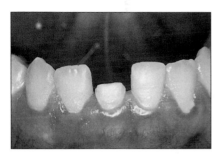

Fig 16-21a Fractured mandibular right central incisor.

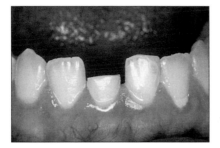

Fig 16-21b Preparation of the fractured mandibular right central incisor for a porcelain veneer.

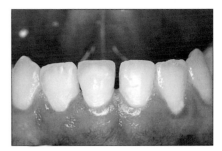

Fig 16-21c Porcelain veneer bonded on the mandibular right central incisor.

missing tooth structure that can be replaced with a porcelain veneer are not known. However, anecdotal evidence seems to indicate that approximately 50% of the clinical crown can be replaced with a porcelain veneer when the preparation on the remaining tooth structure is in enamel. Because the veneered tooth does not require endodontic treatment for restorative reasons or the placement of a post and core, it is a highly desirable alternative to previous methods of restoring the fractured tooth. The preparation for this type of veneer extends to near the gingival crest on both the facial and lingual surfaces.

Noncarious Cervical Lesion

Noncarious cervical lesions due to erosion, abrasion, and/or abfraction provide a poor substrate for bonding due to the sclerotic nature of the dentin.[3,10] Therefore, the best treatment solution is to surgically cover these areas with connective tissue grafting.[1] This results in more natural gingival architecture and allows the gingi-

val margin of the veneer preparation to end on enamel. However, if the surgical option is not chosen, and the esthetic demands require that the root be covered with a veneer, the preparation must extend onto the root surface. In this situation, a dentin bonding agent must be used in the bonding process. In addition, the patient should be advised that the risks of staining, microleakage, and/or veneer fracture in the gingival third are much greater due to the poor bonding substrate.[27]

Impressions

When an impression is made of the maxillary teeth, retraction cord is placed to expose all gingival margins. This step is generally not necessary with mandibular teeth because the preparations are at least 1.0 mm incisal to the marginal gingiva. An accurate impression material, such as polyvinyl siloxane, polyether, or reversible hydrocolloid, is then used to make the final impression.

Provisional Restorations

The placement of provisional restorations over veneer preparations is an integral step in the predictable placement of porcelain veneers. Provisional restorations not only improve interim esthetics and decrease sensitivity but provide essential diagnostic information, including veneer color, shape, length, and incisal edge configuration, that can be obtained in no other way. When provisional restorations are being placed on one or two teeth, the procedure is best accomplished with freehand placement of composite. A small area in the incisal third of each tooth is etched with phosphoric acid for 15 seconds, washed, and dried. Adhesive is placed over the entire preparation and light cured. A large increment of resin composite is then patted into place with correct contours, the gingival margins are smoothed with an explorer tip, and the provisional restoration is light cured. There should be no overhanging resin composite at the margins, and the provisional restoration should require virtually no adjustment.

When provisional restorations are being placed on multiple teeth, it is preferable to use a clear matrix made on a preoperative diagnostic cast. A diagnostic waxup is commonly required to change tooth length, alignment, and/or incisal edge configuration (Figs 16-22a and 16-22b). The diagnostic waxup is duplicated, and the clear matrix is fabricated (Fig 16-22c). The clear matrix may be made of a plastic stent material or a clear polyvinyl siloxane bite-registration material. The teeth are spot etched with 30% to 40% phosphoric acid in the incisal third (Fig 16-22d), washed, and air dried. The entire preparation is covered with adhesive, which is then light cured (Fig 16-22e). The facial and incisal areas in the clear matrix are filled with resin composite (Fig 16-22f), and the matrix is placed over the prepared teeth (Fig 16-22g). The gingival two thirds of the matrix is shielded from the polymerization light, and the incisal one third is polymerized with the light for 10 seconds per tooth (Fig 16-22h). The gingival two thirds is then lightly cured for 0.5 to 1 second per tooth (Fig 16-22i). The matrix is gently teased away from the tooth at the gingival margin to ensure that the resin composite does not stick to the matrix (Fig 16-22j). If the resin composite sticks to the matrix, the matrix is returned to place and the gingival two thirds is polymerized again for 0.5 second per tooth. The matrix is removed, and the excess partially cured resin composite is first removed proximally and lingually with a No. 12 scalpel blade (Fig 16-22k). Floss and a floss threader are then used

in each gingival embrasure to ensure patency and to ensure that there are no overhangs (Fig 16-22l). The gingival margins are then carved with the No. 12 scalpel blade. If small areas of resin composite are chipped during the finishing process, adding additional resin composite easily repairs these areas. The incisal and facial embrasures are opened with a thin separating disk (Fig 16-22m), the occlusion is adjusted, and the provisional restorations are smoothed and polished (Figs 16-22n to 16-22p). Finally, the provisional restorations are coated with an adhesive (Fig 16-22q), and the entire restoration is light cured for 30 seconds per tooth (Figs 16-22r and 16-22s).

At the appointment for placement of the definitive veneers, the provisional restorations are removed, and the resin composite over the small area of etched enamel in the incisal third of the facial surface is lightly removed with a diamond bur, cutting dry. If water is used, it is very difficult to determine the interface between the provisional composite and the tooth structure. The remaining resin composite is flicked off with a spoon excavator. If a veneer does not go to place during the try-in, there is probably resin composite from the provisional restoration remaining in the etched area. The preparation should be closely inspected to ensure that all the resin composite has been removed.

Alternatively, the provisional restoration may be made in the laboratory. After the veneer preparations are completed, an impression is made and poured in fast-setting die stone (Snap Stone, Whipmix). The cast is separated from the impression in 5 minutes and covered with a separating medium; the provisional restoration is constructed with the same matrix technique as previously described. The provisional restoration, which is constructed from either acrylic or resin composite, can then be cemented with polycarboxylate cement or temporarily bonded with a resin composite as previously described (Figs 16-23a to 16-23d).

Placement

The anatomy of a porcelain veneer is illustrated in Fig 16-24. The inner surface of the veneer must be etched with hydrofluoric acid. This step is usually accomplished in the laboratory. (For a detailed description of the steps in veneer placement, see Procedures for Porcelain Veneers, page 448). The veneers are first tried in individually for marginal fit. They are then

Figs 16-22a to 16-22s Fabrication of provisional restorations.

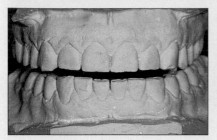

Fig 16-22a Preoperative casts.

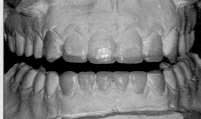

Fig 16-22b Diagnostic waxup.

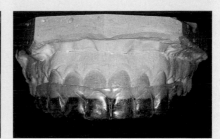

Fig 16-22c Clear stent made from duplicate cast of diagnostic waxup.

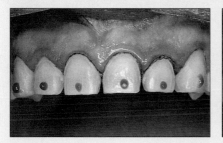

Fig 16-22d Prepared teeth are spot etched with 30% phosphoric acid on the incisal third.

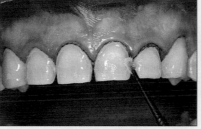

Fig 16-22e The entire surface of each prepared tooth is coated with resin adhesive and light cured.

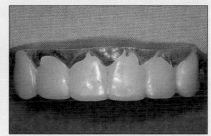

Fig 16-22f The facial and incisal areas of the clear matrix are filled with resin composite.

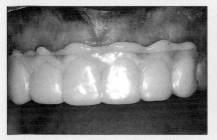

Fig 16-22g The filled matrix is placed over the prepared teeth.

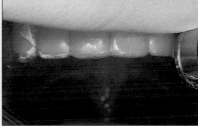

Fig 16-22h The gingival two thirds of the matrix is covered with a finger, while the incisal third is light cured for 10 seconds per tooth.

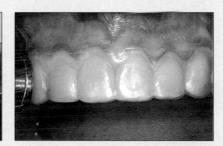

Fig 16-22i The gingival two thirds is lightly cured for 0.5 to 1 second per tooth.

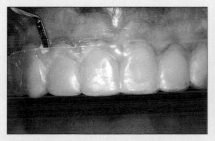

Fig 16-22j The matrix is gently teased away from the preparations to ensure that the resin composite does not stick to the matrix.

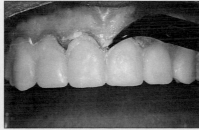

Fig 16-22k A No. 12 scalpel blade is used to remove the partially cured resin composite from proximal and lingual surfaces.

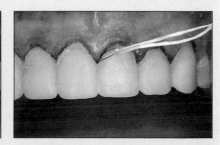

Fig 16-22l Floss and a floss threader are used in each gingival embrasure to ensure patency and overhang-free margins.

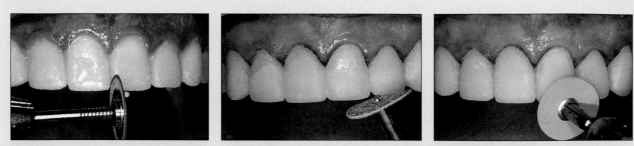

Fig 16-22m Facial and incisal embrasures are refined with a thin diamond disk.

Figs 16-22n and 16-22o A series of composite finishing disks are used to finish the facial surfaces.

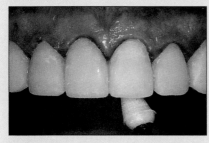
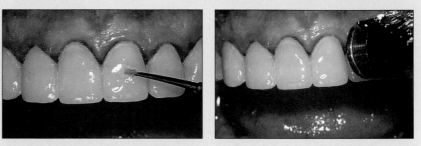

Fig 16-22p A composite polishing point is used to smooth and polish the lingual surfaces.

Figs 16-22q and 16-22r The facial surfaces of the provisional restorations are coated with an adhesive resin and light cured.

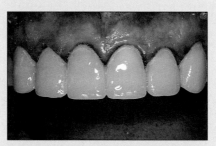

Fig 16-22s Completed provisional restorations.

tried in together to ensure that interproximal contacts are correct. Finally, one veneer (or more) is filled with resin composite luting cement or try-in paste and taken to the mouth for the color try-in. The value of the veneer is almost always lower with the try-in resin or paste, because the natural color of the underlying tooth is transmitted through the veneer to the surface. If the color is acceptable to the patient, the dentist proceeds with the bonding procedure as outlined in Procedures for Porcelain Veneers.

There are many resin luting cement kits available with differing degrees of translucency and viscosity (Figs 16-25a and 16-25b). Translucent cements are indicated as the standard material for veneer bonding. The more opaque cements tend to block the natural

tooth color, resulting in a less natural veneer. The opaque cements are more commonly used to help block the darkness of discolored teeth. However, the use of these cements can result in a monochromatic appearance and an opaque line at the thin gingival margin of the veneer (Figs 16-26a and 16-26b). It is preferable to block the darkness of discolored teeth with a layer of masking dentin, and/or with porcelain modifiers, in the body of the veneer rather than with opaque cement (Fig 16-27).

The second major difference in veneer luting cements is their viscosity. Initially, most resin cements had a low viscosity so that the veneers could be placed with minimal pressure, thereby decreasing the risk of fracture. However, the low-viscosity resins

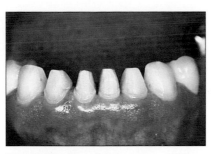

Fig 16-23a Porcelain veneer preparations on the mandibular anterior teeth. The gingival margins are located 1.0 mm above the gingival crests.

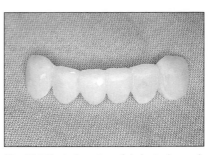

Fig 16-23b Laboratory-fabricated provisional restoration.

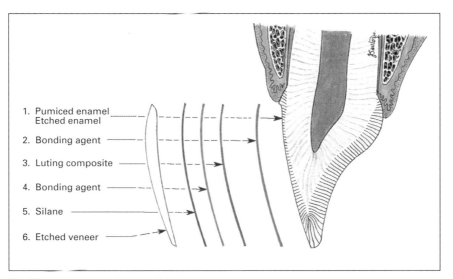

Figs 16-23c and 16-23d Provisional restoration in place.

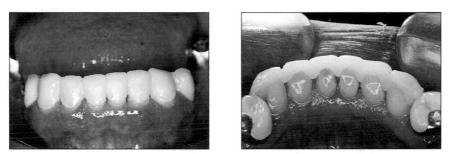

1. Pumiced enamel
   Etched enamel
2. Bonding agent
3. Luting composite
4. Bonding agent
5. Silane
6. Etched veneer

Fig 16-24 Anatomy of a porcelain veneer.

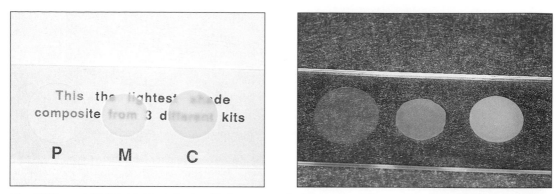

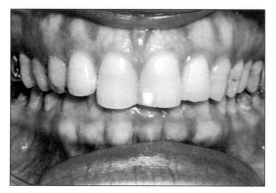

Figs 16-25a and 16-25b Lightest shade of luting composite from three different kits placed between two glass slides. The same materials are shown against two different backgrounds. Note the differences in translucency. (Fig 16-25a from Robbins.[21])

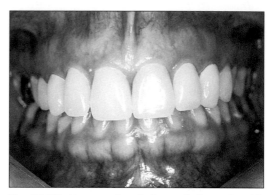

Fig 16-26a Moderately dark, tetracycline-stained teeth prior to veneer preparation.

Fig 16-26b Veneers bonded on dark teeth with opaque resin cement. Note the opaque gingival margins on the right and left canines.

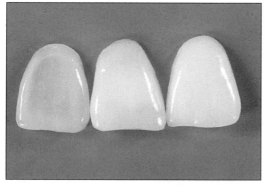

Fig 16-27 Veneers displaying different amounts of translucency. The left veneer is made from a very translucent porcelain and allows most of the underlying tooth color to show through. The center veneer has a base layer of masking dentin porcelain, which is used to block dark underlying tooth color yet maintain some degree of polychromicity. The right veneer has a layer of opaque resin cement bonded to the inner surface of the veneer. The opaque resin is very reflective and results in a displeasing, monochromatic appearance.

have some disadvantages: *(1)* Because of their honey-like consistency, it is more difficult to ensure correct veneer placement, especially when the veneers have no positive stop, ie, no incisal overlap; *(2)* cleanup of excess resin is more difficult; and *(3)* at least theoretically, the physical properties are compromised because of the increased proportion of resin matrix. The major indication for the low-viscosity luting resin is the all-ceramic crown or a veneer that covers most of the tooth surfaces. Because of friction, high-viscosity luting resins will not allow complete seating of these restorations. Recently, interest in the higher viscosity luting resins has increased because they overcome most of the disadvantages of the low-viscosity luting resins.

Friedman[7] has described a technique for using the highly filled resin composite from a standard restorative resin composite kit. The material is brought to room temperature and placed into the veneer in a thin layer through a ribbon tip. The thixotropic properties

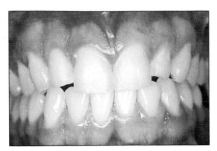

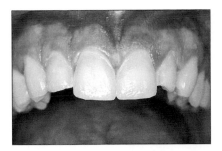

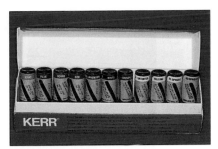

Fig 16-28a Veneer preparations on the maxillary central and lateral incisors. (From Robbins.[20])

Fig 16-28b Placement of yellow resin tint in the gingival third and blue resin tint in the incisal third. (From Robbins.[20])

Fig 16-28c Kit of resin tints and opaques. (From Robbins.[20])

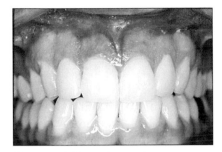

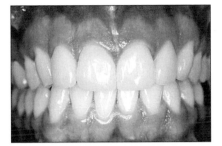

Fig 16-28d Monochromatic appearance of veneers tried in with try-in paste but without the use of resin tints. (From Robbins.[20])

Fig 16-28e Polychromatic appearance of bonded veneers after the placement of resin tints. (From Robbins.[20])

of the resin composite allow the highly filled material to flow under moderate seating pressure. However, placing the ampule of composite in a hot water bath (160°F) before ejecting the composite is a more effective method of improving the flow characteristics of the resin composite. With this technique, the seating of the veneers can be more accurately controlled, and cleanup is simplified (see Procedures for Porcelain Veneers, page 448).

Color Management and Characterization

A common problem with the porcelain veneer is the lack of color differentiation between the gingival and incisal portions of the restoration. Several methods of color characterization can be used to correct the monochromism.[19–21] The best and most basic method makes the color changes in the porcelain itself. A color diagram that outlines the desired shade and color changes and any other special characterization, such as hypocalcified or hyperchromatic areas, can be

given to the technician. However, the most effective method of communicating color to the laboratory technician is with photographs or slides (see Fig 16-6a). When characterization is incorporated into the veneer, it is there to stay. If the esthetic result is not satisfactory during the try-in, it is difficult, if not impossible, to successfully modify the veneer.

A second commonly used method involves the modification of the color with the underlying luting composite. All porcelain veneer kits have several different shades of luting composite. If an appropriate shade of luting cement is not available, resin tints can be added to the luting composite to effect virtually any desired color of luting cement.

A third and less commonly used method of characterization involves the direct placement of the resin tints on the tooth before placement of the veneer (Figs 16-28a to 16-28e). During the try-in, the desired resin tints are placed on the tooth and light cured. The chosen base shade of luting composite is placed in the veneer, and the veneer is placed on the tooth. A determination is then made regarding the esthetic result. The veneer can be removed, and the cured resin tint on the tooth can be easily scraped off with an explorer, be-

placed in the base of the pulp chamber to protect the cervix from bleach. A paste mixture of sodium perborate and water is placed in the pulp chamber, which is sealed with a temporary cement for 3 to 5 days. This can be repeated for several treatments until the desired result is attained. The mixture is ultimately removed, and the access area is restored with a resin composite restoration. At this point, the tooth is prepared for the porcelain veneer restoration. If the darkness returns in future years, the walking bleach can be accomplished again through the lingual access without disturbing the porcelain veneer restoration.

The success of bleaching vital teeth before veneer placement is not as clear-cut. It is known that vital teeth that have been bleached have the potential to revert toward their original color with time.[9] However, the effect that the placement of porcelain veneers has on this relapse is not known. If color relapse does occur, the veneer restorations will also get darker. There has been some success in bleaching teeth that have veneers bonded to them (see Chapter 15).

Bleaching teeth with 35% hydrogen peroxide[26] or carbamide peroxide[8] immediately before the bonding procedure has a catastrophic effect on the resultant bond strength. Any bonding procedure should be delayed at least 1 week after the completion of bleaching. It is hoped that future research will clarify the effects of bleaching on the success of porcelain veneers.

Crown and Veneer Combinations

When a combination of veneers and crowns is placed, all restorations must be tried in individually and then simultaneously for fit. They must also be tried in for color evaluation with a try-in medium. The final color of the veneers may be modified with the choice of the resin cement. For this reason, the full crowns are bonded first, because it is easier to make minor modifications in the color of the veneers, with the veneer luting resin, to match the crowns than to surface stain the all-ceramic crowns to match the bonded veneers.

Failure

On rare occasions, a porcelain veneer will debond. When this happens, it is important to determine at which bonded interface the failure occurred. If the luting composite remains on the tooth, the failure is likely due to either inadequate etching of the veneer or the use of old silane. The stated shelf life of silane is approximately 1 year when it is refrigerated, but it is known that silane efficacy decreases with time.

If the luting composite remains on the inside of the veneer, then there was a problem with either the bonding materials, the placement technique, or the bonding substrate. Veneers that are bonded to a predominantly dentin substrate have a significantly greater likelihood of debonding than veneers that are predominantly bonded to enamel.[27]

When the luting composite remains on the inner surface of the veneer, it must be removed before the veneer can be rebonded. The veneer is placed in a glazing oven, and the temperature is slowly increased to 600°C and held for 10 minutes to ensure burnout of the luting composite. After the veneer is removed from the oven and cooled to room temperature, it is cleaned with acetone and re-etched with 9.5% hydrofluoric acid for 4 minutes. If 9.5% hydrofluoric acid is not available, 1.23% acidulated phosphate fluoride can be used to etch the porcelain; however, this requires a 10-minute etching time. The veneer is then washed, dried, silanated,[11] and rebonded. The patient must know that there is a significant risk of veneer fracture during removal of the luting composite.

A small percentage of veneers will fracture.[14,18,24] It is possible to repair fractured porcelain. First, the porcelain fracture site is etched with 9.5% hydrofluoric acid for 4 minutes. After the veneer is washed and dried, silane is placed and dried. The repair is then accomplished with conventional bonded resin composite. Because the hydrofluoric acid should not be allowed to contact natural tooth structure or soft tissue, this etching procedure should be performed with rubber dam isolation. Alternatively, the porcelain can be prepared with 1.23% acidulated phosphate fluoride or by air abrasion with 50-μm aluminum oxide.

The most common cause of failure of porcelain veneers is marginal staining and leakage.[18,25] If the marginal stain is superficial, it can be removed by tray bleaching with 10% carbamide peroxide for several days. After the stain has been removed, the margin can be etched with 30% phosphoric acid and rebonded with a dentin bonding agent. If the stain is slightly penetrating at the margin (Fig 16-32), it can be mechanically removed with a small bur and the area restored with conventional bonded resin composite. When there is significant penetration of stain under the veneer, the entire veneer must be removed (Fig 16-33).

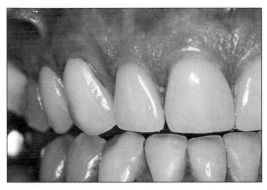

Fig 16-32 Minimally penetrating stain at the mesial margin of the maxillary right canine.

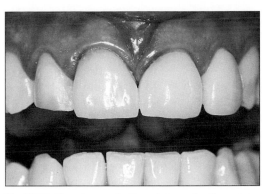

Fig 16-33 Deeply penetrating stain under the porcelain veneer on the right central incisor.

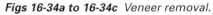

Figs 16-34a to 16-34c Veneer removal.

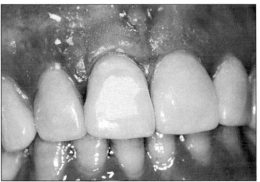

Fig 16-34a Initial removal of porcelain before tooth structure is reached.

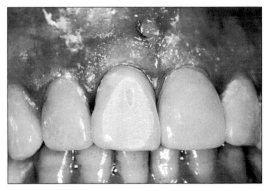

Fig 16-34b Porcelain removed until the first area of enamel is visualized.

Veneer Removal

Removal of porcelain veneers is not only time-consuming, but difficult and technique sensitive, especially if the underlying tooth color is light. The veneer cannot be grooved with a bur and torqued in the same manner that a cemented gold crown is removed. The veneer must be removed with a diamond bur in the same way that enamel is removed during initial tooth preparation.

The dentist starts removing the porcelain in the midfacial area with a back-and-forth sweeping motion with a barrel diamond (Fig 16-34a). This must be done without water spray so that the operator can visualize the subtle color difference between the veneer and the tooth as the interface is reached. Therefore, the dental assistant must cool the tooth with a constant stream of air. Once this interface is apparent (Fig 16-34b), the diamond bur is moved laterally away from the area of exposed enamel toward the periphery of the preparation. Care must be taken to remove as little enamel as possible during this step.

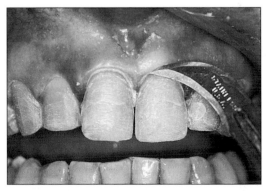

Fig 16-34c Exploring margins with a No. 12 scalpel blade to remove remaining composite and porcelain.

The procedure continues until only a small amount of porcelain remains at the margins. If there has been microleakage at the margins, the remaining marginal porcelain can be removed with a No. 12 scalpel blade. However, if the marginal seal is intact, the remainder of the porcelain must be cautiously removed with the diamond bur.

It is very important that the operator not lose orientation in relation to the porcelain-tooth interface. If this occurs, it is very easy to inadvertently remove all of the enamel. For this reason, one veneer should be completely removed before starting veneer removal on the next tooth.

After all porcelain veneers have been removed, gingival retraction cord is packed to clearly expose all margins. As the final step of veneer removal, all margins are explored with a sharp No. 12 scalpel blade (Fig 16-34c), which commonly results in the removal of additional small areas of residual resin composite and porcelain.

Maintenance

The maintenance of the porcelain veneer restoration is similar to that of the porcelain crown. Devices such as an ultrasonic cleaner, air-abrasive polisher, and prophylaxis cup with pumice must be avoided. Surface stains may be removed from porcelain veneers with aluminum oxide polishing paste or diamond polishing paste on a felt wheel or rubber cup. Proximal stains may be removed with composite polishing strips. When scaling is performed around porcelain veneers, care must be taken not to chip the margins. If a fluoride preparation is needed by the patient, it should have a neutral pH; neither acidulated phosphate fluoride nor stannous fluoride should be used because of their ability to etch porcelain.

The patient should be advised that foods and liquids with a high potential for staining, such as coffee and tea, increase the potential for marginal staining. The patient must also be made aware of the potential for the porcelain to fracture. Activities such as ice chewing and fingernail biting must be absolutely avoided. It is a good idea to make an occlusal guard appliance for all patients who have porcelain veneer restorations. When porcelain veneer restorations will oppose natural teeth or when the patient has a history of a parafunctional habit, a protective appliance should be fabricated to protect both the porcelain veneers and the opposing teeth.

Procedures for Porcelain Veneers

Veneer Try-in

1. Check veneers for fit on dies and transilluminate to check for fracture lines.
2. Try in veneers individually for fit, and then all together. Interproximal contact areas may need to be adjusted with a microfine diamond or disk. Do not make any other adjustments until veneers are bonded.
3. Clean the veneers with acetone. Place silane on the inner surface of each veneer and allow to air dry.
4. Choose a shade of resin composite or water-soluble try-in paste, place on the inside of the veneer, and try in.
5. If water-soluble try-in paste has been used, wash the veneer with water and air dry before loading with the unfilled resin and luting composite. If the shade is correct, skip steps 6 through 13, and proceed with step 14.
6. If the shade is incorrect, remove the try-in composite and select another shade, or customize the shade by adding tint to the luting composite.
7. If characterization (eg, blue in incisal areas, yellow at gingival areas) is required, tints and opaques should be placed only on the tooth and not on the inside of the veneer. The tints and opaques are brushed on the tooth in a thin layer and light cured for 30 seconds. All try-in composite must be removed from the tooth (facial, proximal, and lingual aspects) before curing the tints and opaques. Because the tooth was not etched, the cured tints and opaques can be scraped off easily with an explorer at the end of the try-in.
8. Once a combination of composite, tint, and/or opaque has been determined, note it so that it can be reproduced exactly for final luting.
9. Clean the try-in resin composite from the inside of the veneer with acetone using two different beakers. Clean the bulk of the resin composite with a brush dipped in the first beaker, then transfer the veneer to the second, clean beaker of acetone to remove the remaining resin composite.

Veneer Preparation

10. Place the veneers, etched side down, on a 2 × 2-inch gauze pad in a glass beaker of clean acetone, and place the beaker in an ultrasonic cleaner for 5 minutes.
11. Remove veneers from the acetone and dry.
12. Place silane on the inner surface of the veneers and allow to air dry.
13. Place a thin layer of unfilled resin on the inner surface of all veneers.
14. Place luting composite in the veneers, and cover to protect from light. It is helpful to write the number of each tooth receiving a veneer on a piece of paper and place each veneer on the correct tooth number to avoid placing a veneer on the wrong tooth.

Procedures for Porcelain Veneers (continued)

Tooth Preparation

15. Place retraction cord in the sulcus of each prepared tooth (but not the mandibular incisors if the margins are more than 1.0 mm from the gingival crest).

16. Clean both central incisors with oil-free pumice paste. (This should be done for each tooth just before etching.)

17. Place clear plastic matrix or dead soft metal matrix on the distal aspects of both central incisors.

18. Etch both central incisors with 30% phosphoric acid for 20 seconds, wash for 3 seconds, and air dry to ensure adequate etch of the enamel.

19. Remoisten tooth surface.

20. If using a fourth-generation bonding agent, place several coats of primer and gently air dry until tooth surface is completely dry. Check for uniform shiny surface. If using a fifth-generation bonding agent, place one to two coats and follow manufacturer's instructions for drying and curing.

21. If using a fourth-generation bonding agent, place the dentin adhesive on the tooth surface and the inner surface of the veneer. If using a fifth-generation bonding agent, place the agent on the inner surface of the veneer.

22. If tints or opaques are necessary, place on the predetermined areas and light cure for 90 seconds.

Placement

23. Place light-cured resin composite into each veneer. Operatory light should be turned off at this time.

24. With shimstock (0.0005-inch thickness) between central incisors and clear plastic matrix strips or dead soft metal matrix material on distal aspects of each central incisor, gently place veneers onto both central incisors and tease to place. Ensure that excess resin composite appears at all margins.

25. Remove excess resin composite from veneers with a small brush or explorer, depending on viscosity.

26. Visually inspect, standing in front of the patient to ensure that veneers are placed correctly. Ensure that mesial surfaces are in contact.

27. Lightly press facial surfaces of veneers and light cure from the lingual aspect for 30 seconds; then light cure from the facial aspect for 30 seconds.

28. Remove the excess resin composite only on the distal surfaces of the central incisors with a No. 12 scalpel blade to ensure that the lateral veneers will fit.

29. Visually inspect for voids and repair if possible.

30. Try in the left lateral incisor veneer to ensure correct fit.

31. Repeat steps 16 to 30 for each veneer being placed.

Finishing

32. Remove minimal gingival flash of resin composite with a No. 12 scalpel blade. Move blade from veneer gingivally to avoid chipping the veneer margin. Ensure that all flash is removed on the facial and proximal surfaces.

33. Remove excess resin composite from lingual surfaces with an egg-shaped, 12-fluted carbide bur.

34. Smooth lingual surfaces with Sof-Lex (3M) disks and composite polishing points or disks.

35. Check and adjust occlusion in centric occlusion and in excursions (with special attention to the distal incisal edges of maxillary lateral incisors).

36. Reshape incisal edges and contours while standing in front of the patient.

37. Reshape and contour embrasure surfaces with a finishing diamond or thin separating disk.

38. Gingival margins should be smooth and require no finishing. If gingival margins are rough, smooth them with a finishing diamond or 12-fluted carbide bur. Be careful not to scar cementum.

39. Polish all roughened porcelain with abrasive-impregnated rubber porcelain polishing system (Brasseler or Shofu).

40. Finish proximal areas with finishing and polishing strips.

41. Any visible porcelain that has been finished and smoothed with a rubber point is polished with diamond polishing paste on a wet felt wheel and prophylaxis cup at the gingival margin. Be careful not to polish cementum.

42. With retraction cord still in place, re-etch and re-bond all margins.

43. Remove retraction cord.

44. Have the patient return in 1 week to inspect for excess composite and rough areas. At this time, final esthetic reshaping may be accomplished.

References

1. Allen EP. Use of mucogingival surgical procedures to enhance esthetics. Dent Clin North Am 1988;32:307–330.

2. Andreason FM, Flugge E, Daugaard-Jensen J, Munksgaard EC. Treatment of crown fractured incisors with laminate veneer restorations. An experimental study. Endod Dent Traumatol 1992;8:30–35.

3. Bayne SC, Heymann HO, Wilder AD, et al. One-year clinical study of sclerotic vs. non-sclerotic dentin bonding [abstract 1221]. J Dent Res 1995;74:164.

4. Castelnuovo J, Tjan AHL, Phillips K, et al. Fracture strength and failure mode for different ceramic veneer designs. [abstract 1373]. J Dent Res 1998;77:803.

5. Crispin B. Esthetic moieties. J Esthet Dent 1993;5:37.

6. Fradeani M. Six-year follow-up with Empress veneers. Int J Periodontics Restorative Dent 1998;18:217–225.

7. Friedman M. Multiple potential of etched porcelain laminate veneers. J Am Dent Assoc 1987;122(special issue):83E–87E.

8. Godwin JM, Barghi N, Berry TG, et al. Time duration for dissipation of bleaching effects before enamel bonding [abstract 590]. J Dent Res 1992;71:179.

9. Haywood VB. Nightguard vital bleaching: current concepts and research. J Am Dent Assoc 1997;128(suppl):19s–25s.

10. Heymann HO, Bayne SC. Current concepts in dentin bonding: focusing on dentinal adhesion factors. J Am Dent Assoc 1993;124:27–36.

11. Hsu CS, Stangel I, Nathanson D. Shear bond strength of resin to etched porcelain [abstract 1095]. J Dent Res 1985;64:296.

12. Kihn PW, Barnes DM. The clinical longevity of porcelain veneers. J Am Dent Assoc 1998;129:747–752.

13. Kois JC. The restorative-periodontal interface: biological parameters. Periodontol 2000 1996;11:29–38.

14. Kreulen CM, Creugers NHJ, Meijering AC. Meta-analysis of anterior veneer restorations in clinical studies. J Dent 1998; 26:345–353.

15. Levinson N. Psychological facets of esthetic dental health care: a developmental perspective. J Prosthet Dent 1990;64: 486–491.

16. Magne P, Douglas WH. Design optimization and evolution of bonded ceramics for the anterior dentition: a finite-element analysis. Quintessence Int 1999;30:661–672.

17. Meijering AC, Peters MCRB, DeLong R, et al. Dimensional changes during veneering procedures on discoloured teeth. J Dent 1998;26:569–576.

18. Peumans M, Van Meerbeek B, Lambrechts P, et al. Five-year clinical performance of porcelain veneers. Quintessence Int 1998;29:211–221.

19. Reid JS. Tooth color modification and porcelain veneers. Quintessence Int 1988;19:477–481.

20. Robbins J. Color characterization of porcelain veneers. Quintessence Int 1991;22:853–856.

21. Robbins J. Color management of the porcelain veneer. Esthet Dent Update 1992;3:132–135.

22. Rotstein I, Mor C, Friedman S. Prognosis of intracoronal bleaching with sodium perborate preparation in vitro: 1-year study. J Endod 1993;19(1):10–12.

23. Seghi R, Gritz MD, Kim J. Colorimetric changes in composite resins due to visible light polymerization [abstract 892]. J Dent Res 1988;67:224.

24. Shaini FJ, Shortall ACC, Marquis PM. Clinical performance of porcelain laminate veneers. A retrospective evaluation over a period of 6.5 years. J Oral Rehabil 1997;24:553–559.

25. Strassler HE, Weiner S. Long term clinical evaluation of etched porcelain veneer. [abstract 1017]. J Dent Res 1998; 77:233.

26. Torneck C, Titley K, Smith D, Adibfar A. The influence of time of hydrogen peroxide exposure on the adhesion of composite resin to bleached bovine enamel. J Endod 1990; 16:123–128.

27. Troedson M, Derand T. Shear stresses in the adhesive layer under porcelain veneers—a finite analysis study. Acta Odontol Scand 1998;56:257–262.

28. Van Gogswaardt DC, Van Thoor W, Lampert F. Clinical assessment of adhesively placed ceramic veneers after 9 years [abstract 1178]. J Dent Res 1998;77:779.

Anterior Ceramic Crowns

Jeffrey S. Rouse

The provision of anterior ceramic crowns can be the most valuable and difficult service in dentistry. Protecting the natural dentition and providing an illusion of reality requires the practitioner to choose the correct ceramic system and prepare the site for success. This chapter discusses a systematic approach for selection of the proper ceramic system[115] and development of a foundation for the restoration that enables predictable results.

Decision-Making Factors

There are two common myths pertaining to anterior ceramics: *(1)* strength is the most important decision-making factor, and *(2)* all-ceramic crowns are always more esthetic.

Strength should not be the overriding factor in choosing an anterior ceramic crown system. While it is true that metal-ceramic crowns are stronger than all-ceramic systems, the real question is, how much strength is required? The answer is that the crown must be able to resist fracture under load. Normal incisal bite force averages between 100 and 150 N.[76] The weakest ceramic choice, a luted porcelain jacket crown, has an adequate load value (545 N) for the anterior region. Bonded ceramic crowns, Dicor (Dentsply) (1,583 N) and IPS-Empress (Ivoclar) (2,180 N), have load values an order of magnitude greater than loads generated during normal function.[76] In addition, the ultimate strengths for axial and oblique loads on anterior ceramic systems exceed the maximum normal bite force peaks.[76] Normal functional loads, therefore, should not damage all-ceramic crowns (Table 17-1).

Abnormal bite force peaks are found in patients with parafunctional habits. Parafunction is a physiologically normal activation of voluntary skeletal muscles to produce behaviors that lack functional purpose and are potentially injurious. It occurs cyclically, and because it is mediated by the limbic system, it is harder to control and change.[42] Human bite force on anterior teeth rarely exceeds 200 N, well within the tolerances of most ceramic systems. However, forces generated during a single parafunction episode can exceed the limits of the porcelain system, leading to failure. More damaging to bonded crowns are repeated high loads on anterior teeth from bruxism. These repeated loads can damage the bond to dentin, leading to porcelain fracture. Therefore, the ceramic choice for parafunctional patients becomes more critical.

All-ceramic systems are not always more esthetic. In the hands of an average technician, all-ceramic systems will be repeatably more esthetic simply because of the lack of a metal core[97] (Fig 17-1). However, given proper preparation depths, skilled technicians can mimic natural teeth using a metal-ceramic system (Fig 17-2).

Table 17-1	Comparison of all-ceramic restorative systems			
Product	Flexural strength	Abrasiveness vs natural tooth	Special equipment	Other characteristics
Traditional feldspathic porcelain	110–150 MPa	Varies; higher leucite content yields higher wear	Special refractory die	No core material; uniform translucency and shade throughout; etchable for bonding to tooth
Pressable ceramics				
IPS-Empress (Ivoclar Williams)	160–182 MPa	Comparable to natural tooth except when layered with conventional feldspathic porcelain	Special oven, die material, and molding process	Etchable for bonding to tooth; core material shaded and translucent
Optec pressable ceramic	165 MPa	Same as for IPS-Empress	Same as for IPS-Empress	Same as for IPS-Empress
Empress 2 (Ivoclar Williams)	350 MPa	Less wear than natural tooth	Same as for IPS-Empress	Crown can be cemented or etched to bond; possible to do three-unit fixed partial denture for anterior teeth
Infiltrated ceramics				
In-Ceram (Vident)	450 MPa	Same as for conventional feldspathic porcelain	Special die material; high-temperature oven	Core material is more opaque; not etchable, must be cemented
In-Ceram Spinell (Vident)	350 MPa	Same as for In-Ceram	Same as for In-Ceram	Core material 20% more translucent than In-Ceram; not etchable, must be cemented
Procera (Nobel Biocare)	600 MPa	Same as for In-Ceram	Special die scanner; computer with modem; CAD/CAM machine	Dense translucent core; not etchable, must be cemented

Adapted from Rosenblum and Schulman.[97]

Metal-ceramic crowns are more appropriate for some patients than others. Teeth that are opaque or have high chroma and high value may be easier to match with metal-ceramic than all-ceramic systems. Patients with a low lip line are good candidates for metal ceramics, because the esthetic weakness of metal ceramics is limited to the gingival third where the opacity influences the brightness. The highly reflective opaque ceramic coating used to mask the metal is difficult to disguise when matching teeth with low color saturation or brightness (Fig 17-3). In the anterior region, patients demand a perfect match of crown, tooth, and gingiva. This can be challenging for metal-core crowns. In an attempt to eliminate the gingival opacity, some ceramists reduce the metal substructure up to 2 mm from the shoulder.[74] This removes the highly reflective opacity in the gingival third, decreasing reflection and allowing light pene-

tration into the root, without decreasing the strength of the crown.[103] Light transmission illuminates the gingiva and eliminates the dark gingival shadow sometimes found around metal-ceramic crowns.[103]

If practitioners should not make decisions based solely on the strength of metal-ceramic restorations or the esthetics of all-ceramic systems, then what criteria are appropriate? When esthetic demands are high, an enamel-bonded veneer is the first choice. Adequate enamel must be present, and the patient should have no more than moderate parafunctional habits. It is commonly agreed that enamel-bonded veneers are the most predictable, most esthetic, and strongest restoration for anterior teeth (see Chapter 16). Veneers are, however, contraindicated when less than 50% of the prepared tooth is in enamel; a sound bonding surface is critical to the strength and success of porcelain restorations. In addition, veneers are not recommended

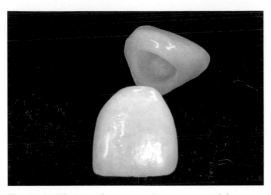

Fig 17-1 All-ceramic crowns have a porcelain core, which facilitates an esthetic match. These crowns provide adequate strength to resist functional loads.

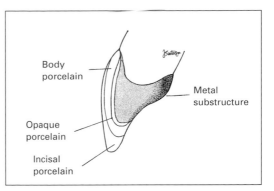

Fig 17-2 Porcelain layered over the metal substructure.

when there is more than 2 mm of unsupported incisal porcelain in bruxers and 3 mm of unsupported incisal porcelain in nonbruxers.[115]

When veneers are contraindicated, choosing the correct anterior ceramic crown system is critical. The choice involves a hierarchy based on the esthetic goals of the patient, the preoperative condition of the tooth, and the load that the tooth will receive. The questions to be asked when deciding on the correct ceramic crown system are: *(1)* What are the esthetic demands, especially in the gingival third? *(2)* What is the quality of the bonding surface? *(3)* Does the patient have parafunctional habits? If so, what is the severity?

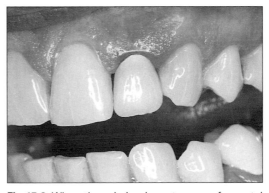

Fig 17-3 When there is inadequate space for metal and porcelain, the opaque porcelain may cause unnatural opacity (maxillary lateral incisor).

Esthetic Demands

An evaluation of esthetics and a diagnosis should be conducted following the guidelines established in Chapter 3. Patient expectations should be addressed before treatment begins. If there are limitations in the treatment, they should be discussed in advance. Diagnostic waxups or computer imaging may help determine what can be achieved with the restorations and aid in patient communication. Elements that affect the esthetic choice of materials include the color of the underlying structures (post and core, discolored dentin, etc) and the importance of the esthetic match in the gingival third.

Veneers bonded to enamel provide some of the most beautiful and dependable restorations for anterior teeth. The thin laminate of porcelain provides an optical refractive index similar to that of translucent enamel, allowing the natural tooth to act as the color substrate. Therefore, when the tooth substrate is an

ideal color, a veneer restoration that is almost imperceptible can be placed (Figs 17-4a and 17-4b).

A ceramic crown can be thought of as a veneer of "enamel" porcelain over a "dentin" ceramic core (Fig 17-5). This "dentin" core material can be feldspathic porcelain, castable glass, heat-pressed leucite-reinforced ceramic, infiltrated alumina, or lithium disilicate.[3,6,45,82] All cores can be laminated with veneering porcelain or stain. The type of core material used in a particular patient depends on the underlying tooth structure (Table 17-2).

Because the core material has a perceptible effect on crown color,[18] the ideal core material should match the natural optical properties of dentin and mask any discoloration present.[17] Today, the feldspathic porcelains most closely mimic the opalescent and fluorescent properties of natural teeth. They are translucent, color stable, brilliant, and natural. Therefore, if the underlying tooth color is acceptable,

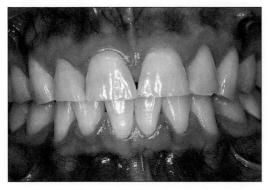

Fig 17-4a An increase in length and alteration of shape is required esthetically. The tooth color is acceptable, there are no restorations, and there is adequate enamel for bonding. Enamel-bonded veneers are the restorations of choice.

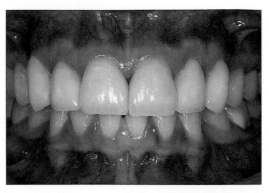

Fig 17-4b When properly planned and constructed, enamel-bonded veneers are almost imperceptible.

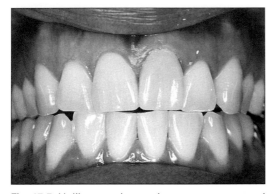

Fig 17-5 Unlike metal-ceramic crowns, cemented all-ceramic restorations are significantly influenced by the underlying color. In this case, an amalgam buildup shows through an all-ceramic crown on the maxillary left central incisor, making it too gray.

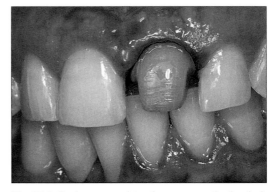

Fig 17-6 Dark prepared teeth are an esthetic challenge for all-ceramic restorations. The correct ceramic core must be chosen to minimize the effect of the discoloration.

full feldspathic crowns produce the most natural result, because they allow the underlying tooth color to show.[99]

If the "dentin" core color must be varied, the ceramic core selection changes (Fig 17-6). IPS-Empress (Ivoclar), Optimal Pressed Ceramic (Jeneric/Pentron), and Finesse All-Ceramic (Dentsply Ceramco) allow broader choices of substrate color with intermediate translucency. In-Ceram (Vident) and Procera (Nobel Biocare) provide a high-strength core that is relatively opaque. In-Ceram, for example, creates a core that is roughly 50% as translucent as dentin.[77] The influence of the core material is most noticeable in the gingival third. The more translucent the core, the more gray it appears as the darkness of the oral cavity shows through. This is most evident with translucent

Optimal Pressed Ceramic. A higher value or brightness is produced by the more opaque, reflective cores found in In-Ceram and metal-ceramic crowns. The esthetic demands on a ceramic system begin with an evaluation of dentin color and the alteration of core color required by the ceramist.

Quality of the Bonding Surface

Anterior crowns can be fixed to the tooth by traditional cementation or by bonding. Traditional cementation utilizes a cement such as zinc phosphate, glass ionomer, or resin-modified glass-ionomer cement. Bonding uses a luting resin or a resin composite and resin adhesive. (In this chapter, the terms *cement* and

Table 17-2 Selection criteria for anterior ceramic crown materials[17]

Shade and appearance of natural teeth	Conventional feldspathic	Veneered Optimal	Colored Optimal	Veneered Empress	Colored Empress	Empress 2	In-Ceram	In-Ceram Spinell	Procera	Metal-ceramic
Vita A-1 to A-2; Low color content, opaceous, high brightness	X							X	X	X
Vita A-3; Moderate color content, translucent body, opaque body	X	X	X	X	X	X	X	X	X	X
Vita A-3.5 to A-4; High color content, translucent or opaque	X	X	X	X	X	X	X	X	X	X
Altering shade from high color to low color			X		X	X	X	X	X	X
Translucent, low brightness, high color		X	X	X	X	X				
Translucent, grayish teeth		X		X						
Translucent, moderately bright teeth	X		X	X	X	X				

cementation will be used, for the most part, to discuss insertion with traditional cements. The terms *resin cement, luting resin, bonding resin,* and *bonding* will be used in reference to resin bonding of restorations.) A traditional cement occupies the space between the restoration and the tooth surfaces but does not provide adhesion between them. In most cases, bonding provides adhesion to both surfaces. Because of this, a bonded crown may not have the same requirements for tooth preparation as a cemented crown. In addition, bonding acts to transfer force from the ceramic to the underlying tooth and strengthens an all-ceramic restoration that would be relatively weak if cemented.

When most all-ceramic crowns are bonded, the ceramic is etched to create micromechanical retention for the resin cement. Bonding procedures, such as described in Chapter 8, are performed on the tooth. When the resin cement is polymerized, it forms a rigid union between the restoration and the tooth. Under function, the dentin bond allows the resin to transfer load to underlying tooth structure.[51] Properly bonded crowns have fracture strengths far greater than human bite force,[13,15,85] but functional and parafunctional forces and the hydrodynamic nature of dentin

may decrease bond strength with time. If the dentin bond is compromised, the porcelain becomes more susceptible to fracture. A study by Neive et al[85] comparing the fracture strength of three ceramic materials reported that bonded IPS-Empress had a higher mean fracture strength than In-Ceram or Procera. However, with a compromised bond, IPS-Empress was significantly weaker than the other systems.

The nature of the dentin surface significantly impacts the strength of the tooth-resin interface (Fig 17-7). The risk of debonding and fracture is magnified when the underlying dentin is less than optimal. Clinicians must recognize differences in dentin composition before planning restorations that depend on long-term dentin bonding.[80] Clinical evidence suggests that loss of cervical bonded restorations is more prevalent in older patients with more sclerotic dentin. Changes in the microstructure of dentin associated with aging have been hypothesized as the cause. Sclerotic dentin has been classified.[54] If no sclerosis is present, the dentin will appear light yellow and opaque (category 1). If there is significant sclerosis, the dentin will have a dark yellow or discolored appearance and will be glossy or translucent (category

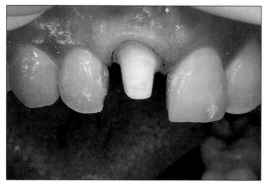

Fig 17-9a When the tooth substrate is acceptable for bonding and color, a bonded, feldspathic all-ceramic crown is indicated.

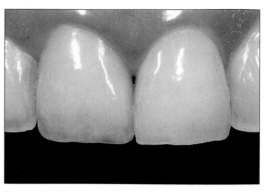

Fig 17-9b The bonded feldspathic crown provides functional predictability and natural esthetics.

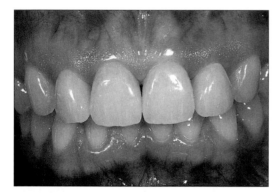

Fig 17-10 The maxillary central and lateral incisors are restored with IPS-Empress crowns. When the tooth color is poor but a reliable bond is available, IPS-Empress is a good choice because several core colors are available.

zation colors on the crown, which is then covered with a glazing powder and fired. The layering technique is the recommended method for anterior ceramics (Fig 17-10). The preparation depth must allow a core reduction such that the substructure resembles a veneer preparation. Enamel and incisal feldspathic porcelains are then veneered on the core. Both techniques provide very promising clinical results.[73,78] IPS-Empress and OPC have comparable flexural strength.[2,14,21] The in vitro margin fit of IPS-Empress has been reported to provide a mean marginal opening of 63 μm with facial and lingual marginal openings being larger than mesial and distal marginal openings.[118] A survival rate for anterior crowns of greater than 95% has been reported through 3 years of observation.[73,109] Heat-pressed ceramics offer the benefit of wear values comparable to those of enamel, whereas most ceramic materials cause accelerated enamel wear.[53,56]

Cemented All-Ceramic Crowns

Indications
1. Moderate to high esthetic demands, especially in the gingival third
2. Poor-quality dentin bonding substrate
3. Mild to moderate parafunction

Cemented all-ceramic crowns are used where esthetics is an overriding concern but the dentin substrate does not provide for proper bonding. Because the core material is very strong, bonding to the underlying tooth structure is not necessary. Cementation requires fewer steps, is less technique sensitive, and has less opportunity for mishaps than do bonding procedures. Because the crown is cemented, the preparation must meet the retention and resistance requirements of any cemented crown. Esthetics is compromised slightly since the ceramic core is less translucent than bonded ceramic restorations and is more opaque than many natural tooth substrates. Because of the high strength of these ceramic materials, cemented ceramic crowns can be placed in patients with moderate or controlled parafunction.

The difference between the ceramic materials that must be bonded versus those that can be used in cemented crowns is found in the composition and processing techniques for the core. For example, In-Ceram is an 85% alumina, glass-infiltrated core fabricated on a resin die.[45,82] In-Ceram Spinell (Vident) is a mixture of alumina and magnesia made on a resin die.[45,82] Procera crowns have a 99% alumina core fabricated on a die designed from digitized specifications made from the master die. Empress 2 is a lithium disilicate–based glass ceramic.

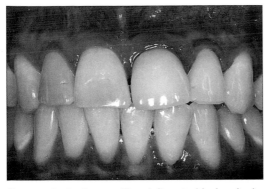

Fig 17-11a Preoperatively, the maxillary left central incisor had a large resin composite restoration. Because composite provides a poor substrate for bonding, a crown material that could be cemented was needed. In-Ceram Spinell was chosen because, unlike a metal-ceramic restoration, it could be made to match the adjacent teeth that were to be restored with porcelain veneers and bonded all-ceramic crowns.

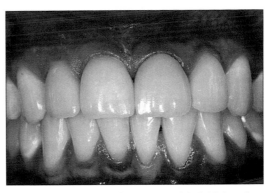

Fig 17-11b In-Ceram Spinell provided high-value, low-chroma restorations.

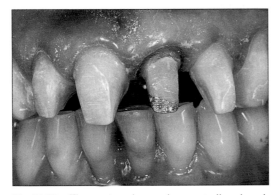

Fig 17-12a The post and core does not allow bonding. A cemented crown is an appropriate choice for the central incisor.

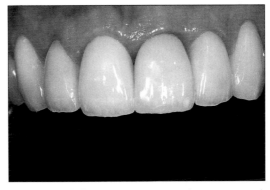

Fig 17-12b A Procera crown was chosen to mask the color of the post and core and to esthetically match the other all-ceramic restorations.

The In-Ceram core is fabricated using a process known as slip casting. A special gypsum die is produced to which an alumina and water mixture or "slip" is applied and shaped. The core is sintered (baked at high temperature) in a furnace, creating an interconnected porous network. The core material is then returned to the porcelain oven, and a lanthanum aluminosilicate glass is infiltrated into the pores of the core to add strength. Aluminous porcelain is then layered over the core to produce the final tooth form. This lengthy process requires at least three separate firings in the porcelain oven. Flexural strengths from 300 to 600 MPa have been reported for In-Ceram.[45,46] Clinical studies of 61 full-coverage single units over 30 months reported no fractures.[63,97]

In-Ceram Spinell is based on the conventional In-Ceram technique, but the core is fabricated from a magnesium-alumina or "spinell" powder. The Spinell core material is more translucent than the regular In-Ceram material, improving the esthetics in the gingival third, but it is not as strong as regular In-Ceram (flexural strength about 350 MPa)[45,82] (Figs 17-11a and 17-11b).

Procera is another system that uses an alumina core (Figs 17-12a and 17-12b). The master die is scanned into a computer, and the surface contour of the die is mapped with the use of over 50,000 measured values. An alumina coping is designed on the computer, and the relief space for the cementing agent is established. The data are then transmitted via modem to a production station where the coping is manufactured with advanced powder technology and a computer-aided design/computer-aided manufacture (CAD/CAM) technique. The coping contains high-purity (99.9%) aluminum oxide powder, which is milled and sintered. A veneering porcelain that is compatible with the coping is layered to develop crown contours

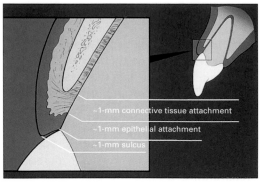

Fig 17-15a The biologic width comprises epithelial and connective tissue attachments. Crown preparations that impinge on the biologic width result in chronic inflammation. (From Robbins JW.[96a] Reprinted with permission.)

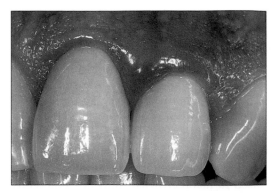

Fig 17-15b This crown preparation impinged on biologic width interproximally. Inflammation had been present for 17 years.

Biologic width describes a vertical measurement of 2.04 mm, the combined width of the connective and epithelial attachments. The total dentogingival complex, biologic width plus sulcus, is approximately 3.00 mm. If the margin of a restoration violates the 2-mm biologic width and impinges on the supracrestal fibers, substantial gingival inflammation often results[62,66,67] (Fig 17-15b).

The difficulty for practitioners is that Garguilo's work presents a "contrived illusion of mathematical precision." The research suggests a vertical measurement of 0.69 mm for the sulcus. Yet, clinically, the depths vary greatly. Not every tooth has the average biologic width of 2 mm and a 1-mm sulcular depth.[57] Each tooth presents unique gingival measurements that must be assessed and used in treatment. Individual measurements of the total dentogingival complex must, therefore, be used in making restorative decisions.[64]

If the goal is to place a restorative margin in the sulcus without violating the biologic width, the base of the sulcus must be identified. But this is extremely difficult. The periodontal literature indicates that the tip of the periodontal probe often penetrates the base of the sulcus and may extend into the connective tissue.[116] The depth of penetration depends on the level of inflammation and pressure used on the probe. Because the sulcus depth can be identified only histologically, the distance from the free gingival margin to the crest of the alveolar bone is the only predictable measurement available to determine intracrevicular margin location. At the crown preparation appointment, the entire dentogingival complex is measured. After the administration of local anesthesia, a round-

ended periodontal probe is pushed through the sulcus until resistance is felt. The probe is kept against the root surface and is pushed hard to the osseous crest. This measurement is taken on the midfacial aspect of the tooth and at both facioproximal line angles.

Measurements on anterior teeth can be categorized into three types of relationships between the free gingival margin and alveolar crest: normal, low, and high[64,67] (Fig 17-16). This relationship will influence margin placement, determine the stability of the attachment levels of the gingiva against the tooth, and influence the need for crown-lengthening surgery prior to restorative procedures. The critical factor in proper management of the soft tissues is accurate location of the alveolar crest, which allows the clinician to avoid impingement on the biologic width.

Normal Crest Relationship

In a normal crest relationship, the measurement from the free gingival margin to the osseous crest is 3 mm facially and 3 to 4.5 mm interproximally (Fig 17-17), which usually results in a gingival scallop of 3 to 4 mm and tissue levels that are stable in relation to the tooth. The normal crest is found on 85% of anterior teeth (Dr John Kois, written communication, April 23, 1998). In the normal crest relationship, restorative margins can be placed 0.5 to 1.0 mm into the sulcus facially and interproximally. The apical limit is 2.0 to 2.5 mm coronal to the osseous crest. The retraction technique is not critical in this crest relationship because the gingival level is stable. Typically, a normal crest relationship should yield no recession and no loss of papilla height following routine inter-

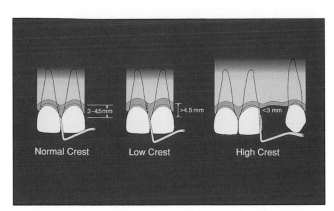

Fig 17-16 Crest classifications are based on the probing depths on the facial and interproximal surfaces from bone to free gingival margin. After the administration of local anesthesia, the probe is forced through the attachment apparatus to bone. This procedure is sometimes called "bone sounding."

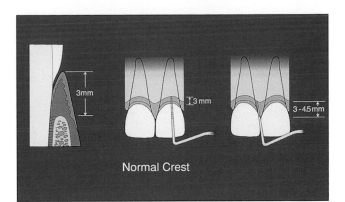

Fig 17-17 Sounding depths of 3.0 mm facially and 3.0 to 4.5 mm interproximally represent a normal crest relationship. The tissue should rebound completely after manipulation.

vention. Van der Velden's[122] research indicates that a normal crest relationship will re-establish itself even if the tissue is completely denuded, although it may take up to 3 years to return to its normal form.

Low Crest Relationship

A low crest relationship is the most difficult of all crest positions to manage and is found in 13% of anterior teeth (Dr John Kois, written communication, April 23, 1998). The relationship of the free gingival margin to the osseous crest is greater than 3 mm facially and greater than 4.5 mm interproximally (Fig 17-18). The gingival scallop does not mimic the osseous crest. Patients with low crests are at high risk for facial recession and loss of papilla height because of the increased distance from the alveolar crest to the gingival margin. The position of the soft tissues on the tooth is not stable in teeth with a low crest relationship and can be easily altered unintentionally during treatment.

If maintenance of the tissue levels is critical during restorative procedures, practitioners have two options. One option is to correct the low crest surgically before tooth preparation, creating a normal crest relationship and thus achieving predictability. This can be accomplished by reducing the tissue height with an internally beveled gingivectomy so that the gingival crest is 3 mm coronal to the osseous crest. However, if the root anatomy, gingival architecture, osseous support, or esthetic demands prevent proactive treatment, the second option is to take great care to avoid damage to the attachment during preparation and impression making. The margin of the preparation

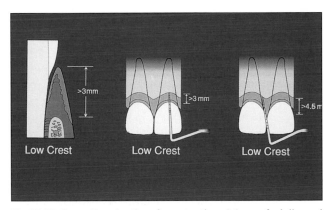

Fig 17-18 Sounding depths of greater than 3.0 mm facially and 4.5 mm interproximally represent a low crest relationship. Tissue response is not predictable after manipulation. Recession and "black triangles" are probable.

should be located at or coronal to the free gingival margin, and there should be minimal, if any, tissue retraction during impression making. The patient should be warned of the possible tissue changes before the preparation begins and have an understanding of the treatment options if tissue loss does occur. While not predictable, thicker tissue seems more resistant to recession following intervention.[102]

High Crest Relationship

Patients with high crests are the least common (2%) and pose the greatest risk for violation of biologic width (Dr John Kois, written communication, April

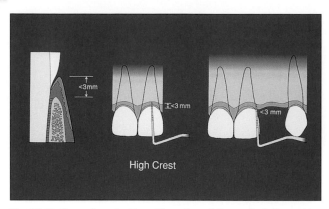

High Crest

Fig 17-19 Sounding depths of less than 3.0 mm facially and interproximally represent a high crest relationship. Intracrevicular preparation is difficult without biologic width violation.

23, 1998). Probing measurements are less than 3 mm facially and interproximally (Fig 17-19). The tissue levels are very stable, and the gingival scallop is flat, less than 3 mm. The high crest sometimes occurs when excessive tissue covers the anatomic crown such as in altered passive eruption,[27] or in patients with toothbrush abrasion or abfraction. However, it is most common adjacent to edentulous spaces where the gingival scallop has flattened. Margin location is determined by the demands of biologic width. High-crest teeth, by definition, will only allow a restorative margin of less than 0.5 mm into the sulcus because of the short distance to the alveolar crest. These teeth are at high risk for biologic width impingement with intracrevicular margin placement. Gingival retraction for impressions should be minimal.

Pulpal Preservation

In one study, irreversible pulpitis occurred in 5.7% of cases in which crowns were placed on vital teeth.[58] Preoperative radiographs and pulp testing are important steps in determining pulp vitality prior to tooth preparation. Unfortunately, pulp testing cannot identify degrees of health. Separately or cumulatively, the effects of large restorations, leaking restorations, caries, deep cracks, pins, etc, increase the chances of pulpal necrosis after tooth preparation. Patients should be made aware of that risk preoperatively.

If the tooth preparation involves an increase of heat to the tooth, pulpal necrosis can occur. In one in

vivo study, pulpal injury occurred in 15% of teeth with a 5.5°C rise in temperature. An 11.1°C rise led to necrosis of the pulp in 60% of the teeth, and a 16.6°C rise caused necrosis of all the teeth tested.[130] Temperature changes have been monitored during complete crown preparation. When an air/water spray coolant was used, a temperature decrease in the pulp chamber from 37°C to 25°C after 4 minutes of exposure occurred. However, when only air coolant was used, the pulpal temperature rose from 37°C to 48°C after 1 minute of continuous exposure.[69] Therefore, continuous air/water coolant is a critical factor in maintaining pulpal health.

Mechanical Principles

During tooth preparation, several mechanical principles must be followed. The preparations must incorporate retention and resistance form, structural durability, and marginal integrity.

Resistance and Retention
Retention is the feature of a crown preparation that resists dislodgment in a vertical direction or along the path of placement. Classic prosthodontic literature indicates that the ideal taper of a preparation is 6 degrees of convergence or 3 degrees on each wall. Jorgensen[60] indicated that there is a 50% reduction in retention when going from 6 to 10 degrees of taper. These tenets are heavily based on clinical empiricism and on two experiments in which crown and abutment analogs were pulled apart along their paths of insertion. The theoretical benefits of preparations with minimal convergence angles do not withstand scrutiny[60,126–128] and are difficult to produce in clinical practice. Divergence from parallel might have to be as much as 12 degrees to be observed and maintained clinically.[91] Routine preparations in practice have been measured at between 15 and 36 degrees without apparent detrimental effect to the longevity of the restorations.[79,89] The minimum convergence value required clinically is unknown, although total convergence up to 20 degrees has been shown to be acceptable.[128]

Resistance is the feature of a tooth preparation that enhances the restoration's stability and resists dislodgment along an axis other than the path of placement.[44] Most retention studies utilize conventional pull-type tests to evaluate preparations and/or cements.[20,124] However, data on functional force vectors in the oral environment strongly suggest that these lift-off type forces are virtually nonexistent in the mouth.[68,83,125] During chewing, teeth are subjected to alternating combinations of buccolingual and occlusogingival forces.[49] These studies indicate that stresses that cause failure of an anterior restoration are repeated, perpendicular, or oblique forces.[125,127] Therefore, as Caputo and Standlee[19] concluded, "Resistance form is the most important factor that must be designed into any restoration if it is to succeed in function."

Resistance clinically is based on preparation taper, height, and cement type. Crowns generally loosen and fail by cleavage of the cement attachment without damaging the abutment or restoration.[128] The cement attachment fails when a portion of the abutment subjected to compressive and shear forces is unable to withstand load application. Attachment failure is a progressive phenomenon linked to increasing abutment taper. Increasing the preparation taper from 10 to 20 degrees creates a broader stress distribution and greater stress within the cement.[128] Clinically, a minimal preparation taper decreases the damaging effects of occlusal stress on the cement attachment, improving a crown's resistance.

The length of the final preparation is also related to resistance.[92] Resistance is increased by lengthening the axial walls of the preparation.[107] The minimum length for resistance on an anterior preparation is 3.5 mm. Two millimeters of the preparation length must be on sound tooth structure to provide a proper ferrule,[34,114,120] and the other 1.5 mm or more can be in either tooth structure or buildup material (Fig 17-20). The ferrule requires a dentin thickness of 1 mm from the external surface of the tooth to the wall of any endodontic preparation.

Resistance is also affected by the mechanical properties of the cement.[128] The limiting threshold of each crown is the cement's resistance to fatigue in compression.[128] The more stress that will be placed on the cement, due to a severe taper and/or lack of preparation height, the more resistant the cement must be. Resin-hybrid cements are more resistant than glass-ionomer cements, which are in turn more resistant than zinc phosphate cements. Most research on resistance and retention data is conducted on cohesively cemented crowns. Today, however, adhesive cements allow the placement of crowns that do not meet standard taper and length requirements. Yet, because the hydrodynamic nature of dentin bonding makes it unpredictable, it is suggested that all preparations meet minimum requirements.[54,80]

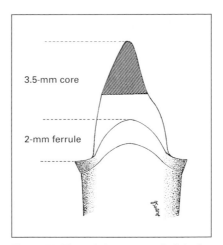

Fig 17-20 The minimum core height for an anterior ceramic crown is 3.5 mm. The cervical 2.0 mm of the facial and lingual aspects must be solid tooth structure for a proper ferrule.

Structural Durability

Structural durability is the relationship between occlusal stress and material strength. It ensures that a restoration does not deform or fracture under load. In a metal-ceramic crown, the minimum metal thickness under porcelain is 0.4 to 0.5 mm for gold alloys and 0.2 mm for base-metal alloys. If the metal is too thin, it will flex under load, resulting in possible porcelain fracture. The minimum porcelain thickness over metal is 0.9 mm (0.2 mm for the opaque material and 0.7 mm for body porcelain). Ceramists prefer a 1.3- to 1.5-mm reduction for the axial surfaces of metal-ceramic crowns and a 2.0-mm reduction incisally/occlusally. The greater the reduction, the easier it is to mask the opaque material in the gingival third of the crown with body porcelain. Most all-ceramic crowns require a minimum thickness of 1.0 mm to provide esthetics and adequate strength.

Marginal Integrity

A completely closed margin is unattainable clinically. Even the finest margins are not sufficiently closed to prevent bacterial ingress. (To place it in perspective, the width of a human hair is 50 µm; bacteria responsible for caries are 4 to 5 µm in diameter.) Because bacteria are constantly passing under restoration margins, patient resistance to disease is more important than the marginal opening of crowns. What, then, is an acceptable marginal opening? One study reported that when the margin of an inlay or onlay

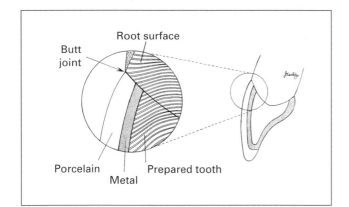

Fig 17-21a In the preferred substructure design for a porcelain facial margin, a uniform thickness of porcelain is carried to the finish line.

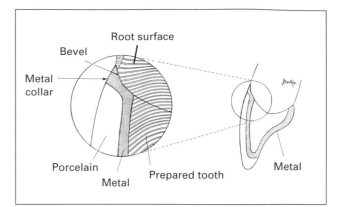

Fig 17-21b The preferred substructure design if a metal facial margin is desired. Metal covers the bevel and forms a butt joint with the porcelain.

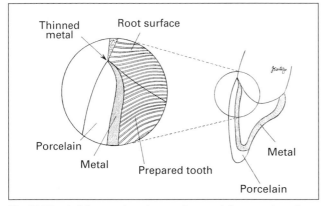

Fig 17-21c A 1.0-mm chamfer can be used for anterior all-ceramic restorations. It is the required finish line for the Procera scanner.

could not be visualized, a marginal discrepancy of 119 μm was found to be acceptable.[25] Bjorn and colleagues reported that 83% of gold and 74% of porcelain crowns exhibited marginal defects; more than half were greater than 200 μm.[9] Yet, defective margins are to blame in only 10% of failed restorations. While all practitioners should strive for the finest margins possible, it is impossible to achieve a closed margin. The best possible margin enables the patient to floss and care for the restoration, minimizing cement dissolution and maximizing the patient's natural resistance factors.

What margin design provides the best marginal integrity? The margin design selected does not have a significant effect on marginal seal.[7,129] Shoulder (Fig 17-21a), shoulder-bevel (Fig 17-21b), and chamfer (Fig 17-21c) finish line preparations all allow accept-

able marginal fit when complete seating is achieved. The shoulder-bevel margin is the least esthetic choice. The bevel should be used only with metal-ceramic crowns and is suited for structurally compromised teeth where additional ferrule is important. If porcelain is placed on a bevel, the cementation process may cause porcelain breakage. In two studies, the geometry exhibiting the least marginal discrepancy after cementation was a shoulder preparation on a die-spaced casting, which was significantly better than that of a shoulder bevel or chamfer.[35,94] The shoulder finish line is thought to be better than the beveled shoulder because it allows the cement to escape more readily. The shoulder design exhibits less marginal distortion than a chamfer because of the crown's thickness adjacent to the margin. Stress analysis of various margin finish lines showed that chamfer and internally rounded shoulder preparations had the lowest stress concentration when loaded vertically, minimizing the risk of catastrophic ceramic failure under load.[33,39]

Proper die spacing is more important than margin design in ensuring complete seating of crowns and closure of margins. In a study by Carter and Wilson,[20] marginal seating of crowns cemented with zinc phosphate was measured on preparations with no die spacing or up to eight layers of die spacer. The mean crown elevation decreased from 547 μm with zero die spacing to 38 μm with eight layers. The mean removal force increased with increasing layers of die spacer from 250 N (zero layers) to 375 N (eight layers). Therefore, marginal integrity improves more with proper die spacing, ensuring complete seating, than with altering preparation design.

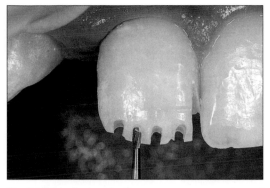

Fig 17-22 Incisal reduction grooves are made and interproximal contact is broken with a 330 carbide bur with a 2.0-mm cutting-head length.

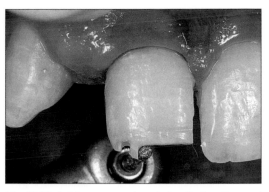

Fig 17-23 A 1.2-mm round-ended cylinder diamond completes the incisal reduction.

Esthetic Design

Porcelain margins must provide an esthetic transition from tooth to crown, preventing the margin from becoming the visual focal point. Such margins are easier to fabricate and more predictable when they are fabricated on a 90-degree shoulder preparation. This is true for metal-ceramic and most all-ceramic systems.[1,41,93,121] A chamfer requires minimal axial reduction and is appropriate for conservative all-ceramic restorations. It is the required finish line for the Procera scanner. It does not, however, provide an adequate reduction for metal-ceramic crowns. The opaque material used to mask the metal at the margin will show through the more translucent porcelain and will compromise the esthetics in the gingival third. A 90-degree shoulder between 1.0 and 1.5 mm in depth allows for a precise margin, maximum seating, and good esthetics. This preparation can be used for porcelain butt margins of metal-ceramic crowns or for all-ceramic crowns.

Functional Crown Preparation Technique

With a complete understanding of the key components of intracrevicular tooth preparation, practitioners can achieve predictability with a standardized, controlled, and functional crown preparation.[65] This preparation design works for any type of anterior ceramic crown. This technique also minimizes the number of burs, bur changes, and cost. Only four burs are used in the technique sequence described below.

Incisal Reduction

The amount of incisal edge reduction is dictated by the planned final incisal edge position. There should be a 2.0-mm reduction from that point. This requires that a diagnostic waxup be completed before tooth preparation if the original incisal edge position is not acceptable. A 2.0-mm reduction allows the technician space to develop incisal translucency and halo effects without a loss of fracture strength of the porcelain.[123] Initial depth cuts are made with a 330 carbide bur that has a 2.0-mm cutting-head length (Fig 17-22). This same carbide bur can be used to open proximal contacts and is also excellent for use in occlusal reduction of posterior teeth. A 1.2-mm-diameter round-ended cylinder diamond is used to remove the remaining incisal-edge tooth structure to the level of the incisal depth cuts (Fig 17-23). This diamond is also used for facial and cervical reduction.

Facial Reduction

Viewed from the proximal aspect, anterior teeth have three facial planes: cervical, midfacial, and incisal. The incisal plane is removed in the first step with a 1.2-mm-diameter round-ended cylinder diamond. The facial reduction focuses only on the facial plane, not the cervical. Depth cuts are prepared to the full depth of the diamond (Fig 17-24), which is aligned with the facial plane, not the cervical plane (Fig 17-25). This approach ensures the necessary reduction for any core-supported porcelain. At this time, the cervical plane should receive almost no reduction. If the bur is

apical migration of junctional epithelium.[4,52,101] The secondary cord should be removed wet to prevent renewed hemorrhage. The preparation is washed and dried to evaluate tissue displacement and hemorrhage control.

If the field is not dry, ferric sulfate can be used to cauterize the tissue. Ferric sulfate provides minimal tissue injury, and healing is more rapid than with aluminum chloride. It must be placed directly against the cut tissues because it coagulates blood so quickly. Otherwise, the ferric sulfate is washed away by the extraneous blood, leaving a bleeding site. There have been reports of the tooth absorbing the ferric ion. In vitro tests, however, have failed to show corrosive effects or staining.[30] A disadvantage to the use of ferric compounds is that they inhibit the setting of polyether impression materials. If a dry field cannot be achieved rapidly, the sulcus width will decrease, increasing the risk of defects in the impression. New chemical agents and secondary cord should be replaced and the retraction attempted again.

Only after the field is acceptable is the impression material mixed. All impression materials are accurate enough to produce well-fitting restorations.[26,32,75] Polyether and polyvinyl siloxane impression materials work well for multipurpose use and provide good soft and hard tissue detail.[36,96] Polyvinyl siloxane materials provide good elastic recovery, are dimensionally stable for indefinite periods, and are clean, odorless, and tasteless.[22] The disadvantage of polyvinyl siloxane is that because it is hydrophobic, it requires an absolutely dry field; even casual contact of the teeth or soft tissues with latex gloves can cause an inhibition of polymerization intraorally.[23,29,61]

Polyether impressions are not affected by latex gloves. They are inherently hydrophilic, so small amounts of blood or saliva do not affect accuracy. Polyether is affected by ferric solutions and some disinfecting solutions. Because of its rigid set, it can be difficult to remove from the mouth, and it has a bad taste and smell.[26,32] The impression material can be used in a custom or stock tray, and studies have shown no difference in accuracy.[47,100] The working and setting times of the impression material must be identified and followed precisely.

Shade

Success of an anterior ceramic crown depends on how well critical information is communicated between the dentist and laboratory. At least 75% of all remakes are caused by poor communication.[84] It is the dentist's challenge to predictably and accurately convey what is visualized in clear terms, allowing the technician to develop the "illusion of reality" in the ceramic material. The dentist must be able to perceive the color, understand and quantify the characteristics, and convey the information.

The experience of seeing color in teeth is dependent on six elements.[131]

1. *Light source:* Light is the basic necessity for vision. In order to see a color, it must be present in the light source. For practitioners to perceive color, the operatory lighting should duplicate natural light as closely as possible. Full-spectrum lighting must emit the correct wavelengths, warmth, and intensity (150 to 250 foot candles) at the operating level. Eight 4-foot long, full-spectrum light tubes should be positioned directly overhead. The spectral composition and warmth of the light can be measured with appropriate measuring devices.
2. *Amount of light:* As the amount of light decreases, the practitioner's ability to see color decreases.
3. *Sensitivity of the eye:* Fourteen percent of males are color blind to one or more colors. Color blindness is rare in females. The condition increases progressively with age. Annual monitoring is appropriate for practitioners who need to perceive color predictably.
4. *The brain's interpretation of color:* Color must be perceived, not merely viewed. Any distortion of the stimulus by the receptor results in an error. Therefore, the light must be constant and controlled, viewing conditions standardized, and the eye and brain trained through repetition.
5. *Optical properties of the tooth:* Natural teeth are translucent; all the light entering is reflected or refracted. The amount of translucency depends on the structure and thickness of the enamel and dentin. The dentin is the primary source for color, and the enamel regulates the brightness.
6. *Condition of tooth and setting:* Factors that affect the interpretation include the color of the operatory walls, the patient's and dentist's clothes, and patient napkin, lipstick, and skin tone. Once those factors are neutralized, the eye's ability to see yellow-orange improves color selection. Surrounding

the tooth with a blue-colored material or looking at blue during shade selection is one way to increase the dentist's ability to detect small differences in the spectral composition of the tooth. With an understanding of color perception and tooth anatomy, practitioners can begin to describe tooth color composition.

A logical place to begin solving the shade-selection dilemma is with an understanding of the four dimensions of color. Artists describe color in terms of three dimensions: hue, chroma, and value. *Hue* is the basic color of an object. It is determined by the wavelength of the reflected light. Dentin is responsible for a tooth's hue. *Chroma* is a further refinement of the hue. It is a measurement of the dilution or saturation of the hue, from pale to intense. *Value* is a measure of the amount of light reflected by a tooth. It is also called *luminance* or *brightness*. It measures the gray scale from black (low value) to white. The thickness and character of enamel affects brightness. Teeth with thick enamel tend to be lower in value because the gray enamel masks the brighter dentin underneath. Teeth have a fourth dimension of color known as *maverick*. Maverick colors are concentrated areas of color in the dentin of most teeth that differ from the overall color. They combine with the basic dentin color and project their resultant effect through the enamel. Maverick colors follow no set rules or pattern, appearing in different areas of the dentin and representing different color families in several degrees of concentration.

Once the four dimensions have been visualized, the components and perceptions must be translated into the language of dental ceramics.[84] Each individual dimension of color should be measured separately. A measuring device must be used to standardize the information provided to the technician. Commercial or customized tooth color guides incorporate much of the information required. Two guides should be used, one set up for value and the other for hue-chroma. The value can be selected first. Color should play no role in its selection. Practitioners should squint when picking value. This will lower the amount of light entering the eye and decrease color perception. Next, hue-chroma is detected. All teeth are yellow; only the chroma varies. Chroma defines the color below the enamel. Commercial guides categorize hue-chroma as Vita A, B, C, and D families. The color family is determined by comparing the tooth to the fully saturated tab (A4, B4, C4, and D4). Second, the exact dilution within the family (1, 2, 3, 4) is measured.

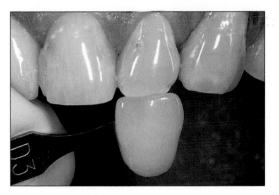

Fig 17-30 Photographs for shade matching should be made at an angle to avoid excess glare on the tooth surface. The shade tab should be held in line with the long axis of the tooth.

Custom shade guides can provide a more reliable means for measuring tooth color dimensions.[50] Each tab is a sample of what the ceramist is capable of producing with a given porcelain and technique (Fig 17-30). Maverick shades are the last to be selected. The family colors are narrow in spectrum (yellow, honey yellow, light and dark brown) but vary in concentration. The maverick guide is constructed of body modifiers and neutral porcelains.[84] Concentrations are determined as with chroma shades. After the dimensions are determined, the information is conveyed to the ceramist.

Communication between the dentist and laboratory can occur in three ways: *(1)* Diagrams: A representation of the tooth may be drawn. While this can be helpful for communicating difficult contours and characteristics, it is difficult for the technician to interpret and very time-consuming. *(2)* Custom stain tabs: Painting colors on a shade tab can display chroma but cannot represent value. In addition, customizing is extremely time-consuming. *(3)* Photographs: Taking photographs of the teeth being restored along with matching shade guides is the most efficient and cost-effective method of shade selection. Photographs must provide an accurate representation of nature. A 35-mm camera with neutral slide film (EPN 100, Kodak) maximizes the ceramist's ability to mimic reality. The more photographs that are taken, the more information the technician can obtain. If the anterior ceramic crown does not match at try-in, more photographs should be taken of the crown to allow the ceramist to modify it correctly. Personal contact between the ceramist and patient would be ideal, but this is often not possible.

Restoration Placement

The classification of anterior ceramic crowns is based on whether the prosthesis is adhesively retained or cemented. Veneer and bonded crowns rely on the formation of a resin bond between the dentin and porcelain. Cemented all-ceramic and metal-ceramic crowns are luted with traditional cements rather than bonded to the preparation. Therefore, the placement protocol will vary significantly between the types of crowns.

Resin Bonding of All-Ceramic Crowns

The goal of adhesive bonding is to provide a marginal seal of the crown and adhesively retain it to the tooth. Resin bonding is extremely technique sensitive and demands proper preparation of ceramic and tooth surfaces. It has been demonstrated that a strong, dependable bond between resin and ceramic can be achieved. The ceramic is etched with hydrofluoric acid to create micromechanical retention sites.[112] Silane is added to the etched surface shortly before bonding and allowed to air dry. Silane coupling agents improve the resin bond to porcelain.[117]

The dentin-resin bond is less dependable than the resin-ceramic bond. Because hemorrhage and crevicular fluid flow may interfere with dentin bonding, teeth should be isolated with retraction cord before cementation. Preparations should be cleaned with pumice or antimicrobial solutions, such as chlorhexidine. Because light polymerization decreases with increasing porcelain thickness[12] and because polymerization of the adhesive before cementation may result in resin pooling and incomplete seating, a chemically activated adhesive system should be applied according to manufacturer's instructions.[11] This includes an etchant, primer, and dual-cure adhesive. A dual-cure resin cement is recommended for bonding of the crown for the same reason. Dual-cured resins have a slow, chemically activated autocure component and a light-activated component. The inside of the crown is painted with adhesive before addition of the luting resin. The crown is gently placed and excess cement removed with a brush. Then the crown is seated with additional pressure or lightly tapped to extrude excess luting resin at the margins. The luting resin is light cured through the facial and lingual aspects for 1 minute each. Excess resin is removed with a No. 12 scalpel blade. The occlusion is adjusted with 15-μm and 8-μm diamonds under water spray. Finally, the porcelain is polished with a porcelain polishing kit.

Cementation of Nonbonded Crowns

The goals of cohesive cementation are complete seating of the crown and maximization of the physical properties of the cement. The preparation should be thoroughly cleaned with pumice or an antimicrobial solution. If the soft tissue interferes with complete seating, retraction cord should be placed. The cement should be mixed according to the manufacturer's instructions, loaded into the crown, and seated. If the crown has metal margins, the patient should bite on an orangewood stick or cotton roll; the stick can be moved up and down and back and forth for a few seconds. This technique, called dynamic seating, results in more complete seating of the crown.[98] Every effort should be made to keep the crown dry during the initial setting phase, that is, the first 5 minutes after cementation.[28] The physical properties of most cements deteriorate if they become wet during setting. The final step is careful removal of the excess set cement with an explorer or scaler.

References

1. Abbate MF, Tjan AHL, Fox WM. Comparison of the marginal fit of various ceramic crown systems. J Prosthet Dent 1989;61:527–531.
2. AbdelHalim T, Lyzak WA, Campbell SD, Wen Z. Effects of pressing programs on optimal pressable ceramic strength [abstract 2064]. J Dent Res 1997;76:271.
3. Andersson M, Razzoog ME, Oden A, et al. Procera: a new way to achieve an all-ceramic crown. Quintessence Int 1998;29:285–296.
4. Azzi R, Tsao TF, Carranza FA, Kenney EB. Comparative study of gingival retraction methods. J Prosthet Dent 1983;50: 561–565.
5. Baharav H, Laufer BZ, Langer Y, Cardish HS. The effect of displacement time on gingival crevice width. Int J Prosthodont 1997;10:248–253.
6. Bello A, Jarvis RH. A review of esthetic alternatives for the restoration of anterior teeth. J Prosthet Dent 1997;78:437–440.
7. Belser UC, MacEntee MI, Richter WA. Fit of three porcelain-fused-to-metal marginal designs in vivo: a scanning electron microscope study. J Prosthet Dent 1985;53:24–29.
8. Benson BW. Tissue displacement methods in fixed prosthodontics. J Prosthet Dent 1986;55:175–181.
9. Bjorn AL, Bjorn H, Grkovic B. Marginal fit of restorations and its relation to periodontal bone level. Part I: metal fillings. Part II: crowns. Odontol Revy 1969;20:311–321.
10. Block PL. Restorative margins and periodontal health. J Prosthet Dent 1987;57:683–689.
11. Bowen RL, Cobb EN. A method for bonding to dentin and enamel. J Am Dent Assoc 1983;107:734–736.
12. Boyer DB, Chan KC. Curing light activated composite cement through porcelain [abstract 1289]. J Dent Res 1989;68:476.
13. Burke FJT. Fracture resistance of teeth restored with dentin-bonded crowns: the effect of increased tooth preparation. Quintessence Int 1996;27:115–121.

14. Burke FJT. Fracture resistance of dentin-bonded crowns constructed in a leucite-reinforced ceramic [abstract 1608]. J Dent Res 1999;78:306.

15. Burke FJT, Qualtrough AJE, Wilson NHF. A retrospective evaluation of a series of dentin-bonded ceramic crowns. Quintessence Int 1998;29:103–106.

16. Campbell SD. A comparative strength study of metal-ceramic and all-ceramic materials: modulus of rupture. J Prosthet Dent 1989;62:476–479.

17. Campbell SD. Clinical selection criteria for esthetic full crown restorations. Presented at the American Academy of Restorative Dentistry; February 23, 1999; Chicago, IL.

18. Campbell SD, Tu SJ, Lund PS. Translucency of a new ceramic crown material [abstract 395]. J Dent Res 1997;76:63.

19. Caputo AA, Standlee JP. Biomechanics in Clinical Dentistry. Chicago: Quintessence, 1987:128.

20. Carter SM, Wilson PR. The effect of die spacing on crown retention. Int J Prosthodont 1996;9:21–29.

21. Cattell MJ, Knowles JC, Clarke RL, Lynch E. The biaxial flexural strength of two pressable ceramic systems. J Dent 1999;27:183–196.

22. Chee WWL, Donovan TE. Polyvinyl siloxane impression materials: a review of properties and techniques. J Prosthet Dent 1992;73:419–423.

23. Chee WWL, Donovan TE, Kahn RL. Indirect inhibition of polymerization of a polyvinyl siloxane impression material: a case report. Quintessence Int 1991;22:133–135.

24. Chiche GJ, Harrison JD. Impression considerations in the maxillary anterior region. Compend Contin Educ Dent 1994;15:318–327.

25. Christensen GJ. Marginal fit of gold inlay castings. J Prosthet Dent 1966;16:297–305.

26. Ciesco JN, William MS, Sandrik JL, Mazur B. Comparison of elastic impression materials used in fixed prosthodontics. J Prosthet Dent 1981;45:89–94.

27. Coslet JG, Vanarsdall R, Wiesgold A. Diagnosis and classification of delayed passive eruption of the dentogingival junction in the adult. Alpha Omegan 1977;10:24–28.

28. Curtis SR, Richards MW, Meiers JC. Early erosion of glass-ionomer cement at crown margins. Int J Prosthodont 1993; 6:553–557.

29. de Camargo LM, Chee WWL, Donovan TE. Inhibition of polymerization of polyvinyl siloxanes by medicaments used on gingival retraction cords. J Prosthet Dent 1993;70:114–117.

30. Donovan TE, Gandara BK, Nemetz H. Review and survey of medicaments used with gingival retraction cords. J Prosthet Dent 1985;53:525–531.

31. Douglas WH. Clinical status of dentin bonding agents. J Dent 1989;17:209–215.

32. Dounis GS, Ziebert GJ, Dounis KS. A comparison of impression materials for complete-arch fixed partial dentures. J Prosthet Dent 1991;65:165–169.

33. El-Ebrashi MK, Craig RG, Peyton FA. Experimental stress analysis of dental restorations. Part III, the concept of the geometry of proximal margins. J Prosthet Dent 1969;22: 333–345.

34. Eismann HF, Radke RA. Postendodontic restoration. In: Cohen S, Burns RC (eds). Pathways of the Pulp. St Louis: Mosby, 1987:640–683.

35. Faucher RR, Nicholls JI. Distortion related to margin design in porcelain-fused-to-metal restorations. J Prosthet Dent 1980; 43:149–155.

36. Federick DR, Caputo A. Comparing the accuracy of reversible hydrocolloid and elastomeric impression materials. J Am Dent Assoc 1997;128:183–188.

37. Felton DA, Kanoy B, Bayne S, Wirthman G. Effect of in vivo crown margin discrepancies on periodontal health. J Prosthet Dent 1991;65:357–364.

38. Flores-de-Jacoby L, Zafiropoulus GG, Ciancio S. The effect of crown margin location on plaque and periodontal health. Int J Periodontics Restorative Dent 1989;9:197–205.

39. Gardner FM, Tillman-McCombs KW, Gaston ML, Runyan DA. In vitro failure load of metal-collar margins compared with porcelain facial margins of metal-ceramic crowns. J Prosthet Dent 1997;78:1–4.

40. Garguilo AW, Wentz FM, Orban B. Dimensions and relations of the dentogingival junction in humans. J Periodontol 1961;32:261–267.

41. Gavelis JR, Morency JD, Riley ED, Sozio RB. The effect of various finish line preparations on the marginal seal and occlusal seat of full crown preparations. J Prosthet Dent 1981;45:138–145.

42. Gear RW. Neural control of oral behavior and its impact on occlusion. In: McNeill C (ed). Science and Practice of Occlusion. Chicago: Quintessence, 1997:59–60.

43. Gibbs CH, Mahan PE, Mauderi A, et al. Limits of human bite strength. J Prosthet Dent 1986;56:226–228.

44. Gilboe DB, Teteruck WR. Fundamentals of extracoronal tooth preparation. Part I. Retention and resistance form. J Prosthet Dent 1974;32:651–656.

45. Giordano RA. Dental ceramic restorative systems. Compend Contin Educ Dent 1996;17(8):779–794.

46. Giordano R, Pelletier L, Campbell S, Pober R. Flexural strength of alumina and glass components of In-Ceram [abstract 1181]. 1992;71:253.

47. Gordon GE, Johnson GH, Drennon DG. The effect of tray selection on the accuracy of elastomeric impression materials. J Prosthet Dent 1990;63:12–15.

48. Gottlieb B. Der epithelansatz am zahne. Dtsch Monatsschr Zahnheilkd 1921;39:142–148.

49. Graf H, Geering AH. Rationale for clinical application of different occlusal philosophies. Oral Sci Rev 1977;10:1–10.

50. Groh CL, O'Brien WJ, Boenke KM, Mora GP. Differences in color between fired porcelain and shade guides [abstract 813]. J Dent Res 1992;71:207.

51. Grossman DG. Photoelastic examination of bonded crown interfaces [abstract 719]. J Dent Res 1989;68:271.

52. Harrison JD. Effect of retraction materials on the gingival sulcus epithelium. J Prosthet Dent 1961;11:514–519.

53. Heinzmann JL, Krejci I, Lutz F. Wear and marginal adaptation of glass-ceramic inlays, amalgam and enamel [abstract 423]. J Dent Res 1990;69(special issue):161.

54. Heymann HO, Bayne SC. Current concepts in dentin bonding: focusing on dentinal adhesion factors. J Am Dent Assoc 1993;124:27–36.

55. Hochman N, Yaffe A, Ehrlich J. Crown contour variations in gingival health. Compend Contin Educ Dent 1983;4(4): 360–365.

56. Imal Y, Suzuki S, Fukushima S. In vitro enamel wear of modified porcelains [abstract 50]. J Dent Res 1999;78:112.

57. Ingber JS, Rose LF, Coslet JG. The "biologic width": a concept in periodontics and restorative dentistry. Alpha Omegan 1977;70:62–65.

58. Jackson CR, Skidmore AE, Rice RT. Pulpal evaluation of teeth restored with fixed prostheses. J Prosthet Dent 1992;67:323–325.

59. Jones DW. Development of dental ceramics—a historical perspective. Dent Clin North Am 1985;29:621–644.

60. Jorgensen KD. The relationship between retention and convergence angles in cemented veneer crowns. Acta Odontol Scand 1955;13:35–40.

61. Kahn RL, Donovan TE. A pilot study of polymerization inhibition of poly (vinyl siloxane) materials by latex gloves. Int J Prosthodont 1989;2:128–130.

62. Kaiser DA, Newell DH. Technique to disguise the metal margin of the metal/ceramic crown. Am J Dent 1988;1:217–221.

63. Kappert HF, Altvater A. Field study on the accuracy of fit and the marginal seal of In-Ceram crowns and bridges [German]. Dtsch Zahnarztl Z 1991;46:151–153.

64. Kois JC. Altering gingival levels: the restorative connection part I: biologic variables. J Esthet Dent 1994;6(1):3–9.

65. Kois JC. New paradigms for anterior tooth preparation: rationale and technique. Contemp Esthet Dent 1996;2(1):1–8.

66. Kois JC. The gingiva is red around my crowns: a differential diagnosis. 1993;4:101–105.

67. Kois JC. The restorative-periodontal interface: biological parameters. Periodontol 2000 1996;11:1–10.

68. Korioth TW, Waldron TW, Versluis A, et al. Forces and moments generated at the dental incisors during forceful biting in humans. J Biomech 1997;30:631–633.

69. Laforgia PD, Milano V, Morea C, Desiate A. Temperature change in the pulp chamber during complete crown preparation. J Prosthet Dent 1991;65:56–61.

70. Laufer BZ, Baharav H, Ganor Y, Cardash HS. The effect of marginal thickness on the distortion of different impression materials. J Prosthet Dent 1996;76:466–471.

71. Laufer BZ, Baharav H, Cardash HS. The linear accuracy of impressions and stone dies as affected by the thickness of the impression margin. Int J Prosthodont 1994;7:247–252.

72. Lee WC, Eakle WS. Possible role of tensile stress in the etiology of cervical erosive lesions of teeth. J Prosthet Dent 1984;52:374–380.

73. Lehner C, Studer S, Brodbeck U, Scharer P. Short-term results of IPS-Empress full-porcelain crowns. J Prosthodont 1997;6:20–30.

74. Lehner CR, Mannchen R, Scharer P. Variable reduced metal support for collarless metal-ceramic crowns: a new model for strength evaluation. Int J Prosthodont 1995;8:337–345.

75. Lin CC, Ziebert GJ, Donegan SJ, Dhuru VB. Accuracy of impression materials for complete-arch fixed partial dentures. J Prosthet Dent 1988;59:288–291.

76. Ludwig K. Studies on the ultimate strength of all-ceramic crowns. Dent Lab 1991;5:647–651.

77. Lund PS, Campbell SD, Giordano RA. Translucency of core and veneer materials for all-ceramic crowns [abstract 2135]. J Dent Res 1996;75:284.

78. Lyzak WA, Campbell SD, Wen Z. Thermal cycling effects on the strength of Optimal Pressable Ceramic [abstract 2062]. J Dent Res 1997;76:271.

79. Mack PJ. A theoretical and clinical investigation into the taper achieved on crown and inlay preparations. J Oral Rehabil 1980;7:255–265.

80. Marshall GW, Marshall SJ, Kinney JH, Balooch M. The dentin substrate: structure and properties related to bonding. J Dent 1997;25(6):441–458.

81. May KB, Russell MM, Razzoop ME, Lang BR. Precision of fit: the Procera AllCeram crown. J Prosthet Dent 1998;80:394–404.

82. McLaren EA. All-ceramic alternatives to conventional metal-ceramic restorations. Compend Contin Educ Dent 1998;19:307–325.

83. Morikawa A. Investigation of occlusal force on lower first molar in function. Kokubyo Gakkai Zasshi 1994;61:250–274.

84. Muia P. Esthetic Restorations: improved Dentist-Laboratory Communication. Chicago: Quintessence, 1993:81–95.

85. Neive G, Yaman P, Dennison JB, et al. Resistance to fracture of three all-ceramic systems. J Esthet Dent 1998;10:60–66.

86. Nementz E, Seibly W. The use of chemical agents in gingival retraction. Gen Dent 1990;3:104–108.

87. Nemetz H, Donovan TE, Landesman H. Exposing the gingival margin: a systematic approach for the control of hemorrhage. J Prosthet Dent 1984;51:647–650.

88. Nevins M, Skurow HM. The intracrevicular restorative margin, the biologic width, and the maintenance of the gingival margin. Int J Periodontics Restorative Dent 1984;4(3):31–49.

89. Nordlander J, Weir D, Stoffer W, Ochi S. The taper of clinical preparations for fixed prosthodontics. J Prosthet Dent 1988;60:148–151.

90. Oden A, Andersson M, Krystek-Ondracek I, Magnusson D. Five-year clinical evaluation of Procera AllCeram crowns. J Prosthet Dent 1998;80:450–456.

91. Ohm E, Silness J. The convergence angle in teeth prepared for artificial crowns. J Oral Rehabil 1978;5:371–375.

92. Owen CP. Retention and resistance in preparations for extra-coronal restorations. Part 2: practical and clinical studies. J Prosthet Dent 1986;56:148–153.

93. Padilla MT, Bailed JH. Marginal configuration, die spacers, fitting of retainer/crowns, and soldering. Dent Clin North Am 1992;36:743–765.

94. Pascoe DF. Analysis of the geometry of finish lines for full crown restorations. J Prosthet Dent 1978;40:157–162.

95. Pospiech P, Kistler St, Frasch C, Rammelsberg P. Clinical evaluation of posterior crowns and bridges of Empress 2: preliminary results after one year [abstract 2714]. J Dent Res 1999;78:445.

96. Pratten DH, Novetsky M. Detail reproduction of soft tissue: a comparison of impression materials. J Prosthet Dent 1991;65:188–191.

96a. Robbins JW. Esthetic gingival recontouring. Quintessence Int 2000;31:553–556.

97. Rosenblum MA, Schulman A. A review of all-ceramic restorations. J Am Dent Assoc 1997;128:297–307.

98. Rosenstiel SF, Gegauff AF. Improving cementation of complete cast crowns: a comparison of static and dynamic seating methods. J Am Dent Assoc 1988;117:845–848.

99. Rouse J, McGowan S. Restoration of the anterior maxilla with ultraconservative veneers: clinical and laboratory considerations. Pract Periodont Aesthet Dent 1999;11:333–339.

100. Rueda LJ, Sy-Munoz JT, Naylor WP, et al. The effect of using custom or stock trays on the accuracy of gypsum casts. Int J Prosthodont 1996;9:367–373.

101. Ruel J, Schuessler PJ, Malament K, Mori D. Effect of retraction procedures on the periodontium in humans. J Prosthet Dent 1980;44:508–515.

102. Sanavi F, Wiesgold AS, Rose LF. Biologic width and its relation to periodontal biotypes. J Esthet Dent 1998;10(3):157–163.

103. Schaffner VB, Jones DW. Light transmission in shoulder porcelain of metal-ceramic restorations. Presented at the Annual Meeting of the Academy of Prosthodontics; May 17, 1994; Orlando, FL.

104. Schweiger M, Holand W, Frank M, et al. IPS Empress 2: a new pressable high-strength glass-ceramic for esthetic all-ceramic restorations. Quintessence Dent Technol 1999;22:143–151.

105. Seghi RR, Sorensen JA, Engleman MJ, et al. Flexural strength of new ceramic materials [abstract 1521]. J Dent Res 1990;89:299.

106. Selby A. Fixed prosthodontic failure. A review and discussion of important aspects. Aust Dent J 1994;39(3):150–156.

107. Shillingburg HT, Hobo S, Whitsett LD. Fundamentals of Fixed Prosthodontics, ed 2. Chicago: Quintessence, 79–96.

108. Sicher H. Changing concepts of the supporting dental structures. Oral Surg 1959;12:31–35.

109. Sorensen JA, Choi C, Fanuscu MI, Mito WT. IPS Empress crown system: three year clinical trial results. J Calif Dent Assoc 1998;26:130–136.

110. Sorensen JA, Sultan E, Condon JR. Three-body in vitro wear of enamel against dental ceramics [abstract 909]. J Dent Res 1999;78:219.

111. Sorensen JA, Berge HX. In vivo measurement of antagonist tooth wear opposing ceramic bridges [abstract 2942]. J Dent Res 1999;78:473.

112. Sorensen JA, Kang SK, Avera SA. Porcelain-composite interface microleakage with various porcelain surface treatments. Dent Mater 1991;7:118–121.

113. Sorensen JA, Torres TJ, Kang SK, Avera SP. Marginal fidelity of ceramic crowns with different margin designs [abstract 1365]. J Dent Res 1990;(special issue)69:279.

114. Sorensen J, Engleman M. Ferrule design and fracture resistance of endodontically treated teeth. J Prosthet Dent 1990;63:529–536.

115. Spear FM, Winter RR. Esthetic alternatives for anterior teeth. Presented at the Annual Meeting of American Academy of Restorative Dentistry; February 22, 1997; Chicago, IL.

116. Spray JR, Garnick JJ, Dloles LR, Klawitter JJ. Microscopic demonstration of the position of periodontal probes. J Periodontol 1978;49:148–152.

117. Stangel I, Nathanson D, Hsu CS. Shear strength of the composite bond to etched porcelain. J Dent Res 1987;66:1460–1465.

118. Sulaiman F, Chai J, Jameson LM, Wozniak WT. A comparison of the marginal fit of Inceram, IPS Empress and Procera crowns. Int J Prosthodont 1997;10:478–484.

119. Tarnow DP, Stahl SS, Magner A. Human gingival attachment response to subgingival crown placement. J Clin Periodontol 1986;13:563–569.

120. Trabert KC, Cooney JP. The endodontically treated tooth: restorative concepts and techniques. Dent Clin North Am 1984;28:423–451.

121. Vahidi F, Egloff ET, Panno FV. Evaluation of marginal adaptation of all-ceramic crowns and metal-ceramic crowns. J Prosthet Dent 1991;66:426–431.

122. Van Der Velden UJ. Regeneration of the interdental soft tissues following denudation procedures. Clin Periodontol 1982;9:455–459.

123. Wall JC, Reisbick MH, Johnston WM. Incisal edge strength of porcelain laminate veneers restoring mandibular incisors. Int J Prosthodont 1992;5:441–446.

124. Wilson AH, Chan DC. The relationship between preparation convergence and retention of extracoronal retainers. J Prosthet Dent 1994;3:74–78.

125. Wiskott A, Belser U. A rationale for a simplified occlusal design in restorative dentistry: historical review and clinical guidelines. J Prosthet Dent 1995;75:169–183.

126. Wiskott A, Nicholls JI, Belser UC. The effect of abutment length and diameter on resistance to fatigue loading. Int J Prosthodont 1997;10:207–215.

127. Wiskott A, Nicholls JI, Belser UC. The relationship between convergence angle and resistance of cemented crowns to dynamic loading. Int J Prosthodont 1996;9:117–130.

128. Wiskott HWA, Krebs C, Scherrer SS, et al. Compressive and tensile zones in the cement interface of full crowns: a technical note on the concept of resistance. J Prosthet Dent 1999;8(2):80–91.

129. Wright WE. Selection of proper margin configuration. J Calif Dent Assoc 1992;20:41–44.

130. Zach L, Cohen G. Pulpal response to externally applied heat. Oral Surg 1965;19:515–530.

131. Zwimpfer M. Color, Light, Sight, Sense. Philadelphia, PA: Schiffer Publishing, 1988:1–264.

18 Esthetic Inlays and Onlays

J. William Robbins/Dennis J. Fasbinder

There are several treatment options for esthetic Class 1 and Class 2 restorations, in addition to direct resin composite restorations. This chapter discusses tooth-colored inlays and onlays fabricated in resin composite and in ceramic materials. Restorations fabricated with computer-assisted design/computer-assisted manufacture (CAD/CAM), currently referred to as computer-assisted design/computer-integrated machining (CAD/CIM) technology, will also be discussed.

Esthetic inlays and onlays have a number of characteristics in common, whether they are resin, ceramic, or fabricated with CAD/CIM technology.

General Considerations

Preparations

The preparations for ceramic and resin composite inlays and onlays are the same. Preparations for CAD/CIM restorations differ somewhat and are discussed in a later section. Preparations for CAD/CIM inlays and onlays are no different from laboratory-fabricated inlays and onlays with the current Cerec 2 (Sirona Dental Systems) unit.

There is little research to support the efficacy of any preparation design over another.[3] However, based on knowledge of the materials and clinical experience, the divergent, relatively nonretentive preparation is most commonly advocated because of ease of placement

(Fig 18-1). Resistance form may be incorporated with rounded proximal boxes, but grooves should not be used. Resistance and retention form for the restoration are provided primarily by adhesion to enamel and dentin. The walls and floors of the preparation should be smooth and even, and the internal angles should be rounded to enhance adaptation of the restorative material (Fig 18-2). The occlusal reduction should be anatomic and uniformly a minimum of 2 mm for strength[15] (Fig 18-3).

There is no benefit to the placement of bevels at the occlusal or gingival margins; in fact, bevels should be avoided because thin margins of both resin composite and porcelain are susceptible to chipping during function.[85,114] A 90-degree butt joint minimizes the chipping problem but results in a visible demarcation between the tooth and the restoration. Therefore, when the esthetic blend of the restoration and the tooth is important, such as on the facial surface of a maxillary premolar, a long chamfer may be placed (Fig 18-2).

Bases and Liners

The use of bases and liners is somewhat controversial. Initially, glass-ionomer bases were used for dentinal protection and to base the preparation to "ideal" form. However, it has been shown that it is not necessary to protect the dentin from the phosphoric acid etchant.[45] Therefore, glass-ionomer cement is recommended only for routine blocking out of undercuts.

Fig 18-1 Onlay preparation technique.

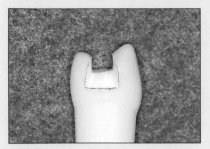

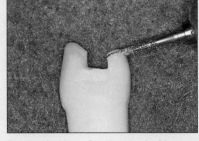

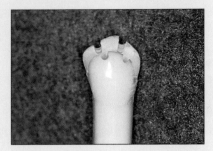

Fig 18-1a Simulation of amalgam preparation after removal of the amalgam.

Fig 18-1b Use of a diamond of known diameter to make the first depth cut of 1 mm.

Fig 18-1c First depth cuts of 1 mm.

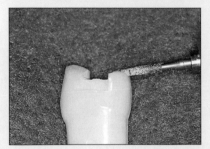

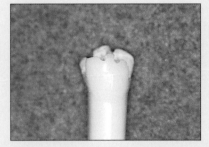

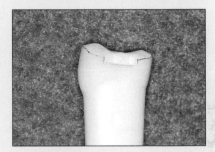

Fig 18-1d Use of a diamond of known diameter to make the second depth cuts of 1.0 mm.

Fig 18-1e Second depth cuts of an additional 1 mm.

Fig 18-1f Occlusal reduction of 2 mm completed; however, sharp line angles remain in the box area.

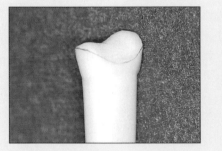

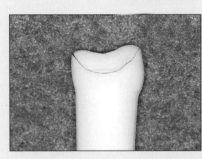

Figs 18-1g and 18-1h Completed smooth, flowing preparation without sharp angles.

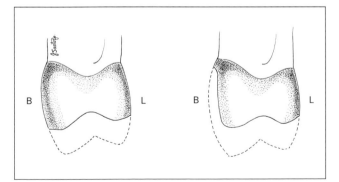

Fig 18-2 Standard onlay preparation *(left)* and modified onlay preparation *(right)* that includes coverage of facial surface to achieve a superior esthetic blend with the natural tooth color. B = buccal; L = lingual.

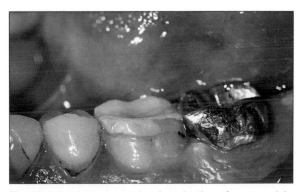

Fig 18-3 Inadequate occlusal reduction for porcelain onlay, resulting in fractured porcelain.

Provisional Restorations

Provisional restorations can be a challenge with esthetic inlays and, particularly, onlays because of the nonretentive design of the preparations. Provisional restorations can be made in the usual manner with acrylic resin or resin composite and cemented with temporary cement. It is commonly stated that a eugenol-containing cement should not be used with the provisional restoration when the final restoration will be bonded with a resin cement.[3,76] However, the literature is equivocal on the deleterious effect of eugenol. Some studies support the hypothesis that eugenol-containing provisional cement inhibits the set of resin cement,[3,55,76] while others show that eugenol-containing provisional cements have no impact on bond strengths.[10,75,92,93,100] Because of the nonretentive design of the onlay preparation, the more retentive polycarboxylate cement is the temporary luting cement of choice. Small mechanical undercuts should be placed on the intaglio surface of the provisional restoration to aid in retention. If adjacent teeth are being restored, the provisional restorations can be connected to improve retention.

For inlay preparations, flexible light-cured materials, such as Fermit (Vivadent) or Barricade (Dentsply), may be used. To provide retention and to decrease sensitivity, a dentin primer can be placed in the preparation and air dried, or a small amount of resin-modified glass-ionomer cement liner can be placed on the pulpal floor and polymerized. The preparation is filled with the provisional material, and the patient is instructed to bite into maximum intercuspation to develop the occlusion. Excess material is removed with an explorer, and the provisional restoration is light cured. This technique is recommended only for short-term use in small preparations.[12]

Adhesive Cementation

Resin luting cement is the only material recommended for this type of restoration because it bonds to enamel, dentin, and the restorative material. Luting resin cement limits microleakage, enhances the strength of the restoration,[21] and provides at least short-term strengthening of the tooth.[17,86] Dual-cured luting resin and dual-cured dentin bonding agents, which combine light-curing and chemical-curing components, should be used to bond all indirect posterior bonded restorations. The light-curing component polymerizes rapidly on exposure to light of the proper wavelength, while the chemical-curing component un-

dergoes a slow polymerization process in those areas to which the light does not penetrate. It is important that the curing light be applied to dual-cured resin for an adequate period of time, because the dual-cure process results in more complete polymerization than is achieved with the chemical polymerization alone.[14,41] The shelf life of dual-cured resins is shorter than that of conventional light-cured resin composites. Therefore, a test batch of dual-cured luting resin should periodically be mixed and allowed to cure in a dark environment to ensure that it will polymerize in the absence of light. It should polymerize in the dark within 10 minutes.

Preparing the Restoration for Bonding

Adhesion is more reliably achieved to ceramic materials than to resin composite. Ceramics can be etched, creating durable micromechanical retention.[2] The ceramic inlay/onlay is prepared for bonding by etching the internal surface, usually with hydrofluoric acid. This is generally done at the laboratory, but may be done chairside. Shortly before bonding,[79,103] silane is applied to the etched surface to enhance wetting by the resin adhesive.

Bonding to resin composite restorations is more difficult. The intaglio surface has no air-inhibited layer and relatively few unreacted methacrylate groups, so a reliable chemical bond does not form between the inlay and the resin cement.[44,64,111] Because the resin composite–cement interface may be the weak link, several procedures have been recommended to enhance the bond to resin. With hybrid resin composite, the intaglio surface should be carefully air abraded with 50-μm aluminum oxide (avoiding the margins)[62] and then cleaned with a steam cleaner or in an ultrasonic bath. The air abrasion provides a rough surface for frictional retention. The cleaned surface should be treated with an agent to allow better wetting by the cement. Silane is generally the preferred wetting agent.[64] Treatment with hydrofluoric acid has also been recommended to etch the glass particles in the hybrid resin composite, but laboratory research does not support the efficacy of this procedure.[44]

Bonding to microfilled resin composite is even more problematic. Neither air abrasion nor hydrofluoric acid etching is effective in preparing the surface for bonding. The placement of Special Bond 2 (Vivadent), a mixture of methacrylates in a solvent, is recommended for placement on the intaglio surface of the microfilled restoration prior to bonding.[22] No method to obtain a true chemical bond to either hybrid or microfilled resin composite inlays and onlays is currently available.

Preparing the Tooth for Bonding

The rubber dam is placed to ensure an isolated field (Fig 18-4a). Silane is placed on the inner surface of the restoration and air dried. Once the restoration is ready for bonding, a decision must be made regarding the type of dentin bonding agent. Fourth-generation light-cured adhesive systems should not be used under indirect posterior bonded restorations. The light-cured adhesive must be air thinned prior to polymerization to ensure that there is no pooling of the adhesive that would prevent complete seating of the restoration. However, it has been shown that air thinning of the light-cured adhesive significantly decreases the bond strength.[40] This leaves fifth-generation, single-bottle systems and fourth-generation dual-cured systems. The technology continues to rapidly change, which makes the discussion of current dentin bonding agents difficult. However, in general terms, the fifth-generation product, with the greatest amount of research support, requires multiple coats for maximum bond strength.[6,41] The placement of multiple coats can potentially result in greater thickness of cured adhesive and areas of pooling, both of which can interfere with complete seating of the restoration.[32] Manufacturers are attempting to overcome these problems with the introduction of fifth-generation products that require only one coat (Prime and Bond NT, Caulk; and Excite, Vivadent)[35] and fifth-generation products that are dual cured (Prime and Bond 2.1 Dual Cure, Caulk).

However, the technique with the most research support employs the dual-cured fourth-generation dentin bonding systems. The enamel and dentin are etched for 15 to 20 seconds, washed for 2 to 3 seconds, and air dried to visually inspect for an adequate enamel etch. The dentin is remoistened, and several coats of primer are applied. One laboratory study indicated that a 30-second application of primer with rubbing resulted in decreased microleakage compared to a 5-second priming.[37] The primer is completely air dried with gentle air pressure. The dual-cured adhesive is placed on the tooth and intaglio surface of the restoration. The dual-cured luting resin is mixed and placed into the preparation and restoration, and the restoration is seated. Excess resin must be completely removed from the interproximal gingival margins with floss and interproximal instruments before polymerization of the luting resin. Some clinicians recommend placement of a clear gel, such as glycerin, on the margins before polymerization to prevent the formation of an air-inhibited layer in the luting resin at the margin.[7] The margins may be finished with microfine diamonds or multifluted carbide finishing burs

and a No. 12 scalpel blade, and can be polished with disks, rubber points, or cups. After removal of the rubber dam, the occlusion is adjusted and the surface is polished to a high shine. The final step is rebonding, as described in Chapter 10, with an unfilled or lightly filled resin (Figs 18-4b to 18-4g and Figs 18-5a to 18-5d).

Maintenance

Maintenance is a very important factor in the longevity of esthetic inlays and onlays. As with all types of restorative dentistry, poor oral hygiene can cause failure of the finest dentistry. Use of devices such as ultrasonic scalers or air-abrasive polishers on these restorations must be avoided, because they can cause surface and marginal damage. Calculus should be removed carefully with hand instruments. When scalers are used around the bonded inlay or onlay, care must be taken not to chip the margins. Surface stain may be removed from a restoration with aluminum oxide polishing paste or diamond polishing paste on a felt wheel or rubber cup. Because of their ability to etch porcelain, neither acidulated phosphate fluoride nor stannous fluoride solutions or gels should be used intraorally in patients with ceramic restorations.

The patient should be advised that foods and liquids with a high potential for staining, such as coffee and tea, increase the potential for marginal staining. The patient must also be made aware of the potential for restoration fracture. Activities such as ice chewing and nail biting must be absolutely avoided. When a patient has a history of a parafunctional habit, a protective appliance should be fabricated to protect both the inlay or onlay and the opposing teeth.

Resin Composite Inlays and Onlays

Inlays and onlays made of resin composite are quite popular in Europe, but have not gained wide acceptance in the United States. These restorations may be fabricated intraorally or on a cast. After polymerization, the restoration is bonded in place with a resin luting cement. Resin composite inlays can be highly esthetic and have certain advantages over direct resin composite and bonded ceramic restorations.

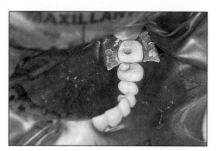

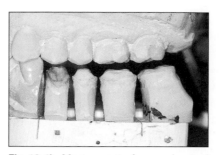

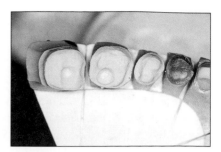

Fig 18-4a Rubber dam isolation for cementation of a quadrant of porcelain onlays.

Fig 18-4b Master cast of a quadrant of porcelain onlay preparations. Note the amount of occlusal reduction.

Fig 18-4c Occlusal view of onlay preparations.

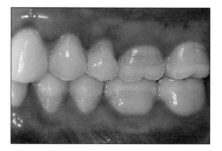

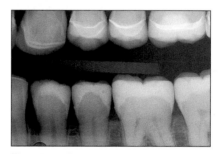

Figs 18-4d and 18-4e Porcelain onlays 2.5 years after placement. (Porcelain onlays created by Gilbert Young, CDT, GNS Dental Laboratory.)

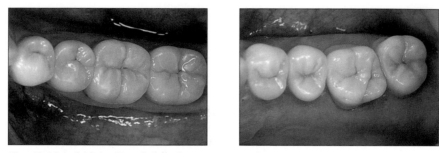

Fig 18-4f Lateral view of the maxillary and mandibular quadrants of porcelain onlays. The esthetic blend on the facial aspect of the maxillary premolars is better because the preparations were taken farther gingivally than on the molars.

Fig 18-4g Bite-wing radiograph at 2.5 years showing porcelain onlays. Note different cement radiopacity in maxillary and mandibular restorations.

Advantages Over Direct Resin Composite Restorations

As discussed in Chapter 10, inadequate proximal contours and open contacts are common problems of direct resin composite restorations. These are rarely problems with resin inlays, because contours and contacts can be developed outside of the mouth. If a contact is inadequate, it can easily be corrected prior to cementation.

Several problems associated with direct resin composite restorations are the result of polymerization shrinkage. During polymerization, resin composite shrinks on the order of 2% to 4%,[28] often causing a gap to form at the least retentive marginal interface, which is usually the gingival margin. Microleakage and bacterial ingress into the marginal gap may cause pulpal irritation and tooth sensitivity.[11] Current dentin adhesives have lessened, but not eliminated, the problem.[88] Polymerization shrinkage can also cause cuspal flexure, which is sometimes associated with craze lines in the enamel and postoperative sensitivity.[49,50]

In theory, polymerization shrinkage should be less of a problem with resin inlays because they are polymerized before cementation. The only polymerization

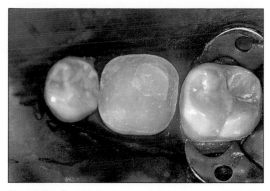

Fig 18-5a Porcelain onlay preparation, mandibular first molar.

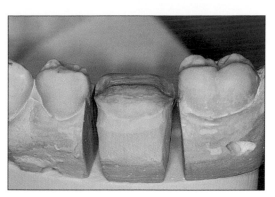

Fig 18-5b Master cast of prepared mandibular first molar for a porcelain onlay.

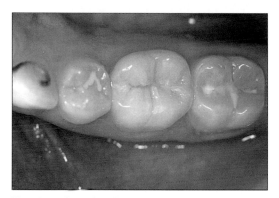

Fig 18-5c Completed porcelain onlay on mandibular first molar.

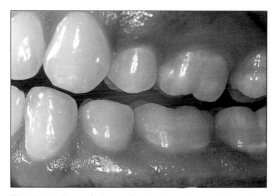

Fig 18-5d Buccal view of completed porcelain onlay on mandibular first molar. (Porcelain onlay created by Gilbert Young, CDT, GNS Dental Laboratory.)

shrinkage that occurs at the time of cementation is in the thin layer of resin cement. Resin inlays are reported to have less microleakage[36,89,95] and greater strength and hardness,[52,108,109] and to result in less postoperative sensitivity than direct resin composite restorations.[104]

Secondary Polymerization

The superior physical properties of resin inlays are primarily due to more complete polymerization resulting from secondary polymerization procedures. Resin composites harden through a process of free-radical polymerization of methacrylate groups. The polymerization reaction is initiated (in most cases) when a molecule within the resin composite (camphorquinone) forms free radicals when exposed to light of the appropriate wavelength (about 470 nm).

The radicals react with a photoreducer (an aromatic or aliphatic amine) to initiate chain formation of the methacrylate groups. As polymerization progresses, the methacrylate chains grow and the material loses its fluidity. A hard surface forms and spreads progressively deeper into the resin composite. The reaction stops when the light is removed, the thickness is too great to allow adequate light penetration, or there are no more reactive molecules in close proximity to each other. Even with long curing times and powerful lights, incomplete polymerization occurs, particularly below the surface.[63]

Light-cured resin composite inlays undergo this initial polymerization, but then are further polymerized in an oven or pressure pot with a combination of intense light, heat, and/or pressure. The postcure can be performed in a postcure unit specifically made for this purpose, in a toaster oven at approximately 250°F for 7 minutes,[52] or with a curing light or light box. Stud-

481

ies[108,109] have shown that the secondary polymerization results in improved physical properties but minimal clinical difference in wear characteristics.[110] The secondary curing procedures are recommended with all indirect resin systems, although they may not be mentioned in all manufacturers' instructions.

While the in vitro data suggest that there are significant advantages to the resin inlay compared to the direct resin composite restoration, this is not corroborated by the in vivo data. In a 5-year clinical study[107] and another 8-year clinical study,[80] no statistically significant difference was found in the success rates for resin inlays compared to direct-placement resin composite restorations. Based on these data, and because of the increased cost of the resin inlay, it is currently difficult to make a strong case in favor of the resin inlay over the direct resin composite restoration.

Many resin composite inlay systems are available. For the purposes of this chapter, they are classified as direct (made on the tooth) or indirect (made on a cast).

Direct Resin Inlays

Inlays can be fabricated directly on the tooth (Fig 18-6). After preparation, a water-soluble separating medium and a matrix are placed on the tooth. The preparation is bulk filled with resin composite and light cured from all directions. The matrix is removed, and the inlay is teased out of the preparation. Because the resin composite shrinks during polymerization, the inlay is slightly smaller than the preparation and will come out easily if no undercuts are present. The inlay is then postcured. Finally, it is tried in, adjusted, and bonded into the preparation (see Direct Resin Inlay Technique, page 486).

Direct/Indirect Resin Inlays

When the direct/indirect method is used, an impression is made of the prepared tooth and a cast is poured (Fig 18-7). Because this technique can be done in one appointment, the master cast must be ready to use in a short period of time (5 minutes). Therefore, the products used must be compatible with the technique. The master die can be made from a silicone material (Mach 2, Parkell), or a master cast made from die stone (Snap Stone, Whip Mix). The restoration is fabricated on the die and usually undergoes a primary (light-cured) and secondary (auxiliary curing unit)

polymerization. This process may be performed in the dental office or at a commercial laboratory.

Indirect Resin Inlays and Onlays

Resin inlays and onlays are also available through commercial laboratories. They can be constructed from either hybrid resin composite or microfilled resin composite. However, there is a newer generation of resin materials that has been termed *ceromers* or *ceramic optimized polymers*.[104] Currently, four ceromer products are widely used: Artglass (Heraeus Kulzer), belleGlass HP (Kerr), Targis (Ivoclar), and Skulptur FibreKor (Jeneric/Pentron). These materials are reported to have greater durability, fracture toughness, wear resistance, esthetics, and repairability.[104] However, in one laboratory study, repaired ceromers were found to be 30% to 60% weaker than the parent material.[65]

There is minimal independent laboratory data available on the physical properties of the ceromer products. Ferracane[29] compared Artglass to the traditional hybrid composite, Charisma (Heraeus Kulzer). The fracture toughness of Artglass was higher than with Charisma; however, the flexural modulus and the hardness were higher with Charisma. Similarly, the physical properties were evaluated for Artglass, Targis, and a traditional hybrid resin composite, Z100 (3M).[87] Targis demonstrated superior strength and Young's modulus compared to the other two products. The ceromer material may be combined with a fiber-reinforced material, which significantly increases fracture resistance.[5] However, flexural strength of fiber-reinforced ceromer has been shown to significantly decrease after storage in water.[4] Ceromer restorations are bonded in the same manner as other indirect resin inlays/onlays (Figs 18-8a to 18-8c).

Posterior Bonded Porcelain Restorations

Ceramic inlays were introduced in 1913,[84] but did not become popular because of difficulties in fabrication and a high failure rate.[3] In the 1980s, the development of compatible refractory materials made fabrication easier, and the development of adhesive resin cements greatly improved clinical success rates.[15]

The modern generation of bonded porcelain restorations was first described in 1983.[42] When it

Fig 18-6 Direct resin composite inlay technique.

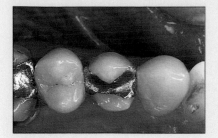

Fig 18-6a Preoperative view of a maxillary first premolar with an amalgam restoration that must be replaced.

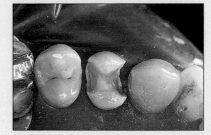

Fig 18-6b Preparation for a direct mesio-occlusodistal resin composite inlay.

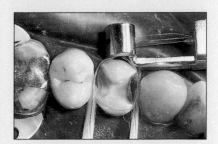

Fig 18-6c Placement of a matrix for a direct resin composite inlay.

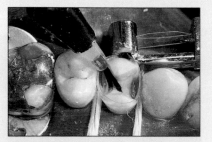

Fig 18-6d Placement of separating medium into the preparation.

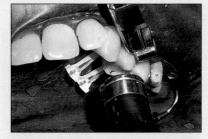

Fig 18-6e Light curing of the resin composite inlay, which was placed in bulk.

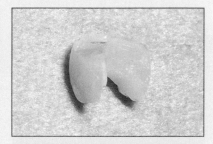

Fig 18-6f Resin composite inlay after it has been removed from the preparation.

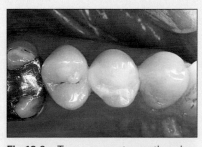

Fig 18-6g Two-year postoperative view of the direct mesio-occlusodistal resin composite inlay in the maxillary first premolar.

became clear that the technique had merit in anterior applications, interest developed in the use of bonded porcelain for posterior applications. In 1986, Redford and Jensen[86] described the strengthening effect of porcelain inlays on the fracture resistance of natural teeth. In 1988, Jensen[51] reported excellent clinical success in a 2-year in vivo study. The technique has since been refined to the point that porcelain inlays and onlays are now an accepted operative modality.

Indications

The indications for posterior bonded porcelain restorations overlap those for direct and indirect posterior resin composite restorations, which have already been described. These restorations are indicated when there is an overriding desire for esthetics and all margins can be placed on enamel. Some clinicians recommend bonded porcelain rather than resin composite for larger restorations.[15]

Direct Resin Inlay Technique

Fabrication

1. Select a shade prior to tooth dehydration.

2. Place rubber dam to isolate the tooth to be restored.

3. Remove restoration and/or carious tooth structure and make preparation with 8 to 10 degrees of occlusal divergence. The preparation should be smooth, with rounded line angles and without marginal bevels. Ensure that the gingival margin is on enamel; if not, choose an alternate restoration.

4. Coat preparation with a thin layer of water-soluble lubricant.

5. Place the matrix band and wedge it.

6. Bulk load the resin composite into the preparation and roughly form occlusal anatomy.

7. Light cure for 45 seconds from the occlusal and proximal aspects.

8. Remove wedge(s) and matrix band.

9. Remove resin composite inlay with a spoon or carver. If there are undercuts in the preparation or the composite bonds to the tooth, the inlay will have to be cut out and redone.

10. Postcure the inlay.

Placement

11. Return the inlay to the preparation and check interproximal contacts. Because of postcure shrinkage, a three-surface inlay may not seat completely. When this occurs, lightly reduce the inner (axial) surfaces of both proximal boxes with a microfine diamond. Try the inlay in again, and repeat the process until the inlay seats completely. If interproximal contacts are open, roughen the surface, place a thin layer of unfilled resin, place a thin layer of resin composite, light cure, and readjust the contact(s).

12. Air abrade the inner surface of the inlay with 50-μm alumina to etch it.

13. Place silane on the etched surface of the restoration only and air dry.

14. Place a Tofflemire matrix on the prepared tooth to ensure that the etchant is not in contact with adjacent teeth.

15. Etch the preparation with 30% to 40% phosphoric acid etch gel for 20 seconds, wash for 5 seconds, and air dry to ensure adequate enamel etch.

16. Remoisten dentin and place several coats of dentin primer on damp dentin. Air dry primer, gently at first, until surface is completely dry, and confirm uniform shiny surface.

17. Remove the Tofflemire matrix.

18. Mix and place a dual-cure adhesive, which is not light cured before restoration placement. Similarly, dual-cure adhesive must be placed on the inner surface of the restoration.

19. Mix dual-cure resin composite luting cement and place into the preparation and inner surface of the restoration with a syringe.

20. Gently place the restoration into the preparation and vibrate with a hand instrument to ensure that it is almost fully seated.

21. Remove excess composite luting cement with a brush both occlusally and interproximally.

22. Gently seat the restoration completely with an instrument on the occlusal surface, making sure that a bead of composite luting cement is expressed at all margins. Confirm correct seating with an explorer at the margins.

23. While the assistant is holding the restoration in place, gently clean interproximal margins with floss, an explorer, and a No. 12 scalpel blade, being careful not to cause bleeding. The interproximal margins must be completely finished before the resin composite luting cement polymerizes. Leave excess composite on facial and lingual margins.

24. Cover all accessible interproximal margins with glycerin.

25. Complete polymerization by light curing 90 seconds from the occlusal aspect and 30 seconds from each proximal aspect.

Finishing

26. Finish all margins with 12-fluted carbide burs, finishing disks, and/or composite polishing points.

27. Remove the rubber dam and adjust the occlusion with articulating paper and a fine diamond (gross adjustment) and a 12-fluted, egg-shaped carbide bur (fine adjustment).

28. Complete polishing with composite polishing points and aluminum oxide polishing paste.

29. Etch with 30% phosphoric acid for 5 seconds and rebond.

may not provide in a cuspal-coverage restoration. The stronger bond of resin cement to porcelain is particularly important when cusps are covered. The stronger the bond, the more efficiently forces are transferred from the restoration through the cement and absorbed into the tooth.[21] For these reasons, when even one cusp of a posterior tooth is being covered with an esthetic bonded onlay, the porcelain onlay is preferred.

Porcelain onlays may be used routinely for the esthetic restoration of premolars. They may also be used as cuspal-coverage restorations for molars, although the occlusal forces will be greater in the molar region. Another indication for the porcelain onlay is in the restoration of a molar with a short occlusogingival dimension. In this circumstance, it is difficult to gain axial retention and resistance with a conventional crown preparation. However, the porcelain onlay preparation requires only 2 mm of occlusal reduction and requires no axial reduction for retention and resistance. The short molar, which would have previously required crown-lengthening surgery before placement of a complete-coverage crown, can now be more conservatively restored with the porcelain onlay.

Selection of appropriate patients is paramount in the placement of posterior bonded porcelain restorations. For the greatest long-term predictable success, all margins should be on enamel. Also, the patient and the tooth to be restored should be amenable to rubber dam placement. Ideally, the patient should exhibit no signs of a parafunctional habit. In addition, the restoration should be fabricated so that it contacts in maximum intercuspation but has no contacts on the porcelain in eccentric mandibular positions.

Shade Selection

The shade used for a porcelain inlay or onlay is selected in the same way as for a metal-ceramic crown. Because of the thickness of the porcelain, the underlying tooth color and cement shade have a minimal effect on the shade of the final restoration except at the margins. As with porcelain veneers, use of a translucent resin cement is recommended to improve the esthetic blend at the margins.

Fabrication

The most common method of fabrication of porcelain inlays and onlays utilizes a refractory die. After a master die is poured in die stone, a refractory die is made by duplicating the master die or repouring the impression in a refractory material. The porcelain is baked on the refractory die, recovered, and fit to the master die. Variations in the fit of ceramic inlays and onlays are reported to be related more to technician ability than the type of ceramic material used.[23]

The newer generation of pressed ceramics is fabricated much differently. The restoration is waxed on a stone die in the traditional manner and invested in a special investment. The invested wax pattern is burned out as in the traditional lost-wax technique. An ingot of the pressed ceramic material is heated and pressed into the lost-wax pattern space. After cooling, the investment is removed and the ceramic restoration is retrieved and finished in the same manner as a feldspathic porcelain restoration.

Isolation

It is universally acknowledged that strict isolation is necessary for bonding of posterior adhesive restorations. This is best accomplished with a well-placed rubber dam. If it is not possible to isolate the tooth with a rubber dam, an adhesive restoration should not be placed (see Porcelain Onlay Technique, page 488).

Resin Composite vs Porcelain

Wear

There is a significant difference in the wear characteristics of resin composite and porcelain. Wear is not a significant factor in a porcelain restoration,[15,16] but traditional feldspathic porcelain is highly abrasive and can cause significant wear of the opposing dentition. A newer generation of low-fusing porcelains has been shown to cause significantly less wear of enamel than traditional feldspathic porcelain.[66,97] The new class of pressable ceramics, described previously, has become popular, in part because they are less abrasive to opposing teeth. These include Empress (Ivoclar), Empress 2 (Ivoclar), Optimal Pressed Ceramic (OPC, Jeneric/Pentron), and Finesse All-Ceramic (Dentsply). The first generation of Empress showed decreased wear of opposing enamel compared to traditional and low-fusing porcelains, in vitro.[43] However, the newer generation, Empress 2, has shown almost no wear of

Porcelain Onlay Technique

Preparation

1. Select a shade prior to tooth dehydration.
2. Make a stent for fabrication of a provisional restoration.
3. Remove existing restoration.
4. Ensure that gingival margins are on enamel and that the tooth can be isolated with a rubber dam; if not, choose an alternate restoration.
5. After completion of the preparation, there should be room for at least a 2-mm thickness of porcelain. All internal line angles should be rounded and walls divergent occlusally. There should be no grooves or boxes.
6. Make an impression, using retraction cord if required.
7. Make a custom provisional restoration using the stent. Place undercuts in the intaglio surface of the provisional restoration.
8. Cement with a strong provisional cement; because the preparation has minimal resistance form, polycarboxylate is the provisional cement of choice.

Placement

9. Check restoration on die for fit and check for fracture lines with transillumination.
10. Place the rubber dam.
11. Remove the provisional restoration and clean cement from the preparation with an ultrasonic scaler or a slow-speed diamond and pumice with a brush.
12. Try in the porcelain restoration; adjust interproximal contacts with coarse Sof-Lex disks (3M), and polish with porcelain polishing points.
13. Clean the onlay with acetone and air dry.
14. Place silane on the etched surface of the onlay only and air dry.
15. Place a Tofflemire matrix on the prepared tooth to ensure that the etch is not in contact with adjacent teeth.
16. Etch the tooth with 30% to 40% phosphoric acid etch gel for 20 seconds, wash for 5 seconds, and air dry to ensure adequate enamel etch.
17. Remoisten dentin and place several coats of dentin primer on damp dentin. Air dry the primer, gently at first, until the surface is completely dry and confirm a uniform shiny surface.
18. Remove the Tofflemire matrix.
19. Mix and place a dual-cure adhesive, which should not be light cured before placement of the restoration. Similarly, dual-cure adhesive must be placed on the inner surface of the restoration.
20. Mix dual-cure resin composite luting cement and place into the preparation and the inner surface of the restoration with a syringe.
21. Gently place the restoration into the preparation and vibrate with a hand instrument to ensure that it is almost fully seated.
22. Remove excess resin composite luting cement with a brush both occlusally and proximally.
23. Gently seat the restoration completely with an instrument applied to the occlusal surface, making sure that a bead of composite is expressed at all margins. Confirm correct seating with an explorer at the margins.
24. While the assistant holds the restoration in place, gently clean interproximal margins with floss, an explorer, and a No. 12 blade, being careful not to cause bleeding. The interproximal margins must be completely finished before the composite polymerizes. Leave excess composite luting cement on facial and lingual margins.
25. Cover all accessible interproximal margins with glycerin.
26. Complete polymerization by light curing 90 seconds from the occlusal aspect and 30 seconds from each proximal aspect.

Finishing

27. Finish all margins with 12-fluted carbide burs, finishing disks, and/or composite polishing points.
28. Remove the rubber dam and adjust the occlusion with articulating paper and a fine diamond.
29. Complete polishing with rubber porcelain polishing points.

---

opposing enamel, both in vitro[97] and in vivo at 6 months.[98] If long-term clinical studies confirm the low wear of opposing enamel, this will be a significant advance in ceramics.

The data concerning wear of resin composite materials have been somewhat contradictory.[13,34,106] Enamel is reported to wear at a rate of 20 to 40 µm per year.[61] Most modern resin composite materials fall within that range.[29,106] Ferracane[29] reported that the wear of the traditional resin composite, Charisma, was lower than that for the ceromer, Artglass. Similarly, Reich et al[87] evaluated the wear of Artglass, Targis, and a traditional resin composite, Z100. Although Targis demonstrated superior physical properties, Z100 had the highest wear resistance. In another laboratory study,[101] the wear of three commercially available ceromer materials was compared to a gold control. Targis demonstrated the greatest wear, followed by Artglass; Skulptur FibreKor demonstrated the least wear, which was approximately equal to that of gold. Similarly, the wear rates for Artglass and Targis were evaluated in a two-body wear test.[56] Targis demonstrated wear similar to that of enamel, and Artglass had significantly higher wear than enamel.

Longevity

Results of short-term clinical studies of resin inlays are encouraging, but there are few long-term data. Bishop[9] reported one failure of 92 resin inlays that had been in place for 7 months to 4 years. A Swedish study[8] reported that 29 of 30 resin inlays were excellent or acceptable at 17 months, while another study[24] reported good marginal integrity at 5 years. One American study[112] reported no failures among 60 resin inlays after 3 years, while another American study[38] reported that 10 of 145 resin inlays failed at 3 years. However, it is still not clear whether the resin inlay offers any advantages in terms of longevity over the direct-placement resin composite restoration. Two clinical studies reported no significant differences between resin inlays and direct resin composite restorations at 5 years[107] and at 8 years.[80]

There has been little clinical research on the longevity of the newer generation ceromer restorations. One clinical study[78] of an experimental ceromer, now marketed as belleGlass, reported 5-year results of 24 inlays and onlays. All restorations were performing satisfactorily, although 12% had interfacial staining and 58% had slight to moderate marginal degradation.

Several clinical studies have evaluated the performance of ceramic inlays/onlays. The clinical success of traditional feldspathic inlays has been mixed. One 4-year study[33] reported no failures in 50 inlays. However, another study reported that 21 of 145 inlays fractured at 3 years,[68] while another study[83] reported 16% failure at 3 years. In a similar study,[38] 24 of 181 inlays fractured for a failure rate of 13%. If these high failure rates are confirmed by other clinical studies, the utility of the feldspathic porcelain inlay must be questioned.

However, clinical results with the pressed ceramic Empress have been more promising. Several clinical studies[25,30,31,99] have shown excellent clinical success up to 6 years.

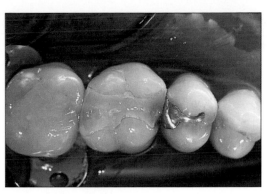

Fig 18-9 Maxillary first molar with a 7-year-old bonded Dicor (Dentsply) inlay demonstrating marginal ditching and a small fracture of the marginal ridge.

Failures

Two types of failure are most common with esthetic inlays and onlays: bulk fracture (see Fig 18-3) and marginal breakdown (Fig 18-9). Bulk fracture sometimes occurs in areas of cuspal coverage, particularly if the restorative material is less than 2.0 mm thick. It also occurs at the isthmus adjacent to marginal ridges, where the porcelain is poorly supported by tooth structure.

Marginal ditching is a common finding in esthetic inlays and onlays.[59,60,78,105] Because resin cements tend not to be heavily filled, they wear more quickly than the adjacent restorations or tooth structure. This is particularly true if the marginal fit is poor.[77,113] Kawai and others[54] demonstrated a linear relationship between wear of resin cement and the horizontal marginal gap. They concluded that reduction of the marginal gap is an important clinical consideration in minimizing the wear of the resin cement. They also found that hybrid resin cements wear faster than microfilled resins. Isenberg and others[47] reported 3-year results of a clinical study of 121 Cerec inlay and onlay restorations. None of the restorations exhibited any evidence of interfacial staining, discoloration, or caries, but about 50% of the restorations exhibited gap dimensions large enough to be detected with an explorer. The rate of wear of the resin composite luting agent was linear over the first year, but no further vertical wear was noted over the course of the investigation. The depth-width ratio of the gap generally did not exceed 50%.

CAD/CIM Ceramic Restorations

A recent addition to the field of dental ceramics has been CAD/CIM technology. Several CAD/CIM systems are available, but the most widely used is the Cerec System (Sirona Dental Systems). The Cerec (*ceramic reconstruction*) System, developed in 1980, was marketed in Europe in 1985, and the first clinical trials took place in 1987.[73] It was introduced in the United States in 1989. With this system, a ceramic inlay, onlay, veneer, or crown is created in a single appointment with the aid of an optical scanner, a computer, and a milling machine. The tooth is prepared, and the preparation is scanned electronically. The image is then manipulated and output to a milling machine, where the restoration is milled from a ceramic block. After adjustments, the restoration is ready for cementation.[70,72,73]

Another CAD/CIM system, the CELAY system (Vident), is also available. A resin or wax pattern of the preparation is made and used as a model for the ceramic restoration. The external surface of the pattern is mechanically traced with a probe, the dimensions are input into the computer and processed by the software, and a ceramic restoration is generated.[26] Although CAD/CIM is not currently widely used, the accuracy to which the restorations can be milled has reached a clinically acceptable level. In both 3-year[47] and 5-year[74] clinical evaluations, CAD/CIM restorations have performed satisfactorily.

Advantages and Disadvantages

The main advantage of CAD/CIM technology is time saved. This technique affords the opportunity to prepare, design, and fabricate a ceramic restoration in a single appointment, without the need for conventional impressions, provisional restorations, or dental laboratory support.

The CAD/CIM technology also offers excellent esthetics, durability, and at least short-term strengthening of the tooth. Roznowski et al[90] compared the fracture resistance of molars restored with various adhesive and nonadhesive restorations and reported that teeth restored with mesio-occlusodistal Cerec inlays were as strong as unprepared, unrestored teeth, while the nonadhesive restorations weakened the tooth.

Many of the problems associated with the original CAD/CAM systems have been overcome with the CAD/CIM systems. Originally, there was no capability for making crowns. However, software (Crown 1.0 and Crown 1.11) is now available to make both anterior and posterior full crowns. Computer design and milling of the occlusal anatomy is significantly improved with the Cerec 2 unit. Advances in the software program allow for preoperative imaging of the occlusal anatomy intraorally or from a preoperative cast or diagnostic waxup for superimposition of the design on the preparation. But because secondary and tertiary anatomy is not duplicated, some occlusal adjustment is still required.

A significant training period is required to achieve proficiency with the system. Participation in a 2- to 3-day initial training course is usually recommended, followed by laboratory practice on an additional 25 to 30 restorations. The cost of the system is considerable, even if shared by several practitioners.

A major concern about CAD/CIM restorations is their precementation marginal fit. Several studies have evaluated marginal openings in CAD/CIM restorations. Molin and Karlsson[67,68] reported that the marginal adaptation of CAD/CIM restorations is inferior to that of traditional ceramic or gold restorations. This study utilized a Cerec 1 unit, which has been shown to mill restorations with a much poorer fit than restorations generated with a Cerec 2 unit. Krejci and others[58] reported precementation marginal openings in the range of 125 to 175 µm. After cementation, they found that more than 90% of enamel-ceramic interfaces had "continuous margins." They found that the quality of the marginal adaptation immediately after cementation does not seem to depend on precementation marginal fit. Peters and Bieniek[82] reported on a clinical study of 22 inlays fabricated with a Cerec 1 unit in which the average marginal gap was 121 µm with a range of 60 to 150 µm. Using the Cerec 1 unit, Wilder[113] reported the average film thickness of cement at the occlusal cavosurface margin to be 89 ± 65 µm. The average thickness at the gingival margin was 105 ± 81 µm. Inokoshi and others[46] evaluated the marginal gap of Cerec inlays with the initial Cerec operating system (COS) 1.0 software (Siemens) and the updated software version, COS 2.0. They reported a mean occlusal marginal gap of 52 µm with the updated software, a significant improvement over that measured when the initial software program was used. Christensen,[19] by comparison, has reported that gold castings can be fabricated with marginal openings of less than 25 µm. Because of the relatively large precementation marginal gaps in restorations produced by CAD/CIM, the exposed resin cement may be the weak link.

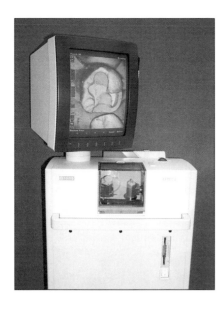

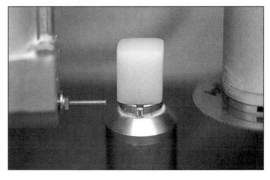

Fig 18-10 Cerec 2 CAD/CIM unit consists of a computer, intraoral camera, video monitor, and milling chamber.

Fig 18-11 Cerec milling chamber with cylindrical diamond and diamond disk milling instruments with ceramic block prior to milling.

Marginal fit of Cerec restorations is directly linked to the unit model (Cerec 1 vs Cerec 2) and the software utilized (COS 4.64, Crown 1.0, or Crown 1.11).

Mörmann and Schug[71] evaluated the marginal fit of CAD/CIM inlays with the improved Cerec 2 unit and the COS 4.01. They reported the overall mean interfacial margin width to be 56 ± 27 µm for Cerec 2 inlays and 84 ± 38 µm for Cerec 1 inlays. They also reported that the grinding precision of the Cerec 2 unit was 2.4 times greater than that of the Cerec 1 unit.

Hardware and Software

The Cerec CAD/CIM system consists of an intraoral camera, a video monitor, a computer, and a milling chamber (Fig 18-10). The computer utilizes software for design and construction of ceramic restorations. Currently available software packages allow fabrication of ceramic inlays, onlays, veneers, and crowns. The Cerec 2 camera has been redesigned with a detachable cover that can be dry-heat sterilized. The pixel size of the camera has been reduced from 54 × 54 µm to 25 × 29 µm, reducing volumetric measurement errors on a typical inlay restoration to less than ± 25 µm. An additional feature is that the computer trackball used for computer graphic design can be removed and disinfected.[69]

The Cerec 2 monitor has been expanded in size and displays the tooth with 12× magnification compared to the Cerec 1 unit, which displayed the tooth at an 8× magnification.[71] A second milling arm has been included in addition to the previous 40-mm-diameter diamond wheel (Fig 18-11). It contains a cylindrical diamond, which comes in 1.2-mm, 1.6-mm, and 2.0-mm diameters. This second milling arm allows six axes of rotation for the Cerec 2 unit compared to three axes of rotation for the Cerec 1 unit. It also accounts for the improved occlusal anatomy of Cerec 2 restorations. The second milling cylinder also overcomes cavity design problems inherent in the Cerec 1 unit and allows the clinician to utilize conventional ceramic inlay and onlay preparation designs.

Inlays

Preparation

The cavity preparation for CAD/CIM inlays is similar to that for a conventional indirect ceramic inlay.[18,20] The occlusal aspect of the tooth being prepared should be reduced to provide at least 2 mm of occlusal depth for the ceramic restoration to impart adequate strength. All cavosurface margins should be well defined and have, as nearly as possible, a 90-degree butt joint. This will allow the camera head to record an accurate image of the cavosurface margin. Bevels and chamfer-style margins should not be used.

Computer-Assisted Design

A dry field is necessary to ensure that the preparation is optically scanned with precision and accuracy. It is also critical to clearly isolate the gingival extent of the preparation from the adjacent soft tissues. For these reasons, the use of a rubber dam is essential.

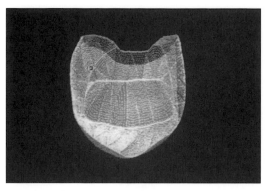

Fig 18-17 Computer software constructing a volume model of the onlay as a guide in milling.

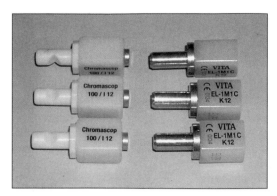

Fig 18-18 Ceramic blocks on stubs for milling chamber. ProCAD (Ivoclar) *(left)* and Esthetic Line (Vita) blocks *(right)*.

sive and more resistant to wear than conventional aluminous and bonded ceramic materials. ProCAD (Ivoclar), introduced in 1998, is a leucite-reinforced ceramic similar to Empress, but with a finer particle size. It is the same material used for the Sonicsys (Ivoclar) ceramic inserts. Both materials can be characterized and glazed with chairside stains and a porcelain oven.

Once the ceramic block has been locked in the milling chamber, the unit is ready to mill the restoration. A diamond disk and cylindrical diamond move into contact with the metallic mounting of the ceramic block, which calibrates the position of the milling head. The ceramic block, rotating as it goes, is fed uniformly across the milling disk (Fig 18-18). Milling occurs in six axes, from mesial to distal; the "sprue" of ceramic material, where the restoration is separated from the ceramic block, ends up on the distal surface. Milling time is a function of the size and complexity of the restoration and ranges, on average, from 10 to 20 minutes.

Try-In and Cementation

Once the ceramic restoration is recovered from the milling chamber, the sprue is removed, and the inlay is tried in (Figs 18-19a to 18-19c). Adjustments may be required for accurate fit. The axiopulpal line angle and the gingival floor of the box are the areas most likely to require adjustment.[113] Should the fit be unacceptable in some area, the design can be reloaded from the program disk and corrected, and a second restoration can be quickly milled.

With the introduction of the Cerec 2 unit, some occlusal anatomy can be programmed into the restoration. However, a moderate amount of occlusal adjustment may be required, depending on the design program selected. The extrapolation option allows the clinician to totally design the occlusal surface. The correlation program allows for the superimposition of the preoperative occlusal anatomy onto the preparation and minimizes the occlusal adjustment required.

The ceramic restoration should be etched and silanated before adhesive cementation. Use of a conventional adhesive cementation technique and a dual-cured resin cement is recommended. Contouring and delineation of anatomy with various microfine diamonds or carbide burs can be accomplished after cementation.[94] Finishing and polishing are completed with abrasive rubber points, disks, and cups with diamond polishing paste as for other ceramic restorations (Fig 18-19d).

Onlays

The computer design of an onlay is essentially the same as that for an inlay, except that one or more cusps are being reconstructed (Fig 18-17). This is accomplished when the marginal ridge is drawn. The software program draws in the marginal ridge as if the onlay were an inlay, resulting in a cuspal height equivalent to that of the marginal ridge. To create a cusp, the marginal ridge is edited in the profile view to elevate that portion of the marginal ridge over the area of the missing cusp. The milling of the restoration occurs in the same manner as for an inlay.

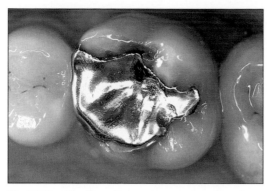

Fig 18-19a Maxillary first molar, preoperative view.

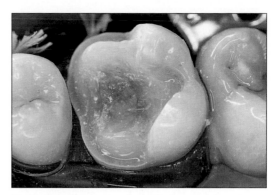

Fig 18-19b Preparation for milled porcelain onlay.

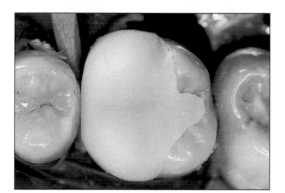

Fig 18-19c Try-in of milled onlay.

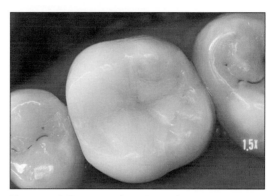

Fig 18-19d Postoperative view of milled porcelain onlay on maxillary first molar. (Photos courtesy of Dr K. Lampe.)

Crowns

The newest feature of the Crown 1.11 software program is the full-crown option for both anterior and posterior all-ceramic crowns. The tooth preparation is the same as that described for other all-ceramic crowns. There must be 2 mm of occlusal clearance and at least 1.2 mm of axial reduction. The computer graphic design process is similar to that of an onlay. The milling process is somewhat longer, and many clinicians choose to characterize the monochromatic shade of the porcelain blocks with shade modifiers and glaze prior to adhesive cementation (Figs 18-20a to 18-20d).

It is also possible to design and mill a coping for a full crown. Aluminum oxide core material is available in block form for the Cerec unit. It can be milled to a predetermined thickness by setting the default parameter in the Cerec unit. After the coping is milled, it can be sent to a dental laboratory where the veneer porcelain is added as with any core-type all-ceramic crown.

An additional preparation design has been suggested for Cerec crowns: the endodontic crown design. This design incorporates the core and short post into the crown as a single restoration (Figs 18-21a to 18-21d) and significantly increases the surface area of the preparation available for adhesive cementation. It is particularly useful in teeth with short clinical crowns. Because this restoration has not been well evaluated clinically, the expected longevity of crowns with this design is unknown.

Longevity/Clinical Studies

Most clinical studies of Cerec restorations have been completed using the Cerec 1 unit, and a good clinical record has been established. Heymann and others[39] reported on a 4-year clinical study of Cerec inlays. They found no significant changes in the 50 inlays during the study period. There were no restoration

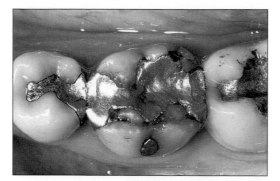

Fig 18-20a Mandibular first molar, preoperative view.

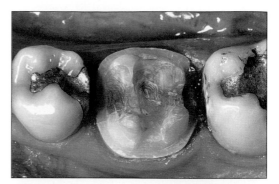

Fig 18-20b Preparation for Cerec full crown.

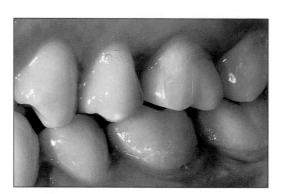

Fig 18-20c Postoperative buccal view of Cerec full crown on mandibular first molar.

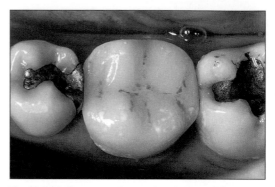

Fig 18-20d Postoperative occlusal view of Cerec full crown on mandibular first molar.

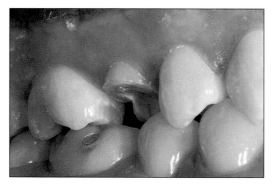

Fig 18-21a Buccal view of endodontically treated maxillary second premolar prepared for a Cerec full crown.

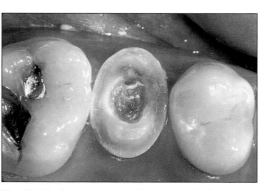

Fig 18-21b Occlusal view of endodontically treated maxillary second premolar prepared for a Cerec full crown.

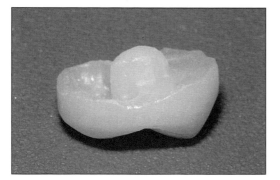

Fig 18-21c Milled Cerec crown.

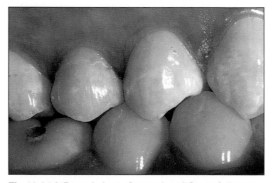

Fig 18-21d Buccal view of completed Cerec full crown on endodontically treated maxillary second premolar.

fractures, nor was any postoperative sensitivity reported. With the improvements in the Cerec 2 unit and software, it is expected that the clinical success of the CAD/CIM technique can only be improved. In a 5-year clinical study of Cerec inlays, Sjogren and others[96] reported that 89% were rated "satisfactory." They reported a 6.1% failure rate, with three inlay fractures, one tooth fracture, and one inlay with dentin exposed at the margin. Zuellig-Singer and Bryant[115] reported on a 3-year clinical evaluation of Cerec inlays with four different luting agents. They found that 94.6% of the inlays had continuous margins and only one inlay fractured. No significant difference was found in continuous margins between the four luting agents, but there was less wear with the microfilled luting agent than with the hybrid composite and the glass-ionomer cement.

References

1. Al-Hyasat AS, Saunders WP, Sharkey SW, et al. Investigation of human enamel wear against four dental ceramics and gold. J Dent 1998;26:487–495.

2. Bailey L, Bennett R. Two year bond results of Dicor ceramic/LA cement system [abstract 1734]. J Dent Res 1989;68:398.

3. Banks RG. Conservative posterior ceramic restorations: a literature review. J Prosthet Dent 1990;63:619–626.

4. Behr M, Rosentritt M, Lang R, Handel G. Flexural strength of fiber-reinforced bars after different types of loading [abstract 2305]. J Dent Res 1999;78:394.

5. BelleGlass Technical Data. Physical properties of indirect composite resins (reference 139AK74). Orange, CA: Kerr Laboratories, 1997.

6. Bergeron C, Guzman S, Vargas MA. Bond strength of single-bottle adhesives: multiple applications [abstract 213]. J Dent Res 1998;77:132.

7. Bergmann P, Noack MJ, Roulet J-F. Marginal adaptation with glass ceramic inlays adhesively luted with glycerine gel. Quintessence Int 1991;22:739–744.

8. Bessing C, Lundqvist P. A one-year clinical examination of indirect resin composite inlays: a preliminary report. Quintessence Int 1991;22:153–157.

9. Bishop BM. A heat and pressure cured composite inlay system: a clinical evaluation. Aust Prosthodont J 1989;3:35–41.

10. Bocangel JS, Demarci FF, Turbino ML, et al. Influence of eugenol on the microleakage and bond strength of two bonding agents [abstract 421]. J Dent Res 1997;76:66.

11. Brännström M. Infection beneath resin composite restorations: can it be avoided? Oper Dent 1987;12:158–163.

12. Burgess JO, Haveman CW, Butzin C. Evaluation of resins for provisional restorations. Am J Dent 1992;5:137–139.

13. Burgoyne A, Nichols J, Brudvik J. In vitro two-body wear of inlay-onlay resin composite restorations. J Prosthet Dent 1991;65:206–214.

14. Burquieres SH, Burgess JD, Ripps A. Bond strength of resin cement to the dentin varying curing modes and light intensity [abstract 2987]. J Dent Res 1999;78:479.

15. Burke FJT, Qualtrough AJE. Aesthetic inlays: composite or ceramic? Br Dent J 1994;176:53–60.

16. Burke FJT, Wilson NHF, Watts DC. The effect of cuspal coverage on the fracture resistance of teeth restored with indirect resin composite restorations. Quintessence Int 1993;4:875–880.

17. Burke FJT, Wilson NHF, Watts DC. The effect of cavity wall taper on fracture resistance of teeth restored with resin composite inlays. Oper Dent 1993;18:230–236.

18. Cerec Operator's Manual. COS 4.3X–CROWN 1.2X. Bensheim, Germany: Sirona Dental Systems, 1999.

19. Christensen GJ. Marginal fit of gold inlay castings. J Prosthet Dent 1966;16:297–305.

20. David SB, LoPresti JT. Tooth-colored posterior restorations using Cerec method CAD/CAM-generated ceramic inlays. Compend Cont Educ Dent 1994;15:802–810.

21. Derand T. Stress analysis of cemented or resin-bonded porcelain inlays. Dent Mater 1991;7:21–24.

22. DeSchepper EJ, Tate WH, Powers JM. Bond strength of resin cements to microfilled composites. Am J Dent 1993;6:235–238.

23. Dietschi D, Maeder M, Holz J. In vitro evaluation of marginal fit and morphology of fired ceramic inlays. Quintessence Int 1992;23:271–278.

24. Dijken JWV, Horstedt P. Marginal breakdown of 5-year-old direct composite inlays. J Dent 1996;24:389–394.

25. Dijken JWV, Hasselroth L, Ormin A, Olofsson AL. Clinical evaluation of extensive dentin enamel bonded all-ceramic onlays and onlay crowns [abstract 2713]. J Dent Res 1999;78:445.

26. Eidenbenz S, Lehner CR, Schärer P. Coping milling ceramic inlays from resin analogs: a practical approach with the CELAY System. Int J Prosthodont 1994;7:134–142.

27. Fasbinder DJ. The effect of powder type and application technique on the precementation die of CAD/CIM inlays. Int J Comput Dent, submitted 1999.

28. Feilzer AJ, de Gee AJ, Davidson CL. Curing contraction of composites and glass ionomer cements. J Prosthet Dent 1988;59:297.

29. Ferracane J. Evaluation of cure, properties, and wear resistance of Artglass dental composite. Am J Dent 1998;11(5):214–218.

30. Fradeani M, Aquilano A, Basseyi L. Longitudinal study of pressed glass ceramic inlays for four and a half years. J Prosthet Dent 1997;78:346–353.

31. Frankenberger R, Rumi K, Kramer N. Clinical evaluation of Leucite reinforced glass ceramic inlays and onlays after 6 years [abstract 1623]. J Dent Res 1999;78:308.

32. Frankenberger R, Sindel J, Kramer N, Petschelt A. Dentin bond strength and marginal adaptation: direct composite resins vs ceramic inlays. Oper Dent 1999;24:147–155.

33. Friedl KH, Schmalz G, Hiller KA, Bey B. In vitro evaluation of a feldspathic ceramic system: 4 year results. J Dent Res 1997;76:163.

34. Gray W, Suzuki M, Jordan R, et al. Clinical evaluation of indirect composite restorations—3 year results [abstract 633]. J Dent Res 1991;70:344.

35. Hammesfahr PD, Sang J, Hayes LC. In vitro shear bond strength study of various adhesives [abstract 3431]. J Dent Res 1999;78:534.

36. Hasegawa EA, Boyer DB, Chan DCN. Microleakage of indirect composite inlays. Dent Mater 1989;5:388–391.

37. Haws SM, Vargas MA, Guzman S, Cobb DS. Effect of primer application on microleakage of composite resins [abstract 403]. J Dent Res 1997;76:64.

38. Hein DK, Christensen RP, Smith SL. 3 year breakage rate of class 2 tooth colored materials [abstract 1200]. J Dent Res 1997;76:163.

39. Heymann HO, Bayne SC, Sturdevant JR, et al. The clinical performance of CAD/CAM generated ceramic inlays: a four year study. J Am Dent Assoc 1996;127;1172–1181.

40. Hilton TJ, Schwartz RS. The effect of air thinning on dentin adhesive bond strength [abstract 243]. J Dent Res 1994;73:132.

41. Hilton TJ, Schwartz RS, Ferracane JL. Fifth generation bonding agent application technique effects on bond strength [abstract 214]. J Dent Res 1998;77:132.

42. Horn HR. A new lamination: porcelain bonded to enamel. N Y State Dent J 1983;49:401–403.

43. Imai, Y, Suzuki S, Fukushima S. In vitro enamel wear modified porcelains [abstract 50]. J Dent Res 1999;78:112.

44. Imamura GM, Reinhardt JW, Boyer DB, Swift EJ. Enhancement of resin bonding to heat-cured composite resin. Oper Dent 1996;21;249–256.

45. Inokoshi S, Iwaku M, Fusayama T. Pulp response to a new adhesive restorative resin. J Dent Res 1982;61:1014–1019.

46. Inokoshi S, Van Meerbeek B, Willems G, et al. Marginal accuracy of CAD/CAM inlays made with the original and the updated software. J Dent 1992;20:171–177.

47. Isenberg BP, Essig ME, Leinfelder KF. Three year clinical evaluation of CAD/CAM restorations. J Esthet Dent 1992;4:173–176.

48. Jedynakiewicz NM, Martin N. CAD-CAM in Restorative Dentistry: The Cerec Method. Liverpool, England: University Press, 1993.

49. Jensen ME, Chan DCN. Polymerization, shrinkage and microleakage. In: Vanherle G, Smith DC (eds). Posterior Resin Composite Dental Restorative Materials. Utrecht, The Netherlands: Szulc, 1985:243–262.

50. Jensen ME, Redford DA, Williams BT, Gardner F. Posterior etched porcelain restorations; an in-vitro study. Compend Contin Educ Dent 1987;8:615–622.

51. Jensen ME. A two-year clinical study of posterior etched-porcelain resin-bonded restorations. Am J Dent 1988;1:27–33.

52. Kanca J. The effect of heat on the surface hardness of light-activated resin composites. Quintessence Int 1989;20:899–901.

53. Karaagaclioglu L, Zaimoglu A, Akoren AC. Microleakage of indirect inlays placed on different kinds of glass ionomer cement linings. J Oral Rehabil 1992;19:457–469.

54. Kawai K, Isenberg B, Leinfelder KF. Effect of gap dimension on resin composite cement wear. Quintessence Int 1994;25:53–58.

55. Kelsey WP, Blankenau RJ, Latta MA. Resin bond strengths to dentin following placement of an adhere liner. [abstract 986]. J Dent Res 1997;76:137.

56. Kern M, Strub JR, Lu XY. Wear of composite resin veneering materials in a newly developed chewing simulator [abstract 2154]. J Dent Res 1998;77:901.

57. Krejci I. Wear of Cerec and other restorative materials. In: Mörmann WH (ed). Proceedings of an International Symposium on Computer Restorations. Chicago: Quintessence, 1991:245–251.

58. Krejci I, Lutz F, Reimer M. Marginal adaptation and fit of adhesive ceramic inlays. J Dent 1993;21:39–46.

59. Krejci I, Lutz F, Reimer M. Wear of CAD/CAM ceramic inlays: restorations, opposing cusps, luting cements. Quintessence Int 1994;25:199–207.

60. Krejci I, Guntert A, Lutz F. Scanning electron microscopic and clinical examination of resin composite inlays/onlays up to 12 months in situ. Quintessence Int 1994;25:403–409.

61. Lambrechts P, Braem M, Vanherle G. In vivo wear of resin composites [abstract S23]. J Dent Res 1988;67:75.

62. Latta M, Barkmeier W. Bond strength of a resin cement and a cured composite inlay material. J Prosthet Dent 1993;72:189–193.

63. Lundin SA. Studies on posterior resin composites with special reference to class II restorations. Swed Dent J 1990;73(suppl):6–33.

64. Lutz F. State of the art of tooth-colored restoratives. Oper Dent 1996;21:237–248.

65. Lyzak WA, Campbell SD, Wen Z. Flexural strength of repaired composite veneer materials for fixed prosthodontics [abstract 1333]. J Dent Res 1998;77:272.

66. Metzler KT, Woody RD, Miller AW, Miller BH. In vitro investigation of the wear of human enamel by dental porcelain. J Prosthet Dent 1999;81(3);356–364.

67. Molin M, Karlsson S. The fit of gold inlays and three ceramic inlay systems. Acta Odontol Scand 1993;51:201–206.

68. Molin M, Karlsson S. A 3-year clinical follow-up study of a ceramic (OPTEC) inlay system. Acta Odontol Scand 1996;54:145–149.

69. Mörmann WH, Bindl A. The new creativity in ceramic restorations: dental CAD/CIM. Quintessence Int 1996;27:821–828.

70. Mörmann WH, Brandestini M, Lutz F, Barbakow F. Chairside computer-aided direct ceramic inlays. Quintessence Int 1989;20:329–339.

71. Mörmann WH, Schug J. Grinding precision and accuracy of fit of Cerec 2 CAD/CIM inlays. J Am Dent Assoc 1997;128(1):47–53.

72. Mörmann WH. Symposium review. In: Mörmann WH (ed). International Symposium on Computer Restorations [proceedings]. Chicago: Quintessence, 1991:17–21.

73. Mörmann WH, Gotsch T, Krejci I, et al. Clinical status of 94 Cerec ceramic inlays after 3 years in situ. In: Mörmann WH (ed). International Symposium on Computer Restorations [proceedings]. Chicago: Quintessence, 1991:355–363.

74. Mörmann W, Krejci I. Computer-designed inlays after 5 years in situ: clinical performance and scanning electron microscope evaluation. Quintessence Int 1992;23:109–115.

75. Murdoch H, Scrabeck J, Dhuru J. The effect of eugenol on the shear bond strength of composite restorative materials [abstract 1012]. J Dent Res 1999;78;232.

76. Nasedkin JN. Porcelain posterior resin-bonded restorations: current perspectives on esthetic restorative dentistry. Part II. J Can Dent Assoc 1988;54:499–506.

77. O'Neal SJ, Miracle RL, Leinfelder LF. Evaluating interfacial gaps for esthetic inlays. J Am Dent Assoc 1993;124:48–54.

78. O'Neal SJ, Givan DA, Suzuki S. Five year clinical performance of heat and pressure cured indirect composite [abstract 1628]. J Dent Res 1999;78:309.

79. Ozden AN, Akaltan F, Can G. Effect of surface treatments of porcelain in the shear bond strength of applied dual-cured cement. J Prosthet Dent 1994;72:85–88.

80. Pallesen U, Qvist V. Clinical evaluation of resin fillings and inlays: 8-year report [abstract 2257]. J Dent Res 1998;77:914.

81. Palmer DS, Barco MT, Pelleu GB. Wear of human enamel against a commercial castable ceramic restorative material. J Prosthet Dent 1991;65:192–195.

82. Peters A, Bieniek KW. SEM-examination of the marginal adaptation of computer machined ceramic restorations. In: Mörmann WH (ed). Proceedings of an International Symposium on Computer Restorations. Chicago: Quintessence, 1991:365–370.

83. Qualtrough AJE, Wilson NHF. A 3-year clinical evaluation of a porcelain onlay system. J Dent 1996;24:317–323.

84. Qualtrough AJE, Wilson NHF, Smith GA. The porcelain inlay: a historical review. Oper Dent 1990;15:61–70.

85. Qualtrough AJ, Cramer A, Wilson NH, et al. An in vitro evaluation of the marginal integrity of a porcelain inlay system. Int J Prosthodont 1991;4:517–523.

86. Redford DA, Jensen ME. Etched porcelain resin-bonded posterior restorations: cuspal flexure, strength, and micro-leakage [abstract 1573]. J Dent Res 1986;65:334.

87. Reich S, Sindel J, Morneburg TH. Wear of prosthetic composites dependent on mechanical matrix properties [abstract 2260]. J Dent Res 1998;77:914.

88. Retief DH. Do adhesives prevent microleakage? Int Dent J 1994;44:19–26.

89. Robinson PB, Moore BK, Swartz ML. Comparison of microleakage in direct and indirect resin composite restorations in vitro. Oper Dent 1987;12:113–116.

90. Roznowski M, Bremer B, Geurtsen W. Fracture resistance of human molars restored with various filling materials. In: Mörmann WH (ed). Proceedings of an International Symposium on Computer Restorations. Chicago: Quintessence, 1991: 559–565.

91. Scherer W, Futter H, Cooper H. Clinical technique for an in-office porcelain modification. J Esthet Dent 1991;3:23–26.

92. Schwartz RS, Davis RD, Mayhew R. The effect of ZOE on the bond strength of resin to enamel. Am J Dent 1990;3:28–30.

93. Schwartz RS, Davis RD, Hilton TJ. Effect of temporary cements on the bond strength of a resin cement. Am J Dent 1992;5:147–150.

94. Shearer AC, Kusy RP, Whitley JQ, et al. Finishing of MGC Dicor material. Int J Prosthodont 1994;7:167–173.

95. Shorthall AC, Baylis RL, Baylis MA, Grundy JR. Marginal seal comparisons between resin bonded Class 2 porcelain inlays, posterior composite restorations and direct resin composite inlays. Int J Prosthodont 1989;2:217–223.

96. Sjogren G, Molin M, van Dijken J. A 5-year clinical evaluation of ceramic inlays (Cerec) cemented with a dual-cured or chemically cured resin composite luting agent. Acta Odontol Scand 1998;56:263–267.

97. Sorensen JA, Sultan E, Condon JR. Three-body in vitro wear of enamel against dental ceramics [abstract 909]. J Dent Res 1999;78:219.

98. Sorensen JA, Berge HX. In vitro measurement of antagonist tooth wear opposing ceramic bridges [abstract 2942]. J Dent Res 1999;78:473.

99. Studer S, Lehner C, Brodbeck G, Scharer P. Short term results of IPS-Empress inlays and onlays. J Prosthodont 1996;5(4): 277–287.

100. Sung E, Caputo A, Dail S. The effect of temporary cements on the composite resin bond strength [abstract 1320]. J Dent Res 1998;77;270.

101. Suzuki S. In vitro wear of indirect resin composite restoratives [abstract 204]. J Dent Res 1998;77:657.

102. Thordrup M, Isidor F, Hørsted-Bindslev P. Comparison of marginal fit and microleakage of ceramic and composite inlays: an in vitro study. J Dent 1994;22:147–153.

103. Thurmond JW, Barkmeler WW, Wilwerding TM. Effect of porcelain surface treatments on bond strengths of composite resin bonded to porcelain. J Prosthet Dent 1994;72:355–359.

104. Trushkowsky RD. Ceramic optimized polymer: the next generation of esthetic restorations—part 1. Compend Cont Educ Dent 1997;18:1101–1112.

105. Van Meerbeek B, Inokoshi S, Willems G, et al. Marginal adaptation of four tooth-coloured inlay systems in vivo. J Dent 1992;20:18–26.

106. Walton JN. Esthetic alternatives for posterior teeth: porcelain and laboratory-processed resin composites. J Can Dent Assoc 1992;58:820–823.

107. Wassell RW, Walls AWG, Van Vogt-Crothers AJR, McCabe JF. Direct composite inlays versus conventional composite restorations: five-year follow-up [abstract 2254]. J Dent Res 1998;77:913.

108. Wendt SL. The effect of heat used as a secondary cure upon the physical properties of three resin composites. I. Diametral tensile strength, compressive strength and marginal dimensional stability. Quintessence Int 1987;18:265–271.

109. Wendt SL. The effect of heat used as a secondary cure upon the physical properties of three resin composites. II. Wear, hardness and color stability. Quintessence Int 1987;18:351–356.

110. Wendt SL, Leinfelder KF. The clinical evaluation of heat treated resin composite inlays. J Am Dent Assoc 1990;120: 177–181.

111. Wendt SL. Microleakage and cusp fracture resistance of heat-treated resin composite inlays. Am J Dent 1991;4:10–14.

112. Wendt SL, Leinfelder KF. Clinical evaluation of a heat treated composite inlay: 3 year results. Am J Dent 1992;5:258–262.

113. Wilder AD. Clinical considerations of Cerec restorations. In: Mörmann WH (ed). Proceedings of an International Symposium on Computer Restorations. Chicago: Quintessence, 1991:141–149.

114. Wilson NHF, Wilson MA, Wastell DG, Smith GA. Performance of Occlusin in butt-joint and bevel-edged preparations: five-year results. Dent Mater 1991;7:92–98.

115. Zuellig-Singer R, Bryant RW. Three year evaluation of computer-machined ceramic inlays: influence of luting agent. Quintessence Int 1998;29:573–582.

19 Cast-Gold Restorations

Thomas G. Berry/David A. Kaiser/Richard S. Schwartz

The cast-gold restoration has lessened in popularity over the past 20 years because of the increased emphasis on esthetics, but it remains an excellent restoration with a long history of success. If used with care, gold is considered to have the greatest longevity of any restorative material used in dentistry. This opinion is generally supported by longitudinal studies,[4,49,53] although it is disputed by other studies.[51,54,86] Cast gold may be used for intracoronal (inlays) or extracoronal (complete-coverage crowns) restorations, or for restorations that are a combination of both (onlays or partial-coverage crowns) (Fig 19-1).

Gold castings present several advantages over direct restorative materials, such as silver amalgam or resin composite. Because castings are fabricated with an indirect technique, it is possible to achieve nearly ideal contours and occlusion.[75] Gold is a strong material that rarely fractures and, when used as an extracoronal restoration, can provide protection to the tooth.[70,81] Gold wears at a rate similar to that of enamel, so it does not cause accelerated wear of the opposing teeth.[13] It casts easily and accurately, and, if a type II or type III gold is used, marginal adaptation can usually be improved after the restoration is cast.

The primary drawback to the use of cast gold rather than direct restorations is higher cost, because castings require at least two appointments for the patient and have associated laboratory costs. For esthetic reasons, gold castings are usually used to restore posterior teeth, which are not as visible. For anterior teeth, preparations are usually designed so that the gold is hidden from direct observation

(Figs 19-2a and 19-2b). This chapter addresses the indications, materials, and clinical steps for the fabrication of cast-gold restorations.

Indications

The indications for a cast-gold restoration range from a tooth with a relatively small caries lesion, restored with an inlay, to a severely weakened and/or malfunctioning tooth, restored with a complete-coverage crown. Cast-gold restorations may be used to restore teeth with carious lesions or to replace existing restorations. They are generally indicated for situations in which other, less expensive materials are not suitable for establishing proper proximal and/or occlusal contacts, creating appropriate axial contours, or protecting the remaining tooth structure. A cast-gold restoration may also be indicated when gold has been used to restore adjacent and/or opposing teeth so that problems arising from use of dissimilar metals do not occur.[11,66]

The morphology of posterior teeth, the number of carious surfaces, the number of restored surfaces, the width and depth of existing restorations,[44] and the occlusal relationships must be considered when the need for a cast restoration is determined. Non–working-side occlusal contacts can be especially important. Hiatt[25] has shown a significant increase in the number of vertical fractures in teeth with non–working-side contacts.

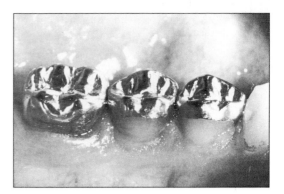

Fig 19-1 Partial and complete-coverage cast restorations.

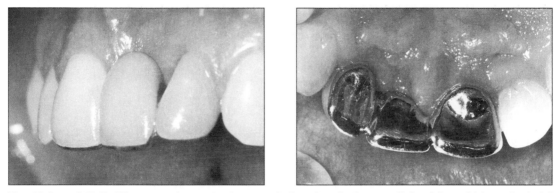

Figs 19-2a and 19-2b These anterior restorations are designed to display very little of the gold from the facial aspect. The incisal gold is angled so that light is not reflected directly back at the viewer.

Basic Principles of Cast Restorations

While there are many acceptable techniques and designs for cast restorations, certain principles always apply.

Conservation of Tooth Structure

Preparations should be made as conservative as possible to maximize the strength of the remaining tooth structure, lessen the likelihood of postoperative sensitivity and pulpal pathosis, and decrease the likelihood of tooth fracture.

Tooth preservation involves more than simply minimizing the removal of tooth structure. Preparations must be designed to protect remaining tooth structure. This may necessitate additional reduction to remove weak tooth structure or it may necessitate cuspal coverage. Studies have shown that, as a cavity preparation gets wider[45,85] and deeper,[6] progressive weakening of the tooth occurs. When an inlay preparation exceeds one third of the intercuspal width, an onlay or another extracoronal restoration should be considered to protect the cusps of the tooth. Because an extracoronal restoration covers both facial and lingual surfaces, it protects the remaining tooth structure to reduce the incidence of tooth fracture.[70]

Retention and Resistance Form

Retention and resistance form are two separate but related features of a preparation. Correctly incorporated, they resist unseating forces that are placed on the restoration during function or parafunction. Retention form resists forces attempting to remove a restoration along the path of insertion. Resistance form resists forces attempting to dislodge a restoration obliquely to the path of insertion. Although retention and resistance are two separate features of the preparation, they are usually closely interrelated and may be difficult to distinguish clinically as separate features.

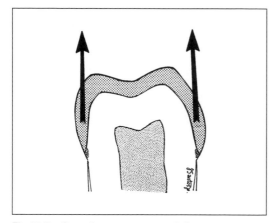

Fig 19-3a Complete-coverage, or full veneer, crowns rely on the opposing external walls to provide retention for the restoration. A slight taper of the walls in the occlusal direction provides a path of insertion.

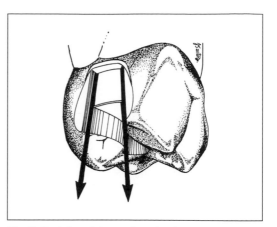

Fig 19-3b Inlays (pictured) and onlays rely on tapering opposing internal walls for retention.

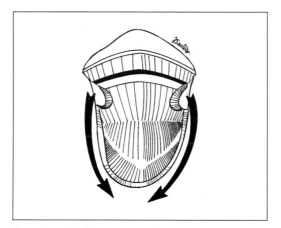

Fig 19-4a Resistance to lingual and rotational forces may be provided by proximal grooves.

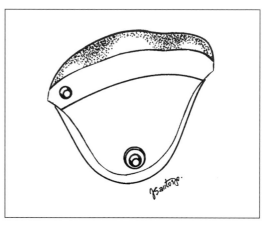

Fig 19-4b Pinholes also provide resistance to lingual displacement.

Retention is gained when two or more walls oppose each other. These walls may be intracoronal, extracoronal, or a combination of the two (Figs 19-3a and 19-3b). The amount of retention created by these opposing walls is determined by several factors. The degree of convergence toward the occlusal (extracoronal walls) or divergence toward the occlusal (intracoronal walls) and the length of the walls are the most important factors. The longer[22] and more nearly parallel the walls, the greater the retention.[35] One long wall opposed by a short wall provides retention equivalent only to that imparted by the short wall. Additionally, the greater the circumference, the greater the retention. Retention and resistance form may also be gained by adding intracoronal walls. Twisting or rotational forces are

countered by the presence of grooves, boxes, or other features such as pins or potholes[23] (Figs 19-4a and 19-4b).

All the preparation types must allow the cast restoration to seat in and/or on the tooth. To allow this seating, the walls of the preparation must taper to some degree. A taper of 3 to 6 degrees of each wall toward the occlusal is considered ideal,[18,51] and a convergence angle of 2.5 to 6.5 degrees has been shown to minimize concentration of stresses.[18] In reality, however, preparations with this degree of parallelism rarely occur. Although a rapid loss of retention occurs as the taper progresses from 5 to 10 degrees for each wall,[15] a total convergence up to 16 degrees still provides adequate retention.[23,90] Insufficient retention is a major cause of failure of fixed prostheses.[86]

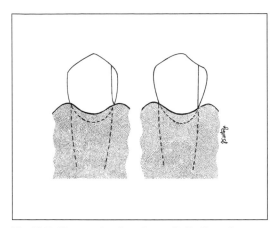

Fig 19-5 Flat proximal surfaces *(left)* allow the easy formation of a chamfered finish line, while bell-shaped anatomy *(right)* makes it difficult to create such a finish line without severe reduction of the proximal surface.

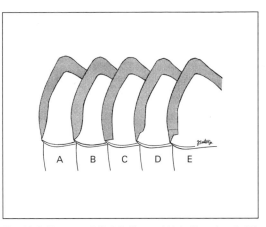

Fig 19-6 Forms of finish lines: (A) knife-edged; (B) chamfer; (C) shoulder; (D) beveled chamfer; (E) beveled shoulder.

Recent developments in luting agents and techniques of metal conditioning allow the cast restoration to be bonded to the tooth, fortifying the resistance to displacement from the preparation. To take advantage of this bonding, the metal may be treated by tin plating and luted with a resin luting cement. The long-term effectiveness of bonded castings is not yet known.

Pulpal Considerations

Tooth preparation for any cast restoration involves dentin and, therefore, affects the pulp. Often, in situations in which a restoration is indicated, the pulp has already been traumatized by caries and/or previous restorations. Prior to tooth preparation, the pulp should be tested for vitality and radiographs should be made. The additional trauma created by tooth preparation can be enough to cause necrosis of an unhealthy pulp. If the vitality of the pulp is in doubt, endodontic therapy should be performed prior to preparation.

Pulpal considerations for cast restorations are the same as those for direct restorations. The best pulpal protection is a thick layer of sound dentin. A thorough discussion of the subject can be found in Chapter 5.

Certain anatomic considerations are critical to the planning of the preparation, especially in younger patients. The pulp horns may be large enough to be exposed during tooth preparation. Examination of preoperative radiographs is imperative to identify po-

tential problems. Because the pulp is narrower in the cervical region of the tooth, pulpal exposures are less likely to occur in this area.

Postcementation thermal sensitivity is sometimes a problem. Several methods to prevent or minimize this problem have been recommended. Some clinicians scrub the preparations with antimicrobial solutions to remove bacterial contamination. Bacterial contamination under restorations is thought to be the major cause of postoperative sensitivity.[7,10] Some clinicians apply a varnish or dentin adhesive to seal the dentin surface prior to cementation to prevent migration of bacteria into the tubules. Techniques vary depending on the cement used.

Finish Lines

The term *finish line* refers to the border of the preparation where the prepared tooth structure meets the unprepared surface of the tooth. The type of finish line depends on the clinical situation. A smooth, well-defined finish line is beneficial, regardless of the design used, to facilitate laboratory procedures and finishing of the restoration. Selection of the type of finish line may be dictated by the shape of the tooth (bell shaped vs flat) (Fig 19-5), the desired location of the finish line, or operator preference. The most common types of finish lines for cast restorations are knife-edged, chamfer, and shoulder. Both the chamfer and the shoulder may be beveled or unbeveled (Fig 19-6).

Knife-edged

A knife-edged finish line requires the least amount of tooth reduction. It is sometimes used when the tooth is bell shaped, because creation of a heavier margin would require excessive removal of tooth structure. Generally, a knife-edged finish line is not desirable because it is more difficult to discern on a die than other finish lines, and it tends to result in overcontoured restorations. It is commonly used, however, on the mesial aspect of a mesially tipped molar.

Chamfer

A chamfer is often the preferred finish line for extracoronal restorations. It creates a sharp, easily identified margin that provides room for adequate thickness of gold without overcontouring the restoration.

Shoulder

The shoulder finish line is chosen primarily in situations where a bulk of material is needed to strengthen the restoration in the marginal areas, as for all-porcelain or metal-ceramic restorations. It is the least conservative of the finish line types for cast gold.

Chamfer or Shoulder with a Bevel

This design is preferred by some clinicians who believe that a beveled margin is easier to detect in an impression and that it makes the margins of the casting more burnishable. A bevel is recommended for proximal boxes.

Gingival Considerations

Gargiulo et al[19] described the dentogingival junction as consisting of the junctional epithelium and the gingival fiber attachment to cementum, coronal to the alveolar crest. In healthy tissue, the average length of each of these zones is approximately 1.0 mm in an apicocoronal direction (Fig 19-7). The combined zones of the junctional epithelium and the supracrestal fibers are often referred to as the *biologic width*.[30] If restorative margins violate the biologic width and impinge on the supracrestal fibers, gingival inflammation results and may lead to loss of periodontal attachment.[16,30,57,99] If possible, finish lines should not be prepared farther than 0.5 to 1.0 mm into the sulcus,[17,56] or closer than 1.0 mm to the base of the sulcus.[101] A more complete discussion of this subject may be found in Chapter 1.

Because gingival health may be adversely affected by subgingival finish lines,[32,58,78,79,88] the finish lines should be placed supragingivally if the situation per-

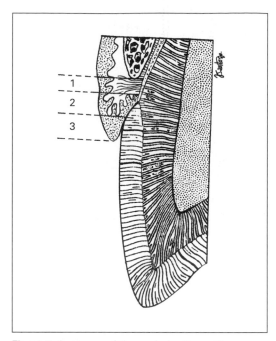

Fig 19-7 Anatomy of the periodontium: (1) connective tissue attachment; (2) junctional epithelium; (3) gingival sulcus.

mits. When it is necessary to place finish lines within the gingival crevice because of caries, existing restorations, fractures, root sensitivity, or short clinical crowns,[40,57] care must be exercised to minimize the damage to gingival tissues. The fragile soft tissue may be reflected by careful placement of retraction cord prior to final preparation of the finish line to avoid damaging these soft tissues.

Contours

The establishment of proper contours of the restoration depends on proper tooth preparation. An overcontoured casting is often the result of an underprepared tooth. If removal of tooth structure is insufficient, the crown has to be overcontoured to obtain sufficient thickness of metal.

Overcontoured crowns have been reported to encourage plaque retention, resulting in gingival inflammation[55,65,103] (Fig 19-8). Even with overcontoured crowns, however, gingival health can be maintained if the patient practices excellent oral hygiene.

Wheeler[91] proposed that convexities be created in the gingival third of artificial crowns to deflect food away from the free gingiva. Herlands et al,[24] however,

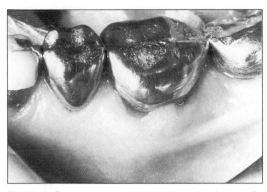

Fig 19-8 Overcontoured restorations lead to problems. Note the loss of normal gingival contours and the edematous appearance of the tissue.

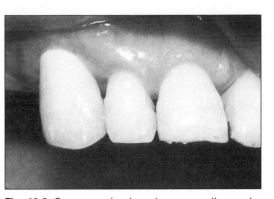

Fig 19-9 Open proximal embrasures allow adequate space for healthy tissues and access for good oral hygiene.

showed that the maximum bulge in the natural crown at its greatest diameter is no more than 0.5 mm greater than at the cementoenamel junction and that the impaction mechanism of gingival injury does not occur. The biologic acceptability of undercontouring is often observed when a provisional crown is lost from a prepared tooth for an extended time without adverse effects on the surrounding gingiva. A natural contour (ie, the exact replacement of the axial and proximal morphology) is the desired form for cast gold restorations when the gingival crest is at a normal level.

When the free gingival margin is more apical because of recession or surgery, a flattened contour best reproduces the contour of the root surface.[103] Flat contours are recommended occlusal to furcations to allow access for cleaning.

Stein[83] described the contour of a restoration adjacent to the gingiva as the *emergence profile*. He stated that the proximal emergence profiles of all natural teeth are either flat or concave. This natural contour provides an open gingival embrasure that promotes good oral hygiene (Fig 19-9).

Occlusion

No restoration, no matter how well crafted, will be successful if it does not function correctly. Satisfactory occlusion is required if the restoration is to achieve adequate function and patient comfort.

Establishing biologically acceptable occlusion starts with careful planning. The teeth opposing the one to be restored (whether in a natural or restored state) should be properly aligned and in the desired

occlusal plane. Occlusal surfaces should be well formed. If these conditions do not exist, the opposing dentition should be recontoured or restored, if possible. Failure to do so may seriously compromise the occlusal relationships and, in turn, the future health and function of the involved teeth[43] as well as the patient's comfort.[3]

Acceptable occlusion has several characteristics. Multiple contact points exist between opposing teeth that come into contact simultaneously during closure. The maximum closure position is referred to as *maximum intercuspation*. Ideally, the facial cusps of the mandibular posterior teeth and the lingual cusps of the maxillary posterior teeth contact the opposing teeth in a fossa or on a marginal ridge so that the occlusal contacts stabilize the teeth in both arches. In most cases, contact of mandibular and maxillary anterior teeth separates the posterior teeth during any eccentric movement of the jaw. This occlusal relationship is referred to as *anterior guidance* or *mutually protected occlusion*. Another occlusal relationship, referred to as *group function*, sometimes exists or is created. In this relationship, several teeth on the functional side share equally in the contact during lateral movements of the mandible.

A major benefit of indirect fabrication of a restoration is the ability to form the wax pattern to fit the desired occlusal relationships. The wax pattern (and ultimately the restoration) must contact its antagonist in the prescribed contact areas at precisely the instant the other teeth contact. A premature contact or a noncentric interference may be uncomfortable, produce loosening or accelerated wear of the restoration or its antagonist, and/or damage the health of the tooth and its supporting structures.

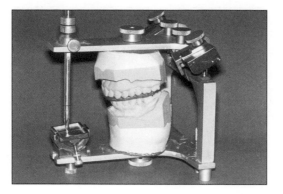

Fig 19-10 The semiadjustable articulator, shown with a jaw relation record in place, simulates mandibular movements more closely than the simple articulators.

Occlusion should be developed with mounted casts on an articulator. For single-unit castings, a simple hinge articulator may be adequate, although it allows accurate reproduction of maximum intercuspation only. Lateral or protrusive interferences must be adjusted in the mouth. In more complicated situations, as for multiple units, use of a more sophisticated semiadjustable articulator may be indicated (Fig 19-10). When casts are mounted on a semiadjustable articulator with a facebow, the lateral and protrusive movements of the mandible may be simulated with reasonable accuracy.[21]

To verify the accuracy of the relationship of the mounted casts, the patient's occlusal contacts should be checked intraorally with shimstock. If a small discrepancy exists between the patient's occlusal contacts and those on the mounted casts, the casts can be corrected with shimstock, thin articulating paper, and a carving instrument. If the discrepancy is great, it will be necessary to remount the casts. If the casts are mounted accurately and the casting is correctly fabricated, minimal adjustment will be necessary at the placement appointment.

Types of Cast Restorations

The variety of cast restorations ranges from inlays (small intracoronal restorations) to complete-coverage castings (restorations that cover the entire coronal surface of the tooth). Onlays and partial-coverage castings are hybrids that possess both intracoronal and extracoronal features. The design chosen should be the one that removes the least sound tooth structure while restoring the missing tooth structure and enabling the tooth to withstand functional and parafunctional forces.

Inlay

The gold inlay is a treatment option for small Class 2 caries lesions. Although used less frequently than in the past, the inlay has a long history of success. It is not uncommon to see a patient who has multiple inlays that are 30 years old and still clinically serviceable.

Inlays are entirely intracoronal restorations, most commonly with occlusal and proximal extensions (Fig 19-11). The preparation should be as conservative as possible to maintain tooth strength. If the occlusal width of the preparation exceeds one third to one half the buccolingual intercuspal distance, a restoration offering more protection for the cusps, such as an onlay, should be planned.[85] The occlusal contacts should be entirely on gold or enamel, not on a margin of the restoration.

Occlusal Preparation

Initial entry is made in the central fossa with a tapered fissure bur to establish the pulpal floor (Fig 19-12). The depth is determined by the extent of existing caries lesions or restorations or the need for additional retention. The occlusal outline is extended mesiodistally along the central groove and stopped just short of the marginal ridge. The bur is kept in the vertical position in the long axis of the tooth throughout the preparation so that its taper provides the 3- to 5-degree divergence toward the occlusal to the facial and lingual walls (total divergence of 6 to 10 degrees) (Fig 19-13).

Proximal Boxes

The tapered fissure bur is used to create proximal boxes mesially and/or distally. A thin layer of proximal enamel is left to protect the adjacent tooth while the proximal box is formed (Fig 19-14). The faciolingual dimension is determined by any existing restora-

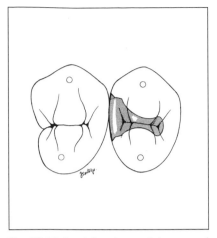

Fig 19-11 An inlay is an intracoronal restoration.

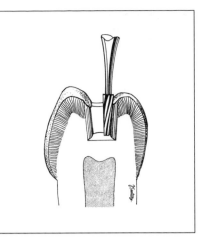

Fig 19-12 The correct pulpal depth for an inlay is established with a tapered fissure bur. It can be used to create the flat floors and well-defined internal angles.

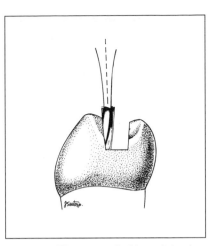

Fig 19-13 The tapered sides of the bur are used to help establish the desired divergence of the walls.

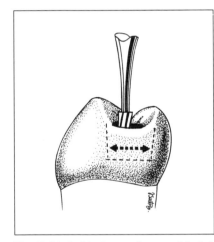

Fig 19-14 A thin layer of enamel is left on the proximal surface to protect the adjacent tooth while the proximal box is being prepared.

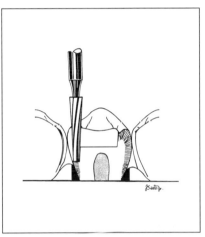

Fig 19-15 A flat gingival floor with a slightly converging axial wall is created. The gingival floor is established occlusal to the gingival tissue, unless otherwise dictated.

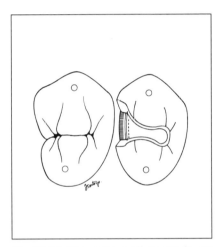

Fig 19-16 The axial wall is made an even depth into the tooth from the facial to the lingual wall.

tion, caries lesion, and the relationship of the proximal surface to the adjacent tooth. The gingival floor of the box should have an axial depth of approximately 1.5 mm. Ideally, the gingival extension should be established occlusal to the height of the papilla (Fig 19-15). However, the presence of caries or an existing restoration, or the need for a longer wall to ensure adequate retention, may require extension to a sub-

gingival location. The contour of the axial wall of the box should follow the faciolingual contour of the external surface of the tooth (Fig 19-16). The box should extend to the facial and lingual borders of the contact area, and the bevels should extend the preparation slightly beyond the box. This extension allows access to the gold margins facially and lingually for finishing with a disk.

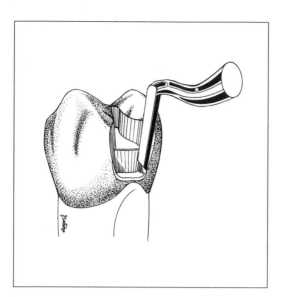

Fig 19-17 A hand instrument, such as an enamel hatchet, is helpful in smoothing the walls of the preparation.

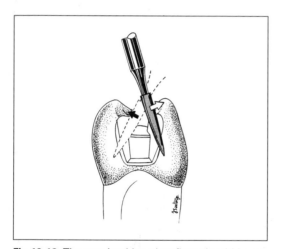

Fig 19-18 The proximal bevel or flare should be established slightly beyond the contact area and is blended with the gingival bevel.

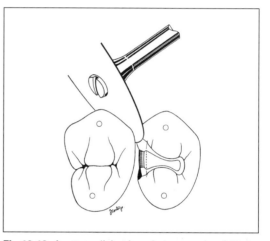

Fig 19-19 A rotary disk, placed at an angle of 45 degrees, can provide a smooth, flat bevel without undercuts.

Refinement

The operator should make certain that all the floors and walls are smooth, that all walls except the axial walls are divergent, that the axial walls are convergent occlusally, and that the internal angles are well defined (see Fig 19-12). It is critical that no undercut area exists that could interfere with placement and withdrawal. All cavosurface margins must be sharply defined (Fig 19-17).

Proximal Bevel

The proximal bevel or flare is established on the facial and lingual walls of the box with a garnet disk, a No. 7901 bur, or a thin diamond bur (Figs 19-18 and 19-

19). A finishing bur or diamond bur must be used carefully to avoid developing an undercut in the facial and lingual walls at the faciogingival or linguogingival line angles. An undercut is less likely to be a problem when a disk is used (Fig 19-19). The walls of the preparation should diverge from the gingival floor in the occlusal direction. The proximal bevel should blend smoothly with the gingival and occlusal bevels.

Horizontal Bevels

A No. 7901 finishing bur or a thin tapered diamond is used to place 0.5-mm-wide occlusal and gingival bevels along the entire cavosurface finish line (Figs 19-18 and 19-20). A gingival margin trimmer may

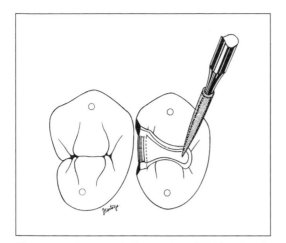

Fig 19-20a A tapered diamond or finishing bur is used to create a short but distinct bevel at the occlusal finish lines.

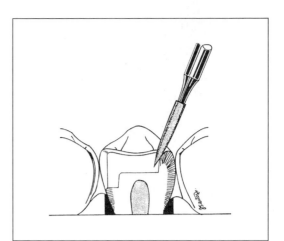

Fig 19-20b The bevel is extended across the entire occlusal margin and blended with the other bevels.

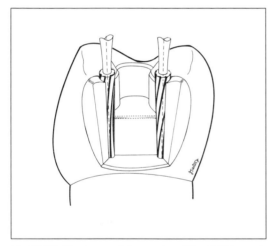

Fig 19-21 The tapered fissure bur (No. 169) is positioned at an angle to give an occlusal divergence for the retentive grooves. The grooves should be at a depth of half the diameter of the bur.

also be used to place the gingival bevels if access is too limited to use a bur. The bevels should be at an angle of approximately 45 degrees to the external surface of the tooth.

Retention Grooves

A No. 169 bur is used to place retention grooves that bisect the facioaxial and linguoaxial line angles (Fig 19-21). The grooves must diverge toward the occlusal aspect in a facial and lingual direction, and the axial walls should converge occlusally.

Onlay

The onlay is essentially an inlay that covers one or more cusps. It incorporates the principles of both extracoronal and intracoronal restorations. Although it is generally more conservative than a partial- or complete-coverage crown, it provides the same protection of the remaining tooth structure (Fig 19-22).

There are several important features of the preparation. All finish lines are beveled. A bevel or flare creates a second plane designed to allow close adaptation of the gold to the tooth. A beveled shoulder is used for the centric cusp and a long bevel or chamfer is used for the noncentric cusp. The gingival margin and the facial and lingual walls of the proximal boxes are designed like those for the inlay with their well-defined bevel or flare. These finish lines are blended to form an uninterrupted finish line around the entire preparation. The gingival floor is essentially a beveled shoulder.

The width and depth of the occlusal portion of the preparation and of the proximal boxes are often dictated by the presence of an old restoration and/or a caries lesion. If additional resistance and retention form are needed, retention grooves may be placed at the axiofacial and axiolingual line angles.

A tapered fissure bur is recommended for preparing the outline form because its taper helps to establish the desired occlusal divergence of 6 to 10 degrees for the internal walls.

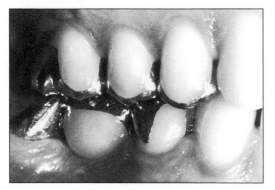

Fig 19-22 Onlays on the maxillary premolars and first molar provide protection to the facial cusps.

Fig 19-23 Ideally, opposing walls diverge 6 to 10 degrees for the inlay preparation.

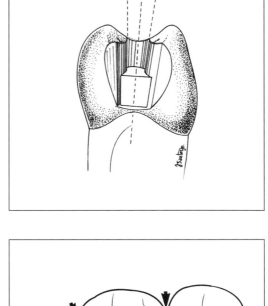
6–10 degrees

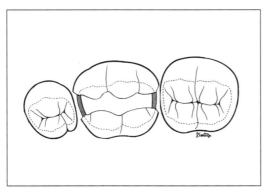

Fig 19-24 The proximal box is extended to or slightly beyond the contact area. Bevels will provide the desired proximal clearance.

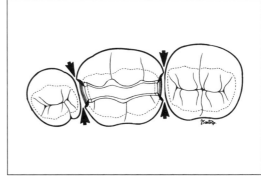

Fig 19-25 After the bevels are placed, there is access for completing the preparation's finish lines and the margins of the restoration.

Occlusal Preparation

The initial entry is made in the central fossa to a depth of approximately 1.0 mm into dentin (total depth of approximately 2.5 mm in the tooth). In some cases, it may be necessary to extend some portions of the preparation to a greater depth because of caries or a previous restoration or for additional retention. The occlusal outline form is extended by moving the bur laterally, cutting with the side of the bur. The occlusal outline form should be as conservative as the carious lesion or old restoration permits. The bur is kept in the long axis of the intended path of insertion so that the taper of the bur provides the desired 3- to 5-degree divergence for each internal cavity wall.

Proximal Boxes

The boxes are created on the proximal surfaces. The facial and lingual walls should exhibit a combined divergence of 6 to 10 degrees from each other as was provided in the occlusal area of the preparation (Fig 19-23). The faciolingual dimension is likely to be determined by the presence of a restoration, caries lesion, and/or the relationship of the proximal surface to the adjacent tooth (Fig 19-24). The bevels will extend the preparations slightly beyond the proximal contact area so that the margins of the restoration will be accessible for finishing with a disk (Fig 19-25).

Cuspal Reduction

A carbide or diamond bur is used to reduce the cusps. Depth cuts of 1.5 to 2.0 mm are made for the centric (vertical holding) cusp(s), and cuts of 1.0 to 1.5 mm are made for the noncentric cusp(s) (Fig 19-26). A bur with a measured diameter is used to gauge the depth of the cuts. The side of the bur is angled at the same angle as the cuspal inclines to make the depth cuts. After the

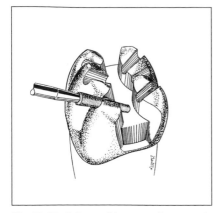

Fig 19-26 A bur of known diameter is used to establish depth cuts to guide the correct reduction of the cusps.

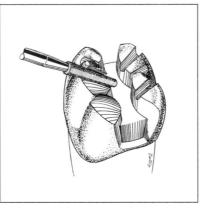

Fig 19-27 The cusps are reduced in accordance with the occlusal anatomy of the tooth.

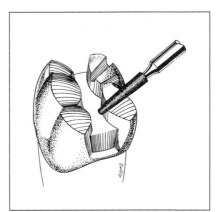

Fig 19-28 The lingual cusps of the mandibular teeth require less reduction because they are not holding cusps.

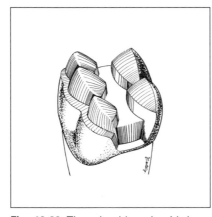

Fig 19-29 The shoulder should have precise line angles.

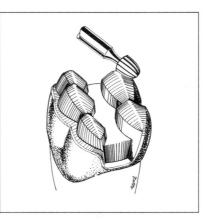

Fig 19-30 A barrel-shaped bur can be used to create the chamfer on the noncentric cusp.

depth cuts are placed, a uniform reduction of the cusps that parallels the general anatomic contours of the occlusal surface is made. The cuspal heights are reduced to the full extent of the depth cuts (Fig 19-27). The noncentric cusp(s) is reduced in the same fashion, but only to a depth of 1.0 to 1.5 mm (Fig 19-28). Reduction for the centric cusps generally needs to be greater than that for the noncentric cusps because less occlusal force tends to be exerted against a noncentric cusp.

Shoulder Preparation

A shoulder is prepared on the external surface of the centric cusp to provide a band of metal (ferrule) to protect the tooth. The bur is held parallel to the ex-

ternal surface of the tooth, and a shoulder about 1.0 mm in height and 1.0 mm in axial depth is cut. The finish line should extend gingivally at least 1.0 mm beyond any occlusal contacts. The occlusoaxial line angles are rounded (Fig 19-29). There must be adequate (1.0- to 1.5-mm) clearance in all eccentric mandibular movements.

Noncentric Cusp

A chamfer or long bevel may be used instead of a shoulder on the noncentric cusp(s). The bur is positioned at an angle of approximately 45 degrees to the axial surface (Fig 19-30). This provides a ferrule effect for additional protection of the cusp.

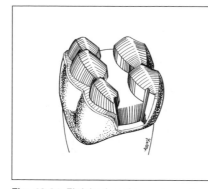

Fig 19-31 Finished onlay preparation. Internal angles are precise, occlusal line angles are rounded, the walls have the correct taper, the grooves are correctly positioned, and all the finish lines are smooth and continuous.

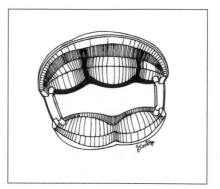

Fig 19-32 The retention grooves are placed at the linguoaxial and facioaxial line angles but do not undermine the enamel.

Gingival Bevel

A smooth and distinct bevel is established on the gingival margins with a No. 7901 finishing bur, a thin tapered diamond, or a gingival margin trimmer. This bevel should be approximately 0.5 mm in width and at an angle of approximately 45 degrees to the external surface of the tooth.

Shoulder Bevel

A 1.0-mm bevel is placed on the shoulder with a No. 7901 or fine diamond bur. This bevel is blended with the proximal bevels. Any corners or sharp angles at the junction of the various bevels and across the occlusoaxial line angles are eliminated (Fig 19-31).

Proximal Bevels

The proximal bevel or flare is established with a garnet disk, a fine tapered diamond, or a No. 7901 bur. Creation of an undercut at the faciogingival or linguogingival line angles must be avoided. Divergence is established from the gingival floor occlusally. The proximal bevel should blend smoothly with the gingival bevel and the buccal and lingual bevels.

Retention Grooves

If retention grooves are needed, grooves are placed in both proximal boxes. A No. 169 bur is used to bisect the facioaxial and linguoaxial line angles. The grooves must diverge toward the occlusal aspect faciolingually and be aligned with the internal path of insertion (Fig 19-32).

Partial-Coverage Crown

The partial-coverage, or partial veneer, crown covers only a portion of the outer circumference of the tooth and completely covers the occlusal surface. Leaving part of the external surface of the tooth uncovered offers several potential benefits. It conserves tooth structure and avoids potential insult to the periodontium on the unrestored tooth surface.[78] Cementation is generally easier and seating is more complete than for a complete-coverage crown because escape of the excess cement is facilitated. The uncovered tooth surface allows for pulp testing.[36] Preservation of the facial surface eliminates the need to match the shade of the adjacent teeth. Because it is not necessary to veneer the casting with a tooth-colored material, the laboratory procedures are simplified.[73]

Retention and resistance of the partial veneer crown are provided by a combination of extracoronal and intracoronal features. The extracoronal retention is created by opposing axial walls on the mesial and distal surfaces that have a combined convergence toward the occlusal of approximately 6 to 10 degrees. This is supplemented with grooves or boxes in the proximal walls that provide not only added retention but resistance to lingual displacement. A slight overlay of the facial cusp protects it from fracture and provides some resistance form.

The extensions of the proximal and facial portions of the preparation can vary in design according to the specific needs. If the tooth is located so that the facial

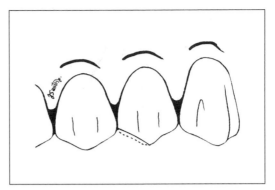

Fig 19-33 Limited reduction of the mesiofacial incline of the facial cusp and greater reduction of the distofacial incline of a maxillary tooth provide some protection to the cusp while limiting the display of gold in a partial-coverage restoration.

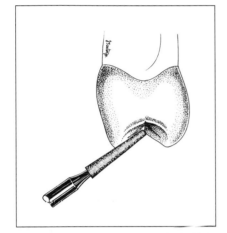

Fig 19-34 The diamond bur is held at the same angle as the natural slope of the cusp to create an even occlusal reduction for partial-coverage crowns.

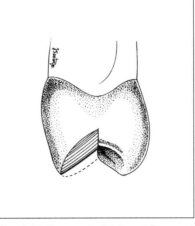

Fig 19-35 Removal of 1.0 to 1.5 mm of tooth structure from the noncentric cusp serves as a guide to reducing the rest of the occlusal surface.

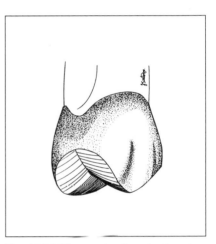

Fig 19-36 The occlusal reduction has followed the original contours of the occlusal surface.

cusps are readily visible, esthetic concerns may dictate a modification of the standard design to conceal the margin. In such cases, the mesial proximal wall is extended toward the facial surface only far enough to barely break contact. The mesial incline of the mesiofacial cusp of molars and the mesial incline of the facial cusp of premolars are left unreduced. The distal incline is reduced to provide protection and the ferrule effect. This more esthetic design is shown in Fig 19-33.

Because partial-coverage crowns are infrequently placed on anterior teeth, this section focuses on the posterior teeth.

Occlusal Reduction

Depth cuts are made by laying the side of the bur (of measured diameter) against the cuspal inclines (Fig 19-34) and reducing them to the desired depth (Fig 19-35). The total reduction of the centric cusp should be 1.5 to 2.0 mm, and that of the noncentric cusp should be 1.0 to 1.5 mm. The remaining occlusal surface is reduced, but the general anatomic contours are maintained (Fig 19-36). As previously mentioned, less reduction may be desirable in some areas for esthetic reasons. The placement of an occlusal channel and the facial bevel are discussed later.

Lingual Reduction

The axial wall of the lingual surface is reduced with a blunt tapered diamond. Close attention must be paid to the desired path of insertion to maintain parallelism. A two-plane reduction of the tooth is needed to maintain natural contours. Because of the anatomic differences in the lingual contours of the maxillary and the mandibular teeth, the second plane

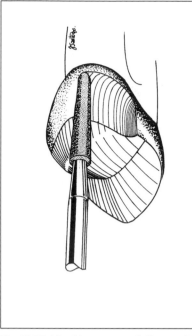

Fig 19-37 The blunt tapered diamond is very effective in creating the proper taper and in creating a chamfer finish line.

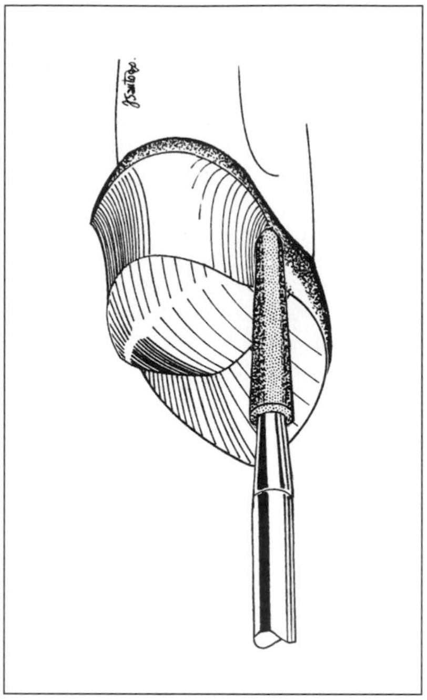

Fig 19-38 The lingual contours and finish line should be carried into the proximal surfaces. Lack of access may require use of a thinner diamond initially.

on the lingual surface of maxillary teeth will be more pronounced. The gingival portion of the lingual surface should have a 3- to 5-degree convergence occlusally to the path of insertion (Fig 19-37), and the second plane should be offset about 30 degrees.

Proximal Reduction

The proximal surfaces are reduced in one plane. A 3- to 5-degree taper is established from the finish line to the occlusoaxial line angle. Space limitations may require use of a thin tapered diamond initially until enough space has been created to·use a blunt tapered diamond bur. The blunt diamond bur has a more appropriate shape to create a chamfer finish line (Fig 19-38).

Finish Lines

The junction of each proximal wall and the lingual wall is blended so that there is a smooth transition. This procedure is especially important at the finish line. The gingival finish lines are placed slightly coronal to the gingival tissue if possible. The presence of caries lesions or existing restorations may alter the level of finish line placement, but, regardless of where the finish line is located, the transition should be smooth and well defined.

Proximal Grooves

The groove is initiated in the proximal areas with a No. 170 bur (or a No. 169 bur for a small tooth). The grooves are located as far facially as possible without undermining the facial enamel. It may be helpful to mark the proposed location of the grooves before they are prepared (Figs 19-39a and 19-39b). Because the grooves must have a path of draw compatible with each other and with the axial walls, their angulation is carefully planned before they are begun. As a general rule, the grooves should be parallel to the long axis of the tooth in posterior teeth (Fig 19-40a). The axial walls of the two grooves should converge occlusally. Failure to align the grooves correctly will result in a preparation that does not have an acceptable path of insertion (Figs 19-40b and 19-40c).

The axial depth of the groove is made equal to or slightly greater than the diameter of the No. 170 bur (Fig 19-41). The groove on the opposing wall is then prepared in the same fashion so that it aligns with the first groove and the axial walls. The grooves may be enlarged, and the internal walls may be left rounded or more acutely refined to form boxes. In many cases, boxes are present after the removal of existing restorations. These may be modified and incorporated in the preparation in lieu of grooves (Fig 19-42).

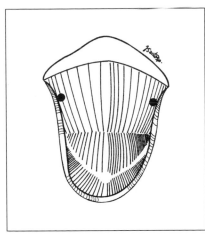

Fig 19-39a Before the proximal grooves are prepared, their desired location is marked with a pencil or an indentation made by a bur. This aids in obtaining the correct faciolingual location.

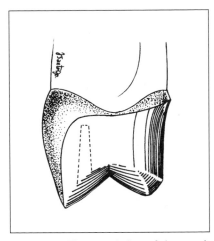

Fig 19-39b The angulation of the proximal groove is equally important, so visualization is critical.

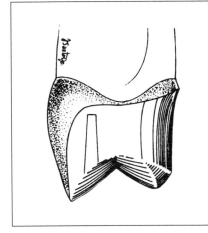

Fig 19-40a Alignment of the proximal groove with the long axis of the tooth provides the best compatibility with the rest of the preparation design.

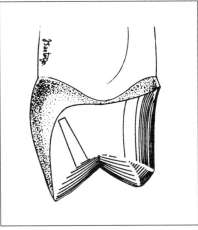

Fig 19-40b This proximal groove is angulated too much toward the lingual surface and will not provide resistance to lingual rotation.

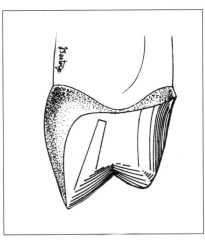

Fig 19-40c This proximal groove is angulated too much toward the facial surface, creating an undercut in relation to the lingual surface of the preparation.

Occlusal Channel

The resistance form and strength of the restoration can be enhanced by preparation of an occlusal channel. A channel may already exist if an occlusal restoration has been removed. If not, it may be prepared. A tapered carbide or diamond bur is used to cut the channel or to remove undercuts in an existing channel. The channel allows the space for a "staple" of thicker metal in the restoration that resists lingual displacement and that helps the restoration resist deformation under pressure (Fig 19-43).

Facial Bevel

Placement of the facial finish line differs in the maxillary teeth and the mandibular teeth. Because the maxillary facial cusp is usually the noncentric cusp, only a 1.0-mm layer of metal and a short bevel are required to protect the cusp (Fig 19-44). Placement of a shoulder and a bevel are recommended for the facial cusp of mandibular teeth to help restorations withstand the forces directed on a centric cusp. A shoulder extending 1.0 mm long occlusogingivally and 1.0 mm deep axially is placed into the facial surface across the fa-

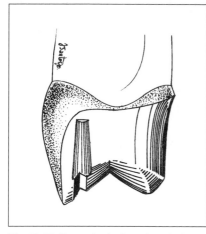

Fig 19-41 Properly designed and placed proximal groove.

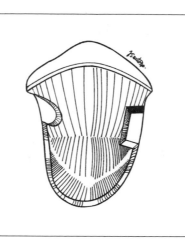

Fig 19-42 A groove is located on one proximal surface and a box on the other. Both meet the requirements for divergence of the facial and lingual walls and convergence of the axial wall toward the opposite proximal wall. The groove has a lingual "lip" to provide resistance to lingual displacement.

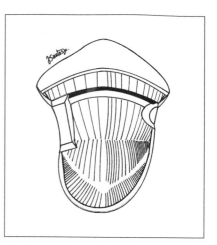

Fig 19-43 The occlusal channel follows the general contours of the facial surface rather than cutting straight across the tooth to the opposite wall. Note the inadequate proximal groove, which provides little resistance to lingual displacement.

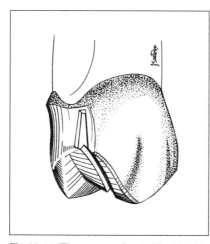

Fig 19-44 The preparation in Fig 19-43 is shown from another view. Note the shape of the occlusal channel as it comes across the occlusal surface to connect to the proximal groove. Also note the small facial bevel.

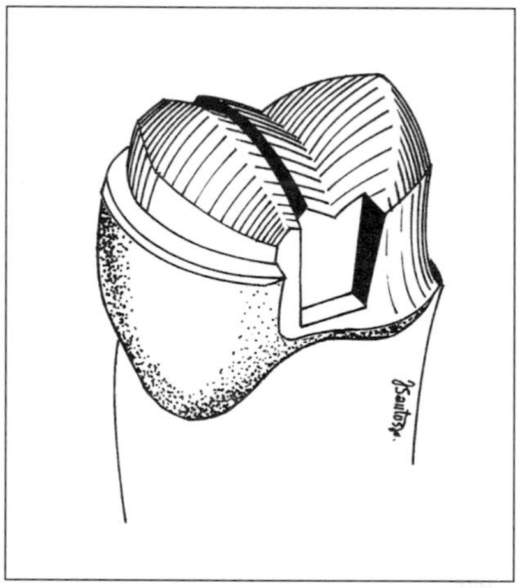

Fig 19-45 In the mandible, the centric holding cusp requires a facial design similar to that of the onlay preparation.

cial cusp with a straight fissure bur held parallel to the external surface of the tooth (Fig 19-45). A 0.5- to 1.0-mm-wide bevel is placed with a fine diamond or a finishing bur. The finish line should be placed gingival to any occlusal contacts.

Final Refinement

All the sharp external angles of the preparation are rounded. Sharp angles make it more difficult to pour the stone into the impression without bubbles. Even if the die is poured without bubbles, it has fragile edges that are easily abraded during laboratory procedures. After all the angles of the preparation are rounded, the surfaces are smoothed with a fine-grit diamond bur (Figs 19-46a and 19-46b).

Figs 19-46a and 19-46b Preparations for partial-coverage crowns require the same refinement of walls, floors, and bevels as are needed for inlay and onlay preparations.

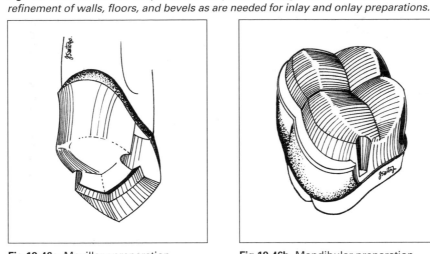

Fig 19-46a Maxillary preparation.

Fig 19-46b Mandibular preparation.

Complete-Coverage Gold Castings

The complete-coverage, or full veneer, casting, as the name implies, includes coverage of the entire coronal portion of the tooth. Extensive loss of tooth structure is the most common indication for complete coverage. For esthetic reasons, this restoration tends to be limited to molars. Because the restoration involves the entire circumference of the tooth, control of occlusal and proximal relationships allows improvements in occlusion and proximal contacts. Correction of tooth malpositioning is sometimes possible.

Retention is provided primarily or entirely by the extracoronal walls. A complete-coverage crown is the most retentive of the casting designs.[47,67] One or more grooves or boxes can be added to the preparation if additional retention and resistance form are needed.

Proximal Reduction

A thin tapered diamond bur is placed at either the facial or lingual embrasure and used to cut proximal tooth structure toward the opposite embrasure (Figs 19-47a and 19-47b). The bur should be extended cervically to the desired location of the gingival finish line. Unless a caries lesion or an old restoration dictates otherwise, the gingival finish line should be established at least 0.5 mm supragingivally. The reduction must be at the expense of the tooth being prepared to avoid damage to the enamel of the adjacent tooth. The reduction, when completed, should taper occlusally 3 to 5 degrees toward the opposing proximal wall. The opposing wall is prepared in the

same manner. Once enough space has been created to permit access, a blunt tapered diamond is used to complete the proximal reduction and place a gingival chamfer.

Occlusal Reduction

A series of depth cuts is made on the occlusal surface with a diamond or a fissure bur. Both the facial and lingual cuspal inclines are cut to a depth of at least 1.5 mm. The 1.5-mm reduction allows an adequate thickness of metal for strength and wear. An even reduction that follows the original anatomic contours allows the development of the appropriate occlusal anatomy in the restoration. The corrugated preparation form adds strength to the crown.

Facial and Lingual Reduction

The facial and lingual surfaces are each reduced in two planes. The first plane, extending occlusally from the gingival finish line, should have a 3- to 5-degree taper to the path of insertion (Fig 19-48). The second plane should be angled at 30 to 45 degrees to the first plane to allow natural facial and lingual contours to be re-established (Fig 19-49). This second plane should begin at the occlusal third of the wall for the centric cusp and the occlusal fourth of the noncentric cusp. A blunt tapered diamond is used to make these reductions.

Refinement

The parts of the preparation are blended to eliminate indefinite areas of the finish line, irregularities in the walls, and sharp corners. A finish line that is distinct

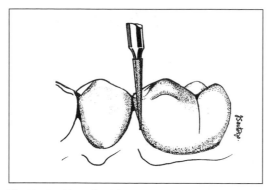

Fig 19-47a Use of a thin tapered diamond is recommended to initiate the proximal reduction of the preparation for a complete-coverage restoration.

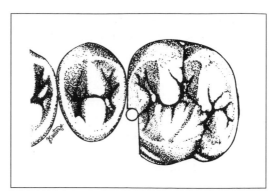

Fig 19-47b The reduction is kept within the original contours of the tooth so that abrasion of the adjacent tooth is avoided.

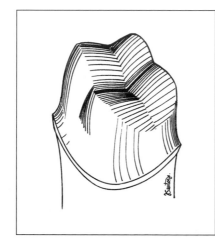

Fig 19-48 Reduction of the axial walls for a complete-coverage restoration is identical to that for the partial-coverage crowns, except the facial wall is also included. At this stage, the facial and lingual walls are each in one plane.

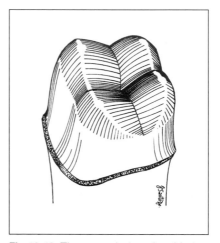

Fig 19-49 The second plane is added to the facial and lingual walls. The second plane should be at a 30- to 45-degree angle to the long axis and involves the occlusal third of the centric holding cusp and the occlusal fourth of the noncentric cusp.

around the whole preparation is established. The areas at the facioproximal and linguoproximal line angles often need to be rounded and distinctly defined. All of the sharp corners of the preparation, such as the occlusoaxial line angles, are rounded. The surfaces of the preparation should be relatively smooth. A fine-grit diamond or a rubber polishing cup may be used. The preparation is carefully viewed from more than one angle to ensure that there are no undercuts within any wall, between the walls, or in relationship to an adjacent tooth.

 Try-In

Before the casting is fitted to the prepared tooth, it should be adjusted to fit the master die. The casting is inspected under magnification for bubbles or other imperfections,[20,62] which can be removed with a small round bur. The die is checked for defects or abraded areas. The casting should not be forced onto the die. If the casting does not seat easily, the die should be sprayed with a disclosing medium and the crown should then be gently reseated. The disclosing medium should mark areas that are binding on the inside of the casting. These areas can be relieved with a bur (No. 2 or No. 4 round bur). This process is repeated until the casting is fully seated.

Once the casting is fully seated on the die, the interproximal contacts are checked and necessary adjustments made. This is best accomplished on a solid cast, especially if there are multiple castings. The occlusion is adjusted until the restoration holds a shim equally with the adjacent natural teeth. The location and size of the occlusal contacts are marked with articulating paper. A stone or abrasive disk is used to make any modifications needed. If these steps are done with precision before the patient arrives, minimal chair time should be required for adjustments.

The internal surface of the casting is carefully air abraded with aluminum oxide, avoiding the margins, in preparation for the clinical try-in. Air abrasion provides a dull, matte finish. Any area that binds during intraoral seating of the casting will create a bright, burnished mark.

Once adjustments have been made on the cast, the casting is tried on the tooth to determine the fit. Adjustments to the proximal contacts are made if needed. The internal surface is inspected for shiny spots. The shiny spots are adjusted, and the casting is reseated. The casting is removed and reinspected for new shiny spots. This process may need to be repeated several times until the casting is fully seated.

Any alternative method to seat castings requires disclosing media. Disclosing media include chloroform and rouge, disclosing pastes or waxes,[37] and impression materials.[20] Whatever the choice, the medium is placed on the internal surface of the casting, which is then seated. The casting is removed and inspected for abrasion of the disclosing medium that allows the gold to show through. These areas are adjusted as needed, more disclosing medium is placed, and the casting is reseated. This process is continued until the casting is fully seated.

The fitting process is completed when the margins are flush against the finish lines of the preparation and there is no binding when the restoration is seated. The casting should go passively to place. A tight fit usually means the casting is not fully seated. Use of a die spacer, placed prior to wax pattern fabrication, will usually simplify the process of fitting a casting.[87]

Marginal Finishing

Marginal finishing is done prior to cementation to thin and/or smooth margins already determined to be satisfactory. The goal is to develop a margin that is adapted to the tooth, extends to, but not beyond, the finish line, and blends with the contours of the tooth.[38] The casting must be fully seated before an attempt can be made to adapt and finish the margins.

Marginal location determines whether any finishing can be done on the tooth. Subgingival and/or interproximal margins are very difficult to reach without damaging the soft tissue, bone, or the tooth itself. In such cases, all finishing must be done on the die. Easily accessible margins can be finished while the casting is seated on the tooth (Fig 19-50). If the margin is tightly adapted but slightly overcontoured or undercontoured, a white stone or abrasive disk can be used in a low-speed handpiece to reduce the protruding surface, whether it is gold or enamel. When finished, the gold margin should be flush with the tooth structure, and adjacent contours of the restoration should be continuous with natural tooth contours. The stone or disk should be rotated from the metal to the tooth or parallel to the margin, but never from tooth to gold. Rubber points or fine-grit abrasive disks may be used to produce a high luster if access permits. Care must be exercised to avoid damage to the soft tissue or abrasion of the tooth surface.

Marginal adaptation can sometimes be improved by hand burnishing, both on the die and on the tooth prior to cementation. Well-controlled pressure is applied with a beavertail or ball burnisher held adjacent and moved parallel to the gold margin (Fig 19-51). The burnisher should not be placed directly on the margin. Pressure should be applied with a back-and-forth motion that moves slowly closer to the margin. Because a small area of the burnisher is contacting the gold, a great deal of pressure (force per unit area) is applied. The casting is stabilized during the burnishing process to ensure that it does not change position. It is also critical to have good finger rests to ensure that the burnisher does not slip off the tooth and injure the soft tissue or the tooth itself if the burnishing is done in the mouth. Some additional benefit may be achieved by burnishing the margins of the casting on the tooth during the cementing procedure, before the cement sets.

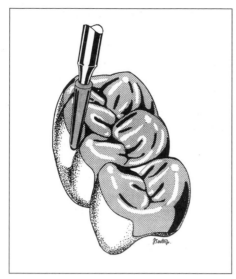

Fig 19-50 A fine diamond bur or finishing stone is held perpendicular to the margin and moved parallel to the margin to reduce small discrepancies in the marginal area.

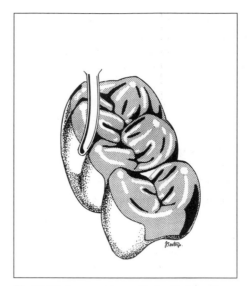

Fig 19-51 Pressure is applied with the side or tip of the burnisher, moved parallel to the marginal area to adapt it more tightly to the tooth.

Cementation

The final step in the process is luting or cementation of the casting. Cement failure has been shown to be the second[71] or third[89] most important factor in failure of cast restorations. A thin layer of the luting agent (cement) is placed in the casting and on the walls of the preparation, and the casting is then seated on or in the tooth. The cement hardens within a few minutes, and the excess is removed. The luting agent fills the gap between the casting and tooth to provide retention and to minimize leakage at the margin. Some luting agents, such as zinc phosphate cement, provide retention entirely from frictional resistance to displacement. Others, such as the adhesive resin cements, bond to the casting and/or the tooth to provide adhesion in addition to frictional resistance.

Selection of a Luting Agent

The primary luting agents in use today are zinc phosphate, glass-ionomer, polycarboxylate, resin, and resin-modified glass-ionomer cements.[14] A survey of 10,000 dentists conducted in 1990 revealed that glass-ionomer cements were used most frequently for cementation of crowns (42%), followed by polycarboxylate (33%), zinc phosphate (22%), resin cement

(2%), and zinc oxide–eugenol (1%) cements.[9] Since that time, resin cements and resin-modified glass-ionomer cements have gained in popularity, with much of the current research in the area of cements focused on these two materials. Because the indications and procedures for the use of each luting agent are different, they are discussed separately.

Zinc Phosphate Cement

Zinc phosphate cement consists of a powder containing 90% zinc oxide and 10% magnesium oxide, which is incorporated into a liquid containing approximately 67% phosphoric acid.[11] Among the many luting agents available, zinc phosphate has the longest record (over 100 years) of successful use.[1] It has good compressive strength and low film thickness and is easy to manipulate.[11] Excess cement is easily removed after it has set. It has a coefficient of thermal expansion similar to that of tooth structure, and its setting shrinkage is minimal. Relatively high compressive and tensile strengths make zinc phosphate a good choice for long-span fixed partial dentures.[74] In a study of zinc phosphate cement samples taken from castings that had been in service for up to 48 years, the cement was found to have maintained a stable chemical structure.[48]

Zinc phosphate cement is slightly soluble in oral fluids, allows relatively high levels of microleakage,[97] and is sometimes associated with postoperative sensitivity.[59,93] Despite these drawbacks, it is not unusual to see patients with gold castings that were cemented more than 30 years ago with zinc phosphate cement.

Zinc phosphate cement is usually mixed on a chilled glass slab. The powder is mixed into the liquid in small increments over a large area of the glass slab. This method dissipates the heat released during the exothermic setting reaction and provides a longer working time. The slower the mix and cooler the glass slab, the longer the working time. A cool glass slab also allows more powder to be incorporated into the liquid, resulting in improved physical properties.[80] Powder is added until the mixed material adheres to the spatula to form a 1-inch string when the spatula is lifted from the glass slab. The mixing should be completed within 90 seconds after initiation. If the mixing is prolonged beyond approximately 90 seconds, the hardening of the cement caused by the setting reaction may be confused with having achieved the proper powder-liquid ratio.[61] Its relatively long working time makes zinc phosphate cement a good choice when multiple castings are luted at the same time.

Glass-Ionomer Cement

Glass-ionomer luting cement is a modification of the glass-ionomer restorative material. It consists of a powder containing aluminum fluorosilicate glass particles that are incorporated into a liquid containing polyalkenoic acids. In some products, these acids are freeze-dried and included in the powder, which is mixed with water.[27] It bonds to tooth structure by formation of ionic bonds to hydroxyapatite crystals in enamel and dentin[27] and has the potential to prevent caries because of fluoride release. It has a low film thickness (20 to 25 μm) and better physical properties than zinc phosphate cement.[11,92,95] It may be hand mixed or is available in preweighed capsules that allow mixing in an amalgamator. Persistent reports of excessive postoperative sensitivity associated with glass-ionomer luting agents have not been borne out in clinical studies.[33,34,41,64]

Glass-ionomer cement is very sensitive to early moisture contamination. If exposed to external moisture during the setting reaction (usually 5 minutes), the reaction is interrupted, resulting in a cement with high solubility and poor physical properties.[84] Therefore, glass-ionomer cement should not be used when bleeding is present or isolation is a problem. As with the restorative material, dehydration is also a problem.[26] Excess cement should not be removed from the margins for at least 5 minutes after the crown is seated.

Leaving a bead of excess cement in place protects the underlying layers of cement from moisture contamination.[12] Because glass-ionomer cement bonds to the tooth surface, excess cement is somewhat difficult to remove once set, particularly in the interproximal areas.

When glass-ionomer cement is mixed by hand, the powder is incorporated into the liquid in bulk as quickly as possible with a premeasured amount of powder and liquid. Most manufacturers now offer the encapsulated form, which results in properly proportioned cement thoroughly mixed in a few seconds. Glass-ionomer cement has a relatively short working time, so a single mix should be limited to luting no more than two or three units. If additional units have to be luted, a new mix of cement should be used.

Resin Luting Agents

The resin cements are especially designed for use with bonded porcelain restorations, but they may also be used with cast restorations. They are generally supplied as a dual paste system that is mixed at the time of use. Polymerization may by initiated by chemical reaction or a combination of light and chemical reactions. Resin cements differ from resin composite restorative materials primarily in their reduced filler content,[31] which results in better flow and reduced film thickness, desirable properties for a cement.[2] Some resin cements contain fillers that are capable of providing fluoride release,[8] although there is questionable therapeutic effect due to the low levels and short duration of fluoride release.[52]

Resin cements have the best physical properties of all of the cements.[76,95,96] They are virtually insoluble in oral fluids and have the highest compressive and tensile strengths of all the cements. They also exhibit less microleakage[5] than other luting agents. If used in combination with a dentin adhesive system, they bond to tooth structure and some metals.[80] For this reason, they are often recommended for less retentive preparations.[28,42,63]

There are several potential problems associated with resin cements. There is great variation in the physical properties and handling characteristics among resin cements,[94] which can cause confusion for clinicians. The film thickness tends to be greater than that of other cements,[46,82,94] so incomplete seating of the casting can be a problem. This is especially true when a dentin adhesive is used, which tends to pool in the internal angles of the preparation. Resin cements require the most clinical steps if used with an adhesive system and can be technique sensitive. Resin cements are relatively new, so there are no long-term clinical studies to determine if the high retention values and low microleakage are long lasting.

Resin-Modified Glass-Ionomer Cements

Like the resin cements and glass-ionomer cements, the resin-modified glass-ionomer cements are modified restorative materials. The combination of resin and glass-ionomer chemistries overcomes some of the problems with moisture contamination and dehydration experienced with glass-ionomer cements[99] and eliminates many of the steps necessary for resin cements.[14] In addition, they release fluoride, providing potential anticaries activity.[100] They have physical properties between those of conventional glass ionomer and resin cements.[95] Their adhesive properties to tooth structure are similar to glass ionomers,[77] and they have adequately low film thickness.[94,98] They absorb fluids during and after setting, causing a net expansion.[39,102] For this reason, they are not recommended for all-ceramic restorations.

Polycarboxylate and Zinc Oxide–Eugenol Cements

Polycarboxylate and zinc oxide–eugenol cements are no longer widely used with cast restorations. Their properties are generally inferior to those of the cements previously discussed. Historically, some clinicians have used them if a tooth has had a history of sensitivity. They have also been used as temporary luting agents and with stainless steel crowns.

Preparing the Tooth for Cementation

Although some materials are more strongly affected by the presence of contaminants than are others, no material fares well if used in the presence of oils, debris, saliva, blood, or other significant contamination. It is important to ensure that the area is cleaned, free of excess moisture, and well isolated. Bleeding and other significant moisture must be well controlled. Temporary cements leave a layer of debris on the dentin surface[72] that should be removed before cementation. This may be accomplished with pumice, detergents, or cleaning agents.

Some clinicians recommend the additional step of disinfecting the preparation with chlorhexidine or other disinfectants. The rationale is that because bacteria are a primary cause of postoperative sensitivity,[7,10] disinfection of the dentin surface will lower the number of microbes and thus lessen the sensitivity. Whether the disinfection has any significant effect is not yet known.

In addition to cleaning and isolating the preparation, specific additional steps are recommended to prepare the tooth to receive certain cements.

Zinc Phosphate Cement

Because zinc phosphate cement exhibits the most microleakage of any cement[94] and has been associated with postcementation sensitivity, several methods have been recommended to prevent sensitivity by "sealing" the dentin prior to cementation. Copal varnish has a long history of use for this purpose with anecdotal reports of success. More recently, use of dentin primers and adhesives to seal the dentin before cementation has resulted in reports of decreased sensitivity. Recent studies[50,68] suggest that dentin primers or desensitizing agents may lessen retention with zinc phosphate cement, however.

Glass-Ionomer Cements

For glass-ionomer cements, the tooth should be clean and slightly moist.[33] No cavity varnish or other coating agent should be placed that might prevent bonding of this luting agent to the tooth surface. The area should be well isolated to prevent moisture contamination during the luting process and for several minutes following the seating of the restoration.

Resin Composite Cements

Most resin composite cements have corresponding dentin adhesive systems that are applied immediately before cementation. In most cases, the preparation is etched and a primer and adhesive are placed. Each adhesive system has specific instructions for its use that must be followed precisely to obtain the best results. Failure to follow the specific directions for both the adhesive and the luting agent can mean the difference between success and failure.

A small amount of the cement should be mixed and observed before cementation procedures are started to confirm that the cement will set. Some autocuring resin cements have short shelf lives and lose their ability to polymerize.

Resin-Modified Glass-Ionomer Cements

One of the advantages of resin-modified glass-ionomer cements is that the cementation procedure is fairly simple. Multiple bonding steps are not necessary, and no special preparation of the tooth surface is performed, other than to make it clean and slightly moist. Removal of excess cement is relatively easy.

Preparing the Casting for Cementation

After adjustments have been made and the external surface of the casting has been polished, the internal surface of the casting should be air abraded with aluminum oxide to produce a uniform, slightly roughened finish. The casting should then be cleaned to remove any contaminants, such as polishing compounds. Ammonia, detergents, or various other cleaning solutions may be used in an ultrasonic bath, or the casting can be cleaned with a steam cleaner.

If an adhesive resin cement is used, additional retention can be obtained by tin plating the inside of the casting.[29,60] A number of inexpensive tin-plating systems that can be used to deposit a thin layer of tin on the surface of the gold alloy are commercially available. This simple process can be done in the laboratory or operatory in a few minutes.[29]

Seating the Casting

The cement is mixed and placed in the casting. Some clinicians also like to place a layer of the cement on the walls of the preparation for intracoronal restorations. The casting should be half filled, and all of the margins should be covered. Once the casting is seated with finger pressure, the patient is instructed to bite on an orangewood stick or other seating instrument. The instrument is moved up and down, and then side to side. This technique, called *dynamic seating*, results in more complete seating of the casting.[69] The margins are checked with an explorer to determine that complete seating has been accomplished.

The excess cement must be removed with proper timing and care. If removal is attempted before the cement is set, thin strands of cement may be dragged from under the margins, thus creating voids. The bead of extruded cement has been shown to protect the cement at the margin from moisture contamination.[12] Therefore, it is important to check the cement to ensure that it has set before the excess is removed. Excess cement may be removed with an explorer or curette and floss or yarn. The gingival crevice should be flushed with water frequently to remove any loose particles. As a final step, an assistant should supply a continuous stream of air to each margin while the clinician reflects the gingiva gently with an explorer to check for any remaining cement. Cement left subgingivally can cause tissue inflammation. A knot is tied in the floss and then the floss is pulled back and forth through the gingival embrasure to remove loose pieces from the interproximal areas.

The occlusion is reevaluated and final adjustments are made, if necessary. The patient is informed of the possibility of postcementation sensitivity and that a minor additional adjustment of the occlusion may be necessary. The patient is instructed in the proper oral hygiene measures to ensure prevention of caries and periodontal problems.

References

1. Ames WB. A new oxyphosphate for crown seating. Dent Cosmos 1892;34:392–393.
2. Aquilino SA, Diaz-Arnold AM, Piotrowski TJ. Tensile fatigue limits of prosthodontic adhesives. J Dent Res 1991;70:208–210.
3. Bell WE. Temporomandibular Disorders: Classification/Diagnosis/Management, ed 2. Chicago: Year Book, 1986:219.
4. Bentley C, Drake EW. Longevity of restorations in dental school clinic. J Dent Educ 1986;50:594–600.
5. Blair KF, Koeppen RG, Schwartz RS, Davis RD. Microleakage associated with resin composite–cemented, cast glass ceramic restoration. Int J Prosthodont 1993;6:579–584.
6. Blazer PK, Land MR, Cochran RA. Effects of designs of class 2 preparations on resistance of teeth to fracture. Oper Dent 1983;8:6–10.
7. Brännström M, Vojinovic O. Response of the dental pulp to invasion of bacteria around three filling materials. J Dent Child 1976;43:83–89.
8. Burgess JO, Norling BK, Cardenas HL. Fluoride release and flexural strength of five fluoride releasing luting agents. J Dent Res 1996;75(special issue):70.
9. Christensen GJ, Christensen R. Use Survey—1990. Clin Res Assoc Newsletter 1990;14:1–3.
10. Cox CF, Suzuki S. Re-evaluating pulp protection: calcium hydroxide liners vs. cohesive hybridization. J Am Dent Assoc 1994;125:823–831.
11. Craig RG. Restorative Dental Materials, ed 6. St Louis: Mosby, 1980:57.
12. Curtis SR, Richards MW, Dhuru VB, Meiers JC. Early erosion of glass-ionomer cement at crown margins. Int J Prosthdont 1993;6:553–557.
13. Delong R, Pintado MR, Douglas WH. The wear of enamel opposing shaded ceramic restorative materials: an in vitro study. J Prosthet Dent 1992;68:42–48.
14. Diaz-Arnold AM, Vargas MA, Haselton DR. Current status of luting agents for fixed prosthodontics. J Prosthet Dent 1999;81:135–141.
15. Dodge WR, Weed RM, Baez RJ, Buchanan RN. The effect of convergence angle on retention and resistance form. Quintessence Int 1985;16:191–197.
16. Donnenfeld OW. Therapeutic end-points in periodontal therapy. Int J Periodontics Restorative Dent 1981;1(4):51–59.
17. Dragoo JR, Williams GB. Periodontal tissue reactions to restorative procedures. Int J Periodontics Restorative Dent 1981; 1(1):9–23.
18. El-Ebrashi MK, Craig RG, Payton FA. Experimental stress analysis of dental restorations IV. Concept of parallelism of axial walls. J Prosthet Dent 1969;22:346–356.
19. Gargiulo AW, Wentz FM, Orban BJ. Dimensions and relations of the dentogingival junction in humans. J Periodontol 1961; 32:261–267.

20. Gerhardt DE. Seating the cast gold restoration. Gen Dent 1987;35:479–480.

21. Gibbs CH, Lundeen HL. Advances in Occlusion. Littleton, MA: PSG, 1982:2–32.

22. Gilboe DB, Teteruck WR. Fundamentals of extracoronal tooth preparation. Retention and resistance form. J Prosthet Dent 1974;32:651–656.

23. Guyer SE. Multiple preparations for fixed prosthodontics. J Prosthet Dent 1970;32:529–553.

24. Herlands RE, Lucca JJ, Morris HL. Forms, contours, and extensions of full coverage restorations in occlusal reconstruction. Dent Clin North Am 1962;6:147–162.

25. Hiatt WH. Incomplete crown–root fracture in pulpal periodontal disease. J Periodontol 1973;44:369–379.

26. Hornsby PR. Dimensional stability of glass-ionomer cements. J Chem Tech Biotechnol 1980;30:595–601.

27. Hosada H. Glass ionomer dental cement—the materials and their clinical use. In: Katsuyama S, Ishikawa T, Fujii B (eds). St Louis: Ishiyaku EuroAmerica, 1993.

28. Hunsaker JK, Christensen GJ, Christensen RP, et al. Retentive characteristics of dental cementation materials. Gen Dent 1993;44:464–467.

29. Imbery TA, Davis RD. Evaluation of tin plating systems for a high-noble alloy. Int J Prosthodont 1993;6:55–59.

30. Ingber JS, Rose LF, Coslet JG. The "biologic width"—a concept in periodontics and restorative dentistry. Alpha Omegan 1977;70:62–65.

31. Jacobson PH, Rees JS. Luting agents for ceramic and polymeric inlays and onlays. Int Dent J 1992;42:145–149.

32. Jameson LM. Comparison of the volume of crevicular fluid from restored and nonrestored teeth. J Prosthet Dent 1979;41:209–214.

33. Johnson GH, Powell LV, DeRouen TA. Evaluation and control of post-cementation pulpal sensitivity: zinc phosphate and glass ionomer cements. J Am Dent Assoc 1993;124:38–46.

34. Jokstad A, Mjor IA. Ten years' clinical evaluation of three luting agents. J Dent 1996;24:309–315.

35. Jorgensen KD. The relationship between retention and convergence angle in cemented veneer crowns. Acta Odontol Scand 1955;13:35–40.

36. Kahn AE. Partial versus full coverage. J Prosthet Dent 1960;10:167–172.

37. Kaiser DA, Wise HB. Fitting cast gold restorations with the aid of disclosing wax. J Prosthet Dent 1980;43:227–228.

38. Kaiser DA. Anatomy of the cast gold margin. J Prosthet Dent 1983;50:437–440.

39. Kanchanavasita W, Pearson S, Pearson GJ. Water sorption characteristics of resin-modified glass-ionomer cements. Biomaterials 1997;18:343–349.

40. Kay HB. Esthetic considerations in the definitive periodontal prosthetic management of the maxillary anterior segment. Int J Periodontics Restorative Dent 1982;2(3):45–59.

41. Kern M, Kleimeier B, Schaller HG, Strub JR. Clinical comparison of post-operative sensitivity for a glass ionomer and a zinc phosphate luting cement. J Prosthet Dent 1996;75:159–162.

42. Krabbendam CA, Ten Harkel HC, Duijesters PPE, Davidson CL. Shear bond strength determinations on various kinds of luting cements with tooth structure and cast alloys using a new testing device. J Dent 1987;15:77–81.

43. Krough-Paulsen WG, Olsson A. Occlusal disharmonies and dysfunction of the stomatognathic system. Dent Clin North Am 1966;10:627–635.

44. Lagouvardos P, Sourai P, Douvitsas G. Coronal fractures in posterior teeth. Oper Dent 1989;14:28–32.

45. Larson TD, Douglas WH, Geistfeld RE. Effects of prepared cavities on the strength of teeth. Oper Dent 1981;6:2–5.

46. Levine WA. An evaluation of the film thickness of resin luting agents. J Prosthet Dent 1989;62:175–181.

47. Lorey RE, Myers GE. The retentive qualities of bridge retainers. J Am Dent Assoc 1968;76:568–572.

48. Margerit J, Cluzel B, Leloup JM, et al. Chemical characterization of in vivo aged zinc phosphate dental cements. J Mater Sci Mater Med 1996;7:623–628.

49. Marynuik GA. In search of treatment longevity—A 30 year perspective. J Am Dent Assoc 1984;109:739–744.

50. Mauser IK, Goldstein GR, Georgescu M. Effect of two dentinal desensitizing agents on retention of complete casting copings using four cements. J Prosthet Dent 1996;75:129–134.

51. Minker JS. Simplified full coverage preparations. Dent Clin North Am 1965;9:355–372.

52. McMillen K, Kerby RE, Thakur A, Johnson WM. Fluoride release of resin-based luting agents. J Dent Res 1996;75:68.

53. Mjör IA. Placement and replacement of restorations. Oper Dent 1981;6:49–54.

54. Mjör IA, Jokstad A, Qvist V. Longevity of posterior restorations. Int Dent J 1990;40;11–17.

55. Morris ML. Artificial crown contours and gingival health. J Prosthet Dent 1962;12:1146–1156.

56. Mount GJ. Crown and the gingival tissues. Aust Dent J 1970;15:253–258.

57. Nevins M, Skurow HM. The intracrevicular restorative margin, the biologic width, and the maintenance of the gingival margin. Int J Periodontics Restorative Dent 1984;4(3):31–49.

58. Newcomb GM. The relationship between the location of subgingival crown margins and gingival inflammation. J Periodontol 1974;5:151–154.

59. Norman RD, Swartz ML, Phillips RW, Vermani RV. A comparison of the intraoral disintegration of three dental cements. J Am Dent Assoc 1969;78:777–782.

60. Olin PS, Hill EME. Tensile strength of air abraded vs tin plated metals luted with three cements [abstract 188]. J Dent Res 1991;70:387.

61. Osborne JW, Wolff MS, Berry JC. Variance in powder-liquid ratio in zinc phosphate cement for luting castings [abstract 468]. J Dent Res 1986;65:778.

62. Ostlund LE. Improving the marginal fit of the cast restorations. J Am Acad Gold Foil Oper 1974;17:56–60.

63. O'Sullivan BP, Johnson PF, Blosser RL, et al. Bond strength of a luting composite to dentin with different bonding systems. J Prosthet Dent 1987;58:171–175.

64. Pameijer CH, Nilner K. Long term clinical evaluation of three luting materials. Swed Dent J 1994;18:59–67.

65. Parkinson CF. Excessive crown contours facilitate endemic plaque niches. J Prosthet Dent 1976;35:424–429.

66. Phillips RW. Skinner's Science of Dental Materials, ed 9. Philadelphia: Saunders, 1991:296.

67. Potts RG, Shillingburg HT, Duncanson MG. Retention and resistance of preparations for cast restorations. J Prosthet Dent 1980;43:303–308.

68. Reinhardt JW, Stephens NH, Fortin D. Effect of Gluma desensitization on dentin bond strength. Am J Dent 1995;8:170–172.

69. Rosensteil SF, Gegauff AF. Improving cementation of complete cast crowns: a comparison of static and dynamic seating methods. J Am Dent Assoc 1988;117:845–848.

70. Salis SG, Good J, Stokes A, Kirk E. Patterns of indirect fracture in intact and restored human premolar teeth. Endod Dent Traumatol 1987;3:10–14.

71. Schwartz NL, Whitsett LD, Berry TG, Stewart JL. Unserviceable crowns and fixed partial dentures: life-span and causes for loss of serviceability. J Am Dent Assoc 1970;81:1395–1401.

72. Schwartz RS, Davis RD, Hilton TJ. Effect of temporary cements on the bond strength of a resin cement. Am J Dent 1992;5:147–150.

73. Shillingburg HT. Cast gold restorations. In: Clark JW (ed). Clinical Dentistry. New York: Harper & Row, 1976.

74. Shillingburg HT, Hobo S, Whitsett LD. Fundamentals of Fixed Prosthodontics. Chicago: Quintessence, 1981:376–377.

75. Shillingburg HT, Jacobi R, Brackett SE. Fundamentals of Tooth Preparation. Chicago: Quintessence, 1987:112.

76. Shinkai K, Suzuki S, Leinfelder KF, Katch Y. Effect of gap dimensions on wear resistance of luting agents. Am J Dent 1995;8:149–151.

77. Sidhu SK, Watson TF. Resin-modified glass-ionomer materials. Part 1: properties. Dent Update 1995;22:429–431.

78. Silness J. Periodontal conditions in patients treated with dental bridges. II. The influence of full and partial crowns on plaque accumulation, development of gingivitis and pocket formation. J Periodont Res 1970;5:219–230.

79. Silness J. Periodontal conditions in patients treated with dental bridges. Part III. The relationship between the location of the crown and margin and the periodontal condition. J Periodont Res 1970;5:225–229.

80. Smith DC. Dental cements. Current status and future prospects. Dent Clin North Am 1983;6:763–792.

81. Sorensen JA, Martinoff JT. Intracoronal reinforcement and coronal coverage: a study of endodontically treated teeth. J Prosthet Dent 1984;51:780–784.

82. Staninec M, Giles WS, Saiku JM, Hattori M. Caries penetration and cement thickness of three luting agents. Int J Prosthodont 1988;1:259–265.

83. Stein RS. Periodontal dictates for esthetic ceramomental crowns. J Am Dent Assoc 1987;Dec(special issue):63E–75E.

84. Um CM, Oilo G. The effect of early water contact on glass-ionomer cements. Quintessence Int 1992;23:209–214.

85. Vale WA. Cavity preparation. Ir Dent Rev 1956;2:33–41.

86. Vanderhaug J. A 15-year clinical evaluation of fixed prosthodontics. Acta Odontol Scand 1991;49:35–40.

87. Van Nortwick WG, Gettlemen L. Effect of internal relief, vibration and venting on the vertical seating of cemented crowns. J Prosthet Dent 1981;45:395–399.

88. Waerhaug J. Histologic considerations which govern where the margins of restorations should be located in relation to the gingiva. Dent Clin North Am 1960;4:161–176.

89. Walton JN, Gardner FM, Agar JR. A survey of crown and fixed partial denture failures: length of service and reasons for replacement. J Prosthet Dent 1986;56:416–421.

90. Weed RM. Determining adequate crown convergence. Tex Dent J 1980;98:14–16.

91. Wheeler RC. Complete crown form and the periodontium. J Prosthet Dent 1961;11:722–734.

92. White SN, Furuichi R, Kyomen SM. Microleakage through dentin after crown cementation. J Endod 1995;21:9–12.

93. White SN, Sorensen JA, Kang SK, Caputo AA. Microleakage of new crown and fixed partial denture luting agents. J Prosthet Dent 1992;67:156–161.

94. White SN, Yu Z. Film thickness of new adhesive luting agents. J Prosthet Dent 1992;67:782–785.

95. White SN, Yu Z. Compressive and diametral tensile strengths of current adhesive luting agents. J Prosthet Dent 1993;69:568–572.

96. White SN, Yu Z. Physical properties of fixed prosthodontic resin composite luting agents. Int J Prosthodont 1993;6:384–389.

97. White SN, Yu Z, Tom JF, Sangsurasak S. In vivo microleakage of luting cements for cast crowns. J Prosthet Dent 1994;71:333–338.

98. White SN, Yu Z, Tom JF, Sangsurasak S. In vivo marginal adaptation of cast crowns lined with different cements. J Prosthet Dent 1995;74:25–32.

99. Wilson AD, Prosser JK, Powis DM. Mechanism of adhesion of polyelectrolyte cements to hydroxyapatite. J Dent Res 1983;62:590–592.

100. Wilson AD. Resin-modified glass-ionomer materials. Int J Prosthodont 1990;3:425–429.

101. Wilson RD, Maynard G. Intracrevicular restorative dentistry. Int J Periodontics Restorative Dent 1981;1(4):35–49.

102. Yap AU. Resin-modified glass ionomer cements: a comparison of water sorption characteristics. Biomaterials 1996;17:1897–1900.

103. Youdelis RA, Weaver JD, Sapkos S. Facial and lingual contours of artificial complete crown restorations and their effect on periodontium. J Prosthet Dent 1973;29:61–66.

Conservative Cast-Gold Restorations: The Tucker Technique

Richard V. Tucker/Dennis M. Miya

The use of gold for restorations in dentistry has declined with the development of composite and porcelain restorations. However, conservative cast-gold restorations continue to be the treatment of choice for restoration of posterior teeth and the distal aspect of canines for many clinicians (Fig 20-1). The primary advantage of a gold casting is its permanence (Fig 20-2); a gold restoration can last a lifetime. A cast-gold restoration maintains the beauty of a natural tooth when cavity design is well considered and when care is given to fabrication of the casting and finishing intraorally (Figs 20-3a to 20-3f).

Although gold castings are relatively technique sensitive and demanding of the operator, this type of restoration, well executed, offers the patient restorative comfort and long-term service.

Dr Richard Tucker has developed techniques for cavity preparations, fabrication, and finishing of conservative gold castings that have become a standard of excellence. His concepts of precise preparation, esthetic outline form, and gold foil–like margins were greatly influenced by Dr George Ellsperman and Dr Gerald Stibbs in the Vancouver Ferrier Gold Foil Study Club. Many study clubs have been established throughout the United States, Canada, and Europe to teach Dr Tucker's techniques for conservative cast-gold restorations.

Characteristics of Gold Restorations

The advantages of gold castings are:

1. Gold alloys do not oxidize and discolor the teeth.
2. A thin layer of gold can protect fragile areas of teeth.
3. The gold restoration itself will not fracture in the isthmus or other areas.
4. The marginal gap at the tooth-gold interface can be nearly imperceptible if handled properly. Reducing the problem of plaque accumulation at the margins should contribute to better tissue health.
5. The cast-gold inlay can be finished to have a highly polished and smooth surface, which is pleasant to the tongue and compatible with the oral tissues. Such a finish is more plaque resistant than a rough surface.
6. Gold castings such as ¾, ⅞, or full crowns can prevent fracture or relieve sensitivity when tiny fractures are present.
7. The dental anatomy can be better reproduced with a casting.
8. A gold inlay or onlay does not become worn to produce a submarginal surface, nor does it chip and fracture at the cavosurface margins.
9. Gold castings have a coefficient of thermal expansion similar to that of tooth structure.

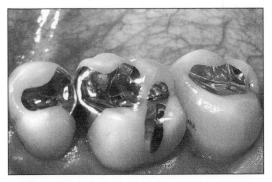

Fig 20-1 Conservative gold inlays in maxillary molars and premolar.

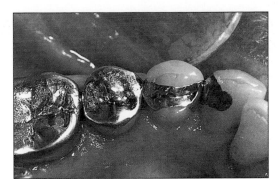

Fig 20-2 The inlays in the canine and first premolar have been in service for 48 years.

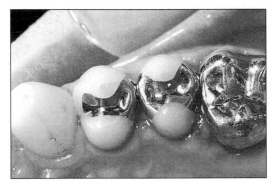

Fig 20-3a Recently placed gold inlays in maxillary premolars.

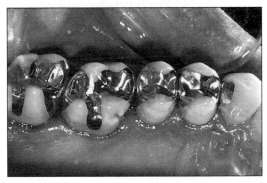

Fig 20-3b Recently placed gold inlays in maxillary molars and premolars.

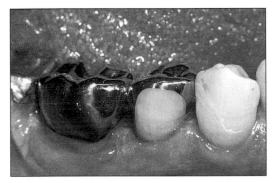

Fig 20-3c A gold onlay on the mandibular right second premolar.

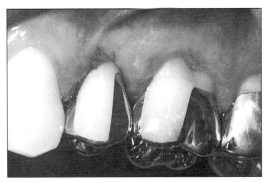

Fig 20-3d Seven-eighths crowns on the maxillary premolar and molar. This design preserves natural esthetics.

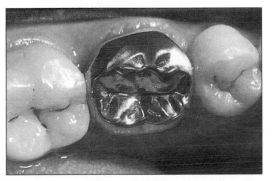

Fig 20-3e Full-coverage crown on a mandibular first molar.

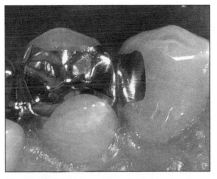

Fig 20-3f Distolingual gold inlay on maxillary canine.

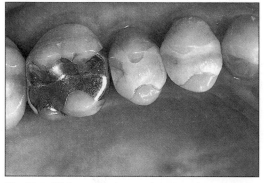

Fig 20-4 Slight reflection at functional margins of gold inlay. Opening and gap formation at functional margins of both porcelain inlays.

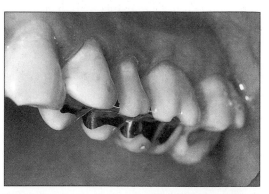

Fig 20-5 Esthetically pleasing restorations of maxillary posterior teeth with conservative outlines following preservation of the buccal enamel.

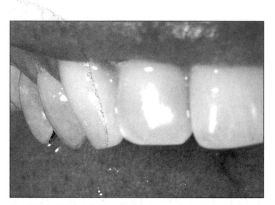

Fig 20-6 Slight gold display at the occlusal aspect of the ⅞ crown of a second premolar.

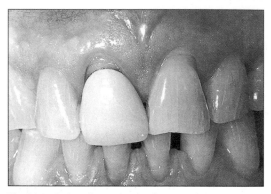

Fig 20-7 Color discrepancy of a porcelain crown as the natural teeth darken with age.

Like other restorative materials, gold castings have disadvantages.

1. Restorative procedures with castings are more time-consuming than those for most other materials.
2. A gold casting is often more expensive for the patient than other types of restorations.
3. A gold casting is somewhat technique sensitive; if not prepared with a real concern for excellence, it is probably less satisfactory than other restorations.
4. Gold can be esthetically unacceptable if placed in certain areas of the mouth, particularly the anterior teeth and the buccal areas of the maxillary posterior teeth.

Occlusion and Marginal Integrity

The marginal integrity of the enamel/gold cavosurface margin is preserved well under occlusal stress. Because the gold and tooth wear at a similar rate and their co-

efficients of expansion are similar, cavosurface margins can be prepared without too much concern for wear of the opposing dentition. The gold margin exhibits only a slight reflection even after many years of function, whereas functional margins of amalgam, composite, and porcelain will eventually open (Fig 20-4).

Esthetics

If conservative gold restorations are properly designed and finished, gold display can be minimal or nonexistent. A tooth can be functionally restored for a lifetime while the esthetics of the original tooth are maintained (Figs 20-5 and 20-6). If a tooth cannot be restored esthetically with a conservative gold restoration, a porcelain restoration might be the treatment of choice. As teeth age and become darker, however, the color of a porcelain restoration will eventually not match the rest of the dentition (Fig 20-7). Therefore, a conservative gold restoration is often the ideal long-term esthetic treatment.

Inlay Preparation

The cavity preparation sequence is as follows:

1. Placement of rubber dam
2. Removal of previous restoration and carious tooth structure
3. Calcium hydroxide liner
4. Resin composite buildup
5. Occlusal preparation
6. Proximal box form
7. Hand instrumentation
8. Occlusal bevel
9. Finishing of proximal walls

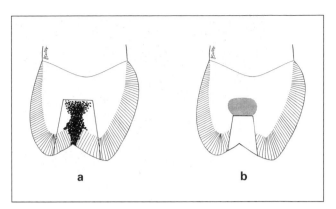

Fig 20-8 Outline without composite buildup (a) and with buildup (b).

Sequence

Rubber Dam

Placement of a rubber dam, a standard procedure for this technique, allows the operator to have the best possible working field. The teeth are isolated, the gingival tissue is slightly retracted, and saliva is eliminated. The tongue, cheek, and lips are eliminated from the operating field, and the patient is not concerned about swallowing any preparation debris. The quality of restorations is enhanced.[1,6,14]

Removal of Existing Restoration and Carious Tooth Structure

The existing restoration is expeditiously removed. Care should be taken not to extend the outline beyond the existing restoration. All remaining carious tooth structure is removed. The operator should not be concerned about the preparation taper at this stage. The remaining tooth structure is then evaluated, and the appropriate restoration is planned. It is helpful to use fiberoptic transillumination during the evaluation of the remaining tooth structure. Some important treatment planning considerations are: amount and quality of remaining tooth structure, occlusion, significant fracture lines or enamel crazing, parafunctional habits, and gold display.

Calcium Hydroxide Liner

A thin film of calcium hydroxide (Dycal, Dentsply) is placed on the internal surfaces of the preparation with a small cotton pellet. It acts as a separator for easy removal of the composite buildup prior to cementation. Retentive pits can be placed in the liner with a No. 2 round bur for composite retention.

Resin Composite Buildup

The use of a resin composite buildup conserves tooth structure because the operator can control the depth of the occlusal and axial walls (Fig 20-8). The preparation outline can be restricted so that it extends only minimally beyond that of the existing restoration. The resin composite buildup allows the operator to cut a precise cavity preparation that has ideal taper, smoothness, and proportions. Such a preparation will facilitate subsequent procedures of impression making, casting fabrication, and seating.

An autocure resin composite can be placed with a packing instrument or a syringe. A matrix band may be used to contain the resin composite buildup.

The buildup is usually entirely removed prior to cementing the casting. The casting often seats more completely because of the absence of the composite pulpal wall, and the area of the previous buildup is filled with luting cement.

Occlusal Preparation

The preparation is cut with a No. 56 straight fissure bur for premolars and a No. 57 straight fissure bur for molars (Fig 20-9a). The occlusal outline and pulpal floor are placed to a depth of 1.5 to 2.0 mm and a uniform inclination of the walls of 3 to 5 degrees[18] (Fig 20-10), resulting in an ideal preparation taper of 6 to 10 degrees[4,8,10,15,20] (Fig 20-11). The No. 56 and No. 57 burs are 4 mm in length and can be used to determine proper depth.

Proximal Box Form

The proximal box form is established next and is blended with the occlusal preparation. The box form

Fig 20-9 Cavity preparation.

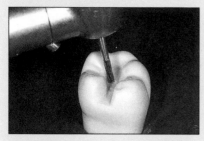

Fig 20-9a Occlusal preparation. No. 57 bur for molars, and No. 56 bur for premolars.

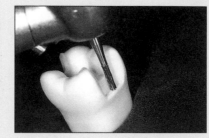

Fig 20-9b Proximal preparation.

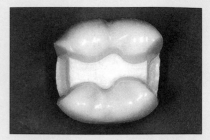

Fig 20-9c Preparation completed with bur.

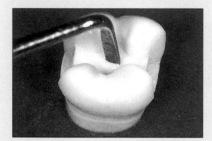

Fig 20-9d Instrument pulpal floor with enamel off-angle hatchet, 42S or 43S.

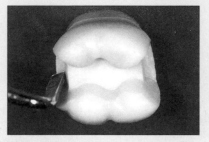

Fig 20-9e Instrument gingival walls (42S and 43S).

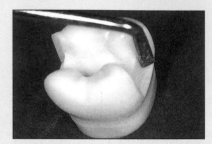

Fig 20-9f Instrument proximal line angles (42S and 43S).

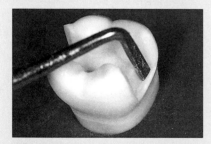

Fig 20-9g Instrument axial walls (42S and 43S).

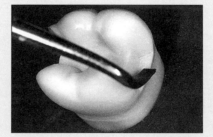

Fig 20-9h Gingival bevel cut with Tucker gingival margin trimmers, No. 232 and No. 233.

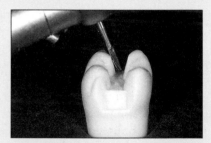

Fig 20-9i Occlusal bevel with fissure bur.

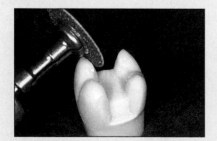

Fig 20-9j Medium garnet disk on proximal and occlusal walls.

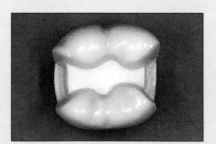

Fig 20-9k Occlusal view of completed preparation.

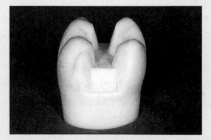

Fig 20-9l Proximal view of completed preparation.

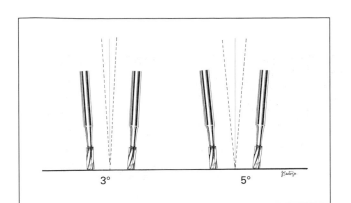

Fig 20-10 Ideal bur inclination.

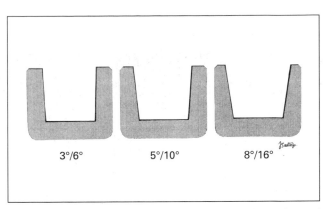

Fig 20-11 Wall inclination/preparation taper (single-wall taper/total-wall divergence).

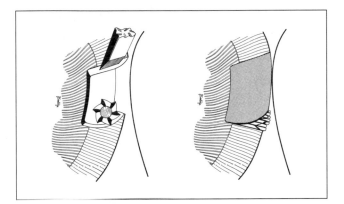

Fig 20-12 Proximal wall enamel rods.

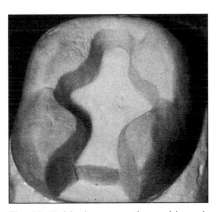

Fig 20-13 Ideal preparation with uniform inclination of walls and taper. There is no reverse curve.

is cut with the same overall taper as the occlusal form (Fig 20-9b). The width of the gingival floor is slightly larger than the diameter of the No. 56 bur for premolars and the No. 57 bur for molars. The buccal and lingual walls must be extended sufficiently (1 mm) beyond the adjacent tooth to be able to finish the casting. A smaller bur (No. 169L) is sometimes convenient to establish the proximal wall extensions without damaging the adjacent tooth.

The proximal walls have a slight flare (approximately 45 degrees) that eliminates unsupported enamel rods (Fig 20-12). Maximizing the use of the bur to cut most of the preparation results in smooth uniform walls and line angles; therefore, very little effort with hand instruments is necessary (Fig 20-13).

Hand Instrumentation

Smooth, precise preparations can be created with minimum effort with very sharp instruments. Instruments should be sharpened before each procedure. The instrumentation sequence is illustrated in Fig 20-14.

1. Pulpal and gingival floors are smoothed with 42S and 43S off-angle hatchets (Figs 20-9d to 20-9f).
2. The proximal axial line angles are ideally formed with one or two strokes. The mesial angles are placed with the 42S (15-10-16) chisel (Fig 20-9e). The distal angles are placed with the 43S (15-10-16) hatchet.
3. Axial wall: The small gouge on the axial wall formed from creating the proximal axial line angle is removed. The rest of the axial wall is smoothed as needed. The distal axial wall is smoothed with a 42S hatchet. The mesial axial wall is smoothed with a 43S hatchet (Fig 20-9g).
4. The gingival bevel is a small bevel 0.5 to 0.75 mm wide. The bevel should be definitive and smooth but not too wide (Fig 20-15). A large bevel offers no advantage. The bevel is created in thirds to prevent the creation of a swale in the middle where it is easiest to cut. The buccal and lingual thirds should be cut by planing toward the proximal walls (Fig 20-9h). The buccal and lingual segments are joined by cutting the middle third of the bevel last.

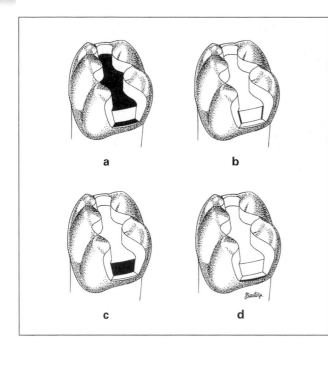

Fig 20-14 Instrumentation sequence: pulpal and gingival floors (a); proximal line angles (b); axial wall (c); gingival bevel (d).

Fig 20-15 Gingival bevel too large (a); ideal bevel (b). Bevels made with Tucker No. 232 and No. 233 gingival margin trimmers, respectively.

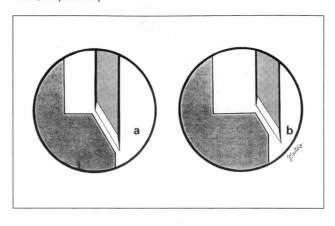

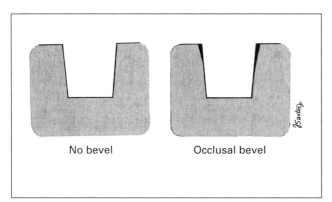

Fig 20-16 Occlusal bevel is only a few degrees more than the occlusal wall. It can include one half to two thirds of the occlusal wall.

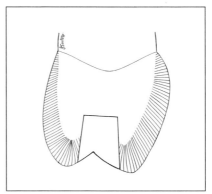

Fig 20-17 No undermined enamel rods are on the occlusal surface.

Gingival margin trimmers that are presharpened by the manufacturer (Suter) at a more acute angle than normal (30 degrees) are marked "Tucker." The No. 232 Tucker (10-98-10-16) gingival margin trimmer is used on the distal aspect. The No. 233 Tucker (10-78-10-16) gingival margin trimmer is used on the mesial aspect.

Occlusal Bevel

The function of the occlusal bevel is to remove fragile enamel rods and any irregularities in the cavosurface margin. It enables the preparation of a smooth, even,

esthetically pleasing outline. This bevel should be placed with the same straight fissure bur (No. 56 or No. 57) used for the rest of the preparation. It is placed with a bur incline of only a few degrees more than that of the occlusal wall (Figs 20-9i and 20-16). Where the existing outline is adequate, no bevel is needed since there are no undermined enamel rods (Fig 20-17).

Finishing of Proximal Walls

A 0.5-inch garnet disk is used to straighten the proximal walls. A 42S or 43S hatchet is used to plane the proximal walls if space is insufficient for the disk.

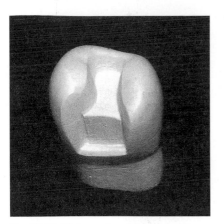

Fig 20-18 Disto-occlusal premolar dovetail and internal bevel.

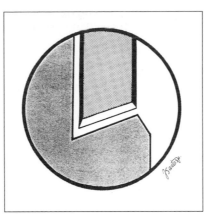

Fig 20-19 Internal bevel made with non-Tucker gingival margin trimmer No. 232 or No. 233.

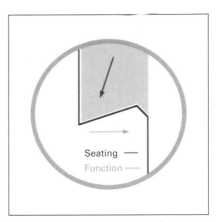

Fig 20-20 Internal bevel functions as a seating guide and provides added retention and resistance form.

Because a two-plane wall is not desirable, the single plane of the proximal wall is maintained. The disk can also be used to blend the box form and the occlusal outline, removing any remnants of a reverse curve (Fig 20-9j). The finished preparation is illustrated in Figs 20-9k and 20-9l.

Special Considerations

The preparation varies depending on the number of surfaces involved.

Disto-Occlusal and Mesio-Occlusal Inlays

A dovetail, the portion of the occlusal preparation made wider than the isthmus to prevent displacement of the casting, is cut on the occlusal aspect for retention and resistance form (Fig 20-18).

For most premolars, an internal bevel is recommended for added resistance and retention form (Figs 20-18 and 20-19). The bevel also acts as a seating guide for these smaller castings during cementation (Fig 20-20). Without this bevel, the cement tends to force the casting away from the axial wall during seating. The entire gingival wall is cut to meet the axial wall at an acute angle using a non-Tucker No. 232 (10-95-10-16) or No. 233 (10-80-10-16) gingival margin trimmer. The bevels on these instruments are less acute (45 degrees) than the ones marked Tucker (30 degrees) (Fig 20-21). The axial wall is instrumented next with an off-angle hatchet to ensure that it is not undercut or irregular at the gingivoaxial line angle. The gingival floor must be cut approximately

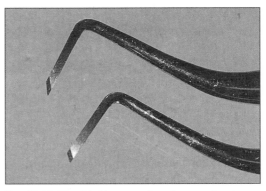

Fig 20-21 The Tucker margin trimmer *(top)* provides a 30-degree gingival bevel. The non-Tucker margin trimmer *(bottom)* provides a 45-degree internal bevel.

0.5 mm wider than usual to accommodate an internal bevel.

Mesio-Occlusodistal Inlay

Mesio-occlusodistal (MOD) inlays are probably the most common preparations made. The opposing mesiobuccal/distolingual proximal walls and the mesiolingual/distobuccal proximal walls are cut approximately parallel to each other. These walls are then retentive against each other and give the preparation symmetry (Fig 20-22). The two axial walls are also nearly parallel to add retentive form to the cavity.[5]

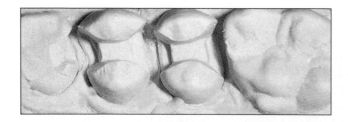

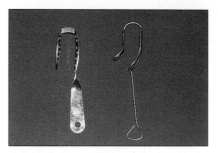

Fig 20-22 Opposing proximal walls of mesial and distal box forms are parallel and retentive with each other. Note the symmetry of the preparations.

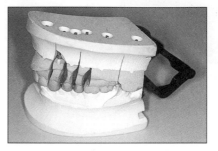

Fig 20-23 Coe (left) and Emery (right) checkbite trays.

Fig 20-24 Quadrant master cast with hinge articulator.

Impression

For one or two crowns or perhaps a quadrant of inlays, the quadrant checkbite is a clinically proven technique.[13] A metal checkbite tray (Coe) is recommended. When the back of this tray does not allow the patient to bite into centric occlusion (maximum intercuspation) comfortably, a smaller wire tray (Emery) is used (Fig 20-23). The impression is made as the patient bites into centric occlusion. The advantage of this procedure is that the impression is made while the teeth are in occlusion, thereby allowing a more precise interocclusal record. In turn, this usually allows the castings to be placed without the need to relieve the occlusion. This more accurate interocclusal registration is probably due to the small amount of movement in the periodontal ligament that allows the teeth to more completely intercuspate as the impression registers their position in function. The quadrant master cast, mounted from the interocclusal record, on a simple hinge articulator is shown in Fig 20-24.

For gingival retraction, a bulky, nonbraided cord (Gingivi-Pak 3, Surgident) is preferred. This cord provides adequate retraction depth below the preparation and adequate sulcus width. A 25% aluminum chloride solution (Hemodent, Premier) is used for hemorrhage control. It is tolerated well by the tissue and leaves no film on the preparation.

One or two cords are placed around the preparation. Two cords are routinely used interproximally. They should be left in place for 3 to 4 minutes. Before the impression is made, the fit of the tray should be checked, and the patient should practice "getting the feel" of biting into centric occlusion with the tray in place. It is important to note the occlusion on the contralateral side as a guide so that it is clear when the patient is biting into centric occlusion.

If a polyvinyl siloxane impression material is chosen, it is advisable to use only the light-bodied material for the entire impression because folds that are unacceptable for inlay impressions can occur at the interface of the light- and heavy-bodied materials. The potential set inhibition due to the rubber dam[12] or latex gloves[2,9] can be counteracted by cleaning the preparation and adjacent teeth with a cotton pellet saturated with diluted hydrogen peroxide, followed by a thorough rinse. Hydrogen gas evolution is a by-product of the polymerization of polyvinyl siloxane impression materials. Small voids in the stone model will result if the impression is poured too soon. Pouring of the impression should be delayed 30 minutes to 2 hours depending on the brand of material.

Before the impression material is mixed, the operating field should be spray washed and dried and the cord slowly removed. A check is performed for adequate retraction and to ensure that there is no hemorrhage. If retraction is inadequate or if there is hemor-

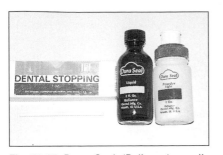

Fig 20-25 Dura Seal (Reliance) acrylic and temporary stopping.

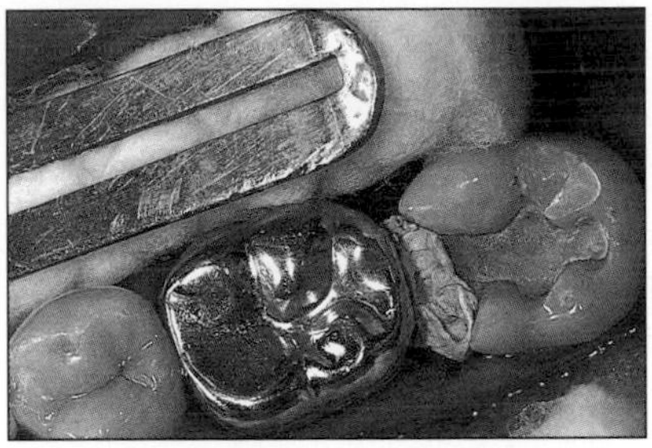

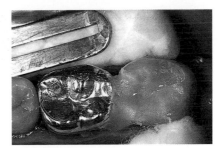

Fig 20-26 Temporary stopping placed.

Fig 20-27 Dura Seal placed.

rhage, repacking is required. If the retraction is satisfactory, the field must remain dry, and the impression material is mixed. Impression material is syringed into the preparation, the checkbite tray is placed, and the patient is asked to bite into maximum intercuspation. The patient may require assistance moving into proper jaw position, which can be provided with gentle pressure on the chin. The patient is monitored and supported for 5 minutes to ensure that there is no distortion in the impression due to patient movement. The impression is removed with a rapid, vertical movement to minimize distortion and tearing.

Temporary Restoration

Armamentarium

Included are a soft fast-set acrylic (Dura Seal, Reliance); temporary stopping (gutta-percha); a large straight brush; a plastic instrument (No. 1-2); two dappen dishes; and a lighter (flame).

A semisoft acrylic (Dura Seal), which is easy and quick to place, is an ideal temporary material for inlays and onlays (Fig 20-25). No cement is used, so it is easily removed and there is no cleanup.

A piece of temporary stopping large enough to cover the gingival two thirds of each box is heated and placed with a plastic instrument (No. 1-2) and an amalgam condenser. The temporary stopping acts like a dam so that the acrylic does not contact the tissue; to accomplish this, the stopping must be placed against the adjacent tooth as well. The stopping should not extend above the contacts to allow the acrylic to be "locked in" at the contacts of the adja-

cent teeth (Fig 20-26). Excess stopping can be contoured and removed with a heated instrument.

The acrylic is placed with the liquid/powder method using a fairly large brush. The acrylic is built up to contour and all margins of the preparation covered. It is important to work quickly so that the patient can bite and go through excursive movements while the acrylic is still soft (Fig 20-27). The acrylic can be molded with moistened fingertips. No attempt is made to refine the occlusion unless there is a gross excess of acrylic. Excess flash can be removed with a cleoid carver or a heated instrument. Multiple preparations can be connected with a single unit of acrylic. In such cases, the patient must be told that he or she will not be able to floss in that region.

While there are more sophisticated methods to fabricate temporary inlays and onlays, this method enables fast and easy placement and removal since no temporary cement is used. Patients tolerate this temporary restoration well, and the gingival response is generally good.

Laboratory Procedures

The skill with which an operator can prepare teeth and seat castings is very important, but unless quality castings are fabricated in the laboratory, it is impossible to provide consistently excellent restorations. A basic understanding of the laboratory procedures is essential for evaluation of castings and communication with the laboratory if refinements are necessary.

As gold is cast and changes from a liquid to a solid, it loses approximately 1.5% of its mass.[7] If nothing is

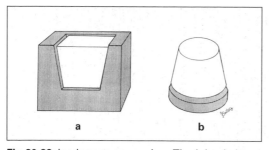

Fig 20-28 Inadequate expansion. The inlay is loose with marginal gaps (a); the crown will not seat completely (b).

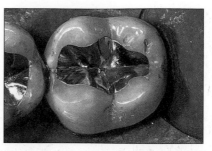

Fig 20-29 Inlay without proper expansion. Note marginal gaps and cement line within the gap at the margins.

Table 20-1	Recommendations for expansion with Novocast		
Restoration	**Water/powder ratio (mL/50g)**	**Oven temperature (°F)**	**Ring liner (no.)**
Crown	15.5	1175	2
¾, ⅞ crowns	18	1150	2
Mesio-occlusodistal buccolingual	18	1150	2
Mesio-occlusodistal	18.5	1150	2
Disto-occlusal, mesio-occlusal, occlusal	15	1175	2

done to compensate for this shrinkage, inlays will fit loosely, with marginal gaps, and crowns will not seat properly (Fig 20-28). The term *expansion* is used to describe methods used to compensate for gold shrinkage.

Is the gold shrinkage clinically significant? The occlusal inlay in Fig 20-29 is an example of an inlay that is too small for the preparation, resulting in marginal gaps that cannot be closed during finishing.

The compensation for gold shrinkage takes place in the investment procedures. Expansion can be increased by decreasing the water in the water/powder ratio; increasing oven temperature; increasing the number of ring liners; and hygroscopic expansion in a water bath (100°F). Recommendations for expansion with Novocast (Whip Mix) investment are shown in Table 20-1.

Cementation Procedures

Castings should be seated after the administration of anesthetic. The temporary restoration is removed, and a rubber dam is placed. The fit of the casting is verified in the preparation, and the contacts are adjusted if necessary. Just prior to cementation, all of the com-

posite buildup should be removed. A high-speed No. 2 round bur can be used to section it. The preparation is cleaned, and a desensitizing agent such as Gluma 3 (Miles) is placed on the dentin.

A slow-setting mix of zinc phosphate cement is prepared by adding small increments of powder slowly to the liquid over a period of 2 minutes until the mixture will just drop freely from the spatula. Cement is placed both in the casting and the preparation. The casting is seated, and considerable pressure is applied with a pointed orangewood stick. The orangewood stick is lightly malleted and held for several seconds until the hydraulic pressure of the cement has dissipated. Excess cement can now be removed.

The Finishing Sequence

Finishing requires disks (½ inch: medium garnet, fine sand, fine cuttle) (Fig 20-30) and powders (slurry of flour of pumice, aluminum oxide with alcohol [15 μm], aluminum oxide dry [1 μm]) (Fig 20-31). Air should be blown on the casting continuously during finishing with disks to dissipate the heat generated.[3]

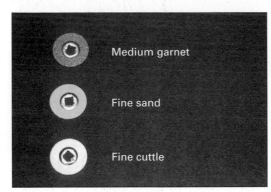

Fig 20-30 Moore ½-inch disks.

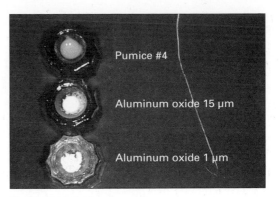

Fig 20-31 Polishing powders.

Enamel and gold are reduced to the same plane, and the margins are burnished with medium garnet disks prior to hardening of the cement. The disks should always be rotated from gold toward the tooth. The garnet disk is the workhorse of the finishing process, and usually several disks are used. All margins can usually be finished with a straight handpiece except in the mesiolingual area, where a contra-angle is used with the grit of the disk toward the handpiece.

After completion with garnet disks, most of the work is achieved so the gold and tooth are merely finished for smoothness. The fine sand disks are used next.

The gingival third of the casting and gingival margins can be finished with finishing strips. After completion with fine sand disks, a narrow, 18-inch medium garnet finishing strip that has been cut to a point is passed under the contact. Usually two or three swipes with the strip will adequately finish this area. Care must be taken not to overcut the relatively soft cementum. A fine cuttle strip should be used next in the same manner.

Fine cuttle disks are used next to remove any remaining scratches and to polish the gold. The key to fine finishing is adequate use of cuttle disks. As disks become used and worn, the scratches they leave become smaller. It has been said that disks have three lives: new, used, and worn. When gold is finished with a "third-life," worn cuttle disk, it can then be polished with powders to a mirrorlike finish. This can be accomplished by finishing the casting a section at a time with all three lives of a single cuttle disk. The life of a disk can be accelerated to a more worn stage by rotating it so that the grit is against a mirror handle.

Difficult access areas might be finished with the smaller ⅜-inch disks. Small finishing diamonds followed by Brownie, Greenie, and Supergreenie points (Shofu) work well for grooves and fissures that are not accessible with disks.

The casting is then ready for polishing. Care must be taken because the powders, especially flour of pumice, cut the tooth and gold at different rates and can open a margin or cause a reflection. Each powder should be used with a clean, ribbed rubber cup on a contra-angle. A slurry of pumice is used to give the gold a uniform finish after use of the disks. A 15-µm aluminum oxide powder with alcohol is used next. The final powder, 1-µm aluminum oxide, is used dry while the assistant provides continuous air and suction.

After the rubber dam is removed, the occlusion is checked with articulating paper. Adjustments are made with a high-speed green stone (Shofu) and polished with high-speed Brownie and Greenie points. Longevity of conservative gold castings requires well-fitting castings that are nicely finished with marginal gaps of less than 50 µm.[16] Keenan et al[11] suggest that a well-finished gold surface accumulates less plaque.

Magnification

The use of magnification for cast-gold restorations facilitates a clinicians' ability to deliver quality restorations. Magnification in the range of 2.0 to 2.5 diopters is recommended.

Variations of Cavity Design

Inlays vs Onlays

The restoration of choice for a posterior tooth is an inlay because it preserves more functional tooth structure and can be predictably fitted and finished. In addition, because most of the enamel can be preserved,

Fig 20-32 Cavity preparation for an onlay.

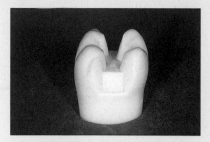

Fig 20-32a Onlay preparation for a mandibular molar. The MOD preparation should be cut first.

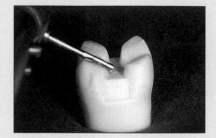

Fig 20-32b Occlusal reduction with a No. 57 bur.

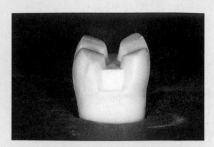

Fig 20-32c Occlusal reduction completed.

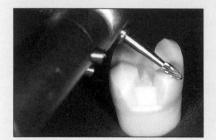

Fig 20-32d Counterbevel is provided on both buccal and lingual aspects with a No. 7404 bur.

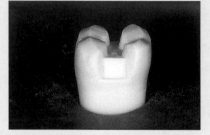

Fig 20-32e Onlay preparation completed.

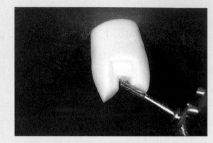

Fig 20-32f Onlay preparation for a maxillary premolar. Occlusal reduction is performed with a No. 56 bur.

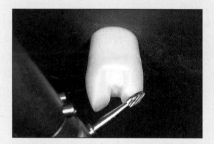

Fig 20-32g Lingual counterbevel with a No. 7404 bur.

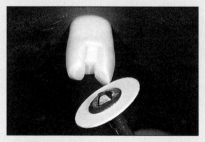

Fig 20-32h Microbevel buccal cusp with a fine cuttle disk.

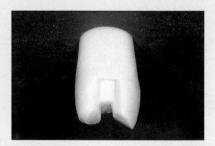

Fig 20-32i Maxillary premolar onlay completed.

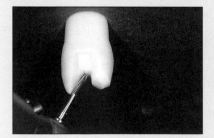

Fig 20-32j "Invisible" onlay for maxillary premolar: bucco-occlusal reduction to pulpal floor.

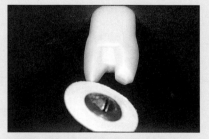

Fig 20-32k Microbevel with a fine cuttle disk.

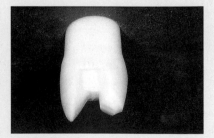

Fig 20-32l "Invisible" onlay preparation completed.

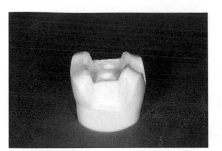

Fig 20-33 Proximal view of an onlay preparation for a mandibular molar.

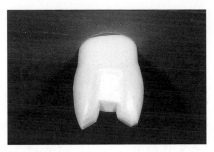

Fig 20-34 Proximal view of an onlay preparation for a maxillary premolar.

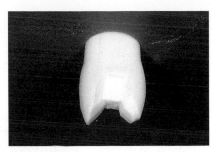

Fig 20-35 Proximal view of an "invisible" onlay preparation for a maxillary premolar.

it is esthetic. It is the experience of the authors that cusp fracture of a tooth restored with an inlay is rare. An onlay restores the strength of a tooth but destroys more tooth structure and the gold display can be unesthetic.

When insufficient sound tooth structure remains to support an inlay, an onlay is indicated. The basic technique is to cut the MOD preparation first and then prepare the cusps as the final step. When there is a question about whether the remaining tooth structure can support an inlay, an onlay is generally advisable since predictable longevity is the goal. If there is sufficient tooth structure, only the weakened portion of the tooth need receive an onlay. However, in most cases, both buccal and lingual cusps are onlayed to distribute the occlusal forces over a broader surface. A tooth with an onlay can be stronger than the original nonrestored tooth. Cusp reduction for a functional cusp is about 1.5 to 2.0 mm, and nonfunctional cusps can be reduced less. The appropriate bevels are placed with a No. 7404 bur. The resulting hollow grind (concave) bevel provides bulk of gold at the bevel and a good margin for waxing and finishing. Step-by-step procedures for onlays are shown in Fig 20-32.

Mandibular Onlay

In the mandibular onlay, both cusps are reduced and counterbeveled. The counterbevel on the buccal functional cusp is larger than that on the nonfunctional lingual cusp (Fig 20-33).

Maxillary Onlay

The nonfunctional buccal cusp is reduced about 1 mm, and a microbevel is placed with a fine cuttle disk. The lingual functional cusp is reduced 1.5 to 2.0 mm, and a counterbevel is placed (Fig 20-34).

"Invisible" Onlay

Indication: The "invisible" onlay is a modification of the traditional onlay preparation to minimize gold display on the occlusobuccal aspect of the maxillary premolars (Fig 20-35).

Armamentarium
1. No. 56 bur (straight fissure)
2. Brasseler No. 7404 bur (egg-shaped finishing)
3. Fine cuttle disk

Preparation synopsis
1. The lingual incline of the buccal cusp is reduced steeply from the cusp tip to the level of the pulpal floor. Reduction at the buccal cusp tip can be 0.5 mm if occlusion permits.
2. The increased thickness of gold protects the cusp and allows the gold to be thinned on the buccal aspect so that it is not visible.

Preparation sequence
1. The lingual incline of the buccal cusp is reduced with a No. 56 bur.
2. A fine cuttle disk is used to place a microscopic counterbevel on the buccal cusp.
3. The lingual cusp reduction and counterbevel are cut in the typical manner.

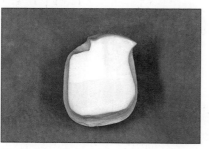

Fig 20-36a Occlusal view of a ⅞ crown preparation for a maxillary molar.

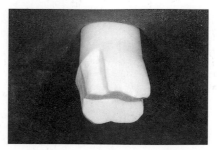

Fig 20-36b Buccal view.

Maxillary Molar ⅞ Crown

Indication: This preparation is indicated when the tooth requires cuspal coverage but a good mesiobuccal cusp remains (Figs 20-36a and 20-36b).

Armamentarium
1. No. 57 bur (straight fissure)
2. 860-012 flame-shaped diamond (1.2-mm diameter)
3. 860-014 flame-shaped diamond (1.4-mm diameter)
4. 42S and 43S off-angle hatchets
5. Medium garnet disk
6. Fine cuttle disk

Preparation synopsis
1. A definitive occlusal center line angle is created as the occlusal aspect is reduced.
2. A minimal taper of the preparation results in parallel walls.
3. The mesial hollow grind (concave bevel) is cut to incline slightly to the lingual aspect. It provides this wall more length, increasing retention.
4. The buccal wall is cut relatively horizontal, and the distobuccal angle of the tooth is left relatively square for added retention. This results in a small, irregular triangle at the distobuccal finish line.
5. The distobuccal wall of the preparation is cut to function in concert with the mesial hollow grind.
6. A definitive distobuccal line angle is created with hand instruments.

Preparation sequence
1. A No. 57 bur is used for the occlusal reduction. There is a definitive occlusal line angle in the center of the occlusal surface.
2. The small, 860-012 flame-shaped diamond may be used to break through the interproximal contacts.

3. The larger, 860-014 flame-shaped diamond is used to cut the rest of the preparation. First, a wall with an accentuated chamfer margin is cut on the mesial aspect. By cutting this area with a slight lingual inclination, the mesiobuccal wall of the preparation can be longer for additional retention. The lingual and distal walls are cut next.
4. The buccal wall is cut fairly straight across, and the distobuccal line angle is quite square for maintenance of a buccal wall. This results in a small triangle or irregularity on the distobuccal finish line, which is left since smoothing this area would result in an undercut.
5. The 42S off-angle hatchet creates a sharp line angle in the back of the mesiobuccal cusp. The 43S is then used to slide down the buccal wall to complete the line angle. This angle should be about 90 degrees.
6. The medium garnet disk is used on the distobuccal wall to sharpen the outline of the preparation.
7. The fine cuttle disk is placed on the occlusal edge of the buccal cusp to slightly bevel and smooth the finish line.

Premolar ⅞ Crown

The premolar ⅞ crown (Figs 20-37a and 20-37b) differs from the molar preparation in the following ways:

1. The small, 860-012 flame-shaped diamond is always used for the initial proximal reduction. Using a larger bur initially could lead to overcutting or damage to the adjacent tooth.
2. The distal wall has a slight hollow grind curve that increases resistance form enough to allow a more conservative reduction of the buccal wall, thus minimizing gold display.

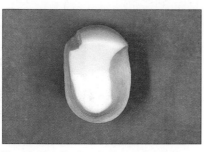

Fig 20-37a Occlusal view of a ⅞ crown preparation for a maxillary premolar.

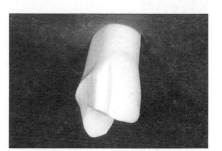

Fig 20-37b Distobuccal view.

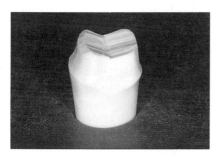

Fig 20-38a Hollow grind crown preparation viewed from the proximal aspect.

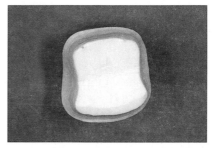

Fig 20-38b Occlusal view.

Full Gold Crown Variations

The full gold crown variations allow the buccal finish line to be kept well coronal to the gingiva for better tissue health. Each variation described has a feature that adds retention and resistance form to the preparation to allow such a buccal finish line. The buccal finish line is finished like an onlay.

Hollow Grind Crown

Indications: This technique is used for mandibular molar full crown preparations where existing restorations or caries would require proximal margins placed far gingivally (Figs 20-38a and 20-38b).

Armamentarium
1. No. 57 bur (straight fissure)
2. 860-012 flame-shaped diamond (1.2-mm diameter)
3. 860-014 flame-shaped diamond (1.4-mm diameter)
4. Brasseler No. 7404 bur (egg-shaped finishing)
5. Fine cuttle disk

Preparation synopsis
1. A gentle buccal to lingual hollow grind curve on both mesial and distal walls provides adequate resistance form.
2. The long mesial and distal walls of the hollow grind that resulted from the increased gingival extension of the preparation enhance retention. They are also cut quite parallel.

Preparation sequence
1. The occlusal reduction is done with a No. 57 bur. A sharp line angle is created in the center of the occlusal aspect.
2. The 860-012 flame-shaped diamond may be used to break the contacts initially.
3. The larger 860-014 flame-shaped diamond is used to cut the bulk of the preparation.
4. The No. 7404 bur is used to finish the buccal margin to provide a sharp, smooth finish line that provides adequate bulk of gold for casting and finishing.
5. A fine cuttle disk is used to smooth the occlusal line angles.

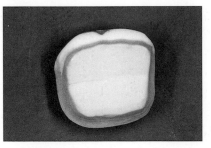

Fig 20-39a Occlusal view of a full-coverage crown with a shoulder.

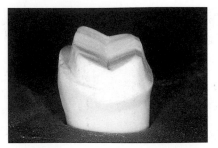

Fig 20-39b Proximal view.

Crown with Shoulder

Indication: Mandibular molar full crown preparations without extensive proximal involvement where a deep concave bevel would be inappropriate (Figs 20-39a and 20-39b).

Armamentarium
1. No. 57 bur (straight fissure)
2. 860-012 flame-shaped diamond (1.2-mm diameter)
3. 860-014 flame-shaped diamond (1.4-mm diameter)
4. Fine cuttle disk

Preparation synopsis
Making a buccal wall more parallel to the other walls by placing a buccal shoulder creates additional retention and resistance form.

Preparation sequence
1. The preparation is cut in the typical manner for a traditional full crown except for the buccal wall.
2. The shoulder is cut with a No. 57 bur and blended interproximally with the 860-014 flame-shaped diamond.

Brasseler No. 7404 Bur Preparation Variations

The Brasseler No. 7404 bur, which is egg-shaped, produces a smooth hollow ground margin that allows good definition and bulk of gold at the margins.[17]

Hollow Grind Marginal Ridge
Indication: Thin, weakened distal marginal ridge, usually on the second molar (Fig 20-40).

Synopsis: The marginal ridge can be expediently included in the preparation without a distal box or hand instrumentation.

Buccal Extension (Bale)

Indication: The fingerlike extension on the buccal aspect of molars is placed when there is extensive breakdown of the lingual cusp. It allows the casting to engage the stronger buccal tooth structure, reducing stress on the lingual aspect (Fig 20-41).

Preparation synopsis
1. The preparation must have adequate length and should not taper too lingually.
2. Adequate depth is necessary for sufficient bulk of gold to prevent bending and distortion.

Occlusolingual Maxillary Molar

Indication: Occlusolingual groove on maxillary molars (Fig 20-42).

Preparation synopsis
1. The entire cavity is cut with the No. 7404 bur.
2. The preparation will have a rounded pulpal floor and no line angles.
3. The shape of the bur creates ideal taper for this preparation.

"Potholes" Made with Midwest No. 7404 Bur

Indication: Wide, open cavity requiring additional retention and resistance form, often a large cavity with a resin composite buildup (Fig 20-43). This type of preparation was named "pothole" by Dr Tucker.

Preparation synopsis
1. A Midwest No. 7404 bur is used because it has increased taper.
2. The depth of the pothole is at least 2 mm. It is deeper if cutting through the entire depth of the

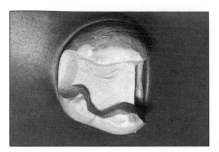

Fig 20-40 The distal aspect of the tooth was prepared with a finishing bur.

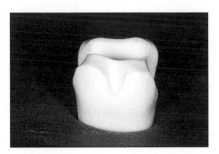

Fig 20-41 Added retention and resistance form were incorporated by extending the preparation onto the buccal surface.

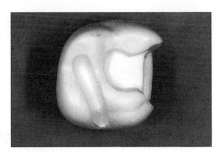

Fig 20-42 The lingual groove was prepared with a No. 7404 finishing bur.

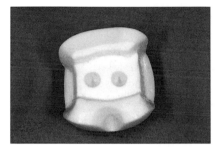

Fig 20-43 Retention and resistance form were added with potholes.

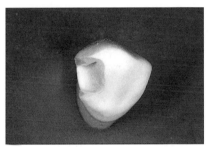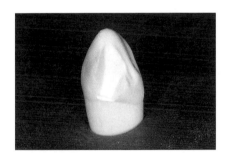

Figs 20-44a and 20-44b Two views of a slot inlay on the distal surface of a maxillary canine.

buildup to dentin is desired. The pothole is made with the end of the No. 7404 bur.
3. The entire resin composite buildup is removed before cementation.

Impression
1. The end of an anesthetic needle is broken to remove the bevel without closing the lumen.
2. The needle is placed in the pothole and impression material ejected from an impression syringe.
3. The needle allows air to escape and thus decreases voids.

Slot Inlay

Indication: Restoration of the distal aspect of a canine with a small lesion or a small existing restoration (Figs 20-44a and 20-44b).[19]

Armamentarium
1. No. 169L fissure bur
2. 44S and 45S off-angle hatchets (10-10-16)
3. Non-Tucker No. 232 and 233 gingival margin trimmers

4. Tucker No. 232 and 233 gingival margin trimmers
5. No. 55 fissure bur

Preparation synopsis
1. Hand instrumentation results in sharp internal line angles.
2. Two-plane labial and lingual walls enhance retention.
3. An internal bevel adds retention and aids in seating of the casting during cementation.
4. A small definitive gingival bevel is placed.

Preparation sequence
1. The cavity is opened with the No. 169L bur, and the labial and lingual extensions and the gingival wall are established. The cavity should look like a crescent.
2. The No. 169L bur is used to enhance the axial line angles labially and lingually for retention, creating the two-plane labial and lingual walls.
3. The narrow 45S off-angle hatchet is used to place the proximal axial line angles, which create sharp retentive walls.
4. The No. 233 margin trimmer is used to place an internal bevel on the gingival wall. It is slid down

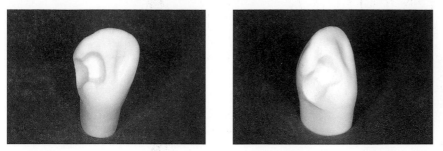

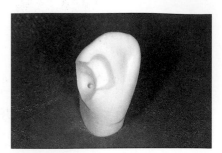

Figs 20-45a and 20-45b The distal aspect of the tooth was prepared with a No. 7404 finishing bur.

Fig 20-46 A pin was added to the preparation in Fig 20-45 to enhance retention and resistance.

both the labial and lingual walls to define the line angles and sharpen the point angles.

5. The axial wall is smoothed with the 44S off-angle chisel since it will be rough from internal bevel instrumentation.

6. A small definitive gingival bevel is placed with the Tucker No. 232 margin trimmer.

7. A No. 55 bur is used for the occlusal bevel, which removes unsupported enamel, smoothes the outline, and creates a "funnel" that aids in seating.

Distal Hollow Grind

Indication: Restoration of a tooth with a large caries lesion or large existing restoration with a lingual dovetail (Figs 20-45a and 20-45b).[19]

Armamentarium
1. No. 56 bur (straight fissure)
2. Brasseler No. 7404 bur (egg-shaped finishing)

Preparation synopsis
1. No hand instruments are used for this preparation.
2. The preparation consists of a lingual dovetail and a distal hollow grind.
3. It has an easy draw to the lingual aspect because there are no sharp internal angles.

Preparation sequence
1. The lingual dovetail is placed with a No. 56 bur. The dovetail draws perpendicular to the lingual cavosurface with equal depth in all aspects.

2. The Brasseler No. 7404 bur is used to place the distal hollow grind. The hollow grind is parallel to the labial surface. The axial wall taper is kept to a minimum.

3. A light occlusal bevel is placed with the No. 7404 bur.

Distal Hollow Grind with a Pin

Indication: Large cavity requiring additional retention and resistance form (Fig 20-46).

Armamentarium
1. No. 6 round bur
2. No. 169L fissure bur

Preparation synopsis
1. Half of distal hollow grind preparations need a pin.
2. The pin is placed as far from the primary retention of the dovetail as possible.

Preparation sequence
1. A countersink is placed with a No. 6 round bur in a high-speed handpiece.
2. The pinhole is placed with a No. 169L bur to a depth of about 1.5 mm and is parallel to the lingual taper of the cavity.

References

1. Christensen GJ. Using rubber dams to boost quality, quantity of restorative services. J Am Dent Assoc 1994;125:81–82.

2. Cook WD, Thomasz F. Rubber gloves and addition silicone materials. Current note no. 64. Aust Dent J 1986;31:140.

3. Cooly RL, Barkmeyer WW, White JH. Heat generation during polishing of restorations. Quintessence Int 1978;9:77–80.

4. Dykema RW, Goodacre CJ, Phillips RW. Johnston's Modern Practice in Crown and Bridge Prosthodontics, ed 4. Philadelphia: Saunders, 1986:24.

5. El-Ebrashi MK, Craig RG, Peyton FA. Experimental stress analysis of dental restorations. Part IV. The concept of parallelism of axial walls. J Prosthet Dent 1969;22:346–353.

6. Gergely EJ. Rubber dam acceptance. Br Dent J 1989;167: 249–252.

7. Hollenback GM, Skinner EW. Shrinkage during casting of gold and gold alloys. J Am Dent Assoc 1946;33:1391–1399.

8. Jorgensen KD. The relationship between retention and convergence angle in cemented veneer crowns. Acta Odontol Scand 1955;13:35–40.

9. Kahn RL, Donovan TE, Chee WWL. Interaction of gloves and rubber dam with poly(vinyl siloxane) impression material: a screening test. Int J Prosthodont 1989;2:342–346.

10. Kaufman EG, Coelho DH, Colin L. Factors influencing the retention of cemented gold castings. J Prosthet Dent 1961;11: 487–502.

11. Keenan MP, Shillingburg HT Jr, Duncanson MG Jr, Wade CK. Effects of cast gold surface finishing on plaque retention. J Prosthet Dent 1980;43:168–173.

12. Noonan JE, Goldfogel MH, Lambert RL. Inhibited set of the surface of addition silicones in contact with rubber dam. Oper Dent 1985;10:46–48.

13. Parker MH, Cameron SM, Hughbanks JC, Reid DE. Comparison of occlusal contacts in maximum intercuspation for two impression techniques. J Prosthet Dent 1997;78: 255–259.

14. Reuter JE. The isolation of teeth and the protection of the patient during endodontic treatment. Int Endod J 1983;16: 173–181.

15. Shillingburg HT, Hobo S, Fisher DW. Preparations for Cast Gold Restorations. Chicago: Quintessence, 1974:16.

16. Skinner EW, Phillips RW. The science of dental materials, ed 6. Philadelphia: Saunders, 1967:473–474.

17. Tucker RV. Variation of inlay cavity design. J Am Dent Assoc 1972;84:616–620.

18. Tucker RV. Class 2 inlay cavity procedures. Oper Dent 1982;7:50–54.

19. Tucker RV. Gold restorations of the distal aspect of cuspid teeth. Signature 1996;Winter:4–9.

20. Tylman SD, Malone WFP. Tylman's Theory and Practice of Fixed Prosthodontics, ed 7. St Louis: Mosby, 1978:103.

Restoration of Endodontically Treated Teeth

J. William Robbins

A great deal of research has been published on the restoration of endodontically treated teeth.[107] However, it is very difficult for the busy practitioner to read all of this information and synthesize it into a logical treatment philosophy. It is the purpose of this chapter to analyze the research and present a logical approach to this subject.

When faced with the challenge of restoring an endodontically treated tooth, the dentist must decide, first, whether a post is required and, second, the type of restoration that is indicated. In the past, a post was thought to strengthen the root of an endodontically treated tooth. This philosophy pervaded dental education until laboratory research began to cast doubts on this assumption. It is widely held today that the primary purpose of post placement is to retain the core buildup material or to reinforce the remaining coronal tooth structure.

It is difficult to discuss the longevity of post-restored teeth because there are many variables to control. Mentink and others[82] reported an 82% success rate in post-restored teeth after 10 years. Torbjorner and others[133] reported a 2.1% failure rate per year. Finally, Nanayakkara and others[88] reported the median survival rate to be 17.4 years.

The long-term clinical success of an endodontically treated tooth is dependent on many factors. It has been reported that the majority of failures are due to inadequate restorative therapy, followed by tooth loss due to periodontal reasons. Relatively few endodontically treated teeth are lost due to failed endodontic therapy.[137] When endodontic therapy fails, the most common reason is inadequate cleaning and obturation of the canal system.[138] However, in recent years, it has become obvious that another important failure mechanism is orthograde contamination, that is, contamination via leakage of oral fluids apically within the root.[4,30] This can be due to the loss of or leakage around a provisional restoration or marginal leakage around a definitive restoration.

The decision to place a post is based on several parameters. These include the position of the tooth in the arch, occlusion, function of the restored tooth, amount of remaining tooth structure, and canal configuration. Each of these considerations will be discussed in detail.

Indications for Placement of Posts

Anterior Teeth

Anterior and posterior teeth function much differently; therefore, they must be evaluated separately. The anterior tooth receives predominately shear forces, which act on both the clinical crown and the root. Although some laboratory studies[57,134] have indicated that a post strengthens an intact anterior endodontically treated tooth, the majority of studies[38,108,136] have suggested that the fracture resistance of these teeth is not affected by, or is decreased with, placement of a post. Therefore, when a complete-coverage restoration is not required for esthetic or functional reasons (eg, to serve as an abutment for a fixed or removable partial denture), a post is not indicated. However, if a complete-coverage restoration is indicated in an endodontically treated anterior tooth for esthetics or function, a post may be indicated.[144] This is especially true for maxillary lateral incisors and mandibular incisors.

With maxillary central incisors and canines, the decision to place a post should be based on the amount of remaining coronal tooth structure, as well as the occlusion and function of the tooth. If there is a significant amount of remaining coronal tooth structure, the crown preparation should be accomplished before the decision regarding post placement is made. Once the axial preparation is completed and the access preparation is cleaned, the dentist can make the decision as to whether the remaining coronal tooth structure needs the reinforcement of a post. If the decision is made, based on the functional requirements of the tooth, that the remaining coronal tooth structure is adequate to support the crown, resin composite can be bonded into the access preparation. However, if there is doubt regarding the adequacy of the resistance form of the coronal portion of the tooth, then a post or post and core is indicated.

Posterior Teeth

For the posterior tooth, the decisions are more clearcut. The forces on posterior teeth are predominately vertical. Therefore, reinforcement of coronal tooth structure is not commonly needed, as it is in anterior teeth. Because of the morbidity associated with post placement (Fig 21-1), a post is indicated in a posterior tooth only when other more conservative retention and resistance features cannot be used for the core. These features include chamber retention, amalgam pins, and threaded pins, all of which have been shown to be exceedingly effective.[106]

In 1980, Nayyar and Walton[91] described the amalcore, or coronal-radicular, restoration. Rather than placing a post, the pulp chamber and coronal 2.0 to 3.0 mm of each canal are used for retention of the buildup material (Figs 21-2a to 21-2c). Subsequently, several authors reported laboratory data on the fracture resistance of the amalcore. Kern and others[60] and Christian and others[15] reported that the placement of a post in the distal canal of a mandibular

molar increases the fracture resistance of the amalcore. However, in these studies the specimens were stressed in compression at 60 degrees and 90 degrees, respectively. This angle of force does not reproduce the vertical forces that molars receive in vivo. In a similar study, Plasmans and others[97] found no statistically significant difference between the amalcore alone and the amalcore with a post when stressed at 45 degrees. Kane and Burgess[56] reported that the placement of two horizontal threaded pins in the buccal and lingual walls of the amalcore restoration provides a significant increase in fracture resistance. In a retrospective clinical study of more than 400 coronal-radicular restorations, Nayyar and Walton[91] reported no failures that could be attributed to the core buildup. The coronal-radicular buildup has proven to be a predictable and cost-effective restorative modality for posterior endodontically treated teeth.

It has been commonly stated that threaded pins should not be placed in endodontically treated teeth because they will cause the teeth to crack. However, no clinical data are available to support this belief. In fact, current data indicate that there is very little difference between the dentin of endodontically treated teeth and vital dentin.[44,115] There is also a move to completely discard traditional retention and resistance features in deference to the adhesively retained core buildup. With regard to core retention, Tjan and others[132] reported that dentin adhesive performed better than mechanical retention with resin composite, while threaded pins performed better with amalgam, in vitro. One 3-year clinical study supports the effectiveness of the adhesively retained complex amalgam without auxiliary retention.[129] However, sufficient long-term clinical data are not available to support the efficacy of using a dentin bonding agent as the sole means of core retention. Therefore, until the efficacy of the adhesively retained buildup can be demonstrated in long-term clinical studies, it would be prudent to use adhesive materials in conjunction with traditional retention and resistance features.

Although a post is not commonly required to retain the core in a posterior tooth, a post may be indicated when the tooth is to serve as an abutment for a removable partial denture.[121] In this circumstance, the forces that play on the tooth are not physiologic, and coronal reinforcement may be necessary (Fig 21-3). In maxillary molars, a post is generally placed only in the palatal canal, and in mandibular molars in the distal canal.

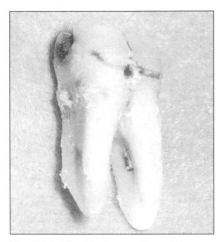

Fig 21-1 Mandibular molar with post perforation in the mesial concavity of the distal root.

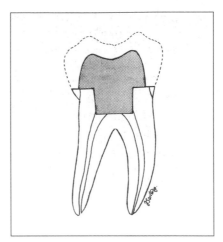

Fig 21-2a Amalcore with adequate chamber retention.

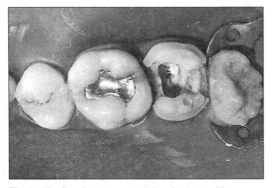

Fig 21-2b Amalcore preparation in a maxillary second molar.

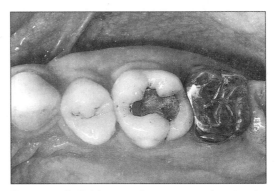

Fig 21-2c Definitive amalcore restoration in the maxillary second molar.

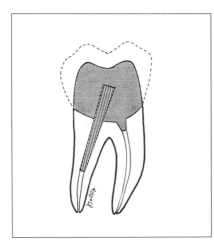

Fig 21-3 Mandibular molar that does not have a large enough pulp chamber for chamber retention of the core buildup. A post is used for retention of the core.

Maxillary premolars are a unique subset of posterior endodontically treated teeth. Because these teeth are subjected to a mixture of shear and compressive forces, the need for a post and core in a maxillary premolar is not as clear. If the remaining coronal tooth structure is inadequate, the clinical crown is tall in relation to its diameter at the point where it enters the alveolar bone, or if the tooth receives significant lateral stress, a post may be indicated (Figs 21-4a and 21-4b). In addition, if the premolar serves as an abutment for a removable partial denture, a post and core may be indicated.[121] Conversely, if the coronal portion of the tooth is relatively short and it functions more like a molar, a post is not usually indicated.

When the decision is made to place a post, the delicate morphologic structure of the maxillary premolar root must be considered during preparation of the post space.[142,147] Posts that necessitate minimal canal

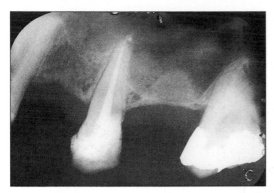

Fig 21-4a Preoperative view of an endodontically treated maxillary second premolar.

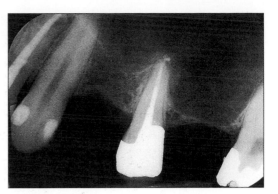

Fig 21-4b Maxillary second premolar after restoration with a tapered prefabricated post and amalgam core. The canal was not enlarged for post placement.

enlargement should be chosen for maxillary premolars. Ideally, after completion of the endodontic obturation, the canal should not be further enlarged. Rather, the post should be modified to fit the canal. This philosophy would commonly dictate the placement of a conservative tapered post in the maxillary premolar (Figs 21-4a and 21-4b).

Considerations in Post Design

Prior to choosing a post system, the dentist must have a clear understanding of the effect of several variables on the post-tooth combination. These variables include post design (Fig 21-5), post length, post diameter, venting, surface roughness, canal preparation, method of cementation, and luting medium.

Post Design

In general, it has been reported that the active threaded post has the greatest retention, followed by the parallel post; the tapered post has the least retention.[18,52,125] Therefore, the post should be chosen, in part, by the amount of post retention that the clinical situation requires. If the canal length is adequate, usually considered to be 7.0 to 8.0 mm, and the canal configuration is normal, either the tapered or parallel post may be selected. However, if the length of post space available is minimal or the canal space is funnel shaped, an active post may be required because of the difficulty in gaining adequate axial retention of the post.

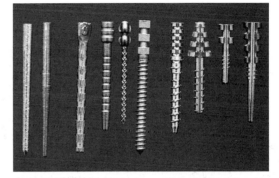

Fig 21-5 Prefabricated posts. (left to right) Passive tapered: Endowel (Star), Filpost (Vivadent); passive parallel: Parapost Plus (Whaledent), BCH (3M), Unity (Whaledent), Boston Post (Roydent); active: Flexipost (Essential Dental Systems), V-Lock (Brasseler), Radix (Caulk), Cytco (Maillefer).

Post Length

Increased post length results in increased retention.[52,125] However, a minimum of 4.0 mm of gutta-percha should be left in the apical portion of the canal space to minimize the risk of apical leakage.[81,92] A passive post should usually be as long as possible without encroaching on the remaining gutta-percha or causing perforation in a curved canal.[119]

Post Diameter

It is commonly stated that endodontically treated teeth are more susceptible to fracture because they exhibit increased brittleness.[12,40] However, more current

549

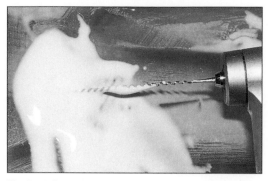

Fig 21-6 Lentulo spiral used to place cement into the canal space.

Canal Preparation

Several methods of preparing the post space and their effect on apical seal have been investigated. These include use of rotary instruments, heated instruments, and solvents.[21,66,74,81,128] The literature is equivocal on preparation of the post space; no method has been shown to be consistently superior. When a rotary instrument is used, care must be taken to ensure that only the gutta-percha is removed. The canal space should not be routinely enlarged. It has also been shown that post space preparation with a rotary instrument can generate large temperature increases on the root surface.[45] Therefore, caution must be exercised during canal space preparation. Immediate preparation (immediately after the endodontic filling) of the post space has been compared to delayed preparation (waiting at least 24 hours).[5,21,74,98,113] Again, neither method has been consistently shown to be superior.

Cementation of Posts

The actual method of post cementation has been investigated,[33,35] including placement of the cement on the post, and/or placement of the cement in the canal with a lentulo spiral, a paper point, or an endodontic explorer. The lentulo spiral is the superior instrument for cement placement (Fig 21-6). The cement may also be placed in the canal with a needle tube, as long as the tip of the tube is inserted to the bottom of the canal space and the cement is extruded from the tip as it is slowly removed from the canal. After the cement is placed in the canal, the post is coated with the cement and inserted. When zinc phosphate cement is used, it has been shown that the placement of an organic solvent (Cavidry, Parkell) in the canal before cementation of the post increases retention.[78]

research questions the validity of this assumption.[44,115] Regardless of the effect of endodontic therapy on the brittleness of a tooth, the dentist has no control over this variable. It is known that the fracture resistance of a restored endodontically treated tooth decreases as the amount of dentin removed increases.[20] Increased post diameter produces minimal, if any, increase in post retention[3,124] and significantly increases internal stresses within the tooth.[79,80] Therefore, increasing the diameter of the post is not the preferred method of increasing its retention. The diameter of the post should be as small as possible, while retaining the necessary rigidity.

Venting

Because of the intraradicular hydrostatic pressure created during cementation of the post,[37] a means for cement to escape must always be provided. Because virtually all prefabricated posts have a venting mechanism incorporated in their design, this factor is most important with the custom cast post. A vent may be incorporated in the pattern before casting or cut into the post with a bur prior to cementation.

Surface Roughness

Surface roughening, such as air abrading or notching, of the post increases post retention.[16,75,105,111,131] Surface texture is usually incorporated in prefabricated posts; however, this feature must be added to the custom cast post and core.

Luting Cements

Cements for posts and post-and-core restorations have been investigated extensively.[7,8,14,65,101,125,143] These include zinc phosphate, polycarboxylate, glass ionomer, and filled and unfilled resin composites. Both zinc phosphate and glass ionomer are commonly used because of their ease of use coupled with their history of clinical success. In recent years, resin cements as well as resin-modified glass-ionomer cements have become popular luting agents. The data are not clear regarding the superiority of one cement

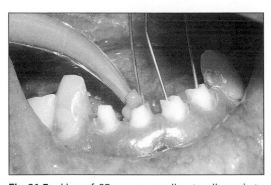

Fig 21-7a Use of 25-gauge needles to allow air to escape from canals during the impression making to ensure a complete impression of the canal spaces.

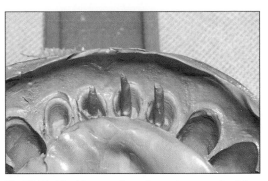

Fig 21-7b Final impression of canal spaces for laboratory fabrication of custom cast posts.

over another. Schwartz and others[114] reported increased retention with zinc phosphate cement over resin cement regardless of whether a eugenol sealer was used. Duncan and Pameijer[24] reported that a resin-modified glass-ionomer cement coupled with a dentin bonding agent had greater retention than either resin composite, glass-ionomer cement, or zinc phosphate cement. Some laboratory studies have shown a significant increase in post retention with resin cements,[34,90,140] but other studies have not confirmed this finding.[94,96,114] There are two problems with the use of resin composite cements. First, resin cement is technique sensitive because of its short working time. Second, it is difficult to remove all of the gutta-percha and eugenol-containing cement from the prepared canal without removing excess tooth structure. This residue in the surface irregularities of the prepared canal prevents adequate conditioning of the dentin and inhibits the set of the polymer.[8,9,85,94,96]

Each cement has distinct advantages and should be chosen based on these advantages in a given situation. However, the choice of luting agent is clearly not the key factor in the longevity of a post-restored tooth. No cement can overcome the inadequacies of a poorly designed post.

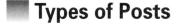

Types of Posts

Custom Cast Post

The custom cast post and core has a long history of success in restorative dentistry. However, laboratory studies[13,72,86,93] have consistently shown that the fracture resistance of teeth restored with custom cast

posts is lower than that of teeth restored with many different prefabricated posts. In addition, retrospective clinical studies[120,133] have shown prefabricated parallel posts to have greater clinical success than custom cast posts. This, coupled with the added expense and extra appointment required to fabricate the custom cast post, makes its routine use questionable.

There are several circumstances when the custom cast post is the post of choice.

1. When multiple post-and-core restorations are planned in the same arch, the laboratory-fabricated custom cast post is the most time- and cost-efficient method. The teeth are prepared for the posts, and the final crown preparations are completed so that all crown margins are on tooth structure. It is important that the crown preparation be completed before the impression for the post and core is made so that the axial contours of the core can be fabricated correctly.

An impression is made with an elastomeric impression material used in an injection technique, which allows the impression material to flow into the total length of the prepared canal space (Figs 21-7a and 21-7b). This can be best accomplished by placing a 25-gauge needle into the canal before the impression is made. The syringe material is then injected into the canal until it begins to flow out the top of the orifice. While the syringe material is being injected, the needle is slowly removed from the canal. The needle serves as an escape channel for the trapped air and allows the elastomeric impression material to reproduce the entire length of the canal space. No reinforcement of the impression material in the canal space is required with the newer impression materials. The impres-

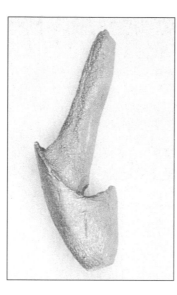

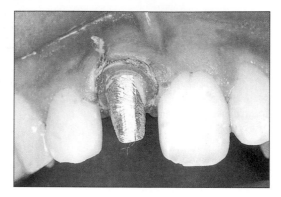

Figs 21-8a and 21-8b Custom cast post to allow a change in the angle of the core in relation to the post.

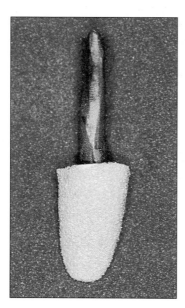

Fig 21-9a Custom cast post with porcelain fired to the core for improved esthetics.

Fig 21-9b Maxillary central incisor with a custom cast post ready to receive an all-ceramic crown.

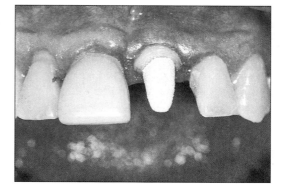

sion is poured, and the custom posts are fabricated in the laboratory. At a subsequent appointment, the posts are cemented and the final impression for the restorations is made without further tooth preparation.

2. When a small tooth, such as a mandibular incisor, requires a post and core, a prefabricated post may be difficult to use. Commonly, there is minimal space around the post for the core buildup material. In this situation, the custom cast post serves well.

3. Occasionally, the angle of the core in relation to the root must be altered. It is not advisable to bend

prefabricated posts; therefore, the custom cast post and core most successfully fulfills this need (Figs 21-8a and 21-8b).

4. When an all-ceramic noncore restoration is placed, it is necessary to have a core buildup that approximates the color of natural tooth structure. Because resin composite is not the core material of choice in high-stress situations, the core of a custom cast post can have porcelain fired to the surface to simulate natural tooth color. The porcelain on the core can be etched, and the all-ceramic crown can be adhesively bonded (Figs 21-9a and 21-9b).

Prefabricated Posts

In recent years, there has been a significant increase in the number of post systems available. Traditional prefabricated posts may be divided into three major groups: passive tapered, passive parallel, and active.

Passive Tapered Post

A goal of all post systems should be minimal removal of tooth structure before post placement. Therefore, the ideal post system requires no further preparation after removal of the gutta-percha. Because the natural shape of the canal is tapered, the passive tapered post best fulfills this criterion (see Fig 21-5). The major advantage of the passive tapered post is that the post can be modified to fit the tapered canal rather than the canal having to be enlarged to fit the post.

The major disadvantage is that the tapered post provides the least retention. This means that the retention must be gained through increased post length. When the root is not long enough to allow for adequate post length (7.0 to 8.0 mm), a more retentive post is indicated. A second commonly stated disadvantage of the tapered post is the alleged wedging effect, which results in increased stress and root fracture. This effect has been demonstrated in laboratory studies[13,86] with custom cast tapered post–core restorations. However, this theoretical wedging effect does not appear to be valid when a passive tapered post is used in conjunction with an acceptable core material and a crown.[105]

The primary indication for the passive tapered post is in teeth with small canals and thin, fragile roots, such as maxillary premolars (see Figs 21-4a and 21-4b). However, it may be used routinely in teeth with normal canal configuration and sufficient canal length to provide the necessary retention.

Passive Parallel Post

The prefabricated post by which all other posts are measured has traditionally been the Parapost (Whaledent)(see Fig 21-5). The success of this post style has been demonstrated clinically,[120,133] as well as in the laboratory.[18,50,52,125] The passive parallel post has greater retention than the passive tapered post. However, a biologic price must be paid for this increased retention. The naturally tapered canal space must be enlarged to accommodate a parallel post. Enlargement of this canal space is not consistent with the ideal of maintaining as much tooth structure as possible. For this reason, use of the passive parallel post is recommended when increased retention is needed and

the parallel canal preparation will not jeopardize the integrity of the root.

Active Post

An active post is one that engages (screws into) the dentin in the canal space. There are several styles of active posts, including those requiring a tap, self-tapping posts, split-shank posts, and hybrid posts, which contain both active and passive features (see Fig 21-5). It is difficult to generalize about active posts because of their design differences. However, the V-Lock (Brasseler) and the Flexipost (Essential Dental Systems) have performed well in the laboratory,[8] and it has been the author's experience that they perform well in clinical use.

Traditionally, the major concern about active posts has been the potential for vertical fracture of the tooth during placement of the post.[10,124] However, many laboratory studies support the use of the newer generation of active posts.[6,11,26,36,109,130] It has been shown that the active post should not be "bottomed out" when it is inserted.[109] After complete seating of an active post, it should be unscrewed one fourth of a turn. This results in decreased residual stress in the root. It has also been shown that, at shorter lengths, the active post produces less stress than other styles of prefabricated posts.[174] Therefore, active posts are indicated when the canal length is insufficient to gain adequate retention with a passive post (eg, in a short canal space or partially occluded canal due to a broken instrument or post) (Figs 21-10a and 21-10b).

Nonmetallic Post Systems

Carbon Fiber Posts

In recent years, a new generation of nonmetallic posts has been developed and marketed as a major advance in technology (Figs 21-11a and 21-11b). The post that has received the most attention is the carbon fiber–reinforced post. The proposed advantages are that the post can be bonded to the tooth with resin cement and that carbon fiber has a modulus of elasticity (rigidity) similar to that of dentin, resulting in greater post flexibility. The major disadvantages of the carbon fiber post are its dark color and radiolucent appearance in a radiograph (Fig 21-11b).

There have been several laboratory investigations of the carbon fiber post; unfortunately, the results are

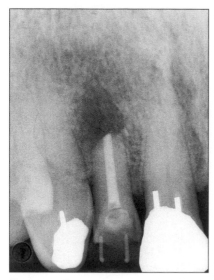

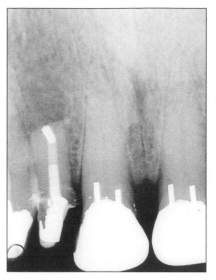

Fig 21-10a Preoperative view of a maxillary lateral incisor with a short canal space.

Fig 21-10b Tooth after restoration with a Brasseler V-Lock active post and amalgam core.

equivocal. These posts are advertised to have a similar modulus to dentin and a much lower modulus than traditional stainless steel. One study supports this claim[99] while another does not.[100] The carbon fiber post was also found to have a 15% decrease in strength and stiffness after soaking in water for 30 weeks.[89] Several in vitro studies investigated the fracture resistance of teeth restored with the carbon fiber post compared to teeth restored with stainless steel or titanium posts. One group of studies found that the teeth restored with the carbon fiber post fractured with significantly less force than those restored with metal posts.[42,77,117,141] Other studies found the fracture strength of the carbon fiber post–restored teeth to be equal to or greater than that of teeth restored with metal posts.[19,49,62] In these fracture resistance studies, there was a significant discussion regarding the nature of the root fractures that occurred at failure. Most studies found the fractures to be more favorable with the carbon fiber post,[19,49,62,77,117] while one study found root fractures to be more favorable with the metal posts.[127]

In vitro retention of the carbon fiber post has also been evaluated. One study found its retention to be greater than that of metal posts when cemented with either resin cement or glass-ionomer cement.[127] Another study found the retention of the carbon fiber post and the metal posts to be equal using a resin cement,[23] while another study found the stainless steel post to be approximately 45% more retentive than

the carbon fiber post bonded with resin cement.[99] Similarly, the retention of the resin composite core to the post head has been evaluated in vitro. Two studies found the retention of the core material to metal posts to be superior to that of carbon fiber post.[84,100] Additionally, one study found the retention of resin composite to a carbon fiber post to be significantly enhanced when the post is first air abraded.[135]

Because the laboratory data do not lead to a clear conclusion regarding the clinical utility of the carbon fiber post, a decision must be made based on an understanding of the tooth-post-core-crown combination. The idea that the post should have the same rigidity as the tooth, resulting in less stress, is appealing for the root. However, this idea disregards the effect of flexibility on the core with a cemented or bonded crown on top of the core. It would seem that a flexible core would ultimately result in marginal breakdown at the crown-tooth interface. In a study utilizing two-dimensional finite element analysis, stresses related to both stainless steel and carbon fiber posts were evaluated.[43] It was found that the use of the carbon fiber post reduced the stresses within the canal but increased the stresses at the restoration margins.

Ultimately, the effectiveness of the carbon fiber post must be confirmed with long-term clinical data. Most of the reported data are retrospective clinical studies. King and Setchell[61] reported a 25% failure rate of the carbon fiber post at 7 years compared to

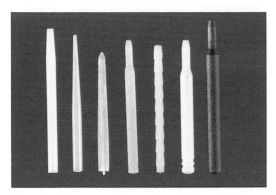

Fig 21-11a Nonmetallic posts. *(left to right)* Cosmopost (Ivoclar), Cerapost (Brasseler), Luscent Anchor (Dentatus), Light-post (Bisco), FibreKor Post (Jeneric/Pentron), Aestheti-Plus (Bisco), and C-Post (Bisco).

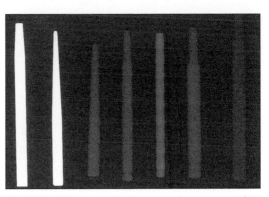

Fig 21-11b Radiograph of nonmetallic posts. *(left to right)* Cosmopost (Ivoclar), Cerapost (Brasseler), Luscent Anchor (Dentatus), Light-post (Bisco), FibreKor Post (Jeneric/Pentron), Aestheti-Plus (Bisco), and C-Post (Bisco).

less than a 10% failure rate with metal posts. The failures occurred at the resin cement–post interface. However, the study sample was small (n = 27) and a gold core was cast to the carbon fiber post. Fredriksson and others[31] reported a retrospective clinical study of 236 teeth restored with the carbon fiber post for a mean duration of 32 months; they reported no failures due to dislodgment or root fracture. Ferrari and others[27] compared the carbon fiber post with the custom cast post over 4 years. They reported no failures in the carbon fiber post group due to the post, while 11% of the cast post group failed due to root fracture and crown dislodgment. In another retrospective study, Ferrari and others[28] reported on the clinical success at 6 years of three types of carbon fiber posts placed in 1,304 teeth. They reported a failure rate of only 3.2%. Finally, in a prospective clinical study, Mannocci and others[76] reported 3-year results comparing the carbon fiber post with the custom cast post. Only one carbon fiber post of 226 placed failed due to post dislodgment. In contrast, 10 of 194 of the custom cast posts failed, all due to root fracture.

Tooth-Colored Posts

A major obstacle to the esthetic restoration of an endodontically treated anterior tooth that requires a post is the dark color of the post, which casts a shadow at the tooth-gingival interface. This is true for both the black carbon fiber post and all-metal posts.

In an attempt to overcome this problem, several other tooth reinforcement methods have been advocated, including zirconium-coated carbon fiber posts, all-zirconium posts, prefabricated fiber-reinforced resin posts (Figs 21-11a and 21-11b), and direct resin composites reinforced with fiber. To conceal the color of the carbon fiber post, one manufacturer has coated the carbon fiber post with white zirconium (Aestheti-Plus, Bisco). One laboratory study found the physical properties of this post to be similar to those of the uncoated carbon fiber post.[42]

The all-zirconium posts, Cosmopost (Ivoclar) and Cerapost (Brasseler), are white, biocompatible,[47] and radiopaque (Figs 21-11a and 21-11b). They are reported to have a higher modulus of elasticity than stainless steel.[83,110] When used in conjunction with a resin composite core material, a very esthetic post and core can be fabricated (Figs 21-12a and 21-12b). However, it is reported that the zirconium post is not etchable with hydrofluoric acid.[110] This means that neither the resin cement nor the resin composite core material would predictably bond to the post. Additionally, Dietschi and others[22] reported a decreased bond between zirconium and composite after fatigue testing. One method used to overcome the problem of bonding resin composite core material to the zirconium post has been described.[63] A leucite-reinforced ceramic (Empress, Ivoclar) is pressed to the prefabricated zirconium post (Figs 21-13a and 21-13b). This reportedly provides an adequate bond between the post and core and provides an excellent substrate for bonding of the final all-ceramic crown.

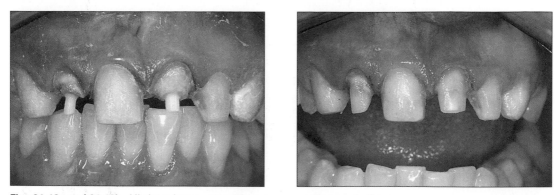

Figs 21-12a and 21-12b All-zirconium posts with resin composite core buildups.

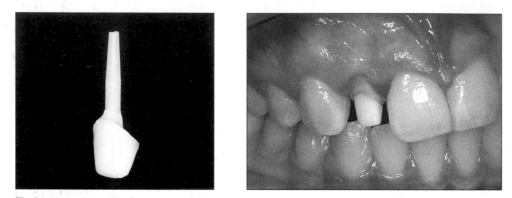

Fig 21-13a and 21-13b Cerapost with leucite-reinforced pressed ceramic core (Empress).

Stresses surrounding the zirconium post were evaluated in a photoelastic study.[118] The zirconium post demonstrated higher stresses at the occlusal emergence location than those recorded for metal posts. Koutayas and Kern[63] recently described the current options for all-ceramic post-and-core systems; however, other than two short-term clinical studies[59,83] and a few case reports,[1,2,145,146] little useful information is available.

Recently, prefabricated fiber-reinforced composite posts, FibreKor Post (Jeneric/Pentron), Luscent Anchor (Dentatus), and Light-Post (Bisco), have become available (see Figs 21-11a and 21-11b). However, very little research is available. One study found the fiber-reinforced resin post to be as strong as the carbon fiber post and approximately twice as rigid.[135] Finally, a technique has been advocated to directly build a post and core in the tooth using composite and a woven polyester bondable ribbon.[58] A laboratory study found the fracture resistance of teeth restored in this manner to be significantly less than that of those restored with carbon fiber posts or metal posts.[42] One laboratory study[32] compared the fracture strength of

teeth restored with several of these tooth-colored post systems. It was found that the Empress post and core was the weakest, followed by the zirconium Cosmopost with a ceramic core (Figs 21-13a and 21-13b). The Vectris (Ivoclar) post and resin composite core was significantly stronger than the all-ceramic post and core but significantly weaker than a prefabricated titanium post with a composite core, which was the strongest.

Removal of this newer generation of bonded nonmetallic posts, in comparison to metallic posts, is reported to be easier with the carbon fiber posts and fiber-reinforced composite posts, and more difficult with the zirconium posts.

At present, the laboratory data regarding the nonmetallic post systems are equivocal. Additionally, few clinical data support the use of any of the tooth-colored post systems. However, there is a growing body of clinical research literature to support the use of the carbon fiber post. Caution in the use of all of the nonmetallic post systems is advised when minimal coronal tooth structure remains and high core strength is required.

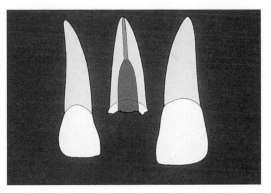

Fig 21-14 Structurally compromised root due to loss of internal radicular tooth structure.

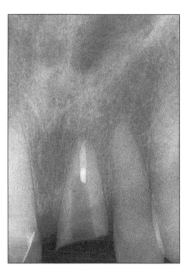

Fig 21-15a Radiograph of a structurally compromised root due to the iatrogenic removal of a broken post.

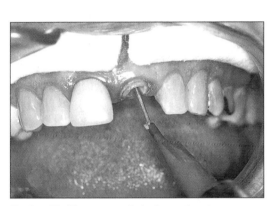

Fig 21-15b Placement of dual-cured resin composite core material into the prepared canal with a needle tube.

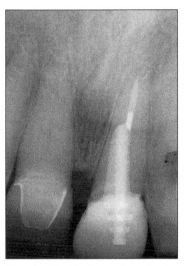

Fig 21-15c Radiograph of the structurally compromised root restored with bonded resin composite and a prefabricated metal post (V-Lock).

Intraradicular Reinforcement of Structurally Compromised Roots

Clinicians are occasionally faced with the difficult task of restoring an endodontically treated tooth in which much of the internal canal dentin has been lost (Fig 21-14). Traditionally, the custom cast post and core has been used in this situation. However, an alternative method of restoring flared canals has been described.[73] The missing internal tooth structure is replaced with bonded resin composite, and a traditional metal post is bonded into the newly created canal space (Figs 21-15a to 21-15c). A laboratory study[112] compared the fracture resistance of teeth restored with the custom cast post to the resin composite–metal post technique. The missing internal tooth structure was replaced with bonded resin composite and cured using a light-conducting plastic post, temporarily inserted during light curing. The resin composite–metal post technique resulted in significantly greater fracture resistance than seen in the custom cast post group. It is postulated that the intimate fit of the custom cast post to the weakened dentin walls results in lower fracture resistance. In a similar but simpler technique, the canal can be prepared for bonding and an autopolymerizing resin composite can be placed in the canal immediately before the insertion of a prefabricated metal post.

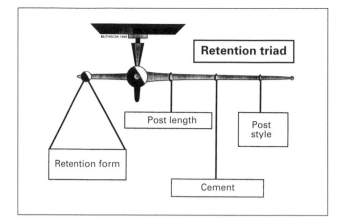

Fig 21-16 Retention triad.

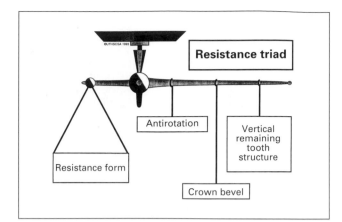

Fig 21-17 Resistance triad.

The Retention Triad

The real difficulty in restoring an endodontically treated tooth is when minimal coronal tooth structure remains. In this circumstance, the dentist must consider both retention of the post and core and resistance of the post-core-crown combination.

Retention is defined as the force that resists a tensile or pulling force. Retention of a post can be gained in three ways (Fig 21-16). The first method to gain retention is through adequate post length in the canal.[52,125] To gain this axial retention, it is imperative that the canal space not be overenlarged iatrogenically or by caries. In an anterior tooth, adequate length is commonly considered to be in the range of 7.0 to 8.0 mm, plus 4.0 mm of gutta-percha that should be left undisturbed at the apex.[92]

The design of the post may be either tapered or parallel. The tapered post requires less removal of tooth structure during preparation of the post space, but exhibits poorer retention than does the parallel post. However, when the parallel post is employed, more tooth structure must be removed, especially at the apical end of the post space. Both of these post designs are acceptable, and the decision should be based on the canal and root configurations, available post space, and the amount of retention required.

The second factor affecting retention is post style. When the decision is made that the canal length is inadequate to retain a passive post, an active post should be selected. This can occur with short clinical roots or because of obstructions in the canal space. An active post can also serve effectively when the

canal space has been overenlarged. The active post can actively engage the dentin in its terminal 2 to 3 mm to gain retention. The weakened coronal portion of the canal space is not engaged, possibly resulting in less stress.

The third part of the retention triad is the luting agent used to cement the post. The idea of bonding a post into the canal with resin cement to increase retention is theoretically appealing. However, the gutta-percha and zinc oxide–eugenol cement smeared in the canal irregularities make the bonded post a dream more than a reality. When technology enables the removal of canal contaminants noninvasively, resin cement will probably be the luting agent of choice. However, until that time, no available cement can overcome the problems created by a poorly engineered post.

The Resistance Triad

The second and most important consideration in the design of the post restoration is the *resistance* of the tooth-post-crown combination. If the resistance requirements are not met, the probability of failure is high, regardless of the retentiveness of the post.[48] Three parameters of resistance must be considered (Fig 21-17). The resistance triad consists of the crown bevel, vertical remaining coronal tooth structure, and antirotation feature(s). These features work in combination; if one of the features is minimal or nonexistent, one or both of the remaining features must be increased.

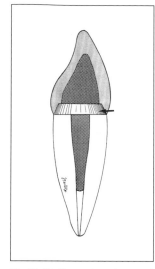

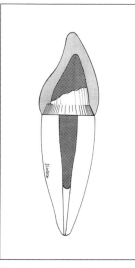

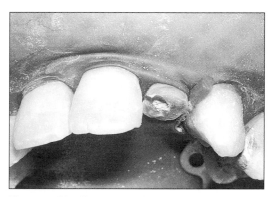

Fig 21-18 Crown bevel around periphery of root surface to increase resistance form.

Fig 21-19 Remaining coronal tooth structure should be left to strengthen the post-core-crown combination.

Fig 21-20 Maxillary lateral incisor that has been unnecessarily flattened prior to placement of the post and core.

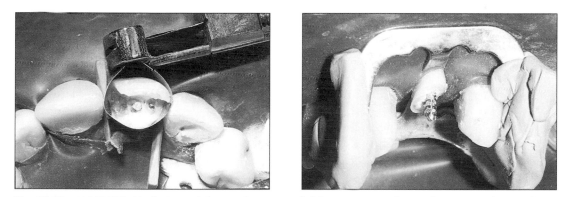

Figs 21-21a and 21-21b Vertical remaining tooth structure left in core preparations to increase resistance form.

The first feature of the resistance triad is the *crown bevel* (Fig 21-18). The bevel is that part of the crown margin that extends past the post-and-core margin onto the natural tooth structure. To be effective, it must encircle the tooth (360 degrees) and ideally extend at least 1.5 mm onto tooth structure below the post-and-core margin.[70] It is not always possible to develop a bevel in every crown preparation. Because all-ceramic crowns and crowns with porcelain labial margins cannot be constructed with a metal collar, it is sometimes not possible to use a bevel with these types of crowns. It may also be difficult to prepare a bevel when the remaining coronal tooth structure is minimal. If tooth structure has been lost to fracture or caries, it is sometimes not possible to gain the neces-

sary bevel because of impingement of the crown margin on the biologic width.

The second feature of the resistance triad is *vertical remaining tooth structure* (Fig 21-19). Traditionally, it was taught that the face of a root should be flattened prior to construction of the post and core (Fig 21-20). However, it has been shown that leaving as much natural vertical remaining tooth structure as possible will significantly increase the resistance of the final restoration (Figs 21-21a and 21-21b).[122] Unfortunately, because of caries, trauma, or iatrogenic removal, vertical remaining tooth structure is not always available.

The third feature of the resistance triad is *antirotation*. Every post and core must have an antirotation feature incorporated in the preparation.[93,111] An elon-

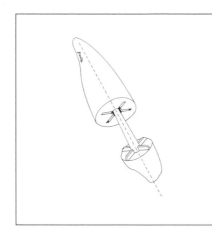

Fig 21-22 Antirotation slots.

gated or oblong canal orifice can provide the antirotation effect for the post and core. However, as the canal becomes more round, the need for incorporation of antirotation features becomes more important. This is especially true for anterior teeth. Auxiliary pins and keyways, prepared in the face of the root before construction of the post, are the most common antirotation devices (Fig 21-22).

The three features of the resistance triad are generally easy to incorporate in the preparations of posterior teeth. If there is not enough tooth structure to allow the placement of a bevel, a simple crown-lengthening procedure will generally expose enough tooth structure to allow for bevel placement after healing. It is also easier to incorporate antirotation features in posterior teeth because of their larger size.

However, the features of the resistance triad are generally more difficult to incorporate into the preparations of anterior teeth. Commonly, not as much vertical tooth structure remains, and it is more difficult to incorporate antirotation features because of the smaller tooth size. If, for reasons related to the biologic width or, more commonly, for esthetic reasons, it is not possible to place a substantial metal margin, a very important part of the resistance triad is absent. If there is also minimal vertical remaining tooth structure, the prognosis for the tooth is guarded unless more vertical tooth structure can be incorporated in the preparation. Because anterior crown lengthening generally results in an esthetically unacceptable gingival discontinuity, the treatment of choice, prior to placement of the restoration, is orthodontic eruption.[126] After forced eruption, there is then sufficient remaining vertical tooth structure to significantly improve both the resistance form and the prognosis.

Buildup Materials

With the increased use of prefabricated posts in recent years, the choice of core material has received much interest. Unfortunately, no material possesses all of the ideal characteristics (see box). In selecting a core buildup material, the dentist must consider both the functional requirements of the core as well as the amount of remaining natural tooth structure. There are currently five widely used core materials: glass ionomer, resin composite, resin-modified glass ionomer, amalgam, and cast metal.

Characteristics of the Ideal Core Material

- Stability in a wet environment
- Ease of manipulation
- Rapid, hard set for immediate crown preparation
- Natural tooth color
- High compressive strength
- High tensile strength
- High modulus of elasticity (rigidity)
- High fracture toughness
- Low plastic deformation
- Inert (no corrosion)
- Cariostatic properties
- Biocompatibility
- Low cost

Conventional glass-ionomer materials have the advantages of fluoride release, ease of manipulation, natural color, biocompatibility, corrosion resistance, and dimensional stability in a wet environment.[17] However, they have the major disadvantage of low fracture toughness, which means that the material is susceptible to propagation of cracks. Unfortunately, the fracture toughness is not improved with the addition of silver reinforcement.[71] Therefore, conventional and silver-reinforced glass ionomers can be recommended only for use in posterior teeth in which at least 50% of natural coronal tooth structure remains.

In recent years, resin-modified glass-ionomer materials have gained popularity as core materials. An initial laboratory study[68] indicated that, in addition to the aforementioned advantages of glass-ionomer cement, resin-modified glass-ionomer cements have physical properties similar to those of resin composite. However, another laboratory study found one resin-modified glass ionomer inferior to resin composite in strength.[69] Until their success can be confirmed with clinical studies, resin-modified glass-ionomer cements should be used cautiously in high-stress situations.

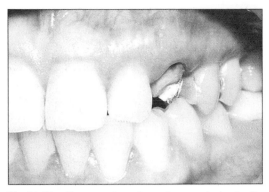

Fig 21-23a Preoperative view of an endodontically treated maxillary canine.

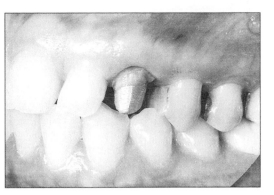

Fig 21-23b Endodontically treated maxillary canine after restoration with a prefabricated post and amalgam core.

Resin composite is the most popular core material because it is easy to use. It is available in light-cure, dual-cure, and autocure formulations. It is provided as both a tooth-colored material to be used as a core material under anterior all-ceramic restorations and as a color-contrast material to be used under metallic restorations. Adequate compressive strength[13,86] and fracture toughness[71] have been confirmed by static load testing. However, resin composite has not performed as successfully when tested with dynamic repeated load tests.[46,64] This type of laboratory test is used to simulate the small, repeated loads of function and parafunction in the oral cavity. It appears that resin composite undergoes plastic deformation under a small repeated load, which may lead to core failure. Another disadvantage of resin composite is that it is not dimensionally stable in a wet environment.[95] As it absorbs water, the buildup expands. This is clinically relevant if a provisional restoration over a resin composite core is lost after the impression has been made for the crown. At delivery, the crown will not fit accurately because of the dimensional expansion of the core.

Resin composite is an adequate buildup material when some vertical tooth structure remains to help support the core buildup. However, it is not recommended for situations in which the entire coronal portion of the tooth is to be replaced with the core material.

Amalgam, as a core buildup material, has several disadvantages. Its early strength is low, necessitating a 15- to 20-minute wait, even when fast-setting spherical alloy is used, until the buildup can be prepared for the crown. It is messy to prepare and can result in ir-

reversible staining of the marginal gingiva during preparation. However, its strength has been confirmed in laboratory studies under both static and dynamic loads.[13,46,64] Therefore, in a high-stress situation in which most of the coronal portion is replaced with the core, either amalgam or custom cast metal is the material of choice (Figs 21-23a and 21-23b).

Definitive Restorations

Multiple materials and techniques are available for the definitive restoration of the endodontically treated tooth. Because the functional requirements are significantly different for anterior and posterior teeth, they are discussed separately.

Anterior Teeth

It has been demonstrated in the laboratory that the endodontically treated anterior tooth has a fracture resistance approximately equal to that of a vital tooth.[38,72,136] Therefore, when a significant amount of coronal tooth structure remains, there is no need to place a post, and a conventional resin composite restoration in the access preparation is the treatment of choice (Fig 21-24). When a moderate amount of coronal tooth structure is missing, but approximately 50% of the coronal enamel remains, the bonded porcelain veneer may be the restoration of choice (Figs 21-25a to 21-25d). Again, there is no need for post placement with the porcelain veneer.

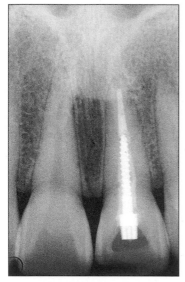

Fig 21-24 Endodontically treated maxillary central incisor that received an unnecessary post.

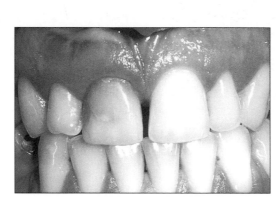

Fig 21-25a Preoperative view of a maxillary right central incisor.

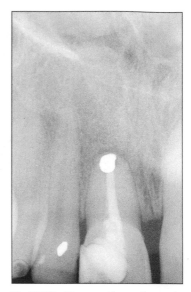

Fig 21-25b Preoperative radiograph.

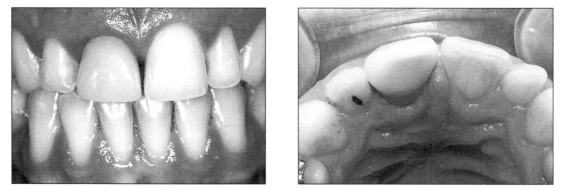

Figs 21-25c and 21-25d Seven-year postoperative views of endodontically treated maxillary right central incisor restored with a porcelain veneer.

When the decision is made to fabricate a crown for an anterior endodontically treated tooth, a post is commonly indicated. This is especially true for maxillary lateral incisors and mandibular incisors. The decision to place a post is based on the amount of remaining coronal tooth structure after completion of the crown preparation and the functional occlusal requirements. Therefore, the tooth should first be prepared for the crown; then the decision is made regarding the need for a post based on the strength of the remaining natural coronal tooth structure. If a post is required, the canal space is prepared, the post cemented, and the core buildup completed.

Posterior Teeth

In posterior teeth, the forces on the occlusal surfaces are more vertical. Laboratory data indicate that the access preparation has a minimal effect on the fracture resistance of posterior endodontically treated teeth.[104] Based on these data, some authors question the need for cuspal-coverage restorations in these posterior teeth. It has also been demonstrated in the laboratory that teeth with mesio-occlusodistal (MOD) preparations can be strengthened to match the values achieved by unprepared teeth if bonded restorations are placed.[51,67,87,103,116,139] In a retrospective clinical

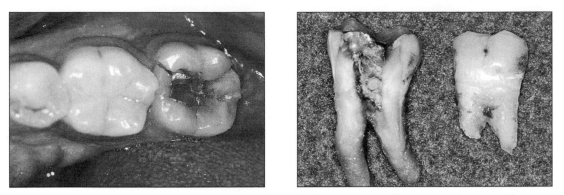

Figs 21-26a and 21-26b Unrestorable, fractured, endodontically treated mandibular second molar with an occlusal amalgam restoration.

study, Kanca[55] reported a high clinical success rate in restoring endodontically treated posterior teeth with resin composite restorations. Other laboratory studies, however, have indicated that MOD resin composite restorations in maxillary premolars have no more strengthening effect than similar MOD unbonded amalgam restorations.[53,54,123] In a retrospective clinical study, Hansen[39] compared the long-term efficacy of resin composite and amalgam in the restoration of endodontically treated premolars. During the first 3 years, teeth restored with amalgam had a greater incidence of cuspal fracture. However, in years 3 through 10, fractures occurred with approximately the same frequency in both groups.

In the face of confusing and contradictory data, it is difficult for the practitioner to develop a treatment philosophy with a sound scientific basis. It seems clear that in wider preparations the strengthening effect of the bonded resin composite restoration is real. However, it has been shown that the strengthening effect diminishes significantly with both thermal cycling[25] and functional loading[29] of the restoration. Because both of these phenomena occur in the oral environment, the long-term strengthening effect of the intracoronal bonded restoration must be questioned. It has also been proposed that a portion of the sensory feedback mechanism is lost when the neurovascular tissue has been removed from the tooth in the course of endodontic therapy, an effect confirmed in an in vivo study.[102] Clinically, this means the patient can inadvertently bite with more force on an endodontically treated tooth than on a vital tooth due to the impaired sensory feedback mechanism (Figs 21-26a and 21-26b).

Both clinical[120] and laboratory[41] studies have demonstrated that the key element in the successful restoration of endodontically treated posterior teeth is the placement of a cuspal-coverage restoration. Although the intracoronal bonded restoration is appealing, based on the current data, the most prudent course of action is to place a restoration that covers all cusps when restoring the endodontically treated posterior tooth. This can be one of a wide variety of restorations, including metal or ceramometal crowns and metal or ceramic onlays.

References

1. Ahmad I. Yttrium-partially stabilized zirconium dioxide posts; an approach to restoring coronally compromised nonvital teeth. Int J Periodontics Restorative Dent 1998;18:455–465.

2. Ahmad I. Zirconium oxide post and core system for the restoration of an endodontically treated incisor. Pract Periodont Aesthet Dent 1999;11(2):197–204.

3. Assif D, Bliecher S. Retention of serrated endodontic posts with a composite luting agent: effect of cement thickness. J Prosthet Dent 1986;56:689–691.

4. Barrieshi KM, Walton RE, Johnson WT, Drake DR. Coronal leakage of mixed anaerobic bacteria after obturation and post space preparation. Oral Surg Oral Med Oral Pathol Oral Radiol Endod 1997;84:310–314.

5. Bourgeois RS, Lemon RR. Dowel space preparation and apical leakage. J Endod 1981;7:66–69.

6. Boyarsky H, Davis R. Root fracture with dentin-retained posts. Am J Dent 1992;5:11–14.

7. Brown JD, Mitchem JC. Retentive properties of dowel post systems. Oper Dent 1987;12:15–19.

8. Burgess JO, Summitt JB, Robbins JW. The resistance to tensile, compression, and torsional forces provided by four post systems. J Prosthet Dent 1992;68:899–903.

9. Burgess JO, Re GJ, Nunez A. Effect of sealer type on post retention [abstract 1356]. J Dent Res 1997;76:183.

10. Burns DA, Krause WR, Douglas HB, Burns DR. Stress distribution surrounding endodontic posts. J Prosthet Dent 1990;64:412–418.

11. Caputo AA, Hokama SN. Stress and retention properties of a new threaded endodontic post. Quintessence Int 1987;18:431–435.

12. Carter JM, Sorensen SE, Johnson RR, et al. Punch shear testing of extracted vital and endodontically treated teeth. J Biomech 1983;16:841–848.

13. Chan RW, Bryant RW. Post-core foundations for endodontically treated posterior teeth. J Prosthet Dent 1982;48:401–406.

14. Chapman KKKW, Worley JL, von Fraunhofer JA. Retention of prefabricated posts by cements and resins. J Prosthet Dent 1985;54:649–652.

15. Christian GW, Button GL, Moon PC, et al. Post core restoration in endodontically treated posterior teeth. J Endod 1981;7:182–185.

16. Colley IT, Hampson EL, Lehman ML. Retention of post crowns. Br Dent J 1968;124:63–69.

17. Cooley R, Robbins J, Barnwell S. Stability of glass ionomer used as a core material. J Prosthet Dent 1990;64:651–653.

18. Cooney JP, Caputo AA, Trabert KC. Retention and stress distribution of tapered-end endodontic posts. J Prosthet Dent 1986;55:540–546.

19. Dean JP, Jeansonne BG, Sarkan N. In vitro evaluation of a carbon fiber post. J Endod 1998;24:807–810.

20. Deutsch AS, Musikant BL, Cavallari J, et al. Root fracture during insertion of prefabricated posts related to root size. J Prosthet Dent 1985;53:782–789.

21. Dickey DJ, Harris GZ, Lemon RR, Luebke RG. Effect of post space preparation on apical seal using solvent techniques and Peeso reamers. J Endod 1982;8:351–354.

22. Dietschi D, Romelli M, Goretti A. Adaptation of adhesive posts and cores to dentin after fatigue testing. Int J Prosthodont 1997;10(6):498–507.

23. Drummond JL, Toepke TR, King TJ. Pullout strength of thermal and loaded cycled carbon and stainless steel posts [abstract 3393]. J Dent Res 1999;78:530.

24. Duncan JP, Pameijer CH. Retention of parallel-sided titanium posts cemented with six luting agents: an in vitro study. J Prosthet Dent 1998;80:423–428.

25. Eakle WS. Effect of thermal cycling on fracture strength and microleakage in teeth restored with a bonded composite resin. Dent Mater 1986;2:114–117.

26. Felton DA, Webb EL, Kanoy BE, Dugoni J. Threaded endodontic dowels: effects of post design on incidence of root fracture. J Prosthet Dent 1991;65:179–187.

27. Ferrari M, Vichi A, Garcia-Godoy F. A retrospective study of fiber-reinforced epoxy resin posts vs. cast posts and cores; a four year recall. Am J Dent (in press).

28. Ferrari M, Mason PN, Mannocci F, Vichi A. Retrospective study of clinical behavior of several types of fiber posts. Am J Dent (in press).

29. Fissore B, Nicholls JI, Yuodelis RA. Load fatigue of teeth restored by a dentin bonding agent and a posterior composite resin. J Prosthet Dent 1991;65:80–85.

30. Fox K, Gutteridge DL. An in vitro study of coronal microleakage in root canal-treated teeth restored by the post and core technique. Int Endod J 1997;30:361–368.

31. Fredriksson M, Astback J, Pamenius M, Arvidson K. A retrospective study of 236 patients with teeth restored by carbon fiber-reinforced epoxy resin posts. J Prosthet Dent 1998;80:151–157.

32. Furer C, Rosentritt M, Behr M, Handel G. Fracture strength of all-ceramic, metal, and fiber reinforced posts and cores [abstract 1489]. J Dent Res 1998;77:818.

33. Goldman M, DeVitre R, Tenca J. Cement distribution and bond strength in cemented posts. J Dent Res 1984;63:1392–1395.

34. Goldman M, De Vitre R, White R, Nathonson D. An SEM study of posts cemented with an unfilled resin. J Dent Res 1984;63:1003–1005.

35. Goldstein GR, Hudis SI, Weintraub DE. Comparison of four techniques for cementation of posts. J Prosthet Dent 1986;55:209–211.

36. Greenfeld RS, Roydhouse RH, Marshall FJ, Schoner B. A comparison of two post systems under applied compressive shear loads. J Prosthet Dent 1989;61:17–24.

37. Gross MJ, Turner CH. Intra-radicular hydrostatic pressure changes during the cementation of post-retained crowns. J Oral Rehabil 1983;10:237–249.

38. Guzy GE, Nichols JI. In vitro comparison of intact endodontically treated teeth with and without endo-post reinforcement. J Prosthet Dent 1979;42:39–44.

39. Hansen EK. In vivo cusp fracture of endodontically treated premolars restored with MOD amalgam or MOD resin fillings. Dent Mater 1988;4:169–173.

40. Helfer AR, Melnick S, Schilder H. Determination of moisture content of vital and pulpless teeth. Oral Surg Oral Med Oral Pathol 1972;34:661–670.

41. Hoag EP, Dwyer TG. A comparative evaluation of three post and core techniques. J Prosthet Dent 1982;47:177–181.

42. Hollis RA, Christensen GJ, Christensen W, et al. Comparison of strength for seven different post materials [abstract 3421]. J Dent Res 1999;78:533.

43. Holmgren EP, Mante FK, Shokoufeh E, Afsharzand Z. Stresses in post and core build-up materials [abstract 934]. J Dent Res 1999;78:222.

44. Huang TG, Schilder H, Nathanson D. Effects of moisture content and endodontic treatment on some mechanical properties of human dentin. J Endod 1992;18(5):209–215.

45. Hussey DL, Biagioni PA, McCullagh JJP, Lamey PJ. Thermographic assessment of heat generated on the root surface during post space preparation. Int Endod J 1997;30:187–190.

46. Huysmans MC, Van Der Varst PG, Schafer R, et al. Fatigue behavior of direct post and core restored premolars. J Dent Res 1992;71:1145–1150.

47. Ichikawa Y, Akagawa Y, Nikai H, Tsuru H. Tissue compatibility and stability of a new zirconia ceramic in vivo. J Prosthet Dent 1992:68:322–326.

48. Isador F, Brondum K, Ravnholt G. The influence of post length and crown ferule length on the resistance to cyclic loading of bovine teeth with prefabricated titanium posts. Int J Prosthodont 1999;12(1):78–82.

49. Isador F, Odman P, Brondum K. Intermittent loading of teeth restored using prefabricated carbon fiber posts. Int J Prosthodont 1996;9:131–136.

50. Isador F, Brondum K. Intermittent loading of teeth with tapered individually cast or prefabricated, parallel-sided posts. Int J Prosthodont 1992;5:257–261.

51. Jensen ME, Redford DA, Williams BT, Gardner F. Posterior etched-porcelain restorations: an in vitro study. Compend Contin Educ Dent 1987;8:615–622.

52. Johnson JK, Sakamura JS. Dowel form and tensile force. J Prosthet Dent 1978;40:645–649.

53. Joynt RB, Wieczkowski G, Klockowoski R, Davis EL. Effects of composite restorations on resistance to cuspal fracture in posterior teeth. J Prosthet Dent 1987;57:431–435.

54. Joynt RB, Davis EL, Wieczkowski GJ, Williams DA. Fracture resistance of posterior teeth restored with glass ionomer–composite resin systems. J Prosthet Dent 1989;62:28–31.

55. Kanca J. Conservative resin restoration of endodontically treated teeth. Quintessence Int 1988;19:25–28.

56. Kane J, Burgess JO. Modification of the resistance form of amalgam coronal-radicular restorations. J Prosthet Dent 1991; 65:470–474.

57. Kantor ME, Pines MS. A comparative study of restorative techniques for pulpless teeth. J Prosthet Dent 1977;38:405–412.

58. Karna JC. A fiber composite laminate endodontic post and core. Am J Dent 1996;9:230–232.

59. Kern M, Simon MHP, Strub JR. Clinical evaluation of all ceramic zirconia posts: a pilot study [abstract 2234]. J Dent Res 1997;76:293.

60. Kern SB, von Fraunhofer JA, Mueninghoff LA. An in vitro comparison of two dowel and core techniques for endodontically treated molars. J Prosthet Dent 1984;51:509–514.

61. King PA, Setchell DJ. 7 year clinical evaluation of a prototype CFRC endodontic post. [abstract 2235]. J Dent Res 1997;76:293.

62. King PA, Setchell DJ. An in vitro evaluation of a prototype CFRC prefabricated post developed for the restoration of pulpless teeth. J Oral Rehabil 1990;17:599–609.

63. Koutayas SO, Kern M. All-ceramic posts and cores: the state of the art. Quintessence Int 1999;30:383–392.

64. Kovarik RE, Breeding LC, Caughman WF. Fatigue life of three core materials under simulated chewing conditions. J Prosthet Dent 1992;68:584–590.

65. Krupp JD, Caputo AA, Trabert KC, Standlee JP. Dowel retention with glass ionomer cement. J Prosthet Dent 1979;41:163–166.

66. Kwan EH, Harrington GW. The effect of immediate post preparation on apical seal. J Endod 1981;7:325–329.

67. Landy NA, Simonsen RJ. Cusp fracture strength in class 2 composite resin restorations [abstract 39]. J Dent Res 1984; 63:175.

68. Lattner ML. Fracture Resistance of Five Core Materials for Cast Crowns [thesis]. San Antonio, TX. University of Texas; 1994.

69. Levartovsky S, Goldstein GR, Georgescu M. Shear bond strength of several new core materials. J Prosthet Dent 1996; 75:154–158.

70. Libman W, Nicholls J. Load fatigue of teeth restored with cast posts and cores and complete crowns. Int J Prosthet 1995; 2:155–161.

71. Lloyd CH, Adamson M. The development of fracture toughness and fracture strength in posterior restorative materials. Dent Mater 1987;3:225–231.

72. Lovdahl PE, Nicholls JI. Pin-retained amalgam cores vs. cast-gold dowel cores. J Prosthet Dent 1977;38:507–514.

73. Lui JL. Composite resin reinforcement of flared canals using light-transmitting plastic posts. Quintessence Int 1994;25: 313–319.

74. Madison S, Zakariasen KL. Linear and volumetric analysis of apical leakage in teeth prepared for posts. J Endod 1984;10: 422–427.

75. Maniatopolous C, Pilliar RM, Smith DC. Evaluation of shear strength at the cement endodontic post interface. J Prosthet Dent 1988;59:662–669.

76. Mannocci F, Vichi A, Ferrari M, et al. Carbon fiber posts, clinical and laboratory studies. The esthetical endodontic posts. In: Proceedings from the Second International Symposium. Reconstruction with Carbon Fiber Posts. Milan, Italy: Hippocrates Edizioni Medico-Scientifiche, 1998:18–19.

77. Martinez-Insua A, Da Silva L, Rilo B, Santana U. Comparison of the fracture resistances of pulpless teeth restored with a cast post and core or carbon-fiber post with a composite core. J Prosthet Dent 1998;80:527–532.

78. Maryniuk GA, Shen C, Young HM. Effects of canal lubrication on retention of cemented posts. J Am Dent Assoc 1984; 109:430–433.

79. Mattison GD. Photoelastic stress analysis of cast-gold endodontic posts. J Prosthet Dent 1982;48:407–411.

80. Mattison GD, von Fraunhofer JA. Angulation loading effects on cast-gold endodontic posts: a photoelastic stress analysis. J Prosthet Dent 1983;49:636–638.

81. Mattison GD, Delivanis PD, Thacker RW, Hassell KT. Effect of post preparation on the apical seal. J Prosthet Dent 1984; 51:785–789.

82. Mentink AGB, Meeuwissen R, Kayser AF, Mulder J. Survival rate and failure characteristics of the all metal post and core restoration. J Oral Rehabil 1993;20:455–461.

83. Meyerberg KH, Kuthy H, Scharer P. Zirconia posts: a new all-ceramic concept for nonvital abutment teeth. J Esthet Dent 1995;7:73–80.

84. Millstein P, Maya A, Freeman Y, O'Leary J. Comparing post and core retention with post head diameter [abstract 1528]. J Dent Res 1999;78:296.

85. Millstein P, Robison B, Rankin C. Effects of EDTA/NaOCL and resin cement on post tooth retention [abstract 1527]. J Dent Res 1999;78:296.

86. Moll JFP, Howe DF, Svare CW. Cast gold post and core and pin-retained composite resin bases: a comparative study in strength. J Prosthet Dent 1978;40:642–644.

87. Morin D, DeLong R, Douglas WH. Cusp reinforcement by the acid-etch technique. J Dent Res 1984;63:1075–1078.

88. Nanayakkara L, McDonald A, Setchell DJ. Retrospective analysis of factors affecting the longevity of post crowns [abstract 932]. J Dent Res 1999;78:222.

89. Narva KK, Lassila LVJ, Vallittu PK. Comparison of mechanical properties of commercial carbon graphite fiber root canal posts [abstract 418]. J Dent Res 1999;78:158.

90. Nathanson D. New views on restoring the endodontically treated tooth. Dent Econ 1993;August:48–50.

91. Nayyar A, Walton RE. An amalgam coronal radicular dowel and core technique for endodontically treated posterior teeth. J Prosthet Dent 1980;44:511–515.

92. Neagley RL. The effect of dowel preparation on apical seal of endodontically treated teeth. Oral Surg Oral Med Oral Pathol 1969;28:739–745.

93. Newburg RE, Pameijer CH. Retentive properties of post and core systems. J Prosthet Dent 1976;36:636–643.

94. Nourian L, Burgess JO. Tensile load to remove cemented posts cemented with different surface treatments [abstract 1788]. J Dent Res 1994;73:325.

95. Oliva RA, Lowe JA. Dimensional stability of silver amalgam and composite used as core materials. J Prosthet Dent 1987; 57:554–559.

96. Paschal JE, Burgess JO. Tensile load to remove posts cemented with different cements [abstract 1362]. J Dent Res 1995;74:182.

97. Plasmans PJJM, Visseren LGH, Vrijhoef MMMA, Kayser FA. In vitro comparison of dowel and core techniques for endodontically treated molars. J Endod 1986;12:382–387.

98. Portell FR, Bernier WE, Lorton L, Peters DD. The effect of immediate versus delayed dowel space preparation on the integrity of the apical seal. J Endod 1982;8:154–160.

99. Purton DG, Love RM. Rigidity and retention of carbon fibre versus stainless steel canal posts. Int Endod J 1996;29:262–265.

100. Purton DG, Payne JA. Comparison of carbon fiber and stainless steel root canal posts. Quintessence Int 1996;27:93–97.

101. Radke RA, Barkhordar RA, Podesta RE. Retention of cast endodontic posts: comparison of cementing agents. J Prosthet Dent 1988;59:318–320.

102. Randow K, Glantz P. On cantilever loading of vital and nonvital teeth. Acta Odontol Scand 1986;44:271–277.

103. Reeh ES, Douglas WH, Messer HH. Stiffness of endodontically treated teeth related to restoration technique [abstract 1510]. J Dent Res 1988;67:301.

104. Reeh ES. Reduction in tooth stiffness as a result of endodontic restorative procedures. J Endod 1989;15:512–516.

105. Richer JB, Lautenschlager EP, Greener EH. Mechanical properties of post and core systems. Dent Mater 1986;2:63–66.

106. Robbins JW, Burgess JO, Summitt JB. Retention and resistance features for complex amalgam restorations. J Am Dent Assoc 1989;118:437–442.

107. Robbins JW. Guidelines for the restoration of endodontically treated teeth. J Am Dent Assoc 1990;120:558–566.

108. Robbins JW, Earnest L, Schumann S. Fracture resistance of endodontically treated cuspids: an in vitro study. Am J Dent 1993;6:159–161.

109. Ross RS, Nicholls JI, Harrington GW. A comparison of strains generated during placement of five endodontic posts. J Endod 1991;17:450–456.

110. Rovatti L, Mason ON, Dallare EA. The esthetical endodontic posts. In: Proceedings from the Second International Symposium. Reconstructions with Carbon Fiber Posts. Milan, Italy: Hippocrates Edizioni Medico-Scientifiche, 1998:12.

111. Ruemping DR, Lund MR, Schnell RJ. Retention of dowels subjected to tensile and torsional forces. J Prosthet Dent 1979;41:159–162.

112. Saupe WA, Gluskin AH, Radke RA. A comparative study of fracture resistance between morphologic dowel and cores and a resin-reinforced dowel system in the intraradicular restoration of structurally compromised roots. Quintessence Int 1996;27:483–491.

113. Schnell FJ. Effect of immediate dowel space preparation on the apical seal of endodontically filled teeth. Oral Surg Oral Med Oral Pathol 1978;45:470–474.

114. Schwartz RS, Murchison DF, Walker WH. Effects of eugenol and non-eugenol endodontic sealer cements on post retention. J Endodont 1998;24:564–567.

115. Sedgley CM, Messer HH. Are endodontically treated teeth more brittle? J Endod 1992;18:332–335.

116. Share J, Mishell Y, Nathanson S. Effect of restorative material on resistance to fracture of tooth structure in vitro [abstract 622]. J Dent Res 1982;61:247.

117. Sidoli GE, King PA, Setchell DJ. An in vitro evaluation of a carbon fiber-based post and core system. J Prosthet Dent 1997;78:5–9.

118. Snyder TC, Caputo AA. Retention and load transfer characteristics of zirconium dioxide endodontic dowels [abstract 1529]. J Dent Res 1999;78:297.

119. Sorensen JA, Martinoff JT. Clinically significant factors in dowel design. J Prosthet Dent 1984;52:28–35.

120. Sorensen JA, Martinoff JT. Intracoronal reinforcement and coronal coverage: a study of endodontically treated teeth. J Prosthet Dent 1984;51:780–784.

121. Sorensen JA, Martinoff JT. Endodontically treated teeth as abutments. J Prosthet Dent 1985;53:631–636.

122. Sorensen JA, Engelman MJ, Mito WT. Effect of ferrule design on fracture resistance of pulpless teeth [abstract 142]. J Dent Res 1988;67:130.

123. Stampalia LL, Nicholls, JI, Brudvik JS. Fracture resistance of teeth with resin-bonded restorations. J Prosthet Dent 1986;55:694–698.

124. Standlee JP, Caputo AA, Collard EW, Pollack MH. Analysis of stress distribution by endodontic posts. Oral Surg Oral Med Oral Pathol 1972;33:952–960.

125. Standlee JP, Caputo AA, Hanson EC. Retention of endodontic dowels: effects of cement, dowel length, diameter, and design. J Prosthet Dent 1978;39:401–405.

126. Starr C. Management of periodontal tissues for restorative dentistry. J Esthet Dent 1991;3:195–208.

127. Stockton L, Williams P. Retention and shear bond strength of 2 post systems. Oper Dent 1999;24:210–216.

128. Suchina JA, Ludington JR. Dowel space preparation and the apical seal. J Endod 1985;11:11–17.

129. Summitt J, Burgess JO, Betty T, et al. Three-year evaluation of Amalgambond Plus and pin-retained amalgam restorations [abstract 2716]. J Dent Res 1999;78:445.

130. Thorsteinsson TS, Yaman P, Craig RG. Stress analyses of four prefabricated posts. J Prosthet Dent 1992;67:30–33.

131. Tjan AHL, Whang SB. Retentive properties of some simplified dowel-core systems to cast gold dowel and core. J Prosthet Dent 1983;50:203–206.

132. Tjan AHL, Munoz-Viveros CA, Valencia-Rave GM. Tensile dislodgment of composite/amalgam cores: dentin adhesives versus mechanical retention [abstract 1355]. J Dent Res 1997;76:183.

133. Torbjorner A, Karlsson S, Odman P. Survival rate and failure characteristics for two post designs. J Prosthet Dent 1995;73:439–444.

134. Trabert KC, Caputo AA, Abou-Rass M. Tooth fracture—a comparison of endodontic and restorative treatments. J Endod 1978;4:341–345.

135. Triolo PT, Trajtenberg C, Powers JM. Flexural properties and bond strength of an esthetic post [abstract 3538]. J Dent Res 1999;78:548.

136. Trope M, Maltz DO, Tronstad L. Resistance to fracture of restored endodontically treated teeth. Endod Dent Traumatol 1985;1:108–111.

137. Vire DE. Failure of endodontically treated teeth: classification and evaluation. J Endod 1991;17:338–342.

138. Weine FS. Endodontic Therapy, ed 5. St Louis: Mosby, 1996:14.

139. Wendt SL, Harris BM, Hunt TE. Resistance to cusp fracture in endodontically treated teeth. Dent Mater 1987;3:232–235.

140. Wong B, Utter JD, Miller BH, et al. Retention of prefabricated posts using three different cementing procedures [abstract 1360]. J Dent Res 1995;74:181.

141. Wong EJ, Ruse ND, Greenfield RS, Coil JM. Initial failure of post/core systems under compressive shear loads [abstract 2269]. J Dent Res 1999;78:389.

142. Yaman P, Zillich R. Restoring the endodontically treated birooted premolar—The effect of endodontic post preparation on width of root dentin. J Mich Dent Assoc 1986;68:79–81.

143. Young HM, Shen C, Maryniuk GA. Retention of cast posts relative to cement selection. Quintessence Int 1985;16:357–360.

144. Zakhary SY, Nasr HH. In vitro assessment of intact endodontically treated anterior teeth with different restorative procedures. Egypt Dent J 1986;32:221–239.

145. Zalkind M, Hochman N. Direct core buildup using a preformed crown and a prefabricated zirconium oxide post. J Prosthet Dent 1998;80:730–732.

146. Zalkind M, Hochman N. Esthetic considerations in restoring endodontically treated teeth with posts and cores. J Prosthet Dent 1998;79:702–705.

147. Zillich R, Yaman P. Effect of root curvature on post length in restoration of endodontically treated premolars. Endod Dent Traumatol 1985;1:135–137.

Index

Page numbers followed by "t" indicate tables; those
followed by "f" indicate figures; those followed by
"b" indicate boxed text.

A

Abfraction, 39, 386, 395
Abrasion, 386
Acid etchants
  classification of, 201t
  demineralization potency of, 201t
  phosphoric, 194
Acid etching
  dentin, 104, 191
  enamel, 5, 6f, 191–194, 215–216
Adhesion
  adhesives. See Adhesives.
  advantages of, 178
  amalgam, 222, 222f
  ceramics, 222, 223f
  chemicals used in, 185b
  conditioning of enamel and dentin
    agents for, 215–216
    compomers, 216–217
    definition of, 198
    self-etch approach, 216
    techniques for, 198–202
  dentin
    adhesives, 195–198
    conditioning. See Adhesion, conditioning.
    demineralization, 198, 200, 206
    description of, 194
    hybridization, 203–206
    primers, 202
    protection considerations, 215
    resin tag formation, 206–207
    wetting, 214
  enamel
    conditioning techniques. See Adhesion,
      conditioning.
    techniques, 191–194
  factors that affect
    biocompatibility, 190–191
    dentin, 181–183
    description of, 180
    enamel, 181–182

polymerization, 188–189
polymerization shrinkage. See Polymerization
  shrinkage.
smear layer, 183–184
stress transmission across restoration-
  tooth interface, 189–190
thermal conductivity and expansion, 189
wetting of adhesive, 185–186
indications, 178–179
isolation technique for, 214–215
primers
  application of, 220
  description of, 202
  principles of, 179–180
  pulp protection during, 215
  resins, 202–203, 220–221
  restorative procedure, 221
  theories regarding, 179
  wet vs. dry bonding, 217–218
Adhesives
  classification of, 207–208
  for Class 5 restorations, 394–395
  glass-ionomer cements, 213, 214f
  resins, 202–203
  self-etching, 210–211, 211f–212f, 216
  smear layer–dissolving, 210–211, 211f–212f
  smear layer–modifying, 208
  smear layer–removing, 209–210, 210b, 216
  types of, 195–198
  wetting of, 180, 185–186
Adhesive sealers, 96
Air abrasion
  commercial units for, 145, 146f, 311f
  post retention and, 550
Amalgam
  advantages of, 307
  antimicrobial properties of, 106
  bonding of, 222, 222f
  carving of, 348–349
  composition of, 306
  concerns regarding, 265
  core material use, 561
  definition of, 306
  disadvantages of, 307
  failure rates, 262f
  history of, 306

longevity of, 261t
properties of, 95t
resistance form, 307–308
sealers for, 96
trituration of, 306, 307f, 345–346
Amalgam carriers, 128, 128f
Amalgam restorations
  bonded
    description of, 222, 222f, 335
    matrices for, 345
  Class 1
    description of, 307
    indications, 308
    outline form, 308, 310, 313f
    resistance form, 310–313
    retention form, 310–313
  Class 2
    carving of, 349
    description of, 307
    facial access, 320–321
    indications, 313
    lingual access, 320–321
    occlusal extensions, 321
    outline form, 314–315, 320f
    resistance form, 316–320
    retention form, 316–320
  Class 5, 394, 394f
  complex
    amalgam placement in, 352, 353f–358f
    carving of, 353f–355f
    condensation of, 353f–355f
    cuspal-coverage, 321–325
    resistance and retention methods
      efficacy of, 333, 334f
      pins, 325–333
    finishing of, 359
    fracture of, 360
    matrices
      bonded restorations, 345
      description of, 336–337
      modeling compound for strengthening,
        342, 344f, 345
      Tofflemire, 337–342
      types of, 342, 343f
    placement technique for
      burnishing, 348, 351–352

carving, 348–349
    in complex restorations, 352, 353f–358f
    condensation, 346–348
    description of, 345
    occlusal adjustments, 350–351
    polishing of, 359–360
    repair of, 360
    root caries and, 372–373
    sealers used with, 336
Amalgapins, 333
Anterior ceramic crowns
    all-ceramic
        bonded, 457–458
        cemented, 458–460
        characteristics of, 452t
        description of, 451
        resin bonding of, 472
    bite forces, 451
    cementation of, 472
    decision-making criteria for
        bonding surface, 454–456
        description of, 451–453
        esthetics, 452–454
        overview of, 455t
        parafunctions, 456
        strength, 451–452
    functional preparation technique
        cervical reduction, 468, 468f
        completion of, 469
        description of, 467
        facial plane reduction, 467–468
        incisal edge reduction, 467, 467f
        lingual reduction, 469
    impression technique for, 469–470
    metal-ceramic
        characteristics of, 460–461
        indications, 452, 460
    placement of, 472
    retraction techniques, 469–470
    shade selection, 470–471
    tooth preparation
        biologic principles that influence, 461–462
        crest relationships, 462–464
        description of, 461
        die spacing, 466
        esthetics, 467
        marginal integrity, 465–466
        pulpal preservation, 464
        resistance and retention form, 464–465
        structural durability considerations, 465
    veneer, 456–457
Anterior guidance, 505
Anterior teeth
    anatomic contour of, 116
    caries lesion. See Caries and carious lesions.
    Class 3 restorations
        finishing and polishing of
            instruments, 255–256
            procedure, 257

glass-ionomer cements, 242, 242f
        guidelines for, 254
        matrices, 251, 251f
        rebonding of, 257
        resin composites
            characteristics of, 240–242, 241f
            curing of, 253
            placement of, 253
    Class 4 restorations
        description of, 242
        guidelines for, 254
        matrices, 251f, 251–252
        rebonding of, 257
        retentive pins, 244, 245f
        treatment considerations, 242–244
    crowns. See Anterior ceramic crowns.
    endodontically treated, 546–547, 561–562
    nomenclature for, 115
    posts, 546–547, 561–562
    resin composite use. See Resin composite.

B

Bases
    definition of, 94
    placement guidelines, 98
    purpose of, 97, 98f
    zinc oxide–eugenol cements, 97
    zinc phosphate cements, 97
Biologic width
    definition of, 21–22, 461–462, 504
    pretreatment evaluations of, 34
Bite block, 168–169
Black, G.V., 118–119
Bleaching. See also Discoloration.
    agents
        carbamide peroxide, 403–404
        hydrogen peroxide, 403–404
        packaging of, 412, 413f
        sodium perborate, 406
    alternatives, 420–422
    at-home
        adverse effects associated with, 409
        description of, 407, 407f
        duration of, 415–416
        extended treatments, 419
        patient instructions, 415–416
        results of, 416, 417f–418f
        soft tissue irritation, 408
        technique, 413–416
        tray fabrication for, 413–415
    bonding effects, 410
    contraindications, 409–410
    dental record, 411
    description of, 401
    discolorations, 402
    factors that affect
        additives, 404–405
        peroxide concentration, 404
        pH, 404

sealed environment, 404
        surface cleanliness, 403
        temperature, 404
        time, 404
    history of, 401
    indications, 409
    in-office
        description of, 407, 407f
        laser-assisted, 412–413
        technique for, 411–413
    longevity of, 405
    modalities, 402–403
    mode of action, 402–403
    nonvital, 405–406
    patient education regarding, 411
    porcelain veneer placement and, 422, 422f–423f, 445–446
    pulpal problems associated with, 408
    restoration effects, 420
    shade selection, 410–411
    soft tissue response, 408
    stains, 402
    systemic effects and responses, 409
    tetracycline-stained teeth, 402, 416, 419–420, 422f–423f
    treatment planning, 410–411
    types of, 403
    vital, 406–407
Bonding
    adhesive systems, 96
    amalgam restorations, 335
    anterior ceramic crowns, 472
    bleaching effects, 410
    dentin as substrate for, 12–13
Buccal corridor, 58
Burnishers, 130, 130f, 348
Burs, 139–141, 142t–145t, 255, 256f

C

CAD/CIM restorations
    crowns, 495
    inlays and onlays
        advantages of, 490
        cavity preparation, 491
        cementation, 494
        clinical studies of, 495, 497
        computer-assisted design, 491–493
        disadvantages of, 490–491
        hardware, 491
        longevity of, 495, 497
        manufacturing process, 493–494
        materials, 493–494
        onlay technique, 494, 494f
        software, 491
        training, 490
        try-in, 494, 495f
Calcium hydroxide
    liner use, 96–97
    properties of, 97

for pulp capping
  description of, 103–104
  disadvantages of, 107
Calcium phosphate, 371
Carbon fiber posts, 553–555
Caries and carious lesions. *See also specific lesion.*
  activity assessments, 78–80
  classification of, 118, 119f
  Class 3 caries lesion
    cavitated, 238–239
    dentinal, 239, 240f
    description of, 238
    incipient, 238
  Class 4 caries lesion
    etiology of, 242
  Class 5 caries lesion
    definition of, 386
    etiology of, 386–388
    illustration of, 387f
  dentinal, 239, 240f, 377
  description of, 70
  detection of, 75–77
  diagnosis of, 77–80
  discolorations associated with, 402
  dyes for disclosing, 100f, 102
  enamel demineralization secondary to, 8
  etiology of, 71–72
  in existing restorations, 35–36
  fluoride use, 73
  multifactorial nature of, 82–83
  occlusal
    activity assessments, 78, 79f
    Class 1 amalgam restoration for, 308, 309f
    illustration of, 31f
    treatment of, 86–87
  pit and fissure
    detection of, 76, 77f
    pretreatment assessment of, 30–31
    treatment of, 87
  predictors of, 73–74, 74t
  preventive approaches, 83–84, 371
  progression of, 74–75, 83, 86
  proximal
    activity assessments, 79
    detection of, 77, 78f
    progression of, 75
  radiographic detection of, 75–76, 77t
  recurrent
    activity assessments, 80
    Class 1 amalgam restoration for, 308
    definition of, 80
    fluoride prevention of, 381, 383
    pretreatment assessment of, 35–36
  restorative materials and, 46
  risk assessments. *See* Caries risk.
  risk factors
    diet, 72
    hyposalivation, 73
    plaque levels, 71–72

    saliva, 73
    socioeconomics, 73, 74t
    time, 72
  root. *See* Root caries.
  schematic representation of, 13, 14f
  secondary, 266–267
  smooth-surface
    activity assessments, 79, 80f
    cavitated, 238–239
    detection of, 77
    incipient, 238
    pretreatment assessment of, 31
    progression of, 75
  treatment of
    algorithms, 84f–85f
    considerations for, 82–83
    decisions regarding, 85–86
    description of, 84–85
    indications, 87–88
    occlusal caries, 86–87
    pit and fissure caries, 87
    preventive, 83–84
Caries risk
  assessment of, 29–30
  factors that determine, 81–82
  purpose of, 81
  reversal of, 86
  salivary flow rate and, 369
Carvers
  design of, 129–130
  sharpening of, 132f–133f
Cast-gold restorations
  advantages of, 500, 526, 527f–528f
  castings, 500, 523
  cementation of
    description of, 520
    glass-ionomer cement, 521–522
    polycarboxylate, 522
    resin cement, 521–522
    resin-modified glass-ionomer cement, 522
    tooth preparations, 522
    zinc oxide–eugenol, 522
    zinc phosphate cement, 520–521
  complete-coverage, 517–518
  considerations in preparing
    contours, 504–505
    finish lines, 503–504
    gingiva, 504
    occlusion, 505–506
    pulpal preservation, 503
    retention and resistance form, 501–503
    tooth conservation, 501
  description of, 500
  disadvantages of, 528
  esthetics of, 528, 528f
  illustration of, 501f
  indications, 500
  inlays
    bevel, 508–509

    indications, 506
    occlusal preparation, 506, 507f
    proximal boxes, 506–507
    refinement, 508
    retention grooves, 509
  marginal finishing of, 519, 520f
  marginal integrity of, 528
  onlays
    bevel, 512
    cuspal reduction, 510–511, 511f
    description of, 509
    noncentric cusp, 511
    occlusal preparation, 510
    preparations for, 509–510
    proximal boxes, 510, 510f
    retention grooves, 512
    shoulder preparation, 511, 511f
  partial-coverage
    bevel, 515–516, 516f
    description of, 512
    finish lines, 514
    lingual reduction, 513–514
    occlusal channel, 515, 516f
    occlusal reduction, 513
    proximal grooves, 514, 515f–516f
    proximal reduction, 514
    refinements, 516, 51/f
    retention and resistance of, 512
  try-in, 518–519
  Tucker technique
    cavity design and preparation
      Brasseler No. 7407 bur variations, 542, 543f
      distal hollow grind, 544
      inlays, 529–533
      onlays, 538f
      "potholes" made using Midwest No. 7404 bur, 542–543
    cementation, 536
    crowns
      full, 541–542
      maxillary molar, 540
      premolar, 540, 541f
    finishing, 536–537
    impressions, 534–535
    inlays
      cavity preparation, 529–533
      disto-occlusal, 533
      mesio-occlusal, 533
      mesio-occlusodistal, 533, 534f
      slot, 543–544
    laboratory procedures, 535–536
    onlays
      cavity preparation, 538f
      "invisible," 539, 539f
      mandibular, 539
      maxillary, 539
    temporary restoration, 535
  wear resistance of, 500
Casts. *See* Diagnostic casts.

Cavity preparation
  Black's steps, 119–120
  classification of, 118
  shape of, 119
Cavity sealers. *See* Sealers and sealants.
Cements. *See also specific cement.*
  for porcelain veneers, 440, 442
  for posts, 550–551
Centigrade scale, 126f–127f, 127
Ceramics
  bonding of, 222, 223f
  crowns. *See* Anterior ceramic crowns.
  silanization of, 223f
Ceromers, 482, 485f
C-factor, 186
C fibers, 17
Chief complaint, 28–29
Chisel
  design of, 122f–123f, 123, 127
  sharpening of, 132f–133f
Chlorhexidine, 84
Class 1 restorations
  amalgam. *See* Amalgam restorations.
  resin composite, 278
Class 2 restorations
  amalgam. *See* Amalgam restorations.
  resin composite
    acid etching, 283
    adhesives for, 261–264
    bevel placement, 279–281
    bonding resin application, 283–284
    finishing of, 293–294
    gingival margins, 281, 282f
    incremental technique for, 286–291
    interproximal contact, 290
    liners, 281–283
    matrices, 284–285
    occlusal margins, 281
    preparations, 279–281
    prewedging, 278–279
    proximal margins, 281
    rebonding of, 295, 296f
    resin-modified glass-ionomer cements, 291
Class 3 restorations
  characteristics of, 240–242, 241f
  curing of, 253
  finishing and polishing of
    instruments, 255–256
    procedure, 257
  glass-ionomer cements, 242, 242f
  guidelines for, 254b
  matrices, 251, 251f
  placement of, 253
  rebonding of, 257
Class 4 restorations
  description of, 242
  finishing and polishing of
    instruments, 255–256
    procedure, 257

  guidelines for, 254b
  matrices, 251f, 251–252
  rebonding of, 257
  retentive pins, 244, 245f
  treatment considerations, 242–244
Class 5 restorations
  dentinal sensitivity associated with, 398
  materials for
    adhesive, 394–395
    amalgam, 394, 394f
    compomers, 397–398
    description of, 392, 394
    glass ionomer, 396–397
    resin composite, 395–396
    resin-modified glass ionomers, 396–397
  retraction methods
    flap surgery, 390, 391f–392f
    gingivoplasty, 389
    miniflaps, 389, 390f
    nonsurgical, 388–389
    surgical, 389–392
  treatment decisions regarding, 392
Color. *See also* Discoloration.
  anterior ceramic crowns, 470–471
  bleaching. *See* Bleaching.
  of enamel, 3
  esthetic considerations, 65
  modifiers of, 65
  resin composite, 250
  terms for describing, 65, 471
Compomers
  Class 5 restorations, 397–398
  enamel and dentin conditioning, 216–217
  setting mechanism, 226t
  wear resistance of, 383
Condensers, 128f, 128–129
Cracked-tooth syndrome, 39
Crown (restorations)
  anterior ceramic. *See* Anterior ceramic crowns.
  bevel of, 559
  CAD/CIM, 495
  Cerec, 495, 496f
  overcontoured, 504, 505f
  porcelain veneers and, 446
Crown (tooth structure)
  bevel of, 559
  definition of, 117
Cutting instruments. *See* Instruments.

D

Dam. *See* Rubber dam.
Demineralization
  acid etchants, 201t
  caries effect, 8
  dentin, 198, 200, 206
  enamel, 8
  fluoride effects, 73
Dental history, 28–29

Dental record
  formats, 51f–52f
  information in, 51
  legal nature of, 53
  purposes of, 50
  SOAP format, 51, 53
Dentin
  acid etching of, 104, 191
  adhesion to
    adhesives, 195–198
    conditioning, 198–202
    demineralization, 198, 200, 206
    description of, 194
    hybridization, 203–206
    primers, 202
    resin tag formation, 206–207
  aging effects, 13–15
  bonding agents for pulp capping
    bond quality and durability, 104
    cellular toxicity, 105
    description of, 103
    microleakage reductions using, 103–104
    pulpal effects, 104–105
    studies of, 103–104
  bonding substrate use, 12–13
  composition of, 8, 9f, 181
  conditioning of, 198–202, 219
  demineralization of, 198, 200, 206
  depth of, 9
  function of, 8
  inner, 9
  intertubular, 8–9
  microabrasion of, 200, 201f
  morphology of, 8–10
  outer, 9, 10f
  peritubular, 9, 10f
  permeability of, 11, 184–185
  physiologic, 13
  pulp capping. *See* Dentin, bonding agents for pulp capping.
  reactionary, 13
  remineralization of, 382
  reparative, 14f, 15, 183
  response, 13
  sclerosis of, 13–15, 182f, 182–183, 455–456
  sensitivity of
    in Class 5 restorations, 398
    description of, 11, 12f
    etiology of, 398
    primers for, 202
  structure of, 181
  support provided by, 8
  surface assessments, 455
  tertiary, 13
  thickness of, 91
  wetness
    adhesion and, 184–185, 214
    evaluation of, 214

Dentinal tubules
  diameter of, 181
  obstruction of, 182f
  structure of, 181, 182f
Dentinoenamel junction, 313
Dentogingival junction, 19–21
Diagnostic casts
  occlusal evaluations using, 506
  porcelain veneers, 428, 429f
  treatment planning uses of, 42
Diastema closure, 246–249
Diet
  caries etiology and, 72
  caries risk based on, 81
Discoloration. *See also* Color.
  aging and, 402
  assessment of, 35
  caries-related, 402
  classification of, 402
  drugs that cause, 402
  masking of, 444–445
  porcelain veneers and, 444
  tetracycline-induced, 402, 416, 419–420, 422f–423f

E

Electrosurgery, 93
Enamel
  acid etching of, 5, 6f, 191–194, 215–216
  aging effects, 2
  anatomy of, 2f
  cavitation of, 3
  color of, 3
  composition of, 1–2, 181–182
  conditioning of, 215–216
  cracks in, 5
  crystal structure of, 5, 6f
  demineralization of, 8
  description of, 1
  faults and fissures in, 4, 5f
  permeability of, 1–2
  resilience of, 8
  structure of, 181–182
  wear of, 4
  yellowing of, 1–2
Enamel rods
  characteristics of, 5
  cleavage lines, 7
  illustration of, 6f
  restoration preparation considerations, 7
Endodontically treated teeth
  anterior teeth, 546–547, 561–562
  description of, 546
  posterior teeth, 547–549, 562–563
  post systems for. *See* Posts.
  with structurally compromised roots, 557
Epithelial attachment, 461
Erosive lesions, 37–38, 386
Esthetics
  of existing restorations, 36

parameters of
  buccal corridor, 58
  color, 65–66
  face height, 56, 57f
  gingival zenith, 62, 63f
  illumination principle, 67–69, 68f
  incisal plane, 57–58, 58f
  interproximal contact areas, 62, 63f
  lip length, 56, 57f
  lip mobility, 56
  lower lip, 59
  mandibular incisal edge shape, 64
  maxillary canines, 65
  maxillary incisors, 60–64
  outline symmetry, 57, 57f, 64
  posterior occlusal plane, 58
  surface texture, 66
  tooth-to-tooth proportions, 66–67
  upper lip, 59, 59f
  pretreatment assessments of, 40
  treatment planning for, 46–47
Examination
  caries
    pit and fissure, 30–31
    risk assessments, 29–30
    smooth-surface, 31
  cracked-tooth syndrome, 39
  diagnostic casts, 42
  elements of, 29b
  esthetics, 36, 40
  existing restorations. *See* Existing restorations,
    examination of.
  nonocclusal contours, 39
  occlusion
    contacts, 37
    interarch space, 38–39
    interferences, 36–37
    wear, 37–38
  periodontal, 40–41
  plaque risks, 29–30
  pulp, 32–33
  radiographic evaluations, 41–42
  reasons for, 27, 29
Existing restorations
  examination of
    anatomic form of, 33
    caries activity, 35–36, 80
    discoloration of, 35
    esthetics of, 36
    interproximal contacts, 34–35
    margins of, 33
    occlusal contacts, 34–35
    periodontal effects, 34
    structural integrity of, 33
  porcelain veneer preparations, 436, 437f
Explorers, 134, 135f

F

Face height, 56, 57f

Filler particles, 236–237
Finishing strips, 256, 256f, 295f
Fissure
  deep, 308
  definition of, 116, 308
  in enamel, 4, 5f
Fissure caries
  detection of, 76, 77f
  pretreatment assessment of, 30–31
  treatment of, 87
Fluoride
  antibacterial effects of, 380–381
  caries prevention, 73–74, 83–84, 371, 381–382
  caries risk and, 81
  description of, 377
  discolorations and, 402
  materials that release
    amount, 382–383
    anticariogenic properties, 380–381
    characteristics of, 378–379
    clinical considerations regarding, 383
    compomers, 378t
    description of, 377–378
    glass-ionomer cements, 378t
    range of, 378–379
    recharging of, 379–380
    resin composites, 378, 378t
  oral retention of, 73
Forceps
  clamp, 154–155
  design of, 136, 136f
Fossa, 116

G

Gingiva
  appearance of, 19, 19f
  attached, 19
  biologic width, 21–22
  cast-gold restoration preparations and, 504
  components of, 19
  dentinal sensitivity and, 398
  dentogingival junction, 19–21
  description of, 18–19
  esthetic considerations, 56, 59, 59f
  fibers of, 20–21
  marginal, 19
  recession of, 365, 398
  restorative dentistry considerations, 21
  zenith of, 62, 63f
Gingival margin trimmer, 124f–125f, 125
Gingivitis, 19
Gingivoplasty, 389
Glass-ionomer cement
  adhesives, 213, 214f
  antimicrobial properties of, 106
  autocured, 397
  base use, 98
  bonding of, 226–227
  cast-gold restorations, 521

characteristics of, 238
classification of, 197t
Class 3 restorations, 242, 242f
Class 5 restorations, 396–397
conventional
    advantages of, 224
    composition of, 224
    disadvantages of, 224–225
    resin-modified glass-ionomer cements and,
        comparisons between, 227
core material use, 560
development of, 224
fluoride release from
    amount of, 382–383
    anticariogenic effects, 382
    description of, 379
    recharging, 379
history of, 224
liner use
    description of, 97
    for indirect pulp capping, 103
mechanical properties of, 378t
moisture contamination of, 521
properties of, 95t, 97
resin-modified
    bonding of, 226–227
    characteristics of, 225
    Class 2 restorations, 291
    Class 5 restorations, 396–397
    clinical uses of, 227–228
    commercial types of, 226t
    conventional glass-ionomer cements and,
        comparisons between, 227
    core material use, 560
    dentin protection using, 215
    description of, 378
    fluoride release, 227, 383
    indications, 383
    post cementation using, 551
    retention rate for, 46
    setting mechanism, 226t
    structure of, 225f
    tooth preparations, 522
    tunnel restorations using, 298
root caries, 373
sandwich technique, 383, 397, 398f
self-adhesive capacity of, 180
tooth preparations for, 522
Gold restorations. See Cast-gold restorations.
Groove, 116, 308

H

Hand instruments. See Instruments.
Handpieces, 138–139, 139f
Hatchet
    design of, 122f, 123
    off-angle, 125
Hemostats, 136, 136f

Hoe
    design of, 123, 124f, 127
    sharpening of, 133f
Hybridization, 203–206
Hydroxyapatite mineral, 1, 5, 6f

I

Illumination principle, 67–69, 68f
Incisal plane, 57–58, 58f
Incisors. See also Teeth.
    mandibular, 64
    maxillary. See Maxillary incisors.
Inlays
    adhesive cementation
        description of, 478
        tooth preparations for, 479, 480f
    bases, 476
    CAD/CIM system
        advantages of, 490
        cavity preparation, 491
        cementation, 494
        clinical studies of, 495, 497
        computer-assisted design, 491–493
        disadvantages of, 490–491
        hardware, 491
        longevity of, 495, 497
        manufacturing process, 493–494
        materials, 493–494
        software, 491
        training, 490
        try-in, 494, 495f
    ceramic. See Inlays, porcelain.
    gold
        bevel, 508–509
        indications, 506
        occlusal preparation, 506, 507f
        proximal boxes, 506–507
        refinement, 508
        retention grooves, 509
    liners, 476
    maintenance of, 479
    porcelain
        bonding to, 478
        fabrication of, 486b, 487
        failure of, 489
        finishing of, 486b
        history of, 482–483
        indications, 483, 485, 487
        longevity of, 489
        placement of, 486b
        resin composite inlay and, comparisons between,
            485
        shade selection, 487
        technique for, 486b, 487
        wear of, 487–489
    preparations, 476, 477f
    resin composite
        bonding to, 478
        description of, 479

direct, 482, 483f
        direct/indirect, 482, 484f
        direct resin composite restorations and, compari-
            sons between, 480–481
        failure of, 489
        indirect, 482, 485f
        light-cured, 481–482
        longevity of, 489
        polymerization shrinkage, 480–481
        porcelain inlay and, comparisons between, 485
        secondary polymerization of, 481–482
        wear of, 487–489
    resistance form, 476
Instruments
    air-abrasion units, 145, 146f
    amalgam carriers, 128, 128f
    burnishers, 130, 130f
    burs, 139–141, 142t–145t, 255, 256f
    carvers, 129–130, 132f–133f
    centigrade scale, 126f–127f, 127
    chisel, 122f–123f, 123, 127
    components of, 120, 121f
    condensers, 128f, 128–129
    description of, 120, 128
    design of, 120, 121f
    diamonds, 141
    explorers, 134, 135f
    forceps, 136, 136f
    gingival margin trimmer, 124f–125f, 125, 532, 532f,
        533f
    grasping techniques for
        description of, 136
        palm-thumb grasp, 138, 138f
        pen grasp, 137, 137f
    handpieces, 138–139, 139f
    hatchet, 122f, 123, 125
    hemostats, 136, 136f
    hoe, 123, 124f, 127, 133f
    magnifiers, 145, 146f
    materials for, 120
    mirrors, 134, 135f
    motions used, 138
    nomenclature, 123
    numeric formulas, 126f, 127
    off-angle hatchet, 125
    periodontal probes, 135, 135f
    plastic instruments, 130–131, 131f
    recommended types of, 127–128, 147
    sharpening of, 131–134
    spatula, 131, 131f
    spoon, 123–125, 124f, 134f
    technique for using, 125
Interproximal contact areas, 62, 63f
Isolation methods and techniques
    absorbent materials, 175, 177
    for adhesion systems, 214–215
    cotton products, 175, 177
    description of, 372
    Hygoformic saliva ejector, 175, 176f

rubber dam. *See* Rubber dam.
Svedopter, 175, 176f

L

Lamina limitans, 181
Lasers, 93
Light curing
    commercial units for, 254–255, 292f
    cure levels using, 271
Line angle, 117
Liners
    calcium hydroxide, 96–97
    Class 2 restorations, 281–283
    definition of, 94
    glass ionomer, 97, 283
    placement guidelines, 98
Lips
    asymmetry of, 60
    esthetic parameters for
        asymmetry, 60
        length, 56, 57f
        mobility, 56
    lower, 59
    upper, 59, 59f
Luting cements. *See* Cements.

M

Macroabrasion, 421–422
Magnifiers, 145, 146f
Mandibular incisors, 64
Marginal ditching, 489
Marginal ridges, 116
Margins
    definition of, 117
    integrity of, 465–466, 528
Matrices
    amalgam restorations, 337–342
    Class 2 restorations, 284–285
    Class 3 restorations, 251, 251f
    Class 4 restorations, 251f, 251–252
    Tofflemire, 337–342
Maxillary incisors
    edge configuration of, 63
    esthetic considerations, 60–64, 65, 66
    facial contour of, 62, 64, 65f
    "halo effect" of, 64
    length of, 66, 67f
    lingual contour of, 62
    post placement, 547
    proportions of, 66–67, 67f
Maximum intercuspation, 505
Microabrasion, 420–421
Miniflaps, 389, 390f
Mirrors, 134, 135f
Modeling compound
    matrix reinforcement using, 342, 344f, 345
    rubber dam retention using, 159, 160f
Monomers, 192f

N

Noncarious cervical lesions. *See* Class 5 restorations.

O

Occlusion
    amalgam restoration adjustments, 350–351
    cast-gold restoration preparations and, 505–506
    casts, 506
    contacts, 37
    interarch space, 38–39
    interferences, 36–37
    pretreatment assessments of, 36–37
    wear, 37–38
Odontoblasts, 17–18
Off-angle hatchet, 125
Onlays
    bases, 476
    CAD/CIM system
        advantages of, 490
        clinical studies of, 495, 497
        disadvantages of, 490–491
        hardware, 491
        longevity of, 495, 497
        software, 491
        technique, 494, 494f
        training, 490
    gold
        bevel, 512
        cuspal reduction, 510–511, 511f
        description of, 509
        noncentric cusp, 511
        occlusal preparation, 510
        preparations for, 509–510
        proximal boxes, 510, 510f
        retention grooves, 512
        shoulder preparation, 511, 511f
    liners, 476
    porcelain, 485, 487, 488b
    preparations, 476, 477f
    provisional restorations, 478
    resin composite, 485, 487
    resistance form, 476
Orthograde contamination, 546

P

Perikymata, 4, 5f
Periodontal pocket, 19
Periodontal probes, 135, 135f
Periodontium
    anatomy of, 504f
    pretreatment evaluation of, 40–41
Pins, for resistance and retention of complex
    amalgam restorations, 325–333, 547
Pit, definition of, 116
Pit caries
    detection of, 76, 77f
    pretreatment assessment of, 30–31
    treatment of, 87

Plaque
    bacterial composition of, 71
    in caries etiology, 71–72
    pH levels, 71–72
    risk assessments, 29–30
Plastic instruments, 130–131, 131f
Point angle, 117
Polymerization
    initiation of, 188–189
    resin composites, 237
    wet-bonding technique effect, 206
Polymerization shrinkage
    compensatory mechanisms
        cervical sealing, 188
        elasticity, 188, 221
        flow increases, 186–187
        hygroscopic expansion, 187
        light curing, 187–188
        prepolymerized inserts, 187
    description of, 186, 395
    in posterior resin composite restorations
        description of, 265–266
        postoperative sensitivity, 267–268
    in resin inlays, 480–481
Porcelain veneers
    anatomy of, 438, 441f
    anterior tooth preparations for
        gingival finish lines, 432–433
        incisal edge, 433–434
        interproximal contact area, 433, 434f
        overlapping teeth, 434
        space closure, 434–435
    color characterization and management methods
        bleaching, 422, 422f–423f, 445–446
        discolored teeth, 444
        masking, 444–445
        principles of, 443–444
    crown and, 446, 456–457
    debonding of, 446, 447f
    failure of, 446, 447f
    finishing of, 449b
    fracture of, 446
    impressions for, 437
    indications, 427
    limitations of, 427
    luting cements, 440, 442
    maintenance of, 448
    multiple, 431–432
    placement of, 438, 440, 441f, 442–443, 449b
    procedures for, 448b–449b
    provisional restorations, 438, 439f–441f
    removal of, 447–448
    single, 431
    tooth preparations for
        anterior teeth. *See* Porcelain veneers, anterior tooth preparations for.
        Class 5 restorations, 437
        existing restorations, 436, 437f

fractured incisal edge, 436–437, 437f
guidelines, 449b
noncarious cervical lesions, 437
premolars, 435–436
treatment planning
computer imaging, 429
face assessments, 427
mock-ups, 428–429, 429f–430f
photographs, 431
smile assessments, 427–428
try-in, 448b
Posterior occlusal plane, 58
Posterior teeth
endodontically treated, 547–549, 562–563
nomenclature for, 115
posts, 547–549, 562–563
preventive resin restorations. *See* Preventive resin restorations.
resin composite restorations
autocured, 265, 271–272, 291
Class 1, 278
Class 2
acid etching, 283
adhesives for, 261–264
bevel placement, 279–281
bonding resin application, 283–284
finishing of, 293–294
gingival margins, 281, 282f
incremental technique for, 286–291
interproximal contact, 290
liners, 281–283
matrices, 284–285
occlusal margins, 281
preparations, 279–281
prewedging, 278–279
proximal margins, 281
rebonding of, 295, 296f
resin-modified glass-ionomer cements, 291
description of, 260
disadvantages of, 265–271
esthetics of, 261, 262f
galvanic current elimination using, 264
indications, 271–272
isolation techniques, 273, 273f
longevity of, 261t
marginal leakage of, 271
mechanical properties of, 270
packable resin composite, 293
polymerization
alternative techniques for, 292
shrinkage, 265–266
postoperative sensitivity of, 267–268
preoperative evaluation, 273
radiopacity benefits of, 265
sealants, 273–274
secondary caries, 266–267
thermal conductivity reductions using, 264
tooth structure adhesion, 264
tooth structure conservation, 261–264

viscosity, 287
water sorption of, 270
wear resistance of, 268–270
tunnel restorations
advantages of, 296
contraindications, 297
description of, 296
disadvantages of, 296–297
indications, 297
longevity of, 297t
preparations, 297, 298f
resin-modified glass-ionomer cements for, 298
Posts
active, 549, 553
anterior teeth, 546–547, 561–562
carbon fiber, 553–555
cementation of
considerations, 550
luting cements for, 550–551
retention considerations, 558
core materials, 560–561
custom cast, 551–552
design considerations
canal preparation, 550
diameter, 549–550
length, 549
overview of, 549
retention, 558
surface roughness, 550
venting, 550
parallel, 549, 553
passive tapered, 553
posterior teeth, 547–549, 562–563
prefabricated, 553
for reinforcing structurally compromised roots, 557
resistance of, 558–560
retention of, 558
tooth-colored, 555–556, 555f–557f
zirconium, 555–556
Potassium nitrate, 408
Premolars. *See also* Teeth.
cast-gold restorations, 540, 541f
porcelain veneers for, 435–436
post placement, 548, 549f
Preventive resin restorations
advantages of, 274
contraindications, 275
history of, 274
indications, 275
sealants used with, 275
technique, 275, 276f–278f
Probes, 135, 135f
Pulp
adhesion considerations, 215
age-related changes, 18
assessment of, 32–33
bleaching effects on, 408
capping. *See* Pulp capping.
cast-gold restorations and, 503

crown preparations, 464
dentin bonding agents effect, 104–105
dentin thickness and, 91
description of, 15
functions of, 15
healing potential of, 18
hydrodynamics of, 94
inflammation of, 17, 92–93
innervation of, 17
instruments for assessing, 91–92
irritation of, 190
morphology of, 15–16
odontoblastic layer, 17–18
pain, 93
pain transmission, 17
restorative dentistry effects, 18, 92–93
sensitivity
bleaching-induced, 408, 419
thermal, 93–94, 503
temperature effects, 18
thermal sensitivity of, 93–94, 503
tissue pressure, 17
tooth preparation considerations, 464, 503
vascular system of, 16–17
vitality testing of, 32
Pulp capping
calcium hydroxide, 103–104, 107
conditions necessary for, 98
definition of, 98
dentin bonding agents
bond quality and durability, 104
cellular toxicity, 105
description of, 103
microleakage reductions using, 103–104
pulpal effects, 104–105
studies of, 103–104
direct
dentin bonding agents. *See* Pulp capping, dentin bonding agents.
description of, 98–99
materials for, 105
schematic representation of, 99f
indirect, 99–103
summary overview of, 106–107

R
Radiographs
caries detection using, 75–76, 77t
treatment planning uses, 41–42
Records. *See* Dental record.
Resin composite
adhesive properties of, 264
antimicrobial properties of, 106
autocured, 271–272
characteristics of, 237
color matching for, 250–251
components of, 236–237, 268
core material use, 561
diastema closure using, 246–249

direct veneers, 245–246, 246f, 248b
elastic deformation of, 270
hybrid, 237, 238f
incremental placement of, 252, 286–291
longevity of, 236
mechanical properties of, 270
microfilled, 237
packable, 293
polymerization
  description of, 237
  shrinkage secondary to. *See* Polymerization shrinkage.
  variable rates of, 270–271
properties of, 106, 264, 270, 522
shade selection, 250
shrinkage of. *See* Polymerization shrinkage.
thermal expansion coefficient of, 237, 270
tooth adhesion of, 264
tooth preparations, 522
visible light–cured, 271–272
water sorption of, 270
wear of, 268–269, 487–489
wedging of, 252
Resin composite restorations
  anterior teeth. *See* Anterior teeth.
  Class 3. *See* Class 3 restorations.
  Class 4. *See* Class 4 restorations.
  Class 5, 395–396
  curing of, 252
  glass-ionomer cements for, 97
  incremental placement of, 252, 286–291
  inlays. *See* Inlays, resin composite.
  posterior teeth. *See* Posterior teeth, resin composite restorations.
  preparations for, 396
  root caries, 373, 373f
Resin-modified glass-ionomer cement. *See* Glass-ionomer cement, resin-modified.
Resins, adhesive, 202–203, 220–221
Resin tags, 206–207
Restorations. *See specific type of restoration.*
Rod sheath, 5
Root caries
  activity assessments, 79, 80f
  appearance of, 365–366, 366f
  definition of, 365
  description of, 365
  diagnosis of, 370
  incidence of, 368
  location of, 366
  microbiology of, 367
  pathogenesis of, 366–367
  pathologic findings, 366–367
  prevalence of, 368
  prevention of, 370–371
  restorative materials
    amalgam, 372–373
    description of, 372
    glass-ionomer cement, 373

gold filling, 372, 372f
  resin composite, 373, 373f
risk factors, 368–370
Rubber dam
  adjustment of, 166
  advantages of, 149
  allergy to, 174
  bite block use, 168–169
  clamp forceps, 154–155
  clamps
    butterfly, 156, 158f
    description of, 155
    floss ligatures, 156, 158
    multiple, 172
    number W8A, 156, 157f–158f
    placement over teeth, 172
    placement techniques, 155
    supplemental types of, 157t
    tooth contact considerations, 156
    winged, 155, 155f
  Class 5 restorations, 388–389
  fixed partial denture, 169, 170f–171f
  floss ligatures, 156, 158, 161
  fluid evacuation methods, 172–174
  gingival relaxation incisions, 172, 173f
  history of, 149
  holders, 152–154
  hole-positioning guides, 150–152
  inversion of
    facilitation methods, 172
    floss use, 167, 168f
    instrument for, 160, 161f, 167
    technique, 167, 167f–168f
  latex allergy considerations, 174, 175f
  lubricant, 161–162
  materials, 150
  modeling compound, 159, 160f
  mouth preparation for, 162, 163f
  napkin
    application of, 166
    description of, 150, 151f
  placement techniques
    dam over clamp, 164, 165f
    overview of, 164
    winged clamp in dam, 166, 166f
    wingless clamp in dam, 166, 166f
  posterior resin composite restorations, 273
  preplacement preparations, 162–164
  protection of, 167
  proximal contact disk, 161, 162
  punch, 150, 151f
  recommendations regarding, 174
  removal of, 168
  retention methods
    alternative types of, 158, 159f
    clamps. *See* Rubber dam, clamps.
    modeling compound, 159, 160f
    root concavity sealing, 174
    second dam use, 174

  thickness of, 150t
  washing of, 167
  wedge, 160, 161f

S
Saliva
  in caries etiology, 73, 82
  flow rate
    caries risk and, 369
    reduction of, 82
Saliva ejector
  fluid evacuation technique using, 172–173
  Hygoformic, 175, 176f
Sclerotic dentin, 13–15
Sealers and sealants
  adhesive, 96
  advantages of, 87, 96
  definition of, 94
  factors that affect, 274
  function of, 95
  indications
    amalgam restorations, 336
    fissure caries, 87
    polymerization contraction, 188
    resin composite restorations
      posterior, 273–274
      preventive resin restorations, 275
  microleakage reduction using, 96
  overview of, 94
  placement guidelines, 98
  retention of, 274
  varnishes, 95
Secondary caries, 266–267
Self-etching adhesives, 210–211, 211f–212f
Sensitivity
  dentin
    in Class 5 restorations, 398
    description of, 11, 12f
    etiology of, 398
    primers for, 202
    posterior resin composite restorations, 267–268
  pulpal
    bleaching-induced, 408, 419
    thermal, 93–94, 503
Shade. *See* Color.
Smear layer
  adhesion strength and, 183–184
  dissolving of, 210–211, 211f–212f
  modification of, 208
  removal of
    agents for, 196, 197t, 208
    description of, 196, 198
Smile, 66
Spatula, 131, 131f
Spoon
  design of, 123–125, 124f
  sharpening of, 134f
Streptococcus mutans
  amalgam prevention of, 106

description of, 71
   fluoride's effects on, 380
Svedopter, 175, 176f

T

Teeth. *See also* Incisors; Premolars.
   age-related characteristics of, 66
   anterior. *See* Anterior teeth.
   bleaching of. *See* Bleaching.
   crown of, 117
   face of, 69
   interface with restoration, 95
   nomenclature for, 113, 114f–115f
   numbering of, 113, 114f–115f
   posterior. *See* Posterior teeth.
   proportion assessments, 66–67
   remaining structure of
      assessment of, 45
      conservation of, 261–264, 501
      post resistance and, 559
   remineralization of, 72
   surfaces, 115–118
   tissue and, interface between, 461
Tetracycline-induced discolorations
   bleaching techniques for, 416, 419–420, 422–423f
   description of, 402
Thermal sensitivity, of pulp
   description of, 93, 503
   etiologic theories, 94
Thermal shock, 94
Tofflemire matrix, 337–342
Tooth. *See* Teeth.

Tooth bleaching. *See* Bleaching.
Tooth stains, 402, 479
Treatment planning
   bleaching, 410–411
   chief complaint, 28–29
   dental history, 28–29
   description of, 42
   endodontic, 33
   esthetic needs, 46–47
   examination. *See* Examination.
   final treatment objective, 47
   functional needs assessment, 45–46
   overview of, 26–27
   problem list, 27, 43f–44f
   problem-oriented, 27
   radiographs, 41–42
   steps involved in, 27
   summary overview of, 53
   tooth structure assessments, 45
Treatment sequence and sequencing
   case study example of, 49–50
   description of, 27–28, 47–48
   factors that influence, 47
   financial effects, 48
   phases of, 28
Tubule wall hybridization, 206
Tucker technique, for cast-gold restorations. *See*
   Cast-gold restorations, Tucker technique.
Tunnel restorations
   advantages of, 296
   contraindications, 297
   description of, 296, 313

   disadvantages of, 296–297
   indications, 297
   longevity of, 297t
   preparations, 297, 298f
   resin-modified glass-ionomer cements for, 298

V

Varnishes, 95, 336
Veneers
   gold, 517–518
   porcelain. *See* Porcelain veneers.

W

Wear
   enamel, 4
   occlusal, 37–38
   porcelain, 487–489
   resin composite, 268–269, 487–489
Wedging, 252, 341
Wetting, 180f
White spot lesion, 3, 4f

X

Xerostomia, 369–370
Xylitol, 371

Z

Zinc oxide–eugenol cements, 97, 522
Zinc phosphate cements
   characteristics of, 97, 520–521
   post cementation using, 551
   tooth preparations, 522